T0254559

Health Informatics

This series is directed to healthcare professionals leading the transformation of healthcare by using information and knowledge. For over 20 years, Health Informatics has offered a broad range of titles: some address specific professions such as nursing, medicine, and health administration; others cover special areas of practice such as trauma and radiology; still other books in the series focus on interdisciplinary issues, such as the computer based patient record, electronic health records, and networked healthcare systems. Editors and authors, eminent experts in their fields, offer their accounts of innovations in health informatics. Increasingly, these accounts go beyond hardware and software to address the role of information in influencing the transformation of healthcare delivery systems around the world. The series also increasingly focuses on the users of the information and systems: the organizational, behavioral, and societal changes that accompany the diffusion of information technology in health services environments.

Developments in healthcare delivery are constant; in recent years, bioinformatics has emerged as a new field in health informatics to support emerging and ongoing developments in molecular biology. At the same time, further evolution of the field of health informatics is reflected in the introduction of concepts at the macro or health systems delivery level with major national initiatives related to electronic health records (EHR), data standards, and public health informatics.

These changes will continue to shape health services in the twenty-first century. By making full and creative use of the technology to tame data and to transform information, Health Informatics will foster the development and use of new knowledge in healthcare.

Gyorgy J. Simon • Constantin Aliferis

Editors

Artificial Intelligence and Machine Learning in Health Care and Medical Sciences

Best Practices and Pitfalls

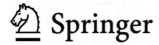 Springer

Editors
Gyorgy J. Simon
Institute for Health Informatics
University of Minnesota
Minneapolis, MN, USA

Constantin Aliferis
Institute for Health Informatics
University of Minnesota
Minneapolis, MN, USA

ISSN 1431-1917   ISSN 2197-3741   (electronic)
Institute for Health Informatics
ISBN 978-3-031-39357-0   ISBN 978-3-031-39355-6   (eBook)
https://doi.org/10.1007/978-3-031-39355-6

This Springer imprint is published by the registered company Springer Nature Switzerland AG
The registered company address is: Gewerbestrasse 11, 6330 Cham, Switzerland

Paper in this product is recyclable.

I am dedicating this book to my wife, Mayuko, and our children, George and Klara, for their love and for their patience with my long hours writing this book. I could not have succeeded either in my career or with this book without Mayuko's dedication and support.

Gyorgy J. Simon

I most affectionately dedicate this work to my wife Alla, for the inspiration she gives me daily and for her love.

Constantin Aliferis

Foreword 1

Imagine a world where you receive treatment that is precisely targeted to give you the best outcome possible, where care is efficient and safe, and where you have guidance in managing your health at home and are a partner in your healthcare. We dream of a world like this, and you as a reader of this book probably see a role for AI in making that dream come true.

Rear Admiral Grace Hopper, developer of the first compiler for a computer language, repeated a motto coined by John Augustus Shedd: "A ship in port is safe; but that is not what ships are built for. Sail out to sea and do new things."[1] As a reader of this book, you are leaving a safe harbor to do something hard and something risky.

I left that safe harbor in 1994 when I pivoted from my humanities university degree in linguistics and Chinese to enroll in a graduate program in medical informatics at the University of Utah. My husband introduced me to the field, and my love of language steered me to the new world of natural language processing. In classrooms, I raised my hand to ask about the meaning of basic words like "algorithm," "heuristic," and "ML," and as the only female in the campus computer lab at 2 am, I sat with my 2-year-old son asleep at my feet trying to get my linked list to compile. I was an outsider in the world of computers and AI, and I was an outsider in the world of healthcare. But like each of you, I brought unique experience, and embracing that, I have been able to both develop methodological innovations and apply those to problems like disease surveillance and creation of research cohorts from electronic health record data.

The department where I studied was chaired by Homer R. Warner,[2] who founded the department in 1964.

> Homer Warner ... developed in 1961 the first computerized program for diagnosing disease. Basing it on 1,000 children with various congenital heart diseases, Warner showed that Bayes' [theorem] could identify their underlying problems quite accurately. "Old cardiologists just couldn't believe that a computer could do something better than a human," Warner recalled.[3]

---

[1] "Grace Hopper: The Youthful Teacher of Us All" by Henry S. Tropp in Abacus Vol. 2, Issue 1 (Fall 1984) ISSN 0724-6722.

[2] https://en.wikipedia.org/wiki/Homer_R._Warner.

[3] https://yalebooks.yale.edu/book/9780300188226/the-theory-that-would-not-die/.

Homer sailed from a safe harbor, and, in doing so, he developed one of the first electronic medical records to collect data not only to improve access to information but ultimately to transform the diagnostic and patient care process through building intelligence into the system.[4]

And now you are here, in this open sea. It has been over half a century since Homer Warner and other pioneers developed and implemented AI systems in healthcare. The age of AI seems to be upon us. The big tech industry sees the opportunity and is making unprecedented investments in healthcare.

So, what is the risk?

When creating innovative healthcare solutions using AI, challenges will arise in at least three steps: development, application, and implementation. In *developing* ML and AI models, you will not be able to fully trust the output of the tools, because the learnings and predictions only represent a potentially deceptive proxy of the real situation,[5] and the algorithms are most likely learning from biased data and biased healthcare delivery practices. In *applying* ML and AI models to healthcare problems, you will encounter unintended consequences—your predictive model may lead to a rapid upsurge in overdiagnoses, for example. In *implementing* your tools, you may discover that the reality does not match the hype: most never even make it to the real world, and when they do, the results are often disappointing.[6] When you put a new technology into the complex system of healthcare, everything around it changes. You will shift relationships, you will shift workflows, and you will shift power differentials. And those changes can cause harm.

Given the risks and the difficulty you will face, should you even launch your boat into the sea of healthcare AI? Yes! We need you. We need the smartest brains tackling problems more consequential than how to get people to click on ads.[7] And that is where this book comes in. *Artificial Intelligence and Machine Learning in Health Care and the Health Sciences: Pitfalls and Best Practices* will be your compass to help you chart a more successful path.

The lead authors of this book have decades of experience teaching and doing research on this topic. Dr. Aliferis has dedicated his career to the responsible use of AI to improve human lives and support scientific discovery. He is an innovator of high-performing and reliable methods with a goal of improving safety and effectiveness. Dr. Simon has extensive experience in data mining, machine learning, statistical analysis, and biostatistics. He has a solid background in hands-on software development in academic and commercial settings. The editors have pulled together a star-studded cast of content contributors with both knowledge and experience.

---

[4] Paul D. Clayton, PhD, Presentation of the Morris F. Collen Award to Homer R. Warner, MD, PhD: "Why Not? Let's Do It!", Journal of the American Medical Informatics Association, Volume 2, Issue 2, March 1995, Pages 137–142, https://doi.org/10.1136/jamia.1995.95261907.

[5] https://www.youtube.com/watch?v=cDAXiq-at5M.

[6] https://khn.org/news/a-reality-check-on-artificial-intelligence-are-health-care-claims-overblown/.

[7] https://web.archive.org/web/20150202014230/http://www.bloomberg.com/bw/magazine/content/11_17/b4225060960537.htm.

Never before has so much wisdom about best practices in health and biomedical AI been compiled into one place.

This book is comprehensive but also extremely practical. It provides diverse and reliable best practices through a wide range of illustrative applications of machine learning and AI. The book will detail specific requirements and adaptations that are necessary to successfully tailor general algorithms and techniques to healthcare and health sciences discovery. Authors describe common pitfalls that plague research and commercial attempts at applying AI to healthcare and will give advice on how to avoid repeating the mistakes of the past. Through this book, you will learn how to develop AI applications that can be trusted and therefore have a higher likelihood of success to achieve the goal of high performance, safety, and cost-effectiveness in healthcare.

Pedro Domingos said, "People worry that computers will get too smart and take over the world, but the real problem is that they're too stupid and they've already taken over the world."[8] If you come from outside of healthcare, you may be surprised at how "stupid" their computers are and how long the path may be to apply your cutting-edge innovation. If you come from within healthcare, you understand why it has taken so long to bring the innovations you see around you to healthcare, but you may not understand the technical aspects well enough to bridge the gap. Studying this book will make us all more informed partners and will accelerate our journey to improved health and discovery through AI.

Digital Health and Informatics   Wendy Chapman
Centre for Digital Transformation of Health
University of Melbourne
Parkville, VIC, Australia

---

[8] Domingos, P. 2015, The master algorithm: How the quest for the ultimate learning machine will remake our world, Basic Books, New York, NY, USA.

Foreword 2

The emergence of advanced technologies impacts healthcare. For several years now, anticipation has been building that artificial intelligence (AI) and machine learning (ML) will lead to a paradigm shift in healthcare, promoting seamless, safe, and convenient access to healthcare services including disease management and prevention. AI/ML technologies can support the diagnosis of complex medical conditions, help clinicians make more informed decisions, and ultimately improve patient outcomes through timely diagnosis and tailored treatment. These technologies can facilitate the collection and analysis of diverse data including clinical data and behavioral, genomic, and environmental datasets that all can provide unique insights into individual healthcare needs in the context of precision health.

In my own work, I have focused on the use of technology to support aging and studied the use of AI and ML in the space of gerontology and geriatrics. I lead the Penn Artificial Intelligence and Technology (PennAITech) Collaboratory for Healthy Aging, which has the goal to identify, develop, evaluate, commercialize, and disseminate innovative technology and artificial intelligence (AI) methods and software to support older adults and those with Alzheimer's disease (AD) and Alzheimer's disease and related dementias (ADRD) in their home environment. These technologies cover a broad spectrum ranging from home-based monitoring technologies and smart home sensors to robotic applications, conversational agents, wearables, and other digital phenotyping tools. The Collaboratory is motivated by the need for a comprehensive pipeline across technology-based monitoring of older adults in the home, collection and processing of monitoring data, integration of those data with clinical data from electronic health records, analysis with cutting-edge AI methods and software, and deployment of validated AI models at point of care for decision support.

In this work, it becomes clear that AI and ML technologies can create new opportunities for monitoring and supporting older adults and their families in a variety of settings. However, for these technologies to be widely adopted and trusted by healthcare providers, patients, and families, it is essential to not only generate solid evidence of their effectiveness but also establish best practices in their development and use.

Such best practices are important to ensure the safety and efficacy of AI and ML technologies in patient care. As has been argued numerous times, AI and ML algorithms are only as good as the data they are trained on, and if the data are biased or inaccurate, the algorithms will produce biased or inaccurate results. The consequences can be significant; incorrect diagnoses can lead to harm or even death, and bias in treatment selection may affect outcomes and exacerbate existing inequities. Informed efforts such as using large, diverse, and representative datasets can in many cases help to mitigate these risks and eliminate algorithmic bias. We have to ensure the transparency and accountability of such technologies. Healthcare providers and patients need to understand how AI and ML technologies "make decisions" and what factors influence these decisions.

Establishing best practices in the development and use of AI and ML technologies in patient care and more broadly in biomedicine is crucial for ensuring the safety, efficacy, transparency, accountability, and ethical use of these technologies. However, to date, data scientists in health sciences, clinicians, and administrators do not have concrete frameworks to help them navigate this landscape. As computational advances accelerate the growth of AI and ML, the healthcare industry appears to try to catch up with methodological, policy, and clinical guidelines. The book by Drs. Simon and Aliferis, "*Pitfalls and Best Practices in AI/ML for Healthcare and Health Science*," addresses this gap as it provides an interdisciplinary perspective and an in-depth insight into reliable AI/ML methods and their properties, approaches for benchmarking, best practices for transparency and dissemination, and broad range of tools allowing data scientists, informaticians, and clinicians to develop or utilize AI/ML while maximizing effectiveness and safety and avoiding well-documented pitfalls. This timely book delves into the application of AI and ML in healthcare, exploring benefits and limitations and providing insights into the future of AI; the book features interdisciplinary and evidence-based perspectives that will lead to more accurate, efficient, and personalized patient care.

Department of Biostatistics, Epidemiology   George Demiris
and Informatics, Perelman School of Medicine
and School of Nursing
University of Pennsylvania
Philadelphia, PA, USA

Preface 1

We are living in an interesting time. Broad adoption of AI is underway with very significant achievements, including chatbots with humanlike language skills and autonomous taxi services operating in many parts of the country, and we are at the cusp of broad adoption of AI in clinical care and health sciences.

AI is not without its risks. We have seen AI dish out bad advice, be racist, and be sometimes utterly incompetent. In the summer of 2019, Constantin and I sat down to write a paper about the "Knowledge Cliff" problem in AI/ML in biomedicine. While researching this paper, we realized that merely pointing out problems with AI, while it is useful, is not particularly constructive or actionable. Drawing on our decades of teaching and research, we refocused the paper into explaining the pitfalls of certain approaches and providing actionable best practice recommendations in six (or so) different areas. As such, one paper had to grow into six. It did not take long to recognize that our goal requires an entire book. We also recognized the dearth of AI/ML textbooks that focus on healthcare, its special characteristics, and requirements, with sufficient technical depth to enable a meaningful discussion about pitfalls and best practices of building AI/ML systems for biomedicine.

This book is meant for a broad audience; virtually anyone can benefit from reading it. Although this book can be read cover to cover in sequential order of the chapters, we aimed to make chapters self-contained (sometimes at the cost of minor repetitions), because certain audiences benefit from some chapters more than others. My recommendations on how to use this book for certain audiences follow.

First, AI/ML professionals with extensive training in computer science and general-purpose AI/ML, who consider getting into healthcare or health sciences. I am a computer scientist who made this transition into biomedicine; thus, the book reflects on my personal experience. For this audience, the book offers overviews of aspects of method and model development that are often neglected in general-purpose AI/ML (Chapters "Principles of Rigorous Development and of Appraisal of ML and AI Methods and Systems" and "The Development Process and Lifecycle of Clinical Grade and Other Safety and Performance-Sensitive AI/ML Models"), an introduction to data design (Chapter "Data Design"), detailed (more detailed than others) description of modeling methods for time-to-event and longitudinal data (Chapter "An Appraisal and Operating Characteristics of Major ML Methods Applicable in Healthcare and Health Science"), introduction to model evaluation from the perspective of health benefits and health economics (Chapter "Evaluation"), description of healthcare standards, terminologies, and ontologies (Chapter "Data Preparation, Transforms, Quality, and Management"), etc. The goal of our book for this audience is to help them transition into healthcare seamlessly.

Second, analysts without a rigorous computer science training who are already building health AI/ML models. To this audience, we cover the foundational concepts in computer science, AI and ML (Chapter "Foundations and Properties of AI/ML Systems"), a 10,000-foot view of a broad range of modeling methods (Chapters "An Appraisal and Operating Characteristics of Major ML Methods Applicable in Healthcare and Health Science" and "Foundations of Causal ML"), and other important aspects of health modeling (Chapters "Principles of Rigorous Development and of Appraisal of ML and AI Methods and Systems," "The Development Process and Lifecycle of Clinical Grade and Other Safety and Performance-Sensitive AI/ML Models", "Regulatory Aspects and Ethical Legal Societal Implications (ELSI)", and "Reporting Standards, Certification/Accreditation, and Reproducibility"). The goal of our book for this audience is to entice and enable them to be more rigorous with their work.

Third, decision makers, who wish to gain a better understanding of the capabilities and limitations of AI in healthcare and health sciences. To this audience, I recommend Chapters "Lessons Learned from Historical Failures, Limitations and Successes of AI/ML in Healthcare and the Health Sciences. Enduring Problems, and the Role of BPs" (historic case studies and lessons learnt), "Characterizing, Diagnosing and Managing the Risk of Error of ML & AI Models in Clinical and Organizational Application", "Regulatory Aspects and Ethical Legal Societal Implications (ELSI)", and "Principles of Rigorous Development and of Appraisal of ML and AI Methods and Systems" for appraising existing methods, and any other chapter that discusses topics that they wish to deepen their knowledge of.

It is my opinion that everybody will find something new. Even readers with minimal technical background will find Chapters "Lessons Learned from Historical Failures, Limitations and Successes of AI/ML in Healthcare and the Health Sciences. Enduring Problems, and the Role of BPs" fascinating, and on the other end, experts in AI/ML may find new nuggets of knowledge in Chapter "Overfitting, Underfitting and General Model Overconfidence and under-Performance Pitfalls and Best Practices in Machine Learning and AI" or about human cognitive biases (Chapter "From 'Human versus Machine' to 'Human with Machine'") or design biases (Chapter "Data Design"). Chapters are self-contained; please feel free to read any chapter you find interesting.

Inspired by my co-author's, mentors', and collaborators' passion for patient care and safety, my ultimate goal with this book, and more broadly with my career, is to promote better patient care, safety, and ethics. This book aims to lay the foundations and instill the scientific rigor necessary for the successful implementation of helpful and safe AI in clinical care and for making fruitful discoveries in health sciences. I wish the reader great success in the exciting and growing field of biomedical AI.

Minneapolis, MN, USA   Gyorgy J. Simon

Preface 2

The promise and challenges of health artificial intelligence (AI) and machine learning (ML). After a long history of exploration and experimentation, brilliant successes interleaved with some striking failures, springs of optimism, and winters of disappointment, AI has arrived and is here to stay. This realization is engraved in the minds of the scientific community and lay public alike.

It is not hyperbolic to recognize that the AI and ML methods and technologies at the service of health sciences and healthcare of our times are nothing short of amazing. As remarkable as the problem-solving tools we have are, in order to be deployed for clinical and other mission-critical tasks, they have to overcome significant gaps in performance and safety, however.

The comparison with other areas of applied technology is both striking and worrisome. Consider a humble and low-tech device such as an oven toaster (or any other electric appliance operating with high voltage): in order to be approved for the consumer market, rigorous testing must be done to ensure that it is not a fire hazard or that it will not electrocute its operator. Bridges are not opened to public use unless the civil engineers that built them provide plans that undergo tremendous scrutiny and establish, for example, how much load they can withstand, what wind forces or earthquakes they can tolerate without collapsing, and what maintenance they need and how often. Similarly, cars, mechanical tools, children's toys, drugs, and so on across the whole gamut of human activity are closely scrutinized and become available for consumer use only when sufficient measures have been established to ensure safe application. Public and individual safety is of paramount consideration and enforced everywhere.

Everywhere, except in health AI and ML, it seems. Poorly constructed, evaluated, deployed, or monitored AI and ML models, apps, and systems have the potential to cause great benefit or grave harm at a massive scale. This is true for healthcare medical applications, healthcare business decisions, and health sciences. Regulation is only now emerging, and AI/ML products have been offered for years (often at huge financial costs) to the trusting healthcare providers and find their ways to profoundly affect human lives, without providing guarantees of effectiveness and safety.

Another related deficiency of the present state of the health AI/ML market is that of efficiency. It would be unthinkable for a car manufacturer to market, for example, a four-passenger automobile for everyday commuting purposes with fuel consumption of 1 mile per gallon. Yet, we routinely see commercial and noncommercial AI/ML offerings that are worse offenders than this example in terms of the computing costs per unit of output when perfectly capable (or better) alternatives exist with orders of magnitude lower costs of use.

From another viewpoint, and to use an electrical engineering analogy, the ML models of today function as components of a larger system that presently lacks protection against overloading the system. Well-designed consumer electrical devices are routinely engineered in such a way that their input and output obey specifications ensuring that a system of interconnected such units will function properly. Nothing like this exists in health AI/ML at present.

But even if a very high standard of accountability was put in place (and steps are being taken recently in this direction by the FDA, NIST, EU, etc. as described in the present volume), it would be of little value, unless we could equip the data scientists and the organizations adopting AI/ML solutions with the technical means by which to achieve (and verify) the standard's expectation.

Pitfalls and Best Practices: A Personal Perspective. This book aims precisely to contributing to solving these problems by providing comprehensive information in the form of identifiable pitfalls and practical best practices supporting the effective, safe, efficient, cost-effective, science-driven, rigorous, informed, rational, de-risked, trust-inspiring, and accountable health AI and ML.

Some of the book's concepts started forming in my mind many years ago when I was a beginning graduate student in AI. I have written elsewhere[1] how my personal journey started and why I believed early on that AI could make medicine more scientific and ultimately more effective. A formative experience of particular relevance to this book has been the NSF-funded ML Pneumonia Prediction project led by my graduate advisor Greg Cooper (connected with the broader Pneumonia Patient Outcomes Research Team (PORT) cohort study). The ML project aimed at exploring many cutting-edge methods of the era to create the most accurate and practical models possible for predicting community-acquired pneumonia mortality. Several word-class labs and AI and machine learning luminaries from the University of Pittsburgh and CMU participated in the effort (i.e., the Bruce Buchanan lab, Greg Cooper lab, Tom Mitchel lab, Peter Spirtes lab, Clark Glymour lab), along with Dr. Michael Fine, the leader of the PORT study, which ended having very significant impact nationally. Everyone strived to produce the best models working off a single discovery dataset. In these circumstances, it would have been very easy to totally overfit the models, but thanks to Greg's scientific foresight and rigor, a nested cross-validation design and other safeguards were put in place to eliminate the risk of overfitting and taught me a career-defining lesson about the value of pursuing high-stakes modeling with utmost rigor.

As I started my career as a faculty, 24 years ago, I placed significant emphasis on the modeling challenges of the very novel at the time gene expression microarray, mass spectrometry, and other high-dimensional data. I was surprised and occasionally dismayed at what appeared to be technical abuse and overinterpretation of

---

[1] https://imia-medinfo.org/wp/history-book/

methods with widespread lack of rigor in the bioinformatics field fueled by exuberant expectations. In one of many memorable incidents during my early faculty career, a cancer biology professor, whom I respected very much for his scientific accomplishments, reached out to me one day and asked me if I could "cluster his gene expression data to predict cancer." I asked how many patients he had assayed, and to my astonishment, he said "three." I asked him what made him believe that clustering three patients in two groups would have any statistical validity and predictive modeling usefulness, and to my continuing amazement, he showed me a recent copy of one of the two most respected biology journals. "Can't you just do it like they did it in this article?" he asked, pointing to the cover article. This incident was representative of the whole field of genomics of the time at the infancy of high-throughput technology and showed me that applying complex AI/ML to genomic datasets had a long way to go in terms of educating many of the key practitioners.

Over the years, I watched many scientific accomplishments and breakthroughs in pure AI and machine learning and followed the numerous applied biomedical advances that they enabled. I also built new methods and put those and every other major technique invented by others to practice, in many NIH-funded projects. I taught students and early-career faculty AI and ML and watched how this knowledge helped them in their careers. I also organized and oversaw at NYU and my current institution, the UMN, institutional-level research support teams and cores that deployed AI and ML via consulting, and team science for hundreds of projects and thousands of consults between 2008 and today. I also gave invited lectures in both academic and industry settings about the dangers inherent in AI and ML when not used with enough rigor and discipline. I followed closely the literature and developments in regulatory frameworks, best practices, and major failures and case studies in AI/ML. Finally, my group conducted some of the largest (and in some cases, I dare say, authoritative) benchmarks of ML in several fields of biomedical research.

Embarking on a long-overdue project. It was thus about time in 2021 to finally put together a book distilling the above information in a format that would be accessible, backed up by all relevant scientific evidence, and practically useful for working scientists, students, administrators, practitioners, and other stakeholders of health AI. With regard to style, a great influence has always been the late Richard Feynman and his monumental *Lectures on Physics,* in which he managed to condense the full range of physics, sparing no difficult subject, in a way that was accessible to first-year college students, without getting vague or sacrificing accuracy. Tom Mitchell, Sholom Weiss, and one of my most respected role models, Casimir Kulikowski, achieved in their corresponding books on ML similar levels of clarity, accuracy, and accessibility. Gyorgy and I used the above three works as inspiration and our "Northern Star" in terms of clarity and accessibility for the present volume.

Best practices imply necessary conditions for success, or necessary and sufficient conditions in some cases. But it also, unavoidably, involves describing sufficient conditions for failure that need to be prevented. Not uncommonly, when the knowledge in some topic is not enough to delineate with absolute certainty what needs to be done, a best practice is no more than the best possible recommendation for how to apply AI/ML given the limited knowledge of the time. In Chapter "Artificial Intelligence (AI) and Machine Learning (ML) for Healthcare and Health Sciences: The Need for Best Practices Enabling Trust in AI and ML", we explain in detail the sources for best practices and pitfalls presented in this work. We decided early on that we should not expunge from this work our personal experiences or hands-on expertise in specific methods and applications. We resolutely decided, however, that this book should not be a summary of our preferred way of developing and applying AI/ML, and our own personal practices would have a place here if and only if they are solidly backed by the scientific evidence in the literature and if they are paradigmatic of the various messages we wish to convey. In many chapters, this decision has worked particularly well, in my view, because we were able to dive deeply into topics that would be hard to present in a clear manner if we did not describe details stemming from in-depth and first-hand experience (Chapter "Principles of Rigorous Development and of Appraisal of ML and AI Methods and Systems" on method development and appraisal is an example whereby we try to "lift the curtain" and show, from the inside, an example of how rigorously-designed and -executed new methods can come to existence).

Regarding helpfulness and defensibility, we realized that such a book should be constructive but not sugarcoat the facts. This is not a volume about presenting on even ground all methods, systems, or efforts, without taking a position on strengths, weaknesses, and relative performance. The result may not be viewed favorably within circles where dogged devotion to this or the other method supersedes objective performance considerations. This is however a book about *pitfalls* and *best practices*. The notion of pitfalls entails dangers, failures, and risk that we should avoid or minimize. It is imperative that all students, teachers, and practitioners of AI/ML embrace its collective history, learn from it, own any mistakes made, and not repeat them again. Showcasing failures in the field is not intended to diminish the people or organizations behind them, but to learn from these case studies how to do AI/ML in a safe and effective manner. Conversely, it is essential to show what can (and does) happen when AI/ML is not done systematically with sufficient scientific and technical rigor. Naturally, it is entirely possible to disappoint people whose methods or practices are criticized. Gyorgy and I took this seriously into account, but we balanced it with the need to present scientific truth (the best way we can grasp it anyway) and above all to protect patients. AI/ML can critically affect the well-being of patients and of society and will increasingly do so in the future, after all.

In terms of scope, we cast a very wide net, first taking a broad look at all types of health science and healthcare applications of AI/ML. We generally refrain in the book from engaging in analysis of methods with only historical significance, except in cases where historical case studies or other works are highly informative for modern-day AI/ML. We retrieved all health AI/ML best practice and guideline papers as well as meta-analyses and systematic reviews of AI/ML methods and model comparisons across all biomedical fields, in PubMed. Chapter "Artificial Intelligence (AI) and Machine Learning (ML) for Healthcare and Health Sciences: The Need for Best Practices Enabling Trust in AI and ML" gives a glimpse of that space. This material was supplemented with our personal collection of AI/ML books and papers, which comprises thousands of entries plus many more that were identified in PubMed and Google Scholar to help with topics outside our usual scope of work. We synthesized and integrated prior best practices, in many cases invisibly to the reader, and in some cases bringing certain preexisting best practices to the forefront of the book because we saw them as very important, or in need of discussion, extensions, etc. Most importantly, we placed a huge emphasis on principles of operation and properties of AI/ML methods for two reasons: on the one hand, these provide the necessary justification for recommended use (or avoidance). On the other hand, method properties can be applied to infinite situations and the readers can tailor them to their own specific projects, which we could not possibly anticipate in full, whereas guidelines and best practices are by necessity more context and problem sensitive. We also worked to modularize the recommended practices to mirror the stages that AI/ML methods are being created, validated, and deployed. This should make reading the material easier. In the end of the book, we provide a collection of all best practices and annotate them as being high or medium impact and as being highly mature or evolving. High-impact recommendations are ones that following or discarding them will have the gravest consequences across most contexts of use. Lower impact ones may have lesser consequences or significant consequences but in a small portion of application areas. Evolving best practices are ones that will likely improve over time as the field's understanding advances, whereas highly mature ones are so foundational that they will almost certainly continue to be applicable far into the future.

Minneapolis, MN, USA   Constantin Aliferis

Acknowledgments

First and foremost, I wish to acknowledge Constantin, with whom I co-authored this book, for convincing me, over a 1-year-plus time period, to write this book. He did a job, worthy of the deepest admiration, with some of the most difficult topics, including lessons learnt and ethics. He managed to keep these difficult chapters, like all other chapters, constructive, actionable, and objective, and I believe that they became the crown jewels of this book. I recommend absolutely everyone to read these chapters. Clearly, this book would not have been possible without his hard work.

Besides co-authoring the book, I owe Constantin a debt of gratitude for his professional mentoring, passion for scientific discovery, and his appreciation of rigor in our work to make those valuable scientific discoveries happen.

I would also like to acknowledge Dr. Vipin Kumar, a well-recognized leader in (general-purpose) data mining and machine learning and a scientific role model to me and many other scientists. I feel fortunate to have had him as my thesis advisor, and he remains one of my professional mentors and collaborators to this day.

At the time I started out as a junior faculty, mentorship for faculty was scarce. I was lucky that Dr. Genevieve Melton-Meaux, a surgeon, NLP expert, and executive at a large health system, offered a helping hand. Drawing on her vast experience in the health system, she channeled my ML knowledge in a direction that is most valuable to clinical care and healthcare delivery research.

Dr. Pedro Caraballo, an MD passionate about patient care and an advocate for ML in clinical decision support, was one of my first collaborators in the ML-based clinical decision support realm who instilled in me the importance of ML in research as well as clinical decision support.

I would also like to thank my past and present co-workers who helped with the book, including Drs. Steve Johnson, Erich Kummerfeld, Sisi Ma, Dennis Murphree, Rui Zhang, Jinhua Wang, Bryan Andrews, Dalton Schutte, Anirudh Choudhary, Puneet Bhullar, and Nneka I. I thank them for the valuable insights they gave me, and especially thank them for the chapters they contributed.

I thank Melissa Malkowski and Beth Madson for their outstanding administrative support and Nithya Sechin from Springer.

Thanks also go to the UMN Office of Academic and Clinical Affairs (Dr. Jakub Tolar) for funding that made the book possible as open access.

I also thank Springer and especially senior editor Grant Weston, who believed and encouraged this project with great passion.

Gyorgy J. Simon

I would be amiss if I did not express my deep gratitude to a number of individuals that made my personal journey in biomedical AI and ML worthwhile and indirectly or directly benefited this book.

The first foundations I received in the data sciences were provided by the late Professor Dimitrios Trichopoulos and his faculty at the University of Athens School of Medicine. Trichopoulos was internationally renowned as an epidemiologist of formidable intellect and scholarship, and he made sure that his students received a wealth of knowledge in research design, biostatistics, and public health methods. Other mentors and collaborators were instrumental in nurturing my curiosity about the quantitative data sciences in the context of several research projects. I am deeply grateful to my former medical school professors and mentors E. Batrinos, E. Geordiadis, N. Katsilambros, and especially E. Georgiou who was my first mentor in biomedical informatics.

Greg Cooper's influence on my AI training was instrumental because of the early formative experience in the years I worked with him as postdoctoral fellow in his Pneumonia Prediction project and the years during which he served as my MS and PhD theses' main advisor. Greg and I became lifelong friends, and he has never stopped giving me valuable guidance for which I am grateful. I am also grateful to all my teachers in the Intelligent Systems Studies Program of the University of Pittsburgh. My other advisors, Bruce Buchanan, Randy Miller, Martha Pollack, Michael Wagner, and Howard Doyle, were outstanding mentors and role models who above all helped me learn to think critically.

I am most grateful to my colleague and co-author Gyorgy Simon for believing that this project could be done, for writing brilliant material, and for working with me in harmony even under a most demanding work schedule and difficult deadlines. Gyorgy is as knowledgeable, and effective, as he is humble and collegial. I thank him for sharing so much of his extensive knowledge in this book and being instrumental in making it a reality.

I am profoundly grateful to Grant Weston, senior editor at Springer, for being a true believer to the need for such a work. His enthusiasm, patience, and support are deeply appreciated.

Frank Harrell has been a great mentor and a fantastic role model both as a distinguished biostatistician and for setting a standard for "speaking the truth that others do not dare say."

Isabelle Guyon has been a wonderful collaborator and inspiring role model in AI/ML. I had the pleasure to work with her as a co-author in several books and papers and in a major ML challenge. I learnt so much from her scientific example and approach to structuring complex tasks and managing teams of diverse competencies.

Perry Miller, Henry Lowe, John Wilbur, and Michael Kahn, along with Greg Cooper, guided me in my early years as informatics leader at NYU and taught me many valuable lessons in leadership. Richard Woodrow, my executive leadership coach at NYU, spent 2 years teaching me how to put honesty above other concerns, and I am very grateful for his wisdom, which I tried to put to practice in this volume. Vivian Lee gave me a big career boost by making me Head of Informatics at NYU Langone and nurtured my developing leadership skills in navigating a complex landscape of avant-garde science in desperate need of high-quality data science and AI/ML modeling. Apostolos Georgopoulos at the UMN has been a most generous mentor and friend and encouraged this volume with great enthusiasm.

Bill Stead and Randy Miller gave me my first faculty academic home at Vanderbilt and enabled my lab there (the Discovery Systems Lab) to exist and make foundational algorithmic advances. I am very grateful for this opportunity. Stead has in addition been an inspiring role model in his unending quest to transform medicine using informatics. I am deeply appreciative of main collaborators in pursuing method development and landmark or other large-scale benchmarking: especially Ioannis Tsamardinos, Alexander Statnikov at Vanderbilt and NYU, and Sisi Ma and Roshan Tourani at the UMN. Had it not been for the extraordinary ability of Alexander Statnikov to execute benchmarking studies of immense complexity and scale in record time, a large body of invaluable benchmarking knowledge would have not existed today. Alexander, my second ever PhD student and later faculty colleague at NYU, has also made very significant methodological contributions with unique capabilities that are discussed in this volume.

I am also thankful to many of my students and mentees who took AI/ML classes from me or sought to receive scientific mentoring because invariably I learnt a lot from them, and they influenced the evolution of my teaching style and provided me with an empirical basis for how certain AI/ML topics can be best conveyed in order to help learners the most. Yindalon Aphinyanaphongs, and Larry Fu in particular, come vividly to mind, in addition, because their work allowed a joint exploration of AI/ML in health information retrieval, scientometrics, translational science, and text categorization that has stood the test of time.

I am also grateful to my extraordinary IP lawyer and friend, Laurence Weinberger, who in the context of preparing >20 patent applications has helped me and other co-inventors immensely toward clarifying and formulating very complicated technical concepts in a way that is accessible to broad audiences. Certainly, the appropriate use of AI/ML comes from theoretical knowledge but equally importantly from successful empirical applications in real-life projects. I have been privileged throughout my career to collaborate with several exceptional clinical, basic, and translational scientists. My main long-term collaborators in AI/ML applications that have most informed the present volume are Glenn Saxe (psychiatry), Boris Winterhoff (cancer precision medicine), Pamala Jacobson (pharmacogenomics), Virginia Kraus (aging and longevity), Bill Kraus (cardiometabolic outcomes), and Laura Niederhoffer (cellular senescence). Several other superb scientists collaborated with me and my lab in shorter term but highly rewarding applied research projects. Marty Blaser (microbiomics), Ed Fisher (atherosclerosis), Steve Abramson (osteoarthritis), and Doug Hardin (text categorization) in particular gave me the opportunity to put AI to good and challenging use in the corresponding fruitful biomedical areas. Our joint work, for which I am grateful, has been a testing lab and proving ground for the principles and practices espoused in the present volume.

Although the majority of this volume was written by Gyorgy Simon and I, we had the good luck to receive wonderful supplemental material by Erich Kummerfeld, Sisi Ma, Bryan Andrews, Jinhua Wang, Steve Johnson, Dalton Schutte, Rui Zhang, Dennis Murphree, Anirudh Choudhary, Puneet Bhullar, and Nneka I. Comfere. I am very appreciative of their expert contributions to this volume.

Melissa Malkowski and Beth Madson provided us with excellent administrative support at the UMN, and Nithya Sechin's, Hashwini Vytheswaran's and the whole editorial support and production teams' work from the Springer side is much appreciated.

The UMN OACA-Office of Academic and Clinical Affairs (led by VP and Dean Dr. Jakub Tolar) and the UMN CTSI (led by Dr. Bruce Blazar and Daniel Weisdorf) provided the Institute for Health Informatics with an environment where we can explore and put novel ideas to test and practice, typically at large scale (across all of the health sciences institutionally and beyond). I am also grateful to OACA for providing financial resources to make this book open access.

Finally, I am grateful to the two eminent colleagues who graciously provided forewords to this volume. Professor Wendy Chapman and Professor George Demiris are distinguished researchers, scholars, innovators, and academic leaders in health AI. They graced this volume with opening remarks that set the stage for the book in intellectually stimulating, compelling, and insightful ways.

It is my hope that the material here will contribute to developing, validating, evaluating, and applying health AI/ML with rigor, leading to performance and safety guarantees for the benefit of patients, science, and the industry. Hopefully, the reader will find the book to be a valuable companion in what is surely going to be a long and exciting journey for the field.

Constantin Aliferis

Contents

Artificial Intelligence (AI) and Machine Learning (ML) for Healthcare and Health Sciences: The Need for Best Practices Enabling Trust in AI and ML

Constantin Aliferis and Gyorgy Simon

Abstract

In the opening chapter we first introduce essential concepts about Artificial Intelligence and Machine Learning (AI/ML) in Health Care and the Health Sciences (aka Biomedical AI/ML). We then provide a brief historical perspective of the field including highlights of achievements of Biomedical AI/ML, the various generations of AI/ML efforts, and the recent explosive interest in such methods and future growth expectations. We summarize how biomedical AI and ML differ from general-purpose AI/ML. We show that pitfalls and related lack of best practices undermine practice and potential of Biomedical AI/ML. We introduce high-level requirements for biomedical AI/ML and 7 dimensions of trust, acceptance and ultimately adoption, which serve as the driving principles of the present volume. We outline the contents of the volume, both overall and chapter-by-chapter, noting the interconnections. We discuss the intended audience, and differences from other AI/ML books. We finally discuss format, style/tone, and state a few important caveats and disclosures.

Keywords

Machine learning (ML) · Artificial intelligence (AI) · Algorithm · Model · AI trust · Acceptance · Adoption

C. Aliferis (✉) · G. Simon
Institute for Health Informatics, University of Minnesota, Minneapolis, MN, USA
e-mail: constantinaibestpractices@gmail.com

What Is Machine Learning? Algorithms, Programs, and Models

A myth that was pervasive in earlier stages of the history of computing was that computers can only solve problems (or perform actions) that a human programmer had specifically instructed them how to tackle. As even the broad lay audience can appreciate circa 2023, computers equipped with Machine Learning (ML) capabilities can learn from data how to perform intelligent tasks and perform complicated problem solving on their own [1–3]. Whereas the ML algorithms are typically programmed by humans, once implemented, these types of software can interpret data in ways that far exceed the capabilities of their human creators, not just in terms of speed but also by making inferences that are qualitatively superior to humans, for example by avoiding human cognitive biases and blind spots and performing inferences that humans do not do at all or are not good at performing (e.g., pattern recognition in very high dimensional spaces sometimes in the 10^6 variables scale or more) [4]. In addition, whereas ML programs are currently typically presented with data prepared by human operators/analysts, it is entirely possible (and in some cases routine) to collect data on their own, or instruct human operators to collect data needed for problem solving [5–7].

> **Definition**
> **Machine Learning (ML)** is the science and technology of computing systems that learn how to solve problems by analyzing data related to the problems.

To go into slightly more detail, ML **algorithms** implemented in ML **programs and systems**, use so-called **training data** from which they build problem-solving **models**. It is useful to understand these important concepts further since there is confusion among the non-technical audience (including biomedical scientists and healthcare providers and administrators).

A *computer program* is a set of instructions that a computer can understand and execute toward performing a task intended by the program [8]. For example, a program written in the language *Python* that instructs a personal computer with the ability to execute Python commands, how to sort a set of numbers into descending order.

A software *computer system* is a complex set of interconnected programs that perform a number of interrelated functions. For example, an Electronic Health Record (EHR) system comprises a set of programs and databases that manage patient data to support patient care, record actions for compliance, perform billing and reimbursement, etc.

A *computer algorithm* is a generalized (programming language-agnostic) set of computer instructions designed to solve a class of problems. Computer algorithms are presented in a form (so called pseudo-code [9]) that is geared towards being interpretable by humans. In contrast, computer programs are written in a computer language that is interpretable by computers. For example, the *"quicksort" number sorting algorithm* is a set of instructions, written in a format meant for human interpretation, that can be translated to any general-purpose computer programming language. Furthermore, the quicksort algorithm needs to be translated by a programmer into a programming language, a process known as *implementing the algorithm,* before it can be executed by a computer. In another ML example, the *ID3 algorithm creates, from previously-diagnosed patient data, decision tree models* that can be used for diagnosing new patients.

An **AI/ML model** is therefore a computable representation of some problem-solving domain so that when informed with a set of inputs describing specific instances of the problem space, outputs solutions to those. These models are created by hand by using AI knowledge and other *knowledge engineering* methods and tools, and in the case of ML fully automatically from training data [10].

Computer algorithms [9, 11] *have a number of distinguishing characteristics from computer programs:*

(a) They (typically, and formally) not need be described in a specific programming language, but in *pseudo-code*, as previously explained.

(b) They represent a potentially infinite set of programs that can be implemented in every applicable programming language and computing environment.

(c) When properly constructed, they have well-defined properties that guarantee performance, error free (or error-acceptable) operation, generalizability etc. (more on this later in the book).

(d) When properly *implemented* (i.e., translated to a specific programming language) they *guarantee that the algorithm properties are imparted in the particular program that implements the algorithm.*

The field of **Design and Analysis of Algorithms** studies the properties of algorithms (and associated **data structures** [9, 11] (i.e., ways to represent and organize data for storage, retrieval and other operations)) and methods to design algorithms for specific problems so that desired operating characteristics (e.g., speed, memory usage, accuracy etc.) are achieved.

> **Pitfall 1.1**
> Very commonly in the commercial healthcare space a computer program or system implements **unspecified, undisclosed or insufficiently-analyzed algorithms,** hence no-one knows what the properties of the program are.

In chapter "Foundations and Properties of AI/ML Systems" but also in several other places of the present volume, we will address the fundamental issue of guaranteed properties of AI/ML systems and best practices enforcing those.

Pitfall 1.2

In healthcare and the health sciences, *clinical algorithms* are often confused with *computer algorithms* (including ML algorithms). A *clinical algorithm* [12, 13] describes diagnostic, risk assessment, preventative, treatment or other actions needed to care for patients with specific diseases, usually in the context of evidence-based guideline-driven medicine. It can be written in human language or specialized *computable languages*. A clinical algorithm is a human-assistive *decision model* and is not an algorithm that can learn how to solve the problem from data. Finally, a model produced by a ML algorithm can serve as a clinical algorithm in a health care setting.

ML algorithms are therefore implemented in ML computer programs that when presented with training data, learn and output decision models. In chapters "An Appraisal of Operating Characteristics of Major Machine Learning Methods Applicable to Healthcare and Health Sciences", and "Foundations of Causal Machine Learning" we will review major ML families of algorithms and describe the types of models they output. In several other chapters of the present volume we will discuss specific algorithms and models and their characteristics and optimal use.

Well-constructed ML models do have general applicability beyond the training data, otherwise they would be just a catalogue of past problem instances and their solutions, without the ability to be used for new problem instances. **Machine Learning theory** [14, 15] provides results and techniques that enable and ideally guarantee the generalization properties of ML models beyond the training data.

Artificial Intelligence (AI); Types of AI and ML Tasks; on the Pervasive Applicability of ML and AI

The language we adopted on ML algorithms as a means of solving problems, has a deeper significance as it relates to the definition of Artificial Intelligence. AI depending on the context, the era and the author, has been viewed as (a) the field of science and technology that investigates the creation of fully autonomous computer systems (i.e., "Intelligent Systems"); (b) exhibiting intelligence capabilities indistinguishable to those of humans (i.e., so-called "hard AI"); (c) providing the empirical means for putting forth and testing under controlled (computer lab) conditions theories of cognition; or (d) creating programs capable of solving hard (computational, mathematical, cognitive, decision, optimization and other inferential) problems [2]. Operationally we will adopt the following view on AI:

Definition

Artificial Intelligence (AI) is the science and technology of computing systems that can autonomously solve hard inferential problems.

Such problems historically have been associated with the prerequisite of "intelligence".

From a perspective of organization of scientific fields and their relationships, ML is one of the fields of AI which, in turn, is a field of Computer Science (CS). At the same time, ML is a core part and arguably the most important component (along with statistics) of the nascent field of *Data Science*.

> **Definition**
> **Data Science** is the field of science and technology that studies the: (a) design and execution of data measurements, sampling/collection; (b) data representation and management, harmonization, secure storage and transmission; (c) analysis, interpretation, and (d) deployment of results in applied problem-solving settings.
>
> Data Science spans and connects several fields including ML and statistics, as well as parts relevant to data sampling and modeling from applied mathematics, operations research, econometrics, psychometrics, decision sciences, information science, scientometrics and bibliometrics, statistical genetics and genomics, etc. [16, 17].

Figure 1 shows the relationship among Computer Science, AI and ML. As can be seen in the figure, both AI and ML are very diverse and developed, comprising many types of research, systems, algorithms, and applications.

An important pitfall (the importance of which will become abundantly obvious in this volume) is to consider one very narrow subfield, for example Deep Learning, as the totality or the main focus/armamentarium of all of ML and AI, or as another example, considering ML as the totality of AI. This has serious consequences as we will see in this book because it prevents users of AI and ML to have the *right perspective in which a plurality of methods can be brought to bear on solving problems by matching the right method to the problems at hand.*

> **Pitfall 1.3**
> Very commonly novice advocates of ML and AI, or vendors promoting certain products will present the whole field as being about one narrow technology or a small set of tools, ignoring the broader spectrum of available options that can solve the problem at hand. The many options available however, have hugely varying performance characteristics that need careful consideration as *no single class of methods is suitable for all biomedical problems.*

In the present book we place a heavy emphasis on data-driven forms versus expert-knowledge-driven AI, for the following reasons: first, modern health AI is predominantly data driven and will continue to be so in the foreseeable future. Second, ML is vastly more scalable than expert knowledge-driven construction of AI systems. Third, ML has many pitfalls and intricacies that require addressing. Fourth, ML is

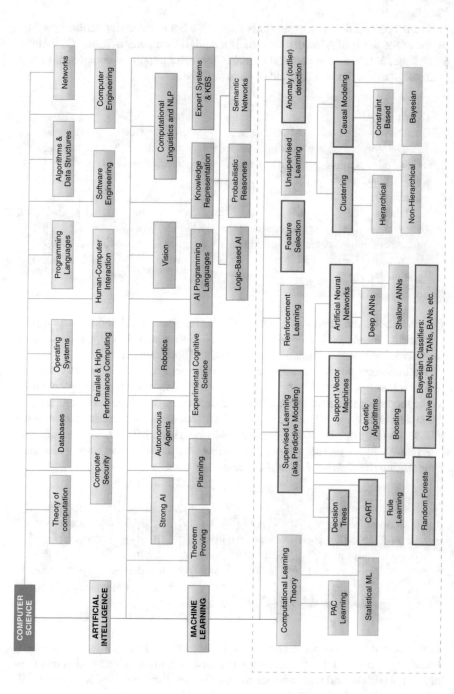

Fig. 1 Relationship and contents of Computer Science, AI and ML. In red rectangles, ML subfields with particular relevance to health sciences and healthcare

also an important component of other forms of AI (e.g., NLP, computer vision, robotics). Finally, the highlighted pitfalls and best practices are often useful for both ML and other forms of AI.

Readers not already deeply familiar with AI/M applications in the health sciences and care delivery are likely to be surprised by the *extraordinarily wide range of applications* of these fields. This *pervasive applicability of ML and AI is not accidental,* however. It can be immediately grasped once one considers that both health sciences and care are fundamentally designed to pursue discovery and application of predictive and causal knowledge. **Predictive modeling** encompasses diagnosis, prognosis, forecasting and general pattern recognition [1–4]. **Causal modeling** [18–20] seeks to discover cause-effect relationships, to quantify their effects, and to choose among various interventions those that will maximize some desired outcome. It encompasses discovery of laws of biology, therapeutics, understanding the factors that drive system and patient-level outcomes such as development, treatment and prevention of disease at the individual level. At the level of the system of care, they encompass intervention on factors that affect quality of care, costs, reimbursements, patient experience and all other desiderata of health systems [21].

Neither General AI/ML, Nor Biomedical AI/ML Are New. Highlights of Achievements of Biomedical AI/ML

The general public became aware of AI and ML as a viable technology in very recent years as a result of the emergence of commercial offerings backed by established corporations as well as numerous startups catering to healthcare systems and health research organizations. The scope of adoption and widespread use of AI and ML, is currently breathtaking and includes: autonomous vehicle navigation (cars, airplanes, industrial robots), cybersecurity, fraud and spam detection, financial applications, internet and e-commerce applications, manufacturing, games, education, legal, and numerous other applications [22].

In healthcare and the health sciences, **examples of successful applications** include automated diagnosis, prognosis, treatment selection (using as inputs: coded clinical data, text reports, images, omics data, etc.) [23]; discovery of gene mutations causing specific forms of cancer or other disease [24]; precision medicine tests (e.g., genes' expression level patterns determining response to a treatment used for treatment selection) [25]; automated evaluation of scientific papers to determine whether the research design was good [26]; annotating genomes and other genetics applications [27]; predicting tertiary & quaternary protein structure from amino acid sequence [28]; predicting drug-drug and drug-food interactions [29]; medical imaging [30] and numerous other applications which we will cover in depth in the present volume.

The advent of **big data** in particular, in healthcare and population health (e.g., EHR, sensor, environmental, social networks) and the health sciences (e.g., genomics, proteomics, metabolomics, microbiomics, copy number variation, and other "bulk" and single cell "omics" data, deep sequencing databases, research consortia data, etc.) has simultaneously demanded the development of high-quality scalable analysis methods and strongly incentivized their deployment at scale [31]. In the last 20 years *there is a synergistic co-evolution of big data generation/capture and ML-driven analysis and discovery* with **key themes of modern health science and health care** such as: rational drug development [32], modern post-sequencing era genomics precision and personalized medicine [25], learning health systems and care cost/quality/experience improvements [33], to mention just some of the key developments that depend on ML and AI and that are foci of the present work.

To give a sense of the immense scope and rapid maturity with respect to health outcomes the following searches[1] return:

(("outcomes" or "health services") and "machine learning")	→ 6255 results (most since 2015)
(("outcomes" or "health services") and "machine learning") and "systematic review"	→ 240 results

These systematic reviews (not cited explicitly here for space, but readily retrievable from PubMed with the stated queries) represent broad application areas with significant and diverse bodies of work. They include predictive, prognostic, diagnostic and etiologic outcomes modeling in:

Neurosurgical outcomes, depression, obesity, surgical outcomes, EEG classification, dermatology, urology outcomes, suicide prevention, Covid mortality, autoimmune disease outcomes, stroke, various cancers, dementias, orthopedic surgery, heart failure outcomes, pregnancy outcomes, imaging and radiomics analysis, sepsis in the ICU, managing covid-19, assessing physician competence, hematopoietic stem cell transplantation (HSCT), various infectious diseases, cardiac surgery, management and treatment of burns, infant pain evaluation, management of heart failure patients, bipolar disorder, degenerative cervical and lumbar spine disease, cardiovascular outcomes from wearable data, psychosocial outcomes in acquired brain injury, acute gastrointestinal bleeding, personalized dosing of heparin, Parkinson's disease, genetic prediction of psychiatric disorders, diabetes, clinical deterioration in hospitalized patients, community-based primary health care, palliative and end-of-life care, hypertension, graft failure following kidney transplantation, outcomes in neonatal intensive care units, degenerative spine surgery, predicting fatal and serious injury crashes from driver crash and offense history data, health care spending, extraction of data from randomized trials, improving medication adherence in hypertensive patients, neighborhood-level risk factors, gait analysis, wearable inertial sensors to quantify everyday life motor activity in people with mobility impairments, outcome prediction of medical litigation, rheumatic and musculoskeletal diseases, analysis of patient online reviews, chronic low back pain, risk of readmission and several other topics.

---

[1] Conducted on June 2, 2022

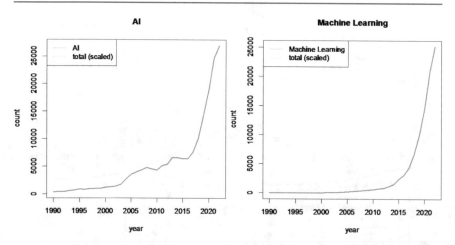

Fig. 2 Number of PubMed publications with MeSH term "Artificial Intelligence" (left) and keyword "Machine learning" (right) in the years between 1990 and 2022. To facilitate the comparison of growth between AI/ML and publications in general, the black dotted line represents (a downward scaled version) of the total number of publications in PubMed

PubMed is also informative on relative literature volumes pertaining to AI/ML methods and applications, and their trends[2]:

Figure 2 illustrates the explosive growth of ML and AI through the number of Pubmed publications over the years between 1990 and 2022. The blue line represents the number of publications for AI [MeSH] (left) and Machine Learning [Keyword] (right); the black dotted line represents the scaled number of total citations (from any field). The rate of growth in AI and ML far outpaces the overall growth rate of publications since 2015.

In Fig. 3, we show how the growth in health AI is distributed over some of its subfields. Machine Learning enjoys most of the growth, with Natural Language Processing (NLP) and Image Analysis following closely. Modern advances in Machine Learning, Deep Learning in particular, serve as an enabling technology for both of these subfields. Other subfields, such as Knowledge Representation exhibited a more modest growth, while Expert Systems appears to have experienced negative growth since they are being replaced by ML. We need to remember that PubMed focuses on biomedicine.

In terms of absolute volume of publications, the following tables provide relevant data (Table 1):

These results are to some degree an artifact of the indexing of articles employed by Pubmed. For example:

"clustering" (which is a form of ML)	→ 489,442 results
"Artificial neural network" (Mesh term)	→ 23,746 results
But:	
"Deep learning" (Mesh term)	→ 40,377 results

---

[2] conducted on June 2, 2022, and using Mesh index terms when available

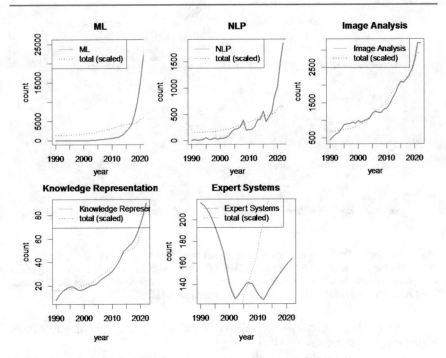

Fig. 3 Trends of publications in various subfields of AI between 1990 and 2022

Table 1 Health AI/ML publication volumes		
	"machine learning" (Mesh term)	→ 89,260 entries
	artificial intelligence (Mesh term)	→ 165,990 results
	("artificial intelligence" or "machine learning") (keywords)	→ 113,531 results

Caveat: Deep Learning is a special type of artificial neural network, which entails that if indexed properly the entries indexed by "artificial neural network" should be a strict superset of the entries indexed by "Deep Learning".

As to articles with key types of ML, in addition to the ones above we see:

"Decision tree" (Mesh)	→ 23,206 results
"Support vector machine" (Mesh)	→ 22,675
"Genetic algorithm" (Mesh)	→ 90,728 results
"Random forest" (Mesh)	→ 23,357 results
"Bayesian network" (Mesh)	→ 10,076 results
"Bayesian classifier" (Mesh)	→ 12,503 results
"Granger causality" (Mesh)	→ 3810 results

With regards to major types of AI in addition to the ML ones mentioned we see:

"Autonomous robot"	→ 2743 results (most since 2005)
"Expert systems"	→ 20,627 results (most since 1990)
"Knowledge representation"	→ 12,526 results (most since 1990)
"Semantic network"	→ 6482 results (most since 2005)
"Natural language processing"	→ 9659 results (most since 2005)

The exponential-rate growth of most of these methods in the biomedical literature started and took place for the most part in the last 15-to 30 years. It is worth noting that in the field of Biomedical Informatics (aka Health Informatics) seminal publications in ML and AI appeared as early as in 1959, however. The 1959 article by Ledley and Lusted [34] is particularly important since it anticipated many of the key themes and methods that were rediscovered (and in some cases ignored) by modern commercial vendors and academic or industry adopters of biomedical AI/ML 63 years later.

Similarly, the 1961 article by Warner et al. is [35] is a seminal paper for the field of Medical Informatics and describes a ML-based approach to improving diagnosis in a significant disease, later expanded to many other diseases in the 60s all the way to the 80s by these and other pioneering investigators.

Another important seminal early work, this time in human expert knowledge-driven AI was the work by Miller et al. [36]. This notable AI system employed heuristic knowledge representation and reasoning that managed to perform at a hard reasoning task (challenging diagnostic cases across all of internal medicine) at a level that matched or in some cases exceeded expert physicians. This system was emblematic of the efforts in the 70 s and the 80 s to create AI that was driven by extracting and representing in computable form human expert problem solving. These efforts were followed by newer ML-based systems with the advent of more capable ML algorithms and representations taking advantage of increasing amounts of training data, such as Bayesian Networks and other sophisticated Bayesian classifiers [37, 38], early multi-layered artificial neural networks [39, 40], decision tree learners and other ML algorithms [1–4] that vastly outperformed in ease of use, cost-effectiveness and accuracy early ML algorithms and human expert knowledge.

The "Perfect Storm" for Biomedical AI/ML

The ability to capture massive Big Data (as indicated above) in the 2000s and onward, fueled the explosive application and refinements in kernel-based nonlinear classifiers (e.g., SVMs) [1–4], boosting algorithms, causal discovery and inference algorithms [18–20], deep artificial neural networks [39, 40, 41], significant extensions to decision trees (Random Forests [42]), regularized versions of statistical regression algorithms [43], and other methods that could now manage tens, hundreds and in some cases millions of variables with modest compute requirements and most importantly with extreme tolerance to low sample sizes without overfitting [44]. These methods exhibited properties that classical statistical science and practice previously considered impossible [4, 14]. Some types of newer algorithms also had the ability to discover causality without experiments which have also been considered previously impossible [18–20] and newer scalable causal algorithms that made application to high dimensional data as well as scalable hybrid predictive and causal modeling feasible [45–48]. This "perfect storm" for biomedical AI/ML led to its current cycle of explosive growth. It is not surprising that the above developments in general AI and ML are closely associated with the work of **9 Turing award recipients** (Marvin Minsky, John McCarthy, Herbert A. Simon, Edward Feigenbaum, Raj Reddy, Judea Pearl, Yoshua Bengio, Geoffrey Hinton, Yan Le Cun), and **7 Nobel Prize recipients** in economics: (Herbert A. Simon, Daniel Kahneman, Clive Granger, Thomas A. Sargent, Christopher A. Sims, Joshua Angirst, Guido Imbens) solidifying thus the scientific credibility and immense importance of these methods.

Yet, despite all of this scientific activity and accomplishments (>three million entries in Google Scholar mentioning ML and > three million mentioning AI as of 2023), these fields have been presented to the general public and the non-experts, as either entirely new, or they have been presented as invented recently in the laboratories of a handful of commercial companies. This brings us to another important pitfall:

Pitfall 1.4
The field of general and biomedical AI and ML is not a new one. Ignoring the vast literature and re-inventing the wheel in some cases, fails to take advantage of a wealth of very substantial prior work that can inform effective, safe and cost-effective use. Methods that have undergone rigorous development, analysis and validation over many years have in general better-understood properties, better performance robustness, and better operating safety characteristics than newer less well-developed methods.

Best Practice 1.1
When considering development or application of AI/ML, ensure that it is informed by the well-developed and evaluated pre-existing science and technology.

Differentiation of Biomedical AI and ML from General-Purpose AI/ML

Another important pitfall we will address in this volume is the distinction between general purpose AI & ML versus biomedically-tailored AI & ML.

Pitfall 1.5

Biomedical AI and ML have specific requirements and adaptations tailored to the goals of healthcare and of health sciences discovery. AI and ML devised and tested in unrelated fields have very different properties and do not ensure the goals of healthcare and health science applications.

A summary of the adaptations and differentiation, to be elaborated further in this volume, is as follows:

Biomedical AI/ML:
(a) Is driven by, and has strong interactions with clinical objectives, health economics, and healthcare delivery within specific health systems.
(b) Requires the ability to handle very large dimensionalities (i.e., number of variables).
(c) Requires the ability to handle very small sample sizes without overfitting.
(d) Must be equipped with the ability to discover and model causality, since it is often necessary to estimate effects of interventions.
(e) Requires specialized data operations and the ability to handle diverse data types including clinical coded data, text, imaging, biomolecular data, and combinations.
(f) Places great emphasis on accuracy, cost-effectiveness, quality control and de-risking.

All of these requirements will be addressed in detail in the present volume.

Future Potential of Biomedical AI/ML

As widespread and rapidly growing biomedical AI/ML is, it has potential for orders of magnitude more growth. For example, compared to classical biostatistics, AI/ML has a smaller data science footprint in biomedical literature as revealed by the following PubMed searches:

"Cox regression" (Mesh)	→ 105,385 results
"Chi square test" (Mesh)	→ 116,546 results
"ANOVA" (Mesh)	→ 522,350 results
"Regression" (Mesh)	→ 1,011,918 results

AI/ML methods are rapidly substituting complex inferential statistics and/or are extending them in substantial ways, however. There are many signals for the forthcoming growth of biomedical AI/ML. We mention a few strong indicators:

(a) In the domain of *molecular profiling for precision medicine* [25], only just a handful of such profiles have been brought to market so far, although, >170,000 molecular signature papers have been published (many of them showing feasibility of clinical signatures). The number of patient-touching precision tests expected to be in use *at any given time* in the future, if estimated as the combination of (*diseases * drugs*), exceeds 100,000.

(b) Other areas where massive biomedical AI/ML growth is expected include *health systems outcomes improvement* [21] with hundreds of thousands of AI/ML models conceivable to be developed and deployed in the future, assuming that at least one model will be deployed for every major decision/disease/outcome combination that is affecting patients, units and systems.

(c) Similarly in the space of *precision clinical trials* [25] currently much less than 1% of all trials are precision trials and migrating to this model of clinical therapeutics validation will necessitate application of AI/ML at scale across the research domain (>20,000 new large new trials annually).

(d) In *radiology*, we can safely expect a massive transition to computer-assisted (and in some cases fully automated) interpretation of clinical or research imaging, across many health science and care domains.

(e) In *single-cell transcriptomics and other omics (including "multiplexed" combinations) and their spatiotemporal extensions*, the use of AI/ML is absolutely necessitated by the immense dimensionalities (> 5000 cells * 10,000 molecular probes with current technology yields dimensionalities of > 50 million variables *per patient/research subject*). Single-cell omics technologies are the successor of bulk deep sequencing technologies (themselves the successor of microarray technologies) and according to all indications, will be driving biological discovery for decades to come. If these precursors are an indication, then 100,000 s of applications of AI/ML single-cell omics are to be expected [49, 50].

(f) The vast majority of models referenced in the hundreds of systematic reviews (covering thousands of modeling studies) mentioned in section "Neither General AI/ML, nor Biomedical AI/ML are New. Highlights of Achievements of Biomedical AI/ML", are pre-clinical or otherwise feasibility efforts as stated in the corresponding systematic reviews. These reviews found very promising results but identified that the models have not yet reached the clinically mature stages needed for broad deployment. Closing this gap will undoubtedly be a large part of the future of health AI/ML.

Pitfalls and Related Lack of Best Practices Undermine Biomedical AI/ML. AI/ML Trust and Acceptance

The strong and sustained trends outlined above in the literature and commercial AI/ML, suggest that *AI/ML will grow to be a science and technology that permanently and irrevocably enables progress across all aspects of health science research and health care delivery. There is an ethical and utilitarian necessity therefore for this science and technology to be executed with an emphasis on meeting performance, safety, and cost-effectiveness requirements.*

Performance requirements entail that AI/ML has to be accurate and minimize false positive and false negative results. For example, the massive application of AI/ML if allowed to generate false positives will drown the research system in noise, rendering the space of scientific investigation a destructively low signal-to-noise environment. Avoidable false negatives due to poorly thought AI/ML represents the space of corresponding opportunity cost.

Safety requirements entail that AI/ML systems applied in clinical care settings as well as preventative policy and other public health settings should not allow for any avoidable errors of either wrong treatment/intervention decisions that incur risk to patients, populations, or systems of care. They should also not allow errors of failing to identify opportunities to improve patient/human subject health (for example, diagnosis of treatable diseases, opportunities to improve cost and quality of the system of care) as such failures translate to decreased life expectancy/quality of life of individuals, populations and negatively affect the health systems that care for them.

Cost-effectiveness requirements entail that AI/ML systems applied in care settings as well as health science discovery should not be wasteful in either time-to-results, or compute requirements, or sample size requirements, or cost of decisions. The costs of such inefficiencies can quickly become unmanageable.

Perspectives on building trust, adoption, and acceptance of technology by humans (as individuals or at the society level) are diverse and encompass performance, economic, legal, accountability, ethical, psychological, social and other factors [51–59]. Operationally we frame the above requirements from the perspective of stakeholders using a Biomedical *AI/ML trust and acceptance framework, comprising the following 7 dimensions:*

1. **Scientific and Technical Trust and Acceptance.** AI/MLmodels must be accurate at deployment (e.g., low error rate, not falling outside their boundaries of strong performance (known as their "knowledge cliff")).
2. **Health System Trust and Acceptance** AI/ML models must be safe, cost-effective and well-embedded in systems of health with clear benefits and without unexpected/unacceptable risks, disruptions or other negative consequences.

3. **System-of-science Trust and Acceptance.** AI/ML models must be safe and cost-effective to operate in the system of science without unexpected/unacceptable risks and consequences.
4. **Beneficiary Trust and Acceptance.** AI/ML models must be accepted by patients and human subjects individually and at the community level.
5. **Delivery and Operator Trust and Acceptance**. AI/ML models must be accepted by clinicians and scientists.
6. **Regulatory Trust and Acceptance.** AI/ML models must be compliant to applicable laws and approved by regulatory bodies.
7. **Ethical Trust and Acceptance.** AI/ML models must be non-discriminatory and must promote health equity and social justice related to health science and care (e.g., by being non-discriminatory on the basis of race, socioeconomic factors, gender, etc.).

In their 2022 program solicitation (NSF 22–502), entitled "*National AI Research Institutes Accelerating Research, Transforming Society, and Growing the American Workforce*", the National Science Foundation (NSF) acknowledged that identifying, prioritizing, and satisfying the fundamental attributes that render an AI trustworthy are open research challenges. Notably the program described trustworthiness through examples from other areas of mature technology such as automobiles or electric lighting. These systems are trustworthy, "*because they are reliable, predictable, governed by rigorous and measurable standards, and provide the expected benefits. Facilitated by basic knowledge of their operation, we are familiar with common faults and how to address them, and there is infrastructure to deal with problems we cannot handle ourselves.*" It's a compelling proposition that health-related AI should have similar characteristics.

The whole purpose of the present volume therefore is to outline a set of **preferred practical requirements and methods ("Best Practices') that will move us forward to biomedical AI/ML that avoids pitfalls and achieves the 7 dimensions of trust, acceptance and eventual adoption**. In order to justify the requirements and assemble/build the proposed best practices we will also need to introduce a body of necessary technical background knowledge.

Intended Purpose and Audience of the Book

AI & ML are extremely popular topics and numerous books are available, generally falling into four categories:

1. *Hands-on instructional texts on how to build a general-purpose AI system*, e.g., using a particular Python software package. Such books are not specific to health care or health sciences and their specific problems; nor do they provide a strong conceptual understanding of how different models work and how this relates to their applicability to different health problems.

2. *General purpose data mining, AI, and ML textbooks.* Such books do not relate to health care or health science and do not give advice on how to develop models specifically for health care or any other area: they focus on a very narrow aspect of model development. Moreover they do not differentiate between feasibility and exploratory analysis from the much more mission-critical clinical and other high-stakes modelling settings that are so prominent in healthcare and the health sciences.

3. *Health care analytics and the promise of AI in health care.* Most works in this category focus on conventional (reporting and compliance) analytics. A few address the new capabilities brought by AI/ML. They are not designed to provide the reader with a deep understanding of what the (primarily) technical challenges are in health care AI, or what the pitfalls are and how specifically and systematically to avoid them.

4. *Bioinformatics and genomics discussing AI/ML approaches in that context.* These are technical books that typically do not focus on systematic methodologies for ensuring appropriateness of various AI/ML methods, or their methodological underpinnings.

From our review of the literature there are more than 100 textbooks in 2023 in press in the above categories. We view them as very useful background for broad fundamentals and/or context of use: from such books readers can learn basic concepts of general machine learning, and can also learn how to build certain types of models; our present effort however focuses on knowledge and practices specific to how health science, clinical, translational, and healthcare AI/ML systems differ from the general-purpose AI/ML. The book aspires to impart comprehensive and in-depth knowledge on how to build robust and safe models for the high-stakes settings in health science and care, and to evaluate the strengths and weaknesses of such models produced by others. We will cover both general (mostly immutable) scientific principles as well as specific technical guidance that may evolve over time.

More precisely, we envisioned the present volume to be the first book in the field to provide guidance for the following concepts/topics:

1. The critical differences between general-purpose AI & ML and medically-applicable AI & ML.
2. Building models that can be applied with minimal risk in high-stakes settings including clinical applications, healthcare system optimization, and discovery of clinical modalities.
3. Models that integrate multi-level, multi-modal clinical and molecular data.
4. The importance of data design and post-modelling safeguards for high-stakes applications.
5. Common limitations and remedies of efforts (commercial and academic) in the field.

6. In-depth presentation of not just predictive but also causal and hybrid causal-predictive methods.
7. A comprehensive summary and critique of operating characteristics of all major AI & ML methods.

This volume emphasizes the need and methods for biomedical AI/ML to:

1. Be intentional, with well-defined and meaningful goals and metrics of success.
2. Effectively manage risk for errors that may affect adversely the health of patients, the effectiveness of health systems, and the effectiveness of the system of science.
3. Operate in real-life (as opposed to idealized and simplified theoretical) health care as well as in health science discovery ecosystems.
4. Develop within a lifecycle that starts from problem statements and needs all the way to successful deployment and continuous iterative improvement.
5. Prevent and overcome the fundamental dangers of over fitting and under fitting as well over confidence in models and under performance of models.
6. Have known properties that guarantee performance and safety.
7. Be based on sophisticated and appropriate data designs.
8. Be differentiated along the levels of systems/stacks, protocols, algorithms, models.

We adopt an interdisciplinary perspective, using and integrating methods from Data Science, Computer science (Machine Learning, AI, predictive analytics), Statistics, Epidemiology (study design), Clinical Decision Support, Bioinformatics, Clinical and Health Informatics, Genomics, Learning Health Systems, and Precision and Personalized Medicine.

Our intended audience comprises all stakeholders to the healthcare and health science ecosystems: (a) *Applied and research Health Data Scientists* working in industry, academia, and healthcare. (b) *Clinicians/Professionals/Practitioners* who are called on to evaluate, select, and use AI&ML based decision support. (c) *Healthcare and translational (e.g. pharmaceutics and biotechnology) industry leaders/ administrators* including but not limited to IT leaders who wish to evaluate and deploy competing technologies in medical AI&ML. (d) *Educators and Students* in informatics, ML & AI, health economics, health business administration, and data science. (e) Funding agency officers. (f) Journals and their editors. (g) Regulatory agency officers. And (h) Community members, representatives and advocates.

We elected to make this book an ***open access*** one, ensuring that all members of our intended audience can access this volume without financial restrictions.

Outline of the Book: Style, Format, and How to Read

The book is organized in three parts (with a total of 18 chapters): Foundations, Modelling, and Implementation. Each chapter typically covers several of the following: technical didactic exposition, case studies (of success and failure varieties), related pitfalls discussion, best practices addressing the pitfalls and serving the trust principles, along with literature references and occasional discussion thereof. We also provide brief chapter abstracts (at the start of each chapter), assignments for classroom use, and recapitulation of concepts, definitions, pitfalls and Best Practices (at the end of each chapter).

Educators may wish to use the book in whole or in part as classroom textbook. Features supporting classroom use include:

1. Consistent structure and tone to the chapters. The two main authors have written the majority of the material and have co-authored or edited the contributing chapters to harmonize the content and style across the volume.
2. Practice questions, discussion topics and assignments. Some of those are more conceptual and open-ended (e.g. appropriate for less technical learners) and some are more technology-oriented (e.g. targeting learners who need to develop technical knowledge and skills).
3. Comprehensive coverage of the topic, not just the methods that the authors have invented, have used, or prefer.
4. In the future we intend to provide an "official" answer key to the assignments and discussion topics of this volume.

Because our intended audience is very diverse, we make every effort to use plain language with minimal jargon and to keep mathematical, statistical and computer science technical details at a minimum. This does not mean that we shy away from presenting formulas, algorithms, and theorems. However, when we do so, we present them only when they are necessary for making sense of the Pitfalls/Best Practices in discussion. We also sought to use the simplest language possible that does not sacrifice validity. We also introduce background we think is required to understand these technical elements and emphasize the intuition and their practical consequences behind them.

The style and level of detail has been ground-tested on our teaching these concepts (for a combined 30+ years) in a variety of settings and audiences (e.g., from undergrad college interns to professional programmers, to graduate students in data science fields, to medical residents, to health sciences faculty, and to national tutorials with mixed health care and health science audiences). As is expected, our writing reflects our own formal training in these fields (spanning 27 years combined). More importantly, both main authors of the present volume are working scientists who have led and are active in many R&D method/technology and applications projects. These have occurred in the health sciences domain (mostly funded by the NIH and the NSF) but also in industry and in health care contexts. These experiences have provided us with a wealth of knowledge about the roadblocks that our intended audience routinely faces, and the ways to overcome them.

At the end, of course, the reader will decide if the approach taken here is as effective as we hope it will be. We caution that audiences with strong technical backgrounds may find the text "hiding" some technical details. We advise these readers to explore the ample references for more technical depth, and to focus their reading of the book on applied aspects that are not covered at all or are not synthesized sufficiently in the primary technical literature.

Audiences without or with incomplete technical backgrounds may find some concepts challenging at first read. Unless otherwise noted, we advise this type of reader to not skip the scientific and technological principles underlying ML/AI, since these are critical for successful use in high stakes tasks and environments.

With regards to the book assignments, we revisit and *incrementally enrich and deepen many of them* as new knowledge is provided by the various chapters. Readers should address them with the knowledge gained up until the chapter they are encountered.

Finally we recommend the independent reader to read the chapters in sequence (possibly only skimming material that the reader has already mastered elsewhere). We made every effort to cross-reference in each chapter concepts with all other parts of the book where they are discussed so even an out-of-sequence reading should be free of confusion.

For in-classroom use, the class instructor is trusted to determine the right components to emphasize or omit, and in the right sequence for her class objectives and learners' background and needs. The incremental structure of assignments and discussion topics is valuable for *developing gradually an increasingly sophisticated understanding of recurring themes and topics*. It can also serve as a record of the students' progress in mastering the related body of knowledge and their ability to integrate and evaluate the material. This will be disrupted unavoidably in any out-of-sequence reading, however, and the instructor has to make adjustments to the assignments in such cases.

We also note that all assignments are motivated by real-life examples of methods development and application challenges. They can be traced to literature and case studies in the public domain as well as to our personal experience as working scientists, teachers, advisors, consultants and administrators. Whenever we felt there was possibility to breach upon privacy or reputation of third parties, we omitted specific references to technology and persons, in all other cases we name methods, products, and scientists, especially when credit was due for important discoveries or other scientific and technological contribution acknowledgment.

Caveats and Disclosures: Sourcing Best Practices

Where Do Best Practices Come from?

The realistic answer is that, circa 2023, biomedical AI/ML Best Practices are not to be found in one place, stated as such, and having fully complete and immutable status. This volume, to the best of our knowledge, is the first book to strive for that goal. Our recommendations originate from a variety of sources and are characterized by different levels of (a) maturity/validation, (b) breadth of applicability, and

(c) technical clarity and depth. We have thus considered and included in the present volume the following sources for the presented Best Practices:

1. **Published guidelines stated as such,** for example the PubMed search ("artificial intelligence" or "machine learning") and "best practices"(e.g., [60]) yields 217 results, several of which contain proposed best practices (of various degrees of validation and usefulness as we will see in subsequent chapters). In some cases important Best Practices and guidelines are contained in articles with a broader scope, for example, guidance issued by the biometrics division of the NCI [61].
2. **Implicit but clear findings and recommendations published by quality control consortia** (e.g., [62]).
3. **Broad and well-designed benchmark studies** that demonstrate the appropriateness and effectiveness of various algorithms in specific settings (e.g., [62, 63]).
4. **AI/ML competitions** (properly designed to prevent biases) e.g., [64].
5. **Criteria used in meta-analytic and systematic review studies** to assess quality, risk of bias etc. (see for example chapter "Reporting standards, Certification/Accreditation & Reproducibility").
6. **Published reporting, regulatory, and certification standards and requirements** (e.g., [65]).
7. **Theoretical properties of AI/ML algorithms, protocols and related methods** that directly suggest proper and improper usage (see for example chapters "Foundations and Properties of AI/ML Systems", "An Appraisal of Operating Characteristics of Major Machine Learning Methods Applicable to Healthcare and Health Sciences", and "Introduction to Causal Inference and Causal Structure Discovery").
8. **Case studies** that inform generalizable types of errors and suggest strategies to avoid them (see for example chapter "Lessons Learnt from Historical Failures, Limitations and Success of Health AI/ML. Enduring Problems and the Role of Best Practices").
9. **Literature reports that have focused on identifying specific types of errors or modeling/analysis problems** and have provided reusable approaches for avoiding or minimizing them (e.g., [66]).

In general this volume avoids offering guidance based on the authors' preferred workflows or methods unless these are falling in one of the above categories.

A key value proposition of the present work therefore is that we have assembled, reviewed, critically analyzed, and synthesized a plurality of sources to inform pitfalls and related best ways currently known for improving AI/ML quality, performance, effectiveness and safety.

We caution the reader that like every other cutting-edge field of scientific endeavor, this is work in progress and some of the currently known Best Practices in ML/AI will undoubtedly improve and be revised as new methods come into play and the field deepens and widens its knowledge. We welcome reader feedback and criticism and we will make every effort to appraise and incorporate all useful suggestions in future editions. See also "Final Synthesis of Recommendations" for discussion about future evolution of Best Practices.

Outline of the Book: Contents Summary by Part and Chapter

Part I: Foundations

This present chapter entitled *"Artificial Intelligence (AI) and Machine Learning (ML) for Healthcare and Health Sciences: the need for Best Practices enabling Trust in AI and ML"*), aims to provide introductory concepts about the field, to motivate the need for best practices in biomedical AI and ML, and to map out the book's scope and contents so that readers are well oriented. A small set of high-level pitfalls and guidelines are also included.

Chapter *"Foundations and Properties of AI/ML Systems"* provides a broad introduction to the foundations of health AI and ML systems and includes: (1) Theoretical properties and formal vs heuristic systems; practical implications of complexity for system tractability. (2) Foundations of AI including logics and symbolic vs non-symbolic AI, Reasoning with Uncertainty, AI/ML programming languages. (3) Foundations of Machine Learning Theory.

Chapter *"An Appraisal of Operating Characteristics of Major Machine Learning Methods Applicable to Healthcare and Health Sciences"* provides an outline of how each method works, and in addition we summarize the intended uses, the usual way it is employed in practice, and its known and unknown properties. Readers who have not delved into ML before, will find a useful introduction and review of key methods. Readers who may already know about some or all of these methods will gain additional insights as we critically revisit the key concepts and add to their prior knowledge summary guidance on *whether and when* each technique is applicable or preferred (or not) in healthcare and health science problem solving.

Chapter *"Introduction to Causal Machine Learning"* covers the important dimension of causality. The vast majority of texts in biomedical AI/ML focuses on predictive modeling and does not address causal methods, their requirements and properties. Yet these are essential for determining and assisting patient-level or healthcare-level interventions toward improving outcomes of interest. Causal methods are also indispensable for discovery in the health sciences.

Chapter *"Principles of Rigorous Development and of Appraisal of ML and AI Methods and Systems"* outlines a comprehensive process, governing all steps from analysis and problem domain needs specification, to creation and validation of AI/ML methods that can address them. The stages are explained and grounded in many existing methods. The process discussed equates to a generalizable Best Practice guideline applicable across all of AI/ML. An equally important use of this Best Practice is as a guide for understanding and evaluating any ML/AI technology under consideration for adoption for a particular problem domain.

Part II: Modelling

Chapter *"The Process and Lifecycle of a Clinical-Grade AI/ML Model"* introduces the notion of "clinical-grade" models and contrasts such models with feasibility, exploratory, or pre-clinical ones. The main tenet of the chapter is that AI/ML systems and models must be designed and deployed in a manner that is aware of, and seamlessly integrated in healthcare systems or discovery processes (for healthcare and health science discovery, respectively). The steps outlined span from requirements engineering to deployment, monitoring and iterative development and continuous improvement. They also emphasize contextual factors that influence success.

Chapter *"Data Design for Biomedical AI/ML"* addresses the critical aspect of data (or research) design and related best practices. This endeavor is foundational to the success of AI/ML for both clinical care and scientific discovery. Yet to the extent of our review of the literature, a systematic and in-depth treatment of this most important aspect receives little attention in the ML literature. In this chapter (a) we present common designs (e.g., retrospective, cohort, case/control, EHR, time series, RCT, hybrid, etc.) and implications of design choices for the success of modelling; (b) we discuss common data biases (e.g., selection bias, assertion bias, confounding bias, Simpson's paradox, etc.).

Chapter *"Data Preparation, Transforms, Quality, and Management"* introduces guidance for performing data preparations so that the goals of modeling are effectively and efficiently accomplished. It also addresses *data quality, mapping, feature engineering, data transformations, clinical and research data warehousing and management.*

Chapter *"Model Selection and Evaluation"* addresses best practices for finding models that are accurate, and generalize well. Estimation of the generalization error is also addressed both in terms of *error estimator* procedures and their interaction with model selection as well as in terms of *error metrics* and their effect on analysis. In addition to general-purpose performance metrics, this chapter also discusses aspects of model evaluation that are unique to biomedical applications, such as evaluating clinical efficacy, the suitability of a model for clinical decision support, and health economic evaluations.

Chapter *"Overfitting, Underfitting and Model Overconfidence and Underperformance in Machine Learning and AI"* makes a deep dive into overfitting and under fitting which are arguably two of the most far-reaching and impactful challenges in AI/ML with high-dimensional data, modest or small sample sizes, and modern high-capacity learners. Avoiding over and under-fitted analyses and models is critical for ensuring high generalization performance. In modern ML/AI practice these factors are typically interacting with error estimator procedures and model selection, as well as with sampling and reporting biases and thus are considered together in context. These concepts are also closely related to statistical significance and scientific reproducibility. We examine several common scenarios where over confidence in model performance and/or model under performance occur as well as recommended practices for preventing, testing and correcting them.

Chapter "From *'Human vs Machine'* to *'Human with Machine'*" addresses: (a) empirical evaluations of healthcare and health science AI/ML decision-making. (b) Empirical comparisons of computer vs human decision making in health sciences and health care. (c) Important human cognitive biases that lead to decision errors.

(d) Summary comparison of human vs computer strengths and limitations that may manifest as errors in medical practice or science discovery settings. (e) Practical considerations in constructing hybrid computer-human problem-solving systems.

Chapter "*Lessons Learned from Historical Failures, Limitations and Successes of Health AI/ML. Enduring Problems, and the Role of Best Practices*" covers a variety of case studies relevant to best practices. Examples include: the infamous "AI winters"; overfitting; using methods not built to purpose; over-estimating the value and potential of early and heuristic technology; developing AI that is disconnected from real-life needs and application contexts; over-interpreting or misinterpreting results from learning theory; failures/shortcomings of literature including the persistence of incorrect findings; failures/shortcomings of modeling protocols, data and evaluation designs; high profile science failures; factors that may render guidelines themselves problematic. These case studies in most cases were followed by improved technology that overcame the limitations. The case studies reinforce, and demonstrate the value of rigorous, science-driven practices for addressing enduring and new challenges.

Chapter "*Characterizing and Managing the Risk of AI/ML Models in Clinical and Organizational Application*" covers practical methods for reviewing the face validity of AI/ML models, and characterizing and managing risk of such models at development and at deployment stages. This chapter also briefly discusses broader methods and practices for detecting and correcting issues with ML modeling and the emerging concept of *debugging* ML models and analyses.

Part III: Implementation

Chapter "*Considerations for Specialized Health AI/ML Modelling and Applications: NLP*" looks into the field- and task-specific best practices for the domain of health NLP.

Chapter "*Considerations for Specialized Health AI/ML Modelling and Applications: Imaging – Through the perspective of Dermatology*" looks into field and task-specific best practices in the specialized domain of Imaging (with a dermatology focus).

Chapter "*Regulatory Aspects and Ethical, Legal, and Societal Implications (ELSI)*" reviews the regulation of AI/ML models, the risk management principles underlying international regulations of clinical AI/ML, discusses the conditions under which AI/ML models in the U.S. are regulated by the Food and Drug Administration (FDA), and reviews FDA's Good Machine Learning Practice (GMLP) principles. In its second part, the chapter provides an introduction to the nascent field of biomedical AI ethics, covering general AI ELSI studies, AI/ML racial bias, and AI/ML health equity principles. The chapter discusses (and gives illustrative examples) of the importance of causality and equivalence classes for practical detection of racial bias in models. It concludes with a series of recommended best practices for promoting health equity and reducing health disparities via the design and use of health AI/ML.

Chapter "*Reporting Standards, Certification/Accreditation & Reproducibility*" covers the interrelated topics enhancing the quality safety and reproducibility of clinical AI/ML via (a) reporting standards; (b) recent efforts for accrediting health care provider organizations for AI readiness and maturity; (c) professional certification; and (d) education and related accreditation of educational programs in data science and biomedical informatics, specific to AI/ML.

Chapter *"Final Synthesis of Recommendations"* presents a consolidated view of the identified pitfalls and recommended practices across the book. We differentiate between macro-, meso- and micro-levels of pitfalls and corresponding best practices-roughly corresponding to high-level principles, concrete differentiations of the above and granular/detailed tools and techniques for implementation. We discuss the non-uniqueness of best practice frameworks and several open problems. The continued development and dissemination of Best Practices for biomedical AI/ML is certain to become in the years to come a field of inquiry with significant growth and value.

Key Concepts Discussed in Chapter " Artificial Intelligence (AI) and Machine Learning (ML) for Healthcare and Health Sciences: The Need for Best Practices Enabling Trust in AI and ML"

Artificial Intelligence (AI) and Machine Learning (ML)
Data Science
Computer program
Computer system
Computer algorithm
AI/ML model
Data Science
Performance requirements
Safety requirements
Cost-effectiveness requirements
Trust, acceptance, and adoption

Key Messages Discussed in Chapter "Artificial Intelligence (AI) and Machine Learning (ML) for Healthcare and Health Sciences: The Need for Best Practices Enabling Trust in AI and ML"

1. AI/ML are long standing disciplines with millions of published articles since the 1960s and with several Turing and Nobel awards linked to them.
2. Biomedical AI/ML has a long history and extensive literature behind them also starting in the 1960s. They have recently exploded in the literature in adoption for discovery and care and as their own fields of study.
3. AI/ML are applied broadly in science and health care because they relate to extremely broad classes of prediction/pattern recognition and causal modeling and problem solving tasks.
4. Biomedical AI/ML has several distinct requirements than general-purpose AI/ML.
5. AI/ML Algorithms, programs and systems must inspire and guarantee trust in their safety, effectiveness and cost effectiveness. Best Practices must be developed, shared and followed to enable trust and acceptance.

6. Known properties are essential for AI/ML trust.
7. Currently known Best Practices originate from a variety of sources, have different levels of maturity or validation and will undoubtedly expand and improve in the future.

Pitfalls Discussed[3] in Chapter "Artificial Intelligence (AI) and Machine Learning (ML) for Healthcare and Health Sciences: The Need for Best Practices Enabling Trust in AI and ML"

Pitfall 1.1: Unspecified, undisclosed or insufficiently-analyzed algorithms.

Pitfall 1.2: In healthcare and health sciences, *clinical algorithms* are often confused with *computer algorithms*.

Pitfall 1.3: Viewing the whole field as being about one narrow technology or a small set of tools, ignoring the broader spectrum of available options.

Pitfall 1.4: Ignoring the vast literature or "re-inventing the wheel".

Pitfall 1.5: Ignoring the specific requirements and adaptations tailored to the goals of healthcare and of health sciences discovery.

Best Practices Discussed in Chapter "Artificial Intelligence (AI) and Machine Learning (ML) for Healthcare and Health Sciences: The Need for Best Practices Enabling Trust in AI and ML"

Best Practice 1.1 When considering development or application of AI/ML ensure that it is informed by well-developed and evaluated existing science and technology.

Classroom Assignments and Discussion Topics[4] chapter "Artificial Intelligence (AI) and Machine Learning (ML) for Healthcare and Health Sciences: The Need for Best Practices Enabling Trust in AI and ML"

1. If *science is self-correcting via reproducibility studies*, what are the dangers/downsides to producing AI/ML systems/methods and related articles with a high proportion of false results?

---

[3] To be further elaborated later in the book, including related Best Practices.

[4] Several of these and similar topics will be clarified and elaborated upon in subsequent chapters. However we recommend to class instructors and self-learners to get a first-pass evaluation of where the reader/classroom is (attitude, knowledge, experience) with regards to such problems.

2. Identify from news sources and business publications articles about past industry failures in health AI/ML. Summarize and draw your conclusions about how to remedy and avoid such problems.

3. What, in your view, is the ideal relationship (i.e., rules of engagement and assignment of responsibilities/foci) of industry and academia in developing and delivering health AI/ML?

4. What are areas where health AI/ML cannot reach human problem solving? What about the reverse?

5. The so-called *No Free Lunch Theorem (NFLT)* states (in simplified language) that all ML and more broadly all AI optimization methods are *equally accurate over all problems on average*. Discuss the implications for choice of AI/ML methods in practical use cases.

6. "It is not the tool but the craftsman". Does this maxim apply to health AI/ML?

7. How would you go about identifying and measuring/documenting the impact that AI/ML has had on specific health science discoveries?

8. Is AI confined to computer systems? Can other artificial intelligent agents such as corporations be viewed as AI? Discuss implications of such a broader view.

9. Construct a "pyramid of evidence" for health AI/ML similar to the one used in evidence based care practice. Consider two pyramids: one focusing on clinical healthcare and another on health science discovery.

10. You are part of a university/hospital evaluation committee for a vendor offering a patient-clinical trial matching AI product. Your institution strongly needs to improve the patient-trial matching process to increase trial success and efficiency metrics.

    The sales team makes the statement that "this is a completely innovative AI/ML product; nothing like this exists in the market and there is no similar literature; we cannot at this time provide theoretical or empirical accuracy analysis, however you are welcome to try out our product for free for a limited time and decide if it helpful to you". The product is fairly expensive (multi $ million license fees over 5 years covering >1000 trials steady-state).

    What would be your concerns based on these statements? Would you be in position of making an institutional buy/not buy recommendation?

11. A company has launched a major national marketing campaign across health provider systems for a new AI/ML healthcare product based on its success on playing backgammon, reading and analyzing backgammon playing books and human games, extracting novel winning strategies from matches, answering questions about backgammon, and teaching backgammon to human players.

    How relevant is this impressive AI track record to health care? How would you go about determining relevance to health care AI/ML? How your reasoning would change if the product was not based on success in backgammon but success in identifying oil and gas deposits? How about success in financial investments?

12. Your university-affiliated hospital wishes to increase early diagnosis of cognitive decline across the population it serves. You are tasked to choose between the following AI/ML technologies/tools:
    (a) AI/ML tool A guarantees optimal predictivity in the sample limit in distributions that are multivariate normal.
    (b) AI/ML tool B has no known properties but is has been shown to be very accurate in several datasets for microarray cancer-vs-normal classification.
    (c) AI/ML tool C is a commercial offshoot of a tool that was fairly accurate in early (pre-trauma) diagnosis of PTSD.
    (d) AI/ML tool D is an application running on a ground-breaking quantum computing platform (Quantum computing is an exciting and frontier technology that many believe has potential to make AI/ML with hugely improved capabilities in the future).
    (e) AI/ML tool E runs on a novel massively parallel cloud computing platform capable of Zettascale performance.

    What are your thoughts about these options?

13. The same question as #12 but with the following additional data:
    (a) AI/ML tool A sales reps are very professional, friendly and open to offering deep discounts.
    (b) AI/ML tool B is offered by a company co-founded by a widely-respected Nobel laureate.
    (c) AI/Ml tool C is offered by a vendor with which your organization has a successful and long relationship.
    (d) AI/Ml tool D is part of a university initiative to develop thought leadership in quantum computing.
    (e) AI/Ml tool E will provide patient-specific results in 1 picosecond or less.

    How does this additional information influences your assessment?

References

1. Hart PE, Stork DG, Duda RO. Pattern classification. Hoboken: Wiley; 2000.
2. Russell, S.J., 2010. Artificial intelligence a modern approach. Pearson Education, Inc.
3. Weiss SM, Kulikowski CA. Computer systems that learn: classification and prediction methods from statistics, neural nets, machine learning, and expert systems. Morgan Kaufmann Publishers Inc.; 1991.
4. Statnikov A. A gentle introduction to support vector machines in biomedicine: theory and methods, vol. 1. world scientific; 2011.
5. Sverchkov Y, Craven M. A review of active learning approaches to experimental design for uncovering biological networks. PLoS Comput Biol. 2017;13(6):e1005466.
6. Statnikov A, Ma S, Henaff M, Lytkin N, Efstathiadis E, Peskin ER, Aliferis CF. Ultra-scalable and efficient methods for hybrid observational and experimental local causal pathway discovery. J Mach Learn Res. 2015;16(1):3219–67.

7. Guyon I, Cawley GC, Dror G, Lemaire V. Results of the active learning challenge. In: Active learning and experimental design workshop in conjunction with AISTATS 2010. JMLR Workshop and Conference Proceedings; 2011, April. p. 19–45.

8. Tanenbaum AS. Structured computer organization. Prentice Hall; 1984.

9. Cormen TH, Leiserson CE, Rivest RL, Stein C. Introduction to algorithms. MIT press; 2022.

10. Brookshear, J.G. Computer science: An overview. Benjamin-Cummings Publishing Co., Inc; 1991.

11. Sedgewick R. Algorithms in c++, parts 1–4: fundamentals, data structure, sorting, searching. Pearson Education; 1998.

12. Margolis CZ. Uses of clinical algorithms. JAMA. 1983;249(5):627–32.

13. Grimshaw J, Russell I. Achieving health gain through clinical guidelines. I: developing scientifically valid guidelines. Qual Health Care. 1993;2(4):243–8.

14. Vapnik, V. The nature of statistical learning theory. Springer science & business media. 1999.

15. Kearns MJ, Vazirani U. An introduction to computational learning theory. MIT press; 1994.

16. Donoho D. 50 years of data science. J Comput Graph Stat. 2017;26(4):745–66.

17. Cao L. Data science: a comprehensive overview. ACM Comput Surv. 2017;50(3):1–42.

18. Spirtes P, Glymour CN, Scheines R, Heckerman D. Causation, prediction, and search. MIT press; 2000.

19. Glymour CN, Cooper GF, editors. Computation, causation, and discovery. AAAI Press; 1999.

20. Pearl J. Causality. Cambridge university press; 2009.

21. Roski J, Bo-Linn GW, Andrews TA. Creating value in health care through big data: opportunities and policy implications. Health Aff. 2014;33(7):1115–22.

22. https://en.wikipedia.org/wiki/Applications_of_artificial_intelligence.

23. Cohen TA, Patel VL, Shortliffe EH, editors. Intelligent Systems in Medicine and Health: the role of AI. Springer Nature; 2022.

24. Szymczak S, Biernacka JM, Cordell HJ, González-Recio O, König IR, Zhang H, Sun YV. Machine learning in genome-wide association studies. Genet Epidemiol. 2009;33(S1):S51–7.

25. Adam T, Aliferis C. Personalized and Precision Medicine Informatics. Health Informatics Series. Basel, Springer Nature Switzerland. 2020.

26. Aphinyanaphongs Y, Tsamardinos I, Statnikov A, Hardin D, Aliferis CF. Text categorization models for high-quality article retrieval in internal medicine. J Am Med Inform Assoc. 2005;12(2):207–16.

27. Libbrecht MW, Noble WS. Machine learning applications in genetics and genomics. Nat Rev Genet. 2015;16(6):321–32.

28. Cheng J, Tegge AN, Baldi P. Machine learning methods for protein structure prediction. IEEE Rev Biomed Eng. 2008;1:41–9.

29. Ryu JY, Kim HU, Lee SY. Deep learning improves prediction of drug–drug and drug–food interactions. Proc Natl Acad Sci. 2018;115(18):E4304–11.

30. Erickson BJ, Korfiatis P, Akkus Z, Kline TL. Machine learning for medical imaging. Radiographics. 2017;37(2):505–15.

31. Andreu-Perez J, Poon CC, Merrifield RD, Wong ST, Yang GZ. Big data for health. IEEE J Biomed Health Inform. 2015;19(4):1193–208.

32. Vamathevan J, Clark D, Czodrowski P, Dunham I, Ferran E, Lee G, Li B, Madabhushi A, Shah P, Spitzer M, Zhao S. Applications of machine learning in drug discovery and development. Nat Rev Drug Discov. 2019;18(6):463–77.

33. Olsen L, Aisner D, McGinnis JM. The learning healthcare system: workshop summary. Institute of Medicine (US). National Academies Press (US); 2007. ISBN 978-0-309-10300-8.

34. Ledley RS, Lusted LB. Reasoning foundations of medical diagnosis: symbolic logic, probability, and value theory aid our understanding of how physicians reason. Science. 1959;130(3366):9–21.

35. Warner HR, Toronto AF, Veasey LG, Stephenson R. A mathematical approach to medical diagnosis: application to congenital heart disease. JAMA. 1961;177(3):177–83.

36. Miller RA, Pople HE Jr, Myers JD. Internist-I, an experimental computer-based diagnostic consultant for general internal medicine. N Engl J Med. 1982;307(8):468–76.
37. Pearl J. Probabilistic reasoning in intelligent systems: networks of plausible inference. Morgan kaufmann; 1988.
38. Shwe MA, Middleton B, Heckerman DE, Henrion M, Horvitz EJ, Lehmann HP, Cooper GF. Probabilistic diagnosis using a reformulation of the INTERNIST-1/QMR knowledge base. Methods Inf Med. 1991;30(04):241–55.
39. Rumelhart DE, McClelland JL, PDP Research Group. Parallel distributed processing, vol. 1. New York: IEEE; 1988. p. 354–62.
40. LeCun Y, Bengio Y, Hinton G. Deep learning. Nature. 2015;521(7553):436–44.
41. Saba L, Biswas M, Kuppili V, Godia EC, Suri HS, Edla DR, Omerzu T, Laird JR, Khanna NN, Mavrogeni S, Protogerou A. The present and future of deep learning in radiology. Eur J Radiol. 2019;114:14–24.
42. Breiman L. Random forests. Mach Learn. 2001;45(1):5–32.
43. Hastie T, Tibshirani R, Friedman JH, Friedman JH. The elements of statistical learning: data mining, inference, and prediction (Vol. 2, pp. 1-758). New York: springer.
44. Aliferis CF, Statnikov A, Tsamardinos I, Mani S, Koutsoukos XD. Local causal and Markov blanket induction for causal discovery and feature selection for classification part I: algorithms and empirical evaluation. J Mach Learn Res. 2010;11(1):171–234.
45. Tsamardinos I, Brown LE, Aliferis CF. The max-min hill-climbing Bayesian network structure learning algorithm. Mach Learn. 2006;65(1):31–78.
46. Tsamardinos I, Aliferis CF, Statnikov AR, Statnikov E. Algorithms for large scale Markov blanket discovery, vol. 2. FLAIRS conference; 2003. p. 376–80.
47. Tsamardinos I, Aliferis CF, Statnikov A. Time and sample efficient discovery of Markov blankets and direct causal relations. In: Proceedings of the ninth ACM SIGKDD international conference on knowledge discovery and data mining; 2003, August. p. 673–8.
48. Aliferis CF, Tsamardinos I, Statnikov A. HITON: a novel Markov blanket algorithm for optimal variable selection. In: AMIA annual symposium proceedings, vol. 2003. American Medical Informatics Association; 2003. p. 21.
49. Wang X, Fan J. Spatiotemporal molecular medicine: a new era of clinical and translational medicine. Clin Transl Med. 2021;11(1):e294.
50. Wu Y, Cheng Y, Wang X, Fan J, Gao Q. Spatial omics: navigating to the golden era of cancer research. Clin Transl Med. 2022;12(1):e696.
51. Glikson E, Woolley AW. Human trust in artificial intelligence: review of empirical research. Acad Manag Ann. 2020;14(2):627–60.
52. Hengstler M, Enkel E, Duelli S. Applied artificial intelligence and trust—the case of autonomous vehicles and medical assistance devices. Technol Forecast Soc Chang. 2016;105:105–20.
53. Siau K, Wang W. Building trust in artificial intelligence, machine learning, and robotics. Cut Bus Technol J. 2018;31(2):47–53.
54. Winfield AF, Jirotka M. Ethical governance is essential to building trust in robotics and artificial intelligence systems. Philos Trans R Soc A Math Phys Eng Sci. 2018;376(2133):20180085.
55. Jacovi A, Marasović A, Miller T, Goldberg Y. Formalizing trust in artificial intelligence: prerequisites, causes and goals of human trust in AI. In: Proceedings of the 2021 ACM conference on fairness, accountability, and transparency; 2021. p. 624–35.
56. Asan O, Bayrak AE, Choudhury A. Artificial intelligence and human trust in healthcare: focus on clinicians. J Med Internet Res. 2020;22(6):e15154.
57. Matheny M, Israni ST, Ahmed M, Whicher D. Artificial intelligence in health care: the hope, the hype, the promise, the peril. Washington, DC: National Academy of Medicine; 2019.
58. Rigby MJ. Ethical dimensions of using artificial intelligence in health care. AMA J Ethics. 2019;21(2):121–4.
59. Bates DW, Auerbach A, Schulam P, Wright A, Saria S. Reporting and implementing interventions involving machine learning and artificial intelligence. Ann Intern Med. 2020;172(11_Supplement):S137–44.

60. Makarov VA, Stouch T, Allgood B, Willis CD, Lynch N. Best practices for artificial intelligence in life sciences research. Drug Discov Today. 2021;26(5):1107–10.
61. Dupuy A, Simon RM. Critical review of published microarray studies for cancer outcome and guidelines on statistical analysis and reporting. J Natl Cancer Inst. 2007;99(2):147–57.
62. Shi L, Campbell G, Jones WD, et al. The MicroArray quality control (MAQC)-II study of common practices for the development and validation of microarray-based predictive models. Nat Biotechnol. 2010;28(8):827–38.
63. Statnikov A, Aliferis CF, Tsamardinos I, Hardin D, Levy S. A comprehensive evaluation of multicategory classification methods for microarray gene expression cancer diagnosis. Bioinformatics. 2005;21(5):631–43.
64. Guyon I, Aliferis C, Cooper G, Elisseeff A, Pellet JP, Spirtes P, Statnikov A. Design and analysis of the causation and prediction challenge. In: Causation and prediction challenge. PMLR; 2008. p. 1–33.
65. https://www.fda.gov/medical-devices/software-medical-device-samd/artificial-intelligence-and-machine-learning-aiml-enabled-medical-devices.
66. Aliferis CF, Statnikov A, Tsamardinos I, Schildcrout JS, Shepherd BE, Harrell FE Jr. Factors influencing the statistical power of complex data analysis protocols for molecular signature development from microarray data. PLoS One. 2009;4(3):e4922.

Foundations and Properties of AI/ML Systems

Constantin Aliferis and Gyorgy Simon

Abstract

The chapter provides a broad introduction to the foundations of health AI and ML systems and is organized as follows: (1) Theoretical properties and formal vs. heuristic systems: computability, incompleteness theorem, space and time complexity, exact vs. asymptotic complexity, complexity classes and how to establish complexity of problems even in the absence of known algorithms that solve them, problem complexity vs. algorithm and program complexity, and various other properties. Moreover, we discuss the practical implications of complexity for system tractability, the folly of expecting Moore's Law and large-scale computing to solve intractable problems, and common techniques for creating tractable systems that operate in intractable problem spaces. We also discuss the distinction between heuristic and formal systems and show that they exist on a continuum rather than in separate spaces. (2) Foundations of AI including logics and logic based systems (rule based systems, semantic networks, planning systems search, NLP parsers), symbolic vs. non-symbolic AI, Reasoning with Uncertainty, Decision Making theory, Bayesian Networks, and AI/ML programming languages. (3) Foundations of Computational Learning Theory: ML as search, ML as geometrical construction and function optimization, role of inductive biases, PAC learning, VC dimension, Theory of Feature Selection, Theory of Causal Discovery. Optimal Bayes Classifier, No Free Lunch Theorems, Universal Function Approximation, generative vs. discriminative models; Bias-Variance Decomposition of error and essential concepts of mathematical statistics.

C. Aliferis (✉) · G. Simon
Institute for Health Informatics, University of Minnesota, Minneapolis, MN, USA
e-mail: constantinaibestpractices@gmail.com

© The Author(s) 2024
G. J. Simon, C. Aliferis (eds.), *Artificial Intelligence and Machine Learning in Health Care and Medical Sciences*, Health Informatics,
https://doi.org/10.1007/978-3-031-39355-6_2

33

Keywords
Properties of AI/ML models · Computational complexity (time, space) · Tractable vs intractable computer solutions · Symbolic and non-symbolic AI · Shallow vs. ontologically rich AI · Bayesian networks · Machine Learning theoretical foundations

Theoretical AI/ML Properties and Formal Vs Heuristic Systems

We will first address a few key concepts regarding studying and understanding, but also designing, AI systems by way of their formal properties. By **formal properties** we mean theoretical properties that are mathematical or computational, and technical and objective in nature.

Computability/Provability and Turing-Church Thesis

The most foundational property for any computer system (not just AI/ML systems) is computability, that is the fundamental question of whether there can even exist a computer program or system that achieves the computation needed for the inferences that we want this system to perform. Goedel [1] proved a theorem that shook the mathematical and computer science worlds.

> **Goedel's celebrated "incompleteness theorem"** shows that any non-trivial mathematical system for making deductive inferences is either complete or consistent but not both. Or stated differently, statements can be formed in this system that are true but cannot be proven if we wish to maintain the correctness of deductions.
>
> A **complete system** is one that can deduce (or prove) from the axioms of the system all statements that are true.
>
> A **consistent system** is one that does not produce contradictory conclusions (which entails false conclusions).
>
> Correspondingly, in the realm of computing there are **functions that are not computable**, that is there is no computer program that can compute them.
>
> These two results (provability and computability) are essentially mirroring each other because there is a close correspondence relationship between a "proof" in a mathematical system and a "program" in an equivalent computing system implementing the mathematical system. Non-computable functions are the ones that cannot be proven and vice versa.

Notice that the existence of *non-computable functions/non-provable statements is with reference to a specific computing system*. A different system may be able to prove certain statements at the expense of not being able to prove others that the first system can. Also, we note that in systems involving a finite number of domain elements, we do not face restrictions in computability. However, this is of small consolation if we realize that even systems as "basic" as common arithmetic, for example, involve many non computable functions.

What is the relationship of computability/provability in the computational/mathematical realm with that in human intelligence and reasoning?

> The **Turing-Church thesis** posits that everything that the human mind can infer can also be inferred by a computer/mathematical system [1]. According to the thesis, there are no special functions of human intelligence that a computer or mathematical system cannot emulate. This thesis is axiomatic, meaning not proven. From what we know so far from neuroscience, cognitive science etc., there is nothing in the human brain that a computer system cannot model in principle, and the vast majority of AI scientists accept the Turing-Church thesis.

Computational Complexity of a Problem, Algorithm of Program

Computational complexity of a program refers to the efficiency of running a computer program that solves a particular problem according to a specific algorithm (that the program implements). In other words, it describes (for problems that can be solved by computer), how expensive is to solve the problem. Computational complexity is in the form of a function that typically takes the **size of the problem instance** as inputs.

Computational complexity of an algorithm applies the same rationale to algorithms instead of programs. Typically we analyze computational complexity at the level of algorithms assuming that programs will be the most efficient implementation of the algorithm (when exceptions happen in practice, we state upfront that a particular implementation of an algorithm is not as efficient as it can be).

Computational complexity of a problem is then analyzed at the level of the most efficient algorithm known (or *that could be devised but not yet known—we will see later how this is accomplished*) for solving this problem.

Space complexity refers to how much space the computer program/algorithm/problem class requires to reach a solution. **Time complexity** refers to how much time the computer program/algorithm/problem class requires to reach a solution. Because different computers differ greatly in the time needed to execute the same basic operation (e.g., one addition or one access of a random access memory location, etc.) we often measure time complexity *not in units of time but in numbers of some essential operation* (and then we can translate these units to time units for available computer systems). Because the differences between computers are within constant factors, this does not make a difference in an asymptotic sense.

Worst, average, and best-case complexity. Often, not all problem instances require the same amount of resources (space or time) to be solved by the same program/algorithm. **Worst case complexity** refers to the cost of the worst (most expensive) instance of the problem when solved by the best possible algorithm (or, alternative for a specific algorithm of interest). **Best case complexity** refers to the cost of the best (least expensive) instance of the problem. **Average case complexity** refers to the cost averaged over all instances of the problem.

Exact complexity refers to a precise complexity for example:

$$Cost(x) = x^2 \tag{1}$$

where x is the size of the ith problem instance. In this example, the cost of solving the problem is exactly the square of the size of the problem instance.

Asymptotic complexity refers to complexity as an asymptotic *growth function, i.e.,* that is how fast the complexity grows as input size grows. For example,

$$Cost(x) = O(f(x)) \tag{2}$$

The **"Big O" notation** *O(f(.))* denotes that there is a problem instance size k, above which the complexity (cost) of all problem instances of size at least as large as k, is bounded from above within a positive constant from the value of function f(.), or more compactly stated:

$$\exists k \text{s.t.}, \forall x \geq k : Cost(x) \leq cf(x)$$

- Where $\exists$ is *the existential oper*ator (denoting that the quantity in the scope of the operator exists)
- $\forall$ is the *universal operator* denoting that for all entities in the scope of the operator a statement that follows is true
- x is the size of the ith problem instance
- *Cost (x)* is the computational cost of running the algorithm for input size x
- k is a input size threshold above which the complexity statement holds
- c is a positive constant
- "S.t." is the common abbreviation "such that".

We often use asymptotic cost complexity for two reasons: (a) It eliminates confusion created by differences in the speeds of various computer systems since in practice these are all within a small constant factor of each other. (b) It shifts the attention to the broad classes of rates of cost growth (e.g. linear, quadratic, exponential, etc.) and not the precise cost formulas that can be convoluted. Mathematical analysis can accordingly be greatly simplified.

To understand the implications of asymptotic growth contrast the polynomial asymptotic complexity of formula (1) with the one below:

$$Cost(x) = O(2^x) \tag{3}$$

The following Table 1 shows how quickly these cost functions grow (assuming, for illustration purposes, $c = 1$). For input sizes above 100, the cost in terms of space and time complexity grows to sizes comparable to the size of the universe

Table 1 Demonstration of the practical significance of asymptotic computational complexity

Size of problem instance	Quadratic Cost	Exponential Cost	Related to complexity $O(2^x)$		
	If cost of computation grows as $O(x^2)$	Cost of computation grows as $O(2^x)$	Moore's Law (here: If speed doubled every 4 years) How many years needed until CPUs catch up starting at size 100 and cost $= 2^{100}$?	Parallelize (linearly by using m CPUs) How many CPUs needed? (within a constant factor)	Other comments
1	1	2	T	2	T
2	4	4	R	4	R
3	9	8	A	8	A
4	16	16	C	16	C
5	25	32	T	32	T
6	36	64	A	64	A
7	49	128	B	128	B
8	64	256	L	256	L
9	81	512	E	512	E
10	100	1024		1024	
20	400	1,048,576		1,048,576	$\geq 10^6$
30	900	1,073,741,824		1,073,741,824	$\geq 10^9$
100	10^4	2^{100}	Wait for 280 years	2^{100} CPUs	Comparable to number of atoms in the universe
1000	10^6	2^{1000}	Wait for 3680 years	2^{1000} CPUs needed	$>>$ than size of known universe
10^6	10^{12}	$2^{1,000,000}$	Wait for ~40 million years	$2^{1,000,000}$ CPUs Needed	universe

(measured in atoms) and quickly becomes much larger than the size of the universe. This means that there is not enough physical space or time to solve these problems!

The fallacy/pitfall that we will "use a big enough cluster" (or other high-performance computing environment) to solve a high-complexity problem is addressed in the parallel column where it is shown that the number of CPUs needed would quickly exceed the size of the universe. The fallacy/pitfall that Moore's law (e.g., computing power doubles every few years) will provide enough power is addressed in the Moore's law column where is shown that millions of years would be needed to address problems of any significant size, and after some point the space and time requirements exceed the size of the known universe.

We will refer to problems, algorithms, programs and systems exhibiting such exorbitant complexities, as **intractable.** The following pitfalls and corresponding best practices need be taken into consideration:

Pitfall 2.1
From a rigorous science point of view, an AI/ML algorithm, program or system with intractable complexity does not constitute a viable solution to the corresponding problem.

Pitfall 2.2
Parallelization cannot make an intractable problem, algorithm or program practical.

Pitfall 2.3
Moore's law improvements to computing power cannot make an intractable problem algorithm or program practical.

Best Practice 2.1
Pursue development of AI/ML algorithm, program or systems that have tractable complexity.

Best Practice 2.2
Do not rely on parallelization to make intractable problems tractable. Pursue tractable algorithms and factor in the tractability analysis any parallelization.

Best Practice 2.3
Do not rely on Moore's law improvements to make an intractable problem algorithm or hard program practical. Pursue tractable algorithms and factor in the tractability analysis any gains from Moore's law.

It is very common in modern AI/ML to be able to address problems that have *worst case* exponential (or other intractable) complexity and routinely tackle, for example, analyses of datasets with $>10^6$ variables for problems with worst-case exponential cost by using a number of strategies that we will summarize below. First we round up the introduction to complexity properties with an overview of complexity classes.

Reduction of Problems to Established Complexity Class

Earlier we mentioned that computational complexity of a problem can be analyzed at the level of the most efficient algorithm known, or *that could be devised but not yet known*. How is this possible? One ingenious way to achieve this was discovered by Cook who proved a remarkable theorem (and received a Turing award for the work) [2]. Karp, based on Cook's result, showed how to prove that several other problems were in the same complexity class (and also won a Turing award for this work) [3].

The above constitute a generalizable methodology, very widely used in computer science and AI/ML, comprising two steps:

1. First establish via mathematical proof that a problem class P1 has an intrinsic minimum complexity regardless of the algorithm or program that has been devised or could be devised to solve it (i.e., intrinsic to the problem and independent of algorithm, in the sense that no Turing machine can exist that could do better). This part does not require the knowledge of a conventional algorithm that solves P1.

2. Second, in order to prove that problem Pi at hand belongs to the same or harder complexity class as P1, it suffices to establish that a **fast reduction** (e.g., with polynomial-time complexity) exists that maps problems and their solutions in P1 to problems and solutions in Pi, such that when a problem solution to a Pi problem instance is found then it can be converted fast to a problem solution for P1.

"Fast" in this context means that: cost of the reduction + cost of solving the P1 version of the Pi problem, will be no costlier (asymptotically) than solving Pi. For example, if Pi has cost $O(2^x)$, a reduction with cost $O(x^2)$ satisfies the requirement since $O(2^x + x^2) = O(2^x)$.

Step 1 has to be accomplished only *once for a prototypical problem class* and is of the greatest mathematical difficulty. Step 2, which is typically considerably easier, is done each time a new method is introduced and is conducted once for the new method, with reference the prototypical problem class.

Cook's discovery provided exactly step 1 and opened the flood gates via the reduction methods of Karp (step 2) for assigning whole problem classes to complexity cost classes *regardless of the algorithm or problem used to solve it and regardless of whether even a single algorithm is currently known for solving the problem.*

AI/ML and computer scientists often use prototypical complexity classes to study and categorize problems and the algorithms solving them, the most common ones being:

The P complexity class: contains problems that can be solved in polynomial time. These are considered as tractable (assuming, as is typically the case, that the polynomial degree is small).

The NP complexity class: contains problems that have the property that a solution can be verified as correct in polynomial time.

The NP-Complete complexity class: These are problems that are in NP and moreover if any of the problems in this class can be solved in polynomial time, then all other problems in the class can also be solved in polynomial time.

NP Hard problems. Are problems that are as hard as those in NP but it is unknown whether they are in NP.

Several other classes exist and are subject to study and exploration (as to what problems belong to them or what relationships exist among them).

The practical significance of the complexity classes is as follows:
- Problems in **P** are considered as tractable (assuming, as is typically the case, that the polynomial degree is small).
- Problems in **NP-Complete** or **NP Hard** classes are considered very hard and it is extremely unlikely that algorithms that solve such problems tractably in the worst case, can be created.

A fundamental property of AI/ML problem solving is that it usually operates in problem spaces belonging to the very high complexity/worst-case intractable classes. Many strategies have been invented to circumvent these theoretical difficulties and guide creation of efficient algorithms and systems, however (discussed later in the present chapter).

A List of Key and Commonly Used Formal Properties of AI/ML (Table 2)

Many **additional special-purpose or ancillary formal properties** can also be studied and established such as: whether performance estimators are biased, statistical decision false positive and false negative errors when fitting models, whether scoring rules or distance metrics used are proper or improper, various measures of statistical certainty, etc. We emphasize that the properties listed in Table 2 have immediate and obvious relationship with, and consequences for, the common

Table 2 Commonly-considered important formal (theoretical) properties that characterize all AI/ML algorithms, programs and systems

1. **Representation power**: Can the models produced by the method represent all problem instances of interest and their solutions?

2. **Semantic clarity and transparency**: Do the programs and the corresponding models exhibit clarity based on precisely understood semantics (i.e., formally defined meaning)? Are the models produced by the method easy to understand (i.e., are they **"transparent box"**) and can they be easily understood by human inspection (i.e., are they human interpretable, aka **explainable**)?

3. **Soundness**: When the methods output a solution to a problem instance, is this solution correct? If there is a degree of error (measured on some scale of loss, risk or other scale) how large is the error and its uncertainty?

4. **Completeness**: Does the method produce correct answers to all problem instances? If only a fraction, how large is the fraction?

5. **Computational complexity.** What is the exact or asymptotic computational complexity of running the method to produce solutions as a function of the input size?

   For AI/ML methods that produce models as intermediate step in producing solutions, we differentiate

   (a) **Computational complexity of producing problem-solving models:** What is the exact or asymptotic computational complexity of running the method to produce models as a function of the input size (e.g., number of variables, or sample size)? And

   (b) **Computational complexity of executing problem-solving models:** What is the exact or asymptotic computational complexity of running the models to produce solutions as a function of the input size (e.g., number of variables, or sample size)?

6. **Space complexity.** What is the exact or asymptotic space complexity of running the method to produce solutions as a function of the input size? For AI/ML methods that produce models as intermediate step in producing solutions we can differentiate:

   (a) **Space complexity of producing problem-solving models:** What is the exact or asymptotic space complexity of running the method to produce models as a function of the input size (e.g., number of variables, or sample size)? And

   (b) **Space complexity of executing problem-solving models:** What is the exact or asymptotic space complexity of running the models to produce solutions as a function of the input size (e.g., number of variables, or sample size)?

7. **Additional cost functions**: For example, *financial costs* to obtain and store input data and run analyses on a compute environment, either at model discovery or at model deployment time? *Compliance risks. Ethical, litigation or reputational risks*, etc.

8. **Sample complexity, learning curves, power-sample requirements**: How does the error of the produced models vary as function of sample size of the discovery data? How much sample size is needed in order to build models with a specific degree of accuracy and statistical error uncertainty, and (separately) to establish statistically superiority to random or alternative models and performance levels?

9. **Probability and decision theoretic consistency**: Is the ML/AI method compatible with probability and utility theory?

objectives of health AI/ML. In the present volume we will refrain from study of properties that do not have strong relevance to the success or failure of AI/ML modeling. For example, the accuracy of a predictive model has immediate consequences for its usefulness. By contrast, the centrality measures of network science models say very little about their predictive (or causal) value. Similarly, the use of perplexity measure to study the degree by which a Large Language Model has learned (essentially the grammar underlying) a text corpus, does not indicate the clinical error severity resuting from output errors made by the model, which may of much higher importance for health applications.

Formal (aka theoretical) properties are "hard" technical properties (i.e., mathematical, immutable). There exist "softer" properties (i.e., less technical, more transient, or even harder to establish objectively) such as compliance to regulatory or accreditation guidance, reporting standards, ethical principles, etc.

An additional category with special significance is that of **empirical performance** properties. These are obtained using methods of empirical evaluation (chapters "Principles of Rigorous Development and of Appraisal of ML and AI Methods and Systems", "The Development Process and Lifecycle of Clinical Grade and Other Safety and Performance-Sensitive AI/ML Models", "Evaluation", and "Characterizing, Diagnosing and Managing the Risk of Error of ML & AI Models in Clinical and Organizational Application").

> **Importance of theoretical and empirical properties.** Taken together these characterizations of AI/ML systems provide an invaluable framework for:
> (a) Understanding the strengths and limitations of AI/ML methods, models and systems;
> (b) Improving them;
> (c) Understanding, anticipating, and effectively managing the risks and benefits of using AI/ML; and
> (d) Choosing the right method for the problem at hand, among the myriad of available methods and systems.

> We will see many examples of these formal, empirical and ancillary properties in the chapters ahead, considered in context. Chapters "Foundations and Properties of AI/ML Systems", "An Appraisal and Operating Characteristics of Major ML Methods Applicable in Healthcare and Health Science", and "Foundations of Causal ML" describe properties of main AI/ML methods and chapter "Principles of Rigorous Development and of Appraisal of ML and AI Methods and Systems" provides a summary table with the main properties of all main health AI/Ml methods.

Principled Strategies to Achieve Practically Efficient Algorithms, Programs and Systems for Worst-Case Intractable Problems

Since most intractability results pertain to worst-case complete and sound problem solving, a number of strategies can be used to achieve tractability, by trading off computational costs with reduction in soundness, completeness or worst-case complexity. Such common example strategies are listed below.

(a) **Focus on portions of the problem space that admit tractable solutions and ignore the portions with intractable solutions.** In problem domains where the worst case complexity diverges strongly form the average case complexity, such an approach is especially appealing. For example, in ML problems, focus on restricted data distributions or target function sub-classes that lead to tractable learning. Or focus on sparse regions of the data-generating processes and ignore dense (and commonly intractable) regions.

(b) **Exploit prior domain knowledge to constrain and thus speed-up problem solving.** For example, in discovery problems, avoid generating and examining many possible solutions that are incompatible with prior biomedical knowledge about the credible solution space. This may viewed as a case of "knowledge transfer" from this or similar problem domains. This is also often called *pruning*, where large branches, that are guaranteed to not contain the correct solution, are eliminated from vast solution search trees.

(c) **Instead of an intractable complete solution, provide a tractable localized part of the full solution that is still of significant value.** For example, when pursuing a causal model of some domain, focus on the partial causal model around some variables of interest (i.e., biological pathway discovery involving a phenotype instead of full network discovery).

(d) **Instead of an intractable complete solution, provide a tractable non-local portion of the full solution that is still of significant value.** For example, when pursuing a causal model of some domain allow discovery of a portion of correct relationships of interest (i.e., biological causal relationship discovery involving factors *across the data generating network* instead of full network discovery; or recovering a correct but unoriented causal network instead of the oriented one).

(e) Instead of producing perfectly accurate but intractable solutions **focus on more tractable but acceptable approximations of the true solutions.**

(f) **Do not solve harder problems than what is needed by your application.** A classic example demonstrating this principle is to prefer *discriminative models over generative ones in predictive modeling.* In plain language, this means that we can often solve a hard problem (e.g., what treatment to give to a patient with a kidney stone?) by building simple decision functions describing only relevant facts and not a full computational theory of the domain (e.g., a full theory of the function of the kidneys from the nephron up, and the interaction of the kidneys with the rest of the body are *not* needed to conclude that removing the stone or breaking it up with ultrasounds will be sufficient for curing the patient with a kidney stone).

(g) **Perform operations on compact representations.** This strategy involves replacing intractable large data structures with declarative and highly compact representations. For example, "every person who suffers from a mental health disorder" encompasses an estimated 10^9 people globally but does not enumerate or even identify them. This approach also involves operating on classes of the problem space simultaneously rather than each member in the class. This is particularly evident in several forms of ML modeling where astronomical numbers of model structures are scored at once and represented compactly.

Best Practice 2.4
When faced with intractable problems, consider using strategies for mitigating the computational intractability by trading off with less important characteristics of the desired solution.

Heuristic and Ad Hoc Approaches and the Prescientific-to Scientif ic Evolutionary AI/ML Continuum

The term **"Heuristic" AI/ML methods or systems** refers to several types of systems or strategies: First, *rules of thumb* that may give a good solution sometimes but do not guarantee this. Second, *functions used inside AI search methods* to accelerate finding problem solutions. Third, *ad hoc* systems, i.e., that are not designed based on a formal frameworks for AI/ML, and do not guarantee strong or safe performance in a generalizable sense. Fourth, methods and systems *applied outside their scope of guaranteed safe, effective, or efficient use* (i.e., hoping that an acceptable solution may be produced).

To clarify these concepts consider the following examples (note: all of the mentioned methods and systems will be thoroughly discussed in this and subsequent chapters):
- "We need at least 10 samples per variable when fitting an ordinary least squares regression model" is an example of the first type of heuristic. Another example of the first heuristic type is "choosing 100 genes at random from a cancer microarray dataset will yield predictor models with very high accuracy for diagnosis, often near the performance of special gene selection algorithms" (for surprised readers, not familiar with such data, this is because there is large information overlap and redundancy among genes with respect to clinical cancer phenotypes).
- The "Manhattan distance" as an estimate for the spatial distance between the current location and the goal location in a robot navigation problem is a heuristic than when used inside the A* search algorithm (see later in present chapter) allows the algorithm to find a path with minimum cost to the goal. This is an example of the second type of heuristic.
- The well-known INTERNIST-I system for medical diagnosis in internal medicine was an example of the third type of heuristic AI. It lacked a formal AI foundation both in knowledge representation and inference. It was shown to be highly accurate in certain tests of medical diagnosis problems, however [4].

- Examples of the fourth type are: (1) using Naïve Bayes (a formal ML method that assumes very special distributions in order to be correct) in distributions where the assumptions are known to not hold, hoping that the error will be small. (2) Using Propensity Score (PS) techniques for estimating causal effects, without testing the distributional assumption that makes PS correct (i.e., "strong ignorability", which is not testable within the PS framework). (3) Using Shapley values, a Nobel-Prize winning economics tool devised for value distribution in cooperative coalitions to explain "black box" ML models (a completely different task, for which the method was not designed or proven to be correct; as we will see later in the present volume, it can fail in a wide variety of models). (4) Using IBM Watson, a system designed and tested in an information retrieval task (Jeopardy game) for health discovery and care (for which it had no known properties of correctness or safety). (5) Using Large Language Models (LLMs), e.g., ChatGPT and similar systems (designed for NLP and conversational bot applications) for general-purpose AI tasks (not supported by the known properties of LLMs).

For the purposes of this book, the third and fourth type are most interesting and we will focus on them in the remainder of this section.

In earlier times in the history of health AI/ML as well as broad AI/ML, proponents of ad hoc (heuristic type 3) systems argued that as long as heuristic systems worked well empirically they should be perfectly acceptable especially if more formally-constructed systems did not match the empirical performance of heuristic systems or if constructing formal systems or establishing their properties was exceedingly hard. Proponents of formal systems counter-argued that this ad-hoc approach to AI was detrimental since one should never feel safe when applying such systems, especially in high-stakes domains. At the same time many proponents of the formal approach engaged in practices of the fourth type of heuristic (not testing assumptions, or using a system designed for task A, in unrelated task B).

From a more modern scientific perspective (with substantial benefit of hindsight) of performant and safe systems operating in high-risk domains such as health, the above historical debate is more settled today than in the earlier days of exploring AI. **Heuristic systems and practices represent pre-scientific approaches** in the sense that a true scientific understanding of their behavior does not exist (yet) and that with sufficient study in the future, a comprehensive understanding of a heuristic system of today can be obtained. In other words, the heuristic system of today will be the well-characterized, scientific, non-heuristic system of tomorrow.

In this book we adopt the sharp distinction:

AI/ML systems with well understood theoretical properties and empirical performance vs. systems that lack these properties (aka Heuristic systems).

A further distinction can be made regarding whether a system is based on formal foundations or being ad hoc. The importance of formal systems is that they make the transition to well-understood systems faster and easier. In the absence of formal foundations, it is hard to derive properties and expected behavior. If formal foundations exist, often many of the properties are immediately inherited from the general properties of the underlying formal framework. In any case, deriving formal properties of methods with strong formal foundations is vastly easier than of ad hoc methods.

In addition, there is a **strong practical interplay between theoretical properties and empirical performance**. If theory predicts a certain behavior and empirical tests do not confirm it, this means that errors likely occurred in how the models/ systems have been implemented and debugging is warranted. Alternatively, it may suggest that we operate in a domain with characteristics that are different from the theoretical assumptions of our model (and we need to change modeling tools or strategy). If model A empirically outperforms model B on a task for which A is not built but B is theoretically ideal, this suggests that there are implementation errors or evaluation data/methodology errors in model B, and so on. In other words, a strong theoretical understanding bolsters, and is enhanced by, the empirical application and validation. What is not working well is lacking one or both of these important components (theoretical base + empirical base). More on the interplay of theorical properties and empirical performance can be found in chapter "Principles of Rigorous Development and Appraisal of ML and AI Methods and Systems".

It is also significant to realize that there is an **evolutionary path** from pre-scientific informally-conceived systems, to partially-understood (theoretically or empirically) systems, and finally to fully-mature and well-understood AI/ML.

In earlier related work Aliferis and Miller [5] discussed the "grey zone" between formal systems with known properties but with untestable or unknown preconditions for correctness in some domain, and ad hoc systems with unknown properties across the board. Their observation was that both classes required a degree of faith (with no guarantees) for future success. This early work can be elaborated taking into account the following parameters: *formal or ad hoc foundation; known theoretical properties or not; whether the known properties are testable and have been tested vs not; known empirical performance or not; and whether empirical performance is satisfactory and what alternatives may exist.*

The following table (Table 3) distills the above multi-dimensional space to its essential cases and describes this landscape and developmental journey from pre-scientific systems (lacking properties, rows 1, 3) to intermediate level systems (with partial properties, rows 2, 4, 5, 6), to mature reliable science-backed systems (with known properties, rows 7, 8). The table also points to pitfalls and BPs of building and using systems of the listed characteristics.

It is worth emphasizing that systems with known properties are not automatically optimal or even suitable for solving a problem. Knowledge of properties of various methods and approaches can be used to find the best solution for a task, however.

Table 3 Classification of AI/ML systems based on their formal foundation and properties. The development spectrum from pre-scientific to mature science-backed systems

	Built on formal theory	Known theoretical properties	Known empirical performance	Comments and further dimensions/considerations
1	No	No	No	• Ad hoc with unknown theoretical properties and performance. • Using such systems is a major pitfall and use should be avoided until they are better understood.
2	No	No	Yes	• Ad hoc with unknown properties but known empirical performance in a number of empirical evaluations. • Using such systems is a major risk and needs to take into account the range of evaluation, how good the performance is, whether the evaluation matches the application domain, and whether better alternatives exist.
3	Yes	No	No	• Systems with formal underpinnings but with unknown theoretical properties and empirical performance. • Examples of those systems are systems built on established mathematical frameworks but being poorly mapped to a biomedical problem of interest. • Using such systems is a major pitfall and should be avoided until they are better understood.
4	Yes	No	Yes	• Systems with some formal underpinnings: built on formal foundations but with unknown properties and known empirical performance. • Examples of those systems are systems built on established mathematical or computational frameworks but being poorly mapped to a biomedical problem of interest. • Using such systems entails major risks and should be avoided until risks are better understood.
5	No	Yes	No	• Systems initially starting as ad hoc that eventually evolved to having known properties but yet unknown empirical performance. • This case is in paractice equivalent to formal systems of type (6).
6	Yes	Yes	No	• Theoretically understood but poorly tested (not yet mature) formal systems. • Lack of empirical performance data leaves open the possibility for misalignment of theory with the application domain. Potentially high risk of empirical failure indicates the need for empirical validation before deployment.
7	No	Yes	Yes	• Systems initially starting as ad hoc that eventually evolved to having known properties and known performance. • This case is in practice equivalent to formal systems of type (8).
8	Yes	Yes	Yes	• Fully-realized, fully mature formal systems with known properties and empirical performance. • They can immediately inform whether they can solve the problem at hand (in absolute terms and compared with alternatives).

Chapters "Foundations of Causal ML" and "Principles of Rigorous Development and of Appraisal of ML and AI Methods and Systems" further elaborate on how these concepts can be implemented in practice during the practical development of performant and safe AI/ML.

> **Pitfall 2.4**
> Believing that heuristic systems can give "something for nothing" and that have capabilities that surpass those of well-characterized systems. In reality heuristic systems are pre-scientific or in early development stages.

> **Best Practice 2.5**
> As much as possible use models and systems with established properties (theoretical + empirical). Work within the maturation process starting from systems with unknown behaviors and no guarantees, to systems with guaranteed properties.

Foundations of AI: Logics and Other Symbolic AI and Non symbolic Extensions

Symbolic vs. Non-Symbolic AI

Logic is a staple of science and the cornerstone of all types of so-called *symbolic AI*.

> By **symbolic AI** we refer to AI formalisms that focus on representing the world with symbolic objects and logical relations, and making inferences using logical deductions.
>
> Symbolic systems typically contain **deep, structured representation of the problem solving domain.**
>
> Examples include *production systems, rule-based systems, semantic networks, deductive reasoners, causal modeling with detailed causal relations,* and other types of systems discussed later in this chapter.

By contrast, **non symbolic AI** encompasses various formal systems that focus on uncertain and stochastic relationships using various forms of inference that either rely on probability theory or can be understood in terms of probability.

Non-symbolic systems are typically **shallow representations** of input-output relationships without a detailed model of the structure of the problem solving domain.

Terminology Caution: Deep Learning neural networks are designated as such because they have many hidden node layers (as opposed to shallow ANNs that have few). However they are both shallow AI systems because they lack a rich representation of the domain and its entities (i.e., they are **ontologically shallow**).

Examples of non-symbolic AI (in the ontological shallowness sense) include connectionist AI that approaches AI from an artificial neural network point of view, probabilistic AI that uses a probability theory perspective, shallow causal models, genetic algorithms that adopt an evolutionary search perspective, reinforcement learning, predominantly within the data-driven ML which is the currently dominant paradigm of AI, and most recently Large Language Models (LLMs).

There exist also **formalisms that transcend and attempt to unify symbolic and non-symbolic AI** such as causal probabilistic graphs, probabilistic logics or ANN-implemented rule systems.

See chapter "Lessons Learned from Historical Failures, Limitations and Successes of AI/ML in Healthcare and the Health Sciences. Enduring problems, and the role of Best Practices" for discussion of this important class of AI/ML.

Propositional Logic (PL)

Propositional logic [1, 6] is the simplest form of logic allowing the construction of sentences like:

$$\left(\begin{array}{l} ((\text{Symptom\_positive\_A} = \text{True}) \wedge (\text{Test\_positive\_B} = \text{False})) \\ \vee \neg (\text{Test\_positive\_C} = \text{True}) \end{array} \right)$$
$$\rightarrow \text{Diagnosis\_Disease1} = \text{True}$$

Or in words, if the patient has symptom A and test B is negative, or if she does not have a positive test C, then she has Disease1.

As can be seen, PL uses *propositions* (statements) that can take values in {*True, False*}, and logical *connectives* (*and, or, implication, negation, equivalence, parentheses*). By combining the above based on the straightforward *syntax* of PL, we create complex sentences that may be valid or not. Other than the (tautological) meaning of the truth values {*True, False*}, the precise meaning (*semantics*) of the propositions is embedded in them (i.e., it is not explicit in the PL language).

A *PL Knowledge Base* (KB) contains a set of sentences that are stated as *axioms* (true propositions or valid complex sentences) by the user and then other sentences can be *constructed and proven* to be valid or not using the **truth table** of a PL sentence. The correspondence between the validity of propositions and sentences in the KB and the real world is provided by the notion of a *model* for that KB which is some part of the world (e.g., a biomedical problem domain) where the KB truth assignments hold. Syntactic operations (e.g., by a computer) on the KB prove the validity of sentences in all models of that KB. Inferring that some manipulation of computer symbols has automatically a valid interpretation in the real world (originating from the validity of axioms) is commonly referred by the expression "the computer will take care of the syntax and the semantics will take care of themselves".

Truth *tables* can be used to show that a sentence is valid or not by examining if the sentence is true for all truth assignments of the propositions involved (hence valid), otherwise it is not valid. Sentences are decomposed to smaller parts in a truth table so that truth values for the sentence can be determined. Commonly-used inference steps are encapsulated in *inference rules* such as *Modus Ponens, And-elimination, And-introduction, Resolution*, etc. These are used to avoid constructing very large/complex truth tables. The computational complexity of proving that a sentence in PL is valid is worst-case intractable but quite manageable in small domains [1].

First Order Logic (FOL)

FOL is a vastly more powerful form of logic than PL and can represent:
- Objects (e.g., patients, genes, proteins, hospital units)
- Properties of objects (e.g., alive, up-regulated, secondary structure, full)
- Relations among objects and terms(e.g., patient 1 has a more severe disease than patient 2, gene 1 determines phenotype 1, protein 1 catalyzes chemical reaction 2, hospital unit 1 is less utilized than unit 2)
- Functions (e.g., BMI of a patient P, length of a gene G, molecular weight of a protein P, bed capacity of a hospital unit U)

The **syntax of FOL uses**:
- Objects,
- Constants,
- Variables,
- Predicates used to describe relations among constants or variables,
- Functions over constants, variables or other functions
- Connectives: equivalent, implies, and, or
- Parentheses
- Negation

- Quantifiers: there exists, for all (defined over objects)
- Terms formed from constants, variables and functions over those
- Atomic sentences defined over predicates applied on terms
- Complex sentences defined using atomic sentences, connectives, quantifiers, negation and parentheses.

For a technical syntax specification see [1].

Higher order logics allow expression of *quantifiers applied over functions and relations* (not just objects). These logics are more powerful, but inference is much harder, thus logic-based AI typically deals with FOL or simpler derivative formalisms.

The application of FOL (or derivatives) to build a Knowledge Base (KB) useful for problem solving in some domain is an instance of **Knowledge engineering**. It involves: (a) **ontology engineering,** that is identifying and describing in FOL (or other appropriate language chosen during ontology engineering) the **ontology** (objects, types of relationships) in that problem domain; and (b) **knowledge acquisition** that is identifying and describing in FOL the relevant axioms (facts) describing key aspects of the domain, and from which inferences can be drawn to solve problems.

In the health sciences and healthcare a number of ontologies have been created and are widely used. A most significant component of those are the common data models used to describe entities and variables. These are of essential value for both symbolic and data driven ML methods and for harmonizing data and knowledge across health care providers, studies, and scientific projects. See chapter "Data Preparation, Transforms, Quality, and Management" for a discussion of the most commonly used common data models and standards.

Knowledge engineering could be substituted for ordinary programming however the fundamental advantage of Knowledge engineering is that it is a **declarative approach to programming** with significant advantages (whenever applicable) such as: ability to represent compactly facts and complex inferences that may be very cumbersome to conventional procedural or functional programming methods. Moreover, once the AI knowledge engineer has constructed the knowledge base, *then a myriad of inferences can be made using the pre-existing inferential mechanisms of FOL.* In other words, no new problem solving apparatus is needed, because it is provided by FOL. Declarative programming needs only a precise statement of the problem.

Logical Inference

FOL has a number of sound inference procedures that differ in their completeness. Such procedures are *Generalized Modus Ponens (that can be used in Forward-Chaining, Backward-Chaining directions), and Resolution Refutation.*

Forward chaining is an algorithm that starts from the facts and generates consequences, whereas Backward chaining starts from what we wish to prove and works backward to establish the necessary precedents. The "chaining" refers to the fact that as new sentences are proven correct, they can be used to activate new rules until no more inferences can be made.

As a very simple example consider a KB with:

Axioms:	A, B
Rules of the type x → y:	A → C, and C ∧ B → D

From this KB,

The **Forward Chaining** algorithm will perform the following sequence of operations:

1. From A and A → C it will infer C and add it to the KB
2. From B, C and C ∧ B → it will infer D and add to the KB
3. Will terminate because no new inferences can be made

The **Backward Chaining** algorithm from the same original KB, and user request to prove D, will:

1. First see that D is not an axiom
2. Identify that C ∧ B → D can be used to try and prove D
3. Will seek to prove C and B separately
4. B is an axiom so it is true
5. C is not an axiom but rule A → C can be used to prove it
6. Will seek to prove A
7. A is an axiom thus true
8. Thus (by backtracking to (5) C is true
9. Thus (by backtracking to (2) D is true
10. Terminate reporting success in proving D

Forward and backward chaining strategies are widely used in biomedical symbolic AI expert systems. They are not FOL-complete however! Recall that Goedel proved that in sufficiently complex reasoning systems (such as FOL) there are true statements that cannot be proven from the axioms of the system. He also proved that if there are provable sentences, then there exists an algorithm to generate the proof. Robinson [7] discovered such an algorithm (Resolution Refutation) which operates by introducing the negation of a sentence we wish to prove in the knowledge base and deriving a contradiction. Resolution Refutation is complete *with respect to what can be proven in FOL.* For technical details of the algorithm refer to [1, 7].

The **Resolution Refutation** algorithm in the KB of the previous example, will:

1. Add ¬ D to the KB
2. From A and A → C it will infer C and add it to the KB
3. From C and C ∧ B → D it will infer D and add to the KB
4. From D and ¬ D it will derive a contradiction and will terminate declaring success in proving D

The above examples are *hugely simplified* by not addressing predicates, variables, functions, quantification, conversion to different canonical forms and their matching, which are all needed for the general case algorithms operation. For technical details see [1, 6, 7]. Nilsson [7] in particular gives a definitive technical treatment of rule-base systems and their properties.

Logic-Derivative Formalisms and Extensions of FOL

FOL is almost never used in its pure form in biomedical AI applications. Instead, it serves as a foundation for other more specialized and invariably simplified formalisms. Occasionally researchers have extended ordinary FOL to accommodate reasoning with probabilities, or time. The following Table 4 lists important FOL derivatives and extensions.

Table 4 Types of logic-based systems (FOL derivatives)

- **Decision Trees** which are very widely used both in the construction of clinical guidelines and as a language for ML (chapter "An Appraisal and Operating Characteristics of Major ML Methods Applicable in Healthcare & Health Science").
- **Rule based systems** for discovery or clinical care based on forward or backward chaining algorithms and extensions for reasoning under uncertainty e.g., the highly influential systems DENDRAL, META-DENDRAL and MYCIN [8, 9]
- **Logic-based programming** e.g., the widely-used PROLOG language [10]
- **Non chaining rule based decision support** e.g., the widely-used ARDEN SYNTAX for clinical decision support [11]
- **Semantic networks/"slot-and-filler" representations, semantic WWW, and taxonomies,** e.g., [12, 13]
- **Boolean networks** e.g., widely used for biological pathway discovery and modeling [14]
- **Symbolic NLP systems** (see chapter "Considerations for Specialized Health AI and ML Modelling and Applications: NLP" for details and references)
- **Ontologies and declarative representations e.g.,** BIOPORTAL [15]
- **Fuzzy logic e.g.,** [16]
- **Non monotonic logic e.g.,** [17]
- **Probabilistic, and temporal logics e.g.,** [18]
- **Planning systems e.g.,** used for therapy planning or for industrial and operations planning purposes [7, 19]

Although FOL is not used without major modifications and simplifications in the above, it remains the most important theoretical framework for understanding the structure, capabilities and limitations of such methods and systems. Chapter "Lessons Learned from Historical Failures, Limitations and Successes of AI/ML In Healthcare and the Health Sciences. Enduring problems, and the role of Best Practicess" discuss present-day concerns in the AI/ML science and technology community that a drastic departure from symbolic AI (e.g., in favor of purely statistical and ontologically shallow input-output representations), does not bode well for the ability of the field to successfully address the full range and complexity of health science and health care problems.

Non-Symbolic AI for Reasoning with Uncertainty

Numerous non-symbolic methods exist and the most important ones in current practice are covered in detail in chapters "An Appraisal and Operating Characteristics of Major ML Methods Applicable in Healthcare and Health Science" and "Foundations of Causal ML". Here we will address two methods of great importance in the modern practice of healthcare and health science research: Decision Analysis and Bayesian networks.

Methods that have predominantly historical significance will not be addressed, in order to preserve reader and book bandwidth and focus more on techniques that are part of modern practices.

Decision Analysis (DA) and Maximum Expected Utility (MEU)-Based Reasoning

Decision Analysis using Maximum Expected Utility stems for the fundamental work of Von Neumann and Morgenstern dating back to 1947. This theory provides a model of *prescriptive* decision making designed to limit the risk of a decision agent facing uncertainty. Whereas the theory may not be universally applicable in all situations involving biomedical decisions with uncertainty, they still describe a powerful model with wide applicability.

The principles of MEU and DA can be readily grasped with a simple example. Consider the hypothetical case of a patient facing the dilemma of whether to undergo a surgery for a condition she has, or to opt for the conservative treatment. Assume that either decision cannot be followed by the other (e.g., a failed surgery precludes improvement by the conservative treatment, whereas the conservative treatment exceeds the time window when the surgery is beneficial).

Furthermore let the probability of success of surgery in such patients be p(surgical success) = 0.9 and probability of success of non-surgical treatment in such patients be p(nonsurgical success) = 0.6. Finally let the quality of life (measured in a *utility scale* ranging in [0,1]) after successful surgery be 0.8, after failed surgery be 0.2, after successful conservative treatment be 1, and under failed conservative treatment be 0.5.

Utility assessment protocols designed to identify a patient's preferences and map them to a utility scale exist. Expected utility defines four axioms describing a rational decision maker: completeness; transitivity; independence of irrelevant alternatives; and continuity [57]. The principle of MEU decision making based on these axioms, designates the optimal decision as the one that maximizes the expected utility over all possible decisions:

$$Optimal\ decision = \text{argmax}_i\ \mathbf{E}\big(U\big(decision_i\big)\big)$$

where

$$\mathbf{E}\big(U\big(decision_i\big)\big) = \sum_j \mathbf{E}\big(U\big(outcome_{ij}\big)\big)$$

and:

- $U\ (decision_i)$ is the expectation of the utility of the ith decision,
- $U\ (outcome_{j,i})$ is the patient-specified utility of the jth outcome based on decision i and
- $E\ (U(outcome_{j,i})$ is the expected patient-specified utility of the jth outcome based on decision i

In our hypothetical example, we can easily see that

$$\mathbf{E}\big(U\big(decision_{surgery}\big)\big) = 0.9*0.8 + 0.1*0.2 = 0.74$$

whereas

$$\mathbf{E}\big(U\big(decision_{conservative}\big)\big) = 0.6*1 + 0.4*0.5 = 0.80$$

The decision that maximizes expected utility is thus the non-surgical treatment.

In graphical form the above scenario is captured by the following **Decision Analysis** Fig. 1.

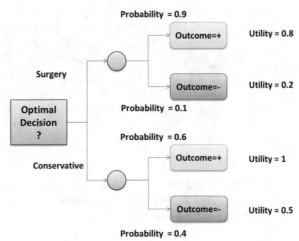

Fig.1 A decision analysis tree augmented with probabilities and utilities corresponding to the hypothetical example in the text

We note that MEU DA, whenever applicable, is a powerful and principled way to make decisions that maximize benefit. Pitfalls in MEU-DA based reasoning are:

Pitfalls 2.5
Decision Analysis (DA) and Maximum Expected Utility (MEU)-based reasoning
1. Errors in the estimation of probabilities for various events.
2. Errors in eliciting utility estimates in a way that captures patients' true preferences (including using the care providers' utilities rather than the patients').
3. The structure or complexity of the problem setting defies analyst's ability to completely/accurately describe it.
4. Developing a DA for one population and applying in another with different structure of the problem, different probabilities for action-dependent and action-independent events, or with different preferences.

The corresponding best practices are addressing these sources of errors that can lead a decision analysis astray.

Best Practice 2.6
Decision Analysis (DA) and Maximum Expected Utility (MEU)-based reasoning
1. Ensure that the structure of the problem setting is sufficiently/accurately described by the DA tree. Omit known or obvious irrelevant factors.
2. Elicit utility estimates in a way that captures patients' true preferences using established utility-elicitation methods.
3. Accurately estimate probabilities of action-dependent events and action-independent events.
4. In most conditions, and whenever applicable, data-driven approaches should be preferred to subjective probability estimates. Use probability-consistent statistical or ML algorithms to estimate the probabilities.
5. Ensure that the decision analysis is applied to the correct population.
6. Conduct sensitivity analyses that reveal how much the estimated optimal decision is influenced by uncertainty in the specification of the model.
7. Whenever possible, produce credible intervals/posterior probability distributions for the utility expectations of decisions.

These cover only the most salient aspects of the art and science of MEU driven decision analysis. A more detailed introduction is given in [20] and a comprehensive applied treatment in [21].

Reasoning with Uncertainty: Probabilistic Reasoning with Bayesian Networks

Bayesian Networks (BNs) are an AI/ML family of models that can describe the probabilistic (or deterministic, or hybrid) relationships among variables. They have extensive usability, range of application, attractive properties and thus high practical value. They can support several use cases and types of problem solving (which can be combined):

- **Use 1:** Overcome the limitations of intractable (brute force Bayes), or unduly restrictive (Naive Bayes), classifiers.
- **Use 2:** They are very economical to describe (i.e., they have space complexity that closely mirrors the distribution complexity).
- **Use 3:** They can be created both from expert knowledge and from data (or with hybrid sources).
- **Use 4:** They can be used for MEU DA (providing probability estimates for DAs or in their "influence diagram" form).
- **Use 5:** They can perform flexible classification and other sophisticated probabilistic inferences.
- **Use 6:** They can be thought of as probability-enhanced logical rules and combine forward and backward, as well as forward-backward inferences in a way that is probabilistically accurate.
- **Use 7:** They can be used (with very mild additional restrictions) to reason causally including: (1) Distinguishing between *observing* passively a variable's value vs. applying interventions that cause the variable to take that value, and reason accordingly. (2) Reasoning from causes to outcomes, from outcomes to causes, and simultaneously in both directions over multiple and overlapping causal pathways.
- **Use 8:** Their causal variants can be used to discover causality, not just perform inferences with existing causal models.
- **Use 9:** They have close relationship to the Markov Boundary theory of optimal feature selection.

Because of these properties we touch upon various forms and derivatives of BNs in several chapters and contexts in this volume: AI reasoning under uncertainty (chapter "Foundations and Properties of AI/ML Systems"), Bayesian classifiers (chapter "An Appraisal and Operating Characteristics of Major ML Methods Applicable in Healthcare and Health Science"), Markov Boundary based feature selection (chapter "An Appraisal and Operating Characteristics of Major ML Methods Applicable in Healthcare and Health Science") and causal discovery and modeling (chapter "Foundations of Causal ML").

We caution that not every graph or every probabilistic graph is a BN and the BN properties derive from very specific requirements. Because there is confusion in parts of the literature (where some authors derive models that are not BNs but present them as such), we will provide here, for clarity, an unambiguous technical description of this family of AI/ML models.

BN Definitions

Definition. Bayesian Network. A BN comprises (1) a directed acyclic graph (DAG); (2) a joint probability distribution (JPD) over variable set V such that each variable corresponds to a node in the DAG; and (3) a restriction of how the JPD relates to the DAG, known as the Markov Condition (MC).

Definition. Directed Graph. directed graph is a tuple $<V,E>$, where V is a set of nodes representing variables 1-to-1, and E is a set of directed edges, or arrows, each one of which connects an ordered pair of members of V.

Definition: Two nodes are **adjacent** if they are connected by an edge. Two edges are adjacent if they share a node.

Definition: A *path* is any set of adjacent edges.

Definition: A **directed path** is a path where all edges are pointing in the same direction.

Definition: A **directed acyclic graph** (DAG) is a directed graph that has no cycles in it, that is, there is no directed path that contains the same node more than once.

Definition: The **joint probability distribution** (JPD) over V is any proper probability distribution (i.e., every possible joint instantiation of variables has a probability associated with it and the sum of those is 1).

Definition: Parents, children, ancestors, and descendants: In a directed graph, if variables X,Y share an edge $X \rightarrow Y$ then X is called the parent of Y, and Y is called the child of X. If there is a directed path from X to Y then X is an ancestor of Y and Y is a descendant of X.

Definition: Spouses: In a directed graph, the spouses of a variable Vj is the set comprising all variables that are parents to at least one of the children of Vj.

Definition: The **Markov Condition (MC)** states that every variable V is independent of all variables that are non-descendants of V given its direct causes.

Definition: If *all dependencies and independencies* in the data are the ones following from the MC, then the encoded JPD is a **Faithful Distribution** to the BN and its graph.

Definition: Degree of a node is the number of edges connected to it. In a directed graph, this can be further divided into **in-degree** and **out-degree**, corresponding to the number of parents (edges oriented towards the node) and children (edges oriented away from the node) that the node has.

Definition: A **collider** is a variable receiving incoming edges from two variables. For example in: $X \rightarrow Y \leftarrow Z$, Y is the collider. A **collider is either "shielded" or "unshielded"** iff the corresponding parents of the collider are connected by an edge or not, respectively. Unshielded colliders give form to the so-called "**v-structures**".

Definition: A **trek** is a path that contains no colliders.

Definition: The **graphical Markov Boundary** of a variable Vj is the union of its parents Pa(Vj), its children Ch(Vj) and the parents of its children Sp(Vj).

Definition: The **probabilistic Markov Boundary** of a variable Vj is the set of variable S that renders Vj conditionally independent of all other variables, when we condition on S, and is minimal.

Key Properties of Bayesian Networks

Unique and Full Joint Distribution Specification. If the Markov Condition (MC) holds, then the conditional probabilities of every variable given its parents specifies a well-defined and unique joint distribution over variables set V.

Any Joint Probability Distribution Can be Represented by a BN. If we wish to model JPD J1 by a BN, we can order the variables arbitrarily, connect with edges every variable Vj with all variables preceding it in the ordering, and define the conditional probability of Vj given the parents in the graph equal to the one calculated from J1. Then the implied JPD J2 of the BN will be J2 = J1. Note: the outline constructive proof presented here is a large sample result. Much more sample-efficient procedures exist for small sample situations.

The Joint Distribution of a BN Can Be Factorized Based on Parents. The joint distribution is factorized as a product of the conditional probability distribution of every variable given is direct causes set

$$probability(V_1, V_2, ..., V_k) = \prod_j probability(V_j \mid Pa(V_j)) \tag{4}$$

Where j indexes the variables in V, and $Pa(V_j)$ is the set of parents of variable V_j.

Because of this factorization, we only need to specify up to |V| conditional probabilities in order to fully specific the BN (where |V| is the number of variables. When all variables have a small number of parents, the total number of probabilities is linear to |V|. By comparison in a Brute Force Bayes classifier we always need specify $2^{|V|}$ probabilities.

Similarly whenever we need to compute the joint probability of Eq. 4, for a particular instantiation of the variables involved, this is a linear time operation in the number of variables.

Definition: D-separation

1. Two variables X, Y connected by a path are d-separated (aka the path is "blocked") given a set of variables S, if and only if on this path, there is
   (a) A non-collider variable contained in S, or
   (b) A collider such that neither it nor any of its descendants are contained in S.

2. Two variables, X and Y, connected by several paths are d-separated given a set of variables S, if and only if in all paths connecting X to Y, they are d-separated by S.

3. Two disjoint variable sets X and Y are d-separated by variable set S iff every pair <Xi, Yj > is d-separated by S, where Xi and Yj are members of X, Y respectively.

Inspection of the Graph of a BN Informs us About all Conditional Independencies in the Data. By inspection **(by eye or algorithmically)** of the causal graph (and application of *d-separation*) we can infer all valid conditional independencies in the data, *without analyzing the data* as follows:

- If variable sets X and Y are d-separated by variable set S then they will be conditionally independent given S in the JPD encoded by the BN.

Inspection of the Graph of a BN Encoding a Faithful Distribution, Informs us about all Conditional Independencies and Dependencies in the Data. A BN encoding a faithful distribution entails that all dependencies *and* independencies in the JPD can be inferred by the DAG by application of the d-separation criterion as follows:

- If variable sets X and Y are d-separated by variable set S in the BN graph, then they will be conditionally independent given S in the JPD encoded by the BN. Otherwise they will be dependent.
- Equivalently:
- Variable sets X and Y are conditionally independent given S in the JPD encoded by the BN, iff they are d-separated by variable set S in the BN graph.

Therefore in faithful distributions, the BN graph becomes a map (so-called **i-map**) of dependencies and independencies in the data JPD encoded by the BN. Conversely, by inferring dependencies and indecencies in the data we can construct the BN's DAG and parameterize the conditional probabilities of every variable given its parents, effectively recovering the unoriented causal process that generates the data. This is a **fundamental principle of operation of causal ML methods** (discussed in more detail in chapter "Foundations of Causal ML").

A Variable in a BN is Independent of all Other Variables Given its Graphical Markov Boundary and Equivalently a variable in a JPD is independent of all other variables given its Probabilistic Markov Boundary in Faithful Distributions.

Relationship of Markov Boundary and Causality. This can be used to obtain optimal feature sets for predictive modeling when the BN is known or is inferred from data. Because the graphical and probabilistic Markov Boundary are identical in faithful distributions, in causal BNs, there is a close connection of the local causal network around a variable and its probabilistic Markov Boundary (see chapter "Foundations of Causal ML").

BNs Allow Flexible Inference

We will illustrate flexible inference with an example depicted in Fig. 2.

In Fig. 2 part (1) we see a BN model for some problem solving domain. In part (2) we query the BN with the question: what is the probability of F (grey node) given that we have observed the values of variables {C, B, H} (green nodes)? The inference algorithms propagate and synthesize information upward (e.g., from C and B to A) and downward from A and B to F. Notice that given B, H is irrelevant to F.

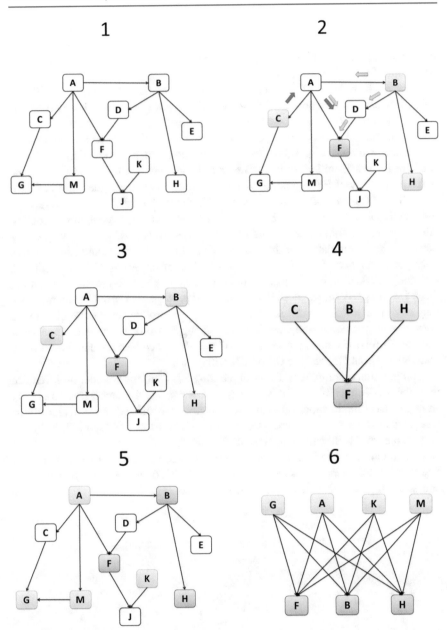

Fig. 2 Flexible predictive modeling and forward/backward reasoning in BNs

If we wish to set up a conventional classifier (of any type, Logistic Regression, Boosting, Deep Learning, SVM, Random Forest etc., it has to obey a fixed input-response structure depicted in (4)); in other words in order to answer this question we need to approximate a function of the probability (F | C, B, H) and train it *from scratch for that query.* The BN (3) requires no modification however.

If we wish to answer next what is the joint probability of {F, B, H} given that we observe {G, A, K, M}, again the same BN (5) can give us the answer. Other predictive modeling methods however (6) will need to be trained *from scratch* to estimate: probability (F, B, H I G, A, K, M).

Because the number of such queries grows exponentially to the number of variables, it is essentially impossible to answer all the answerable queries by a BN by training specialized classifiers. Moreover *any* subdivision of the variables sets as observed, unknown, or query variables is allowed and needs not be known a priori.

We now examine (Fig. 3) how a causal BN (see chapter "Foundations of Causal ML" for formal definitions) can answer causal questions. Consider the query: what is the probability of F (grey node) given that we have observed the values of variables {B, H} (green nodes) and we have manipulated C to take a specific value (via intervention denoted by *do(C)*)? The causal BN (left) knows that when we manipulate a variable, nothing else can affect it. Thus the Arc: A→C is effectively eliminated by the manipulation in the context of the query. Consequently, information does not travel from C to F via A as in the case of observing C. The predictive modeling models lacking causal semantics (e.g., Logistic Regression, Boosting, Deep Learning, SVM, Random Forest etc.) will propagate information from C to F thus arriving at a wrong conclusion. Incidentally this problem cannot be fixed in the conventional predictive modelers by eliminating C from the model, since valid causal/information paths may exist from C to F than need be considered even if we manipulate C (and indeed the causal BN will do so).

Computational complexity for both learning BNs and for conducting inference with them is intractable in the wort case. However highly successful mitigation strategies have led to super-efficient average case or restricted-purpose algorithms (see chapters "An Appraisal and Operating Characteristics of Major ML Methods Applicable in Healthcare and Health Science", and "Lessons Learned from Historical Failures, Limitations and Successes of ML in Healthcare and the Health Sciences. Enduring Problems and the Role of Best Practices" for details). Key references for properties of BNs discussed here are [22–25].

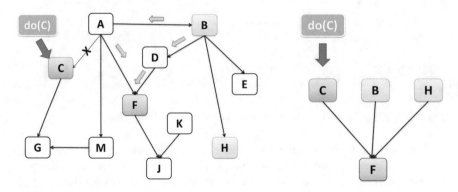

Fig. 3 Causally Consistent Inference with BNs AND Forward/Backward reasoning

AI Search

Search as a General Problem Solving Strategy. Conventional Search Versus AI Search

Search is a general problem solving methodology in which many (if not most) problems can be reduced to. Somewhat similar to physical search of an object or a location inside a physical space, AI search constructs a state space with each state representing a possible solution or partial solution to a problem. The search algorithms then traverse this state space trying to discover or construct a solution. For example, in a ML context, the state space could comprise models fit from data, such that each model has a different structure and corresponding estimated generalization predictivity. AI search in the ML context seeks then to find ML models that achieve the highest or sufficient high predictivity. In an autonomous navigation context, AI search would seek to find a navigation path that achieves smallest traversed distance, smallest cost of trip, or other objectives. In a scheduling context AI search may seek to schedule patients and operating room personnel to operating rooms so that cancelations are minimized. The diversity of problems that can be solved with search is infinite and covers the full space of computable functions.

General AI Search Framework: "Best" First Search (BeFS) Family and Variants

Whereas search is also accomplished outside AI, most notably with linear and non linear optimization methods, ad hoc search algorithms, and Operations Research algorithms, AI search has distinctive qualities:

- AI search can use state spaces that are infinite in size.
- AI search can attempt to solve problems in the hardest of complexity classes.
- AI search admits any computable goal, not just a small space of computable functions.
- AI search can operate with symbolic and non-symbolic representations.

Table 5 outlines a very general framework for AI search.

Table 5 High-level operation of general AI search:

- The general AI search algorithm maintains a priority list of states that will be explored.
- This list is initialized with a starting search state, and an iterative loop begins:
- If the first state in the priority list it is not the goal state then the algorithm
  Creates all successor states from it and updates the list contents and then prioritizes those according to a prioritizing function. Else the algorithms returns the goal state and terminates
- The process will stop iterating when
  – A goal state has been found or
  – No more states can be reached or
  – Another termination criterion is met.
  Each state also stores the path to reach that state and the cost of that solution path. Thus when a goal state is returned, the solution path can be extracted

This prima facie very simple procedure has immense power and flexibility and can be instantiated in a variety of ways leading to different behaviors and properties. For example, the following variants can be had as follows (Table 6):

Table 6 Notable instantiations of general BeFS AI search:

Instantiation of prioritizing function	Resulting type of search	Properties
Ranks states in priority list in ascending order according to order that states were generated (i.e. first in first out, or FIFO)	Depth first search	Will terminate and find a solution if search space is finite and enough computation time and space are allowed Worst case complexity = O (state space size). May not find optimal solution For finite state spaces organized as trees of depth d and breadth b: Worst case time complexity = O (b^d). Space complexity is O (m * b) where m is the maximum depth of a path. Preferable if many optimal solutions are arranged in same search tree depth level
Rank states in priority list in descending order according to order that states were generated (i.e. last in first out, or LIFO)	Breadth first search	Will find a solution and terminate if search space is finite and enough computation time and space are allowed. May not find optimal solution Worst case complexity = O (state space size). For finite state spaces organized as trees of depth d and breadth b: Worst case space and time Complexity = O (b^d) Preferable if many solutions are arranged in same search path
Rank states in priority list in ascending order according to cost of path to each state	Uniform cost search (aka branch and bound)	Will find a solution if search space is finite and enough computation time and space are allowed. Will find optimal solution if path cost is non decreasing Worst case complexity = O (state space size). For finite state spaces organized as trees of depth d and breadth b: Worst case complexity = O (b^d)
Rank states in priority list in ascending order according to estimated cost of state to goal state	Greedy Search (ie., most locally promising next step *with* backtracking)	Will find a solution if search space is finite and enough computation time and space are allowed. May not find optimal solution For finite state spaces with max depth path m: Worst case time complexity = O (b^m) If estimates of cost to goal are good then it may reach a solution very fast

Table 6 (continued)

Instantiation of prioritizing function	Resulting type of search	Properties
Rank states in ascending order according to: Estimated cost of state to goal state. Also eliminate from priority list all but the most locally promising next state.	Hill climbing Search (most locally promising next step *without* backtracking)	May not find a solution or if it finds one it may not be optimal. It may not terminate if search space is infinite For finite state spaces with max depth path m: Worst case time complexity = O (m * b) and space complexity is = 1 Has tendency to be trapped in locally optima that are not globally optimal solutions If, however, search space is convex or concave then it finds the optimal solution with time complexity = depth of solution and space complexity = 1. This fact is exploited by many mathematical convex optimization algorithms [26]
Rank states in priority list in ascending order according to: (cost of path to that state + estimated cost of state to goal state) with the constraint that estimated cost to goal cannot exceed true cost.	A*	Will find a solution if search has finite branching factor, and enough computation time and space are allowed Will find optimal solution No other search algorithm using the same estimated cost to goal state function can outperform A* For max depth path m: Worst case space complexity = $O(b^m)$ Worst case time complexity is polynomial if the error of the heuristic cost estimate to goal state will not grow faster than the logarithm of the "perfect heuristic" h* that returns the true distance to the goal

The fundamental general search algorithm and its instantiations can be readily extended to cope with infinite size search spaces and computing environments with limited space using *depth-limited*, *iterative deepening* and *simplified memory-bounded A** versions. For details see [1].

Other Notable AI Search Methods

In addition to the above "classical" AI search algorithms notable search methods include **Simulated Annealing, Genetic Algorithms, Ant Colony Optimization and search procedures applicable to rule based systems and resolution refutation.**

Simulated annealing [27] is inspired by metallurgy and the annealing process. It comprises a classic hill climbing method modified to incorporate a randomized jump to one of nearby states so that local optima have a larger chance (but no guarantee) of not trapping the algorithm in suboptimal solutions.

Genetic algorithms [28, 29] are inspired by biological evolution which they mimic. Genetic algorithms represent solutions in digital chromosome representation on which they perform, just like evolution does on actual organisms, random mutations and crossover operations. This is their way to generate successor solution states. Multiple states are maintained at each stage of the algorithms with the best-fit ones having a smaller chance to be discarded. The algorithm has the attractive property that an exponentially increasing portion of better performing states are considered in each step. It can be applied in domains where the data scientists now nothing about the domain (i.e., they are "black box optimizers"). On the other hand, they have important limitations: they are not guaranteed to reach an optimal solution (i.e., can be trapped in local optima), it has been proven that they cannot learn certain classes of functions (e.g. epistatic functions); and they are not efficient when compared to non-randomized algorithms solving the same problems.

Ant Colony Optimization (ACO) and **"Swarm intelligence"** is inspired by the foraging behavior of some ant species. These ants deposit pheromone on the ground in order to mark some favorable path that should be followed by other members of the colony. ACO can be used for graph searching, scheduling problems, classification, image recognition and other problems. For several ACOs, convergence has been proven (albeit at an unknown number of iterations). Finally empirical results in >100 NP-hard problems has shown competitive and ocasionaly excellent performance compared to best known algorithms [30].

Specialized search procedures include AO* (suitable for searching AND/OR graphs used in decomposable rule based systems), MINIMAX and ALPHA-BETA search (suitable for game tree search), and Resolution Refutation search strategies (e.g., unit preference, set of support identification, input resolution, linear resolution, subsumption etc.) designed to make the resolution refutation algorithm reach a proof faster [1, 6, 7].

AI/ML Languages

Whereas statement of algorithms and theoretical analysis is typically conducted using *pseudocode*, practical development depends on choice of programming languages. A few languages are particularly suitable for AI/ML and their properties are summarized in the next Table 7:

Table 7 Notable AI/ML Languages

Language	Properties and suggested use
Pseudocode	• Comprises generally-stated data structures, code modularization (e.g., functions, procedures), and control structures that are programming language independent. • May also contain declarative and logical statements that can be implemented in any applicable programming language. For example, a universally quantified statement can be converted to a conventional loop. • It is widely understood by all computer scientists. • Especially appropriate for stating algorithms and conducting theoretical analysis. • They can be passed to programmers that will implement them in a programming language of choice.
LISP	• The most powerful and flexible language for AI and possibly the most powerful programming language ever created. • Systems of immense complexity and capabilities can be implemented very compactly and easily. • Particularly suitable to symbolic AI. • Incorporates procedural, functional, and object oriented paradigms. • Uses lists (with dynamic memory management) as primary data structures. More efficient or special purpose data structures can readily be implemented. • Compiled and interpreted. • LISP programs and data are interchangeable. Programs are themselves data that can be generated or modified by programs. Programs can modify themselves or other programs at runtime or off line. • The language symbols can be assigned to different functions. Thus the language itself can be modified by programs. • These immense powers may create interpretability problems since programmers do not immediately know what a program will do, e.g., they have to understand how the usual language features are modified at runtime.
Prolog	• Designed for symbolic AI. • Uses backward chaining rule-based programming paradigm. • Declarative programming. • (Surprisingly) is resolution-refutation complete. • Not as widely used anymore.

(continued)

Table 7 (continued)

Language	Properties and suggested use
Matlab	• Extremely powerful language and development environment especially suitable for ML. • Uses matrices and matrix operations as fundamental building blocks. • Extremely optimized operations can produce immensely efficient programs. • Very rapid development. • Interpreted and compiled. • Can be interfaced with all major languages. • Numerous toolboxes (libraries) cover all major mathematics, machine learning, engineering, imaging, bioinformatics, etc. types of development project needs. • On the downside it is a commercial product that requires paid educational or commercial licenses.
R	• Flexible and powerful language well suited for statistical and ML development. • Numerous open source libraries. • No license costs. • Many libraries and codes are unoptimized and may also have implementation errors. • Does not scale as well as other languages.
Python	• Flexible language especially well-suited to text processing and ML. • Interpreted and compiled. • Numerous open source, no-cost libraries. • Varying degrees of quality of available free codes.
A sample of other languages commonly encountered in the AI/ML space	• C, C++ and Objective C. • Pascal and variants (e.g. Delphi). • Pearl. • Ruby. • Basic and variants (e.g., Visual Basic). • Older languages (FORTRAN, MODULA, COBOL) are seldomly used for new development. • Assembly language: for specialized applications where speed optimization is of paramount importance. • MUMPS for EHR-focused programming. • SQL: very useful for relational database querying.

Foundations of Machine Learning Theory

AI and ML as Applied Epistemology

Epistemology is the branch of philosophy concerned with knowledge: its generation and sources, nature, its achievable scope, its justification, the concept of belief as it relates to knowledge, and related issues [31]. From the perspective of this volume it is worthwhile to notice first that AI formalizes knowledge so that it can be used in applied settings. AI can also inform what types of knowledge are computable and what inferential procedures can be applied and with what characteristics. ML in particular, by virtue of being able to *generate knowledge from data,* on one hand obtains its justification not just by empirical success but by epistemological principles of science. On the other hand, ML puts to test epistemological hypotheses and theories about how knowledge *is, can, or should* be generated. The following sections provide a concise outline of the key theories that provide the firm scientific ground on which ML is built and in particular for fortifying its performance and generalization properties. They also summarize a few related pitfalls and high level best practices that will be developed further in other chapters.

ML Framed as AI search and the Role of Inductive Bias

We showed earlier in this chapter how AI search can be used to solve hard problems. ML itself can be cast as a search endeavor [29, 32, 33]. In this framework, ML search comprises:

(a) A model language L in which a *family* of ML models can be represented. For example, decision trees, logic rules, artificial neural networks, linear discriminant equations, causal graphs etc. Typically the model language will come with associated procedures that enable models to be built when data D are provided (i.e., model fitting procedure MF).

(b) A data-generating or design procedure DD that creates data (typically by sampling from a population or other data-generating process) from which models are fit.

(c) A hypothesis space S. The language L implicitly defines a space S comprising all models expressible in the language and that can be fit with MF applied on D, with each model M_i representing a location or state in S. For example, the space of all decision trees, neural networks, linear discriminant functions, boosted trees, etc. that can be built over variable set V using MF on D.

(d) A search procedure MLS that navigates the space in order to find a model representing an acceptable solution to the ML problem as defined by a goal criterion. For example, a steepest ascend hill climbing search procedure over the space of decision trees over V *fit by* MF *given data* D.

(e) A goal (or merit) function GM that examines a search state (i.e., a model M_i) and decides whether it is a solution, or how close to a solution it is (its merit function value). For example, whether M_i has acceptable predictivity, uncertainty, generalizability etc. or what is the merit value (e.g., difference of its properties to the goal ones).

The tuple: $< L, MF, DD, S, MLS, GM >$ defines the **architecture of a ML method.**

Every ML method can be described and understood in these terms (although additional perspectives and analytical frameworks are also valuable, and in some cases necessary).

The tuple: $< L, MF, S, GM >$ describes what is commonly referred to as a **ML "algorithm"**, whereas **MLS** describes the **model selection procedure** that ideally will incorporate an **error estimator procedure** for the final (best) model(s) found. **GM** and its estimators from data may or may not be identical to the *error function* and its estimators (see chapter "The Development Process and Lifecycle of Clinical Grade and Other Safety and Performance-Sensitive AI/ML Models").

The tuple: $< L, MF, S, MLS, GM >$ describes the **Inductive Bias** of that ML method.

The inductive bias of a ML method is the **preference ('bias") of that method for a class of models** over other models that are not considered at all or are not prioritized by the method.

Notice that in practice there are *two search procedures* in operation:

MF is a search procedure in the space of model parameter values once a model family and its model family parameter values (aka **"hyperparameters"**) have been visited by the **second (top-level, or over-arching) search procedure MLS which searches over possible model families and their hyper parameters**.

For example, the search procedure in decision tree induction algorithm is a greedy steepest ascent while a hyper parameter may be the minimum number of samples allowed for accepting a new node or leaf. In an SVM model the search procedure is quadratic programming and hyper parameters may be the cost C and the kernel functions and their parameters. The model selection procedure that decides over these two model families and the right hyperparameter values for them may be *grid search* using a cross validation error estimator, or other appropriate model selection process (see chapter "Principles of Rigorous Development and of Appraisal of ML and AI Methods and Systems" for details).

The ML search framework above readily entails important properties of ML:

1. The choice of model language affects most major model properties like error, tractability, transparency/explainability, sample efficiency, causal compatibility, generalizability etc.
2. The data generating procedure implements the principles and practices of data design which is a whole topic by itself (see chapter "Data Design for Biomedical AI/ML"). Because the whole operation of ML as search is so dependent on the data D, the *data design/data generating procedure strongly interacts with the other components and determines the success of the ML model search.*
3. The search space typically has infinite size, or finite but astronomically large size.

4. The ML search procedures MF typically have to find sparse solutions in the infinite/practically infinite search space. Therefore they are often custom-tailored or optimized for the specific ML algorithm.
5. The MLS search procedures are designed to operate over several ML algorithm families and their hyper-parameters. They are typically much less intensive and typically informed by prior analyses in the problem domain of similar data, giving guidance about which hype-parameter ranges will likely contain the optimal values.

Worth noting in particular with respect to the inductive bias:

6. The match of the inductive bias of a ML method to the problem one wishes to solve (hence the data generating function to be modeled and the data design procedure that samples from the data generating function) determines the degree of success of this ML method.
7. It also follows, that if a ML method does not have restrictions on inductive bias, it cannot learn anything useful at all, in the sense that it would accept any model equally as well as any other (i.e., accept good and bad models alike) and in the extreme it would amount to random guess among all conceivable models).
8. At the same time, a successful ML method must not have a too restrictive inductive bias because this may cause lack the ability to represent or find good models for the task at hand.
9. Taken together (6), (7), and (8) show that a successful ML method must find the right level of restriction or "openness" of the inductive bias.

We note that *the inductive bias of ML is a useful bias* and **should not be used as a negative term** (as for example, ethical, social, or statistical estimator biases which are invariably negative).

Pitfall 2.6
Using the wrong inductive bias for the ML solution to the problem at hand.

Pitfall 2.7
Ignoring the fit of the data generating procedure with the ML solution to the problem at hand.

Best Practice 2.7
Pursue ML solutions with the right inductive bias for the problem at hand.

Best Practice 2.8
Create a data generating or design procedure that matches well the requirements of the problem at hand and works with the inductive bias to achieve strong results.

ML as Geometrical Construction and Function Optimization

As will be elaborated in chapter "An Appraisal and Operating Characteristics of Major ML Methods Applicable in Healthcare and Health Science" ML methods are in some important cases cast as geometrical constructive solutions to discriminating between objects. Figure 4 below shows a highly simplified example of diagnosing cancer patients from healthy subjects on the basis of 2 gene expression values. The ML method used (SVMs in the example) casts this diagnostic problem as geometric construction of a line (in 2D space, and hyperplane in higher dimensions) so that the cancer patients are cleanly separated from health subjects (and subject to a maximum gap achieved between the two classes).

Such geometrical formulations of ML can be analytically and algebraically described and then operationalized using linear algebra and optimization mathematical tools and codes. See chapter "An Appraisal and Operating Characteristics of Major ML Methods Applicable in Healthcare and Health Science" for several examples and details on the mathematical formulations and the ensuing properties.

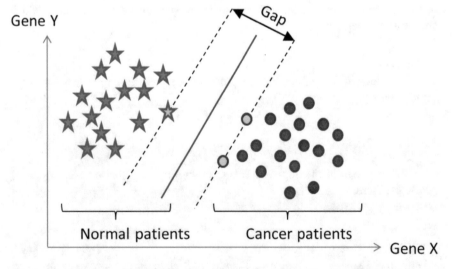

Fig. 4 *Geometrical constructive formulation of ML.* See chapter "An Appraisal and Operating Characteristics of Major ML Methods Applicable in Healthcare and Health Science" for mathematical formulation

Computational Learning Theory (COLT): PAC Learning, VC Dimension, Error Bounds

Computational Learning Theory (COLT) , formally studies under which conditions learning is feasible and provides several bounds for the generalization error depending on the classifier used, the definition of error to be minimized (e.g., number of misclassifications), and other assumptions. While theoretical results in classical statistics typically make distributional assumptions about the data (i.e., the probability distribution of the data belongs to a certain class of distributions), COLT results typically make assumptions only about the class of discriminative model considered. Notice though, that it may be the case that an optimal discriminative model never converges to the data generating function of the data.

COLT research has defined several mathematical models of learning. These are formalisms for studying the convergence of the errors of a learning method. The most widely-used formalisms are the **VC (Vapnik-Chervonenkis) and the PAC (Probabilistically Approximately Correct) analyses**. A VC or PAC analysis provides bounds on the error given a specific classifier, the size of the training set, the error on the training set, and a set of assumptions, e.g., in the case of PAC, that an optimal model is learnable by that classifier. Typical PAC bounds, for example, dictate that for a specific context (classifier, training error, etc.) the error will be larger than epsilon with probability less than delta, for some given epsilon or delta. Unlike bias variance decomposition, COLT bounds are independent of the learning task. From the large field of COLT we suggest [34–36] as accessible introductions.

The VC (Vapnik-Chervonenkis) dimension (not to be confused with the VC model of learning above) is (informally) defined as the *maximum* number of training examples that can be correctly classified by a learner *for any possible assignment of class labels*. The VC dimension of the classifier is a quantity that frequently appears in estimation bounds in a way that all else being constant, higher VC dimension leads to increased generalization error. Intuitively, a low complexity classifier has low VC dimension and vice-versa. An example of VC bound follows: if VC dimension h is smaller than l, then with probability of at least 1-n, the generalization error of a learner will be bounded by the *sum of its empirical error (i.e., in the training data) and a confidence term* defined as:

$$\sqrt{\frac{h\left(\log\frac{2l}{h}+1\right)-\log\left(n/4\right)}{l}}$$

Where $0 < n \le 1$. Notice how this error bound is independent of dimensionality of the problem [37]. The number of parameters of a classifier does not necessarily correspond to its VC dimension. In [38] (examples are given of *a classifier with a single parameter that has infinite VC dimension and classifiers with an unbounded number of parameters but with VC dimension of 1.*

Thus, a classifier with a large number of parameters (but a low VC dimension) can still have low error estimates and provide guarantees of non-over-fitting. In addition, some of these bounds are non-trivial (i.e., less than 1) even when the number of dimensions is much higher than the number of training cases.

Such results prove unequivocally that learning is possible (when using the right learning algortihms) in the situation common in modern health science and healthcare data where the number of observed variables is much higher than the number of available training sample. Many popular classical statistical predictive modeling methods in contrast break down in such situations.

The mentioned COLT results also justify the assertion that over-fitting is not equivalent to a high number of parameters. Unfortunately, many of the estimation bounds provided by COLT are not tight for the number of samples available in common practical data analysis. In addition, COLT results often drive the design of classifiers with interesting theoretical properties, robust to the curse of dimensionality, and empirically proven successful, such as Support Vector Machines (discussed in detail chapter "An Appraisal and Operating Characteristics of Major ML Methods Applicable in Healthcare and Health Science").

ML Theory of Feature Selection (FS)

Traditional ML theoretical frameworks (e.g., PAC and VC frameworks of COLT) focus on generalization error as a function of the model family used for learning, sample size and complexity of models. The theory of feature selection is a newer branch of ML that addresses the aspect of selecting the right features for modeling. It aims to guide the design and proper application of principled feature selection (as opposed to heuristic FS with unknown and suboptimal properties).

Table 8 summarizes key areas and example of results in the theory of feature selection. In the remainder we will discuss two formal feature selection frameworks (i.e., Kohavi-John and Markov Boundary) and will describe certain classes of feature selection problems that are commonly addressed.

The *standard feature selection problem*. Consider variable set V and a data distribution J over V, from which we sample data D. Let T be a variable which we wish to predict as accurately as possible by fitting models from D. The *standard feature selection problem* is typically defined as [40]:

- *Find the smallest set of variables S in V s.t. the predictive accuracy of the best classifier than can be fit for T from D, is maximized.*

Kohavi-John framework for Standard predictive feature selection problem. Kohavi and John [39] decompose the standard feature selection problem as follows:

Table 8 Summary of major topics and examples in the theory of feature selection

Topic	Notes
Filter-wrapper and embedded-explicit feature selection taxonomy	*Wrapper algorithms* conduct a heuristic search in the space of feature subsets and evaluate them using a classifier and loss function of choice. *Filters* examine the data distribution and infer desirable and undesirable features independent of classifier. *Embedded feature selection* removes undesired features as part of fitting a model. The removal may be *implicit* (.e.g. regularization where features with small coefficients may stay in the model but do not influence it much) or *explicit* (i.e., features are dropped out of the model). See [39–41] and chapter "An Appraisal and Operating Characteristics of Major ML Methods Applicable in Healthcare and Health Science" for details.
Ugly duckling and no free lunch theorems	Proofs that the choice of feature selection must be tied to a specific class of target functions, learners and loss functions. See [32, 42] and NFLT section below.
Bespoke characterization of individual FS or classifier models	This body of work examines theoretically (and tests empirically) whether specific ML algorithms and feature selectors are capable of solving specific feature selection problems (e.g., [43–45])
Kohavi-John framework of relevancy	Defines what are necessary/indispensable, or useful but redundant, or useless features in a general sense (without reference to algorithms) [39].
Markov Boundary framework of relevancy (and intersection with other forms of ML)	Defines what are necessary/indispensable, useful but redundant, and useless features in a general sense and leads to construction of specific algorithms. Also allows extensions for causality, equivalence classes, and guided experimentation [24, 41, 46, 47].

A feature X is **strongly relevant** if removal of X alone will result in performance deterioration of the Optimal Bayes Classifier using the feature. Formally:

X is strongly relevant iff: $X \not\perp T \mid \{V - X, T\}$

A feature X is **weakly relevant** if it is not strongly relevant and there exists a subset of features, S, such that the performance of the Optimal Bayes Classifier fit with S is worse than the performance using S U {X}. Formally:

X is weakly relevant iff: X is not strongly relevant and $\exists S \subseteq \{V-S,T\}$ s.t. $X \not\perp T \mid S$.

A feature is **irrelevant** if it is not strongly or weakly relevant.

The strongly relevant feature set solves the standard feature selection problem.

Intuitively, choosing the strongly relevant features provides the minimal set of features with maximum information content and thus solves the standard feature selection problem since a powerful classifier in the small sample or the Optimal Bayes Classifier in the large sample will achieve maximum predictivity. The Kohavi-John framework does not provide efficient algorihms for discovery of the strongly relevant feature set, however.

Markov Boundary framework for Standard predictive feature selection problem. Recall from the section of Bayes Networks (BNs) that a set S is the Markov Boundary of variable T (denoted as S = MB(T)), if S renders T independent on every other subset of the remaining variables, given S, and S is minimal (cannot be reduced without losing its conditional independence property). This is the MB(T) *in the probabilistic sense*. Tsamardinos and Aliferis [24] connected the Kohavi-John relevancy concepts with BNs and Markov Boundaries as follows:

In faithful distributions there is a BN representing the distribution and mapping the dependencies and independencies so that:
1. The strongly relevant features to T are the members of the MB(T).
2. Weakly relevant features are variables, not in MB(T), that have a path to T.
3. Irrelevant features are not in MB(T) and do not have a path to T.

Thus in faithful distributions, the Markov boundary MB(T) is the solution to the standard feature selection problem and algorithms that discover the Markov boundary implement the Kohavi-John definition of strong relevancy.

Local causally augmented feature selection problem and Causal Markov Boundary. In faithful distributions with causal sufficiency (see chapter "Foundations of Causal ML") there is a causal BN that is consistent with the data generating process and can be inferred from data in which: strongly relevant features = members of MB(T), and also comprise the solution to the local causally augmented feature selection problem of finding:
1. The direct causes of T.
2. The direct effects of T.
3. The direct causes of direct effects of T.

Thus in faithful distributions with causal sufficiency, the causal graphical MB(T) set is connected with the probabilistic MB(T). Inducing the probabilistic MB(T) then: 1. Solves the standard predictive feature selection problem, and 2. Solves the *local causally augmented feature selection problem* [24, 41].

Equivalency-augmented feature selection problem and Markov Boundary Equivalence Class. In faithful distributions the MB(T) exists and is unique [22]. However, in non-faithful distributions where variables or variable sets exist that have the same information for the target variable (i.e., target information equivalences exist in (*"TIE distributions"*) and we may have more than one MB(T) [46]). The number of Markov Boundaries can be exponential to the number of variables [46] and in empirical tests with real life genomic data Statnikov and Aliferis extracted tens of thousands of Markov boundaries before terminating the experiments [48].

In TIE distributions:
1. The Kohavi John definitions of relevancy break down since there are no Kohavi-John strongly relevant features any more, only weakly relevant and irrelevant ones. This is because if S1, S2 are both in the MB equivalence class {MBi(T)} then: $S1 \perp T \mid S2$ *and* $S2 \perp T \mid S1$.
2. *The 1-to-1 causal and probabilistic relationship of the probabilistic and graphical MB(T) breaks down.* A variable can be a member in some MBi(T) without having a direct causal or causal spouse relationship with T.
3. The standard predictive feature selection problem is solved by the smallest member in the equivalence class of MBi(T).
4. The *Equivalency-augmented feature selection problem* is to find the equivalence class of all probabilistic MBi(T).

Chapter "An Appraisal and Operating Characteristics of Major ML Methods Applicable in Healthcare and Health Science" provides further details of the above 3 fundamental feature selection problem classes, organizes them into a hierarchy of increasing difficulty, shows examples, and presents and contrasts practical algorithms based on their ability to solve these problems.

Theory of Algorithmic Causal Discovery and of Computational Properties of Experimental Science

The theory of causal discovery extends traditional ML theoretical frameworks that focus on generalization error, by investigating the feasibility, complexity, and other properties of causal discovery algorithms from passive observational data, of experimental interventional approaches (e.g., RCTs, biological experiments, etc.) and hybrid experimental-observational algorithmic approaches. Pearl provides a comprehensive modern theory of causality [49] and Spirtes et al., a historically influential algorithmic framework for its discovery [50]. Chapter "Foundations of Causal ML" presents an extensive introduction to the function of causal discovery algorithms from non-experimental data, and their properties under specific assumptions. Chapter "Foundations of Causal ML" also lists several algorithms used for causal discovery, including more modern and scalable ones. Chapter "An Appraisal and

Operating Characteristics of Major ML Methods Applicable in Healthcare and Health Science" as well as section of "ML Framed as AI search and the Role of Inductive Bias" of the present chapter reference theory and algorithms at the intersection of feature selection and causality. Moreover we mention here selected additional fundamental results that will round the readers' understanding of causal discovery from a theory perspective:

Eberhardt et al. showed that under assumptions: *if any number of variables are allowed to be simultaneously and independently randomized in any one experiment, then log2 (N) + 1 experiments are sufficient and in the worst case necessary to determine the causal relations among N ≥ 2 variables when no latent variables, no sample selection bias and no feedback cycles are present* [51]. Bounds are provided when experimenters can't intervene on more than K variables simultaneously. These results point to fundamental limitations of RCTs and biological experiments conducted with small number of variables manipulated at a time, and is further discussed in chapter "Lessons Learned from Historical Failures, Limitations and Successes of AI/ML In Healthcare and the Health Sciences. Enduring problems, and the role of Best Practices".

The same researchers showed that: *by **combining experimental interventions with causal algorithms** for graphical causal models under familiar assumptions of causal induction, with perfect data, N - 1 experiments suffice to determine the causal relations among N > 2 variables when each experiment randomizes at most one variable* [52]. These results require that all variables are simultaneously measured, however.

Statnikov et al. [47] showed that in TIE distributions (i.e., with multiple equivalent Markov Boundary sets with respect to the response variable T), an algorithm exists that guides experimentation combined with causal discovery from observations, so that at most k single-variable experiments are needed to learn the local causal neighborhood around T where k is the size of the union of all Markov Boundaries of T.

Mayo-Wislon showed [53] that *for any collection of variables V, there exist fundamentally different causal theories over V that cannot be distinguished unless all variables are simultaneously measured. Underdetermination can result from piecemeal measurement, regardless of the quantity and quality of the data.*

The same investigator in [54] found that *when the underlying causal truth is sufficiently complex, there is a significant possibility that a number of relevant causal facts are lost by trying to integrate the results of many observational studies in a piecemeal manner.* Specifically, he shows that as the graph gets large, if the fraction of variables that can be simultaneously measured stays the same, then the proportion of causal facts (including e.g., who mediates what relationships) that can be learned *even with experiments*, approaches 0.

Optimal Bayes Classifier

The optimal Bayes Classifier (or OBC for short) is defined by the following formula:

$$argmax_{(i)} \sum_j P\left(T = i|Mj\right) * P\left(Mj| D\right)$$

Where i indexes the values of the response variable T and j indexes models in the hypothesis space where the classifier operates. In plain language, the OBC calculates the posterior probability that a model has generated the data (i.e., it is the data generating function) given the data, for every model in the hypothesis space. It also calculates for each of the response variable's values, the probability for that value's probability given each model. The predictions are summed over all models, weighted by the probabilities of the models given the data, and the value with the higher value is the one that the classifier outputs.

Because the hypothesis space can be infinite or intractably large, the calculations involved are also intractable. Also, if we calculate the conditional probabilities using Bayes' rule we also have to deal with the problem of prior probability assignment over the model space members; in case of very biased priors, the calculated posteriors will converge slowly to the large sample correct ones. These issues place the application of the OBC outside the realm of the practical. However, it turns out that the error of the OBC is optimal in the large sample. Hence the OBC is a *valuable analysis tool* when we consider the errors of various learning algorithms by comparing them to the OBC error (as we will see in chapter "An Appraisal and Operating Characteristics of Major ML Methods Applicable in Healthcare and Health Science") [29, 32].

No Free Lunch Theorems (NFLTs)

NFLTs is a general class of theorems each one applying to optimization, search, machine learning and clustering (in the last case referred to as Ugly Duckling Theorem or UDT for short) [32, 42].

The crux of these theorems is that under a set of conditions intended to describe all possible application distributions, there is no preferred algorithm, and that by implication the right algorithm should be chosen for the right task, since there is no dominant algorithm irrespective of task. This particular interpretation is commonsensical and useful. It is also stating in different terms essentially the notion that a well-matched inductive bias to the problem at hand will led to better solutions.

This is especially important for clustering algorithms and the UDT. The UDT entails that in the absence of external information, there is no reason to consider two patterns P1 and P2 more or less similar to each other than P3. Over all possible functions associated with such patterns (and the features that define them) any grouping is as good as any other. This implies that similarity/distance functions that define the behavior of clustering algorithms *must be tailored to specific use contexts of the resulting clusters* (which in turn entails a restriction on the class of functions modeled).

The problems with common use of clustering are three-fold: (a) Per the UDT, clustering by algorithm X is as good as random clustering over all possible uses of the clusters. Unless we select or construct a distance/similarity function designed to solve the specific problem at hand, clustering will not provide any useful information. (b) There is no useful unbiased clustering. Researchers who present clustering results as "unbiased" (meaning "hypothesis free" - a practice very common in modern biology research and literature) fail to realize that any practical clustering algorithm has an inductive bias implemented as a distance function and as a grouping/ search strategy. And as we saw, in the absence of (a well-chosen) inductive bias little can be accomplished. (c) Finally *clustering should not be used, for predictive modeling* [55]. Clustering algorithms can only know something about a classification problem, e.g. of response T as T+ or T-, if and only if we design a similarity function that distinguishes between T+ and T- and embed it in the clustering algorithm. But this function is precisely a predictive modeling classifier, rendering the whole clustering-for-prediction endeavor, redundant.

In chapter "An Appraisal and Operating Characteristics of Major ML Methods Applicable in Healthcare and Health Science" we give examples of the above as well as recommendations for goal-specific clustering.

> **Pitfall 2.8**
> Probably more than other theoretical results, the NFLT for ML has the largest risk to be misunderstood and misapplied.

In summary form the NFLT for ML states that *all learning methods have on average the same performance over all possible applications,* as a mathematical consequence of 3 conditions:
(a) The algorithm performance will be judged over all theoretically possible target functions that can conceivably generate data.
(b) The prior over these target functions is uniform.
(c) Off Training Set Error (OTSE) will be used to judge performance [32, 42].

This result has been misinterpreted to suggest that we could use models that have low instead of high accuracy according to unbiased error estimators and do as well as when choosing the high accuracy models. In this (mis)interpretation random classification is as good overall as classification using sophisticated analytics and modeling. The mathematics of the NFLT derivation are impeccable but the results are problematic because of the flaws of the 3 underlying assumptions:
(a) In real life a tiny set of data generating functions among infinite ones are the ones that generate the data. *Nature is highly selective to its distributions.*
(b) The prior distribution over these data generating functions is highly skewed.
    Taken together assumptions (a) and (b) of the NFLT, are *mathematically equivalent with a label random reshuffle procedure* (see chapter "The Development Process and Lifecycle of Clinical Grade and Other Safety and Performance-Sensitive AI/ML Models"). This procedure distorts the relationship between inputs and response variable and creates a distribution of target

functions that on average have zero signal. Because on average there is no signal, this target function space is on average random and thus unpredictable. Therefore no learning algorithm exists that can do better than random and NFLT, naturally, finds and states as much. If such an algorithm existed then the distribution would be predictable and thus non-random. The NFLT for ML then just says that when there is no signal (on average), every algorithm will fail (i.e., will be as good as the random decision rule on average) and thus all algorithms will be equally useless (on average).

(c) In addition, by OTSE excluding the input patters that have been seen by the algorithm during training, an artificially low biased performance estimate is obtained for future applications. By contrast statistical theory and all branches of statistical ML and of science adopt for purposes of validation OSE (Off Sample Error) which is just a random sample from the data generating function.

In the present volume we specifically discussed at some length the dangers in over-interpreting the NFLT for ML because of published claims that the theorem somehow entails that choosing the models with best cross validation error (or best independent validation error, or best reproducibility of error) are just as good as choosing the model with worst reproducibility or independent validation error [42].

Best Practice 2.9
Cross validation and independent data validation, as well as their cousin reproducibility, are robust pillars of good science and good ML practice and are not, in reality, challenged by the NFLT.

Best Practice 2.10
Clustering should not be used for predictive modeling.

Best Practice 2.11
A very useful form of clustering is post-hoc extraction of subtypes from accurate predictor models.

Universal Function Approximators (UFAs) and Analysis of Expressive Power

UFAs are ML algorithms that *can represent any function that may have generated the data*. UAF theorems establish that certain ML algorithms have UAF capability [29].

Pitfall 2.9
If a ML algorithm cannot represent a function class, this outright shows the inability or sub- optimality of this algorithm to solve problems that depend on modeling a data generating function that is not expressible in that algorithm's modeling language.

For example, clustering (i.e., grouping objects or variables into groups according to similarity or distance criteria) does not have the expressive power to represent the causal relationships among a set of variables or entities. Thus the whole family of clustering algorithms is immediately unsuitable for learning causal relationships. Similarly, simple perceptron ANNs cannot represent non-linear decision functions and that places numerous practical modeling goals and applications outside their reach.

By contrast, Decision Trees can represent any function over discrete variables. Similarly, ANNs can represent any function (discrete or continuous) to arbitrary accuracy by a network with at least three layers [29]. BNs can represent any joint probability distribution as we show in the present chapter. AI search can be set up to operate on model languages that are sufficiently expressive to represent any function as well. Genetic Algorithms, being essentially search procedures share this property.

Pitfall 2.10
UAF theorems should not be over-interpreted. While it is comforting that e.g., algorithm A can represent *any function in the function family* F (i.e., the model space and corresponding inductive bias are expressive enough), learning also requires effective (space and time-tractable, sample efficient, non-overfitting etc.) model search and evaluation in that space.

For example, Decision Trees (DTs) do not have practical procedures to search and learn every function in the model space expressible as a DT, since practical (tractable) DT induction involves highly incomplete search of the hypothesis space. Similarly, ANNs can represent any function however, the number of units needed and the time needed for training are intractable and the procedures used to search in the space of ANN parameters are not guaranteed to find the right parameter values.

Generative vs. Discriminative Models

Generative models are typically considered the ones that can model the full joint distribution of the variables in an application domain. Discriminative models, by contrast, are ones that only model a decision function that is sufficient to problem of interest in that domain. Consider as example the SVM hyperplane model in Fig. 4. This model solves the diagnostic problem stated perfectly without modeling the probability distribution of the variables involved.

The optimal choice of generative vs. discriminative model entirely depends on the application domain. For example, for general predictive modeling as well as other pattern recognition such as text categorization, the use of discriminative models confers practical advantages and better performing models than generative models, in many datasets. For causal modeling, simulation, natural language understanding, density estimation, or language generation, generative models are necessary or advantageous. We also wish to clarify a **terminology confusion** (especially in non-technical literature) between generative modeling at large vs "Generative AI". The latter refers to a small number of specific classes of algorithms that generate data (e.g., Generative Adversarial Networks, Large Language Models) with established or unknown properties. Generative modeling on the other hand includes all methods that model the data generating distribution and in typical usage the term refers to algorithms that have guarantees for correct modeling of the data generating distribution (e.g., BNs, Logistic Regression, Density estimator algorithms).

Best Practice 2.12
The choice of generative vs. discriminative modeling affects quality of modeling results and has to be carefully tied to the problem domain characteristics. All else being equal discriminative models confer efficiency (computational and sample) advantages.

Bias-Variance Decomposition of Model Error (BVDE)

The concept of BVDE is one that originates from statistical machine learning but has broad applicability across ML and all of data science. It is pervasively useful, yet not as widely known as it deserves among non-technical audiences, so we will present it here in some detail. A detailed treatment can be found in [56]. While the whole idea of BVDE is that other than noise in measurements (which is intrinsic in the data and independent of modeling decisions) or inherent stochasticity of the data generating function (which is intrinsic in the data generating process and independent of modeling decisions), the remaining modeling error of any ML (or for that matter any statistical or quantitative data science) model has two components: a component due to the inductive bias mismatch with the problem vs. the data at hand; and another component due to sample variation in small sample settings.

In the terminology of BVDE, the error due to inductive bias mismatch is referred to as "bias" with "high bias" indicating a severe mismatch, toward simplicity (aka small complexity, or small capacity) of the model language (and related search and fitting procedures) with respect to the data generating function. The error due to sampling variation is referred to as "variance" with variance increasing as sample size decreases. More precisely, the bias is the error (in the sample limit, relative to the data generating function) of the best possible model that can be fitted within the class of models considered. The variance is the error of the best model (in the small sample, within the class of models considered) relative to the error of the best model that can be fitted in the large sample within the class of models considered. The bias then is a function of the learner used and the data generating function; the variance, for a fixed data generating function, is a function of the learner and the sample size.

Implications for modeling: When the modeling bias is fixed one can reduce total model error by increasing the sample size (reduce variance), and when the sample is fixed one can reduce total error by optimizing the bias. More importantly, when both sources of error are under analyst control, BVDE explains that there is an ideal point of balance of error due to bias and error due to variance. The optimal error will be found when these two sources of error are balanced for a particular modeling setting. Moreover high bias models have smaller variance (i.e., are more stable in low samples) but on average over many samples will approximate the target function worse. Low bias models have higher variance, hence are unstable in small samples but on average(!) approximate the target function better. We now delve into BVDE with a concrete example.

Figure 5 depicts a two-dimensional data set, based on one input variable x, plotted along the horizontal axis and response y along the vertical. The black points

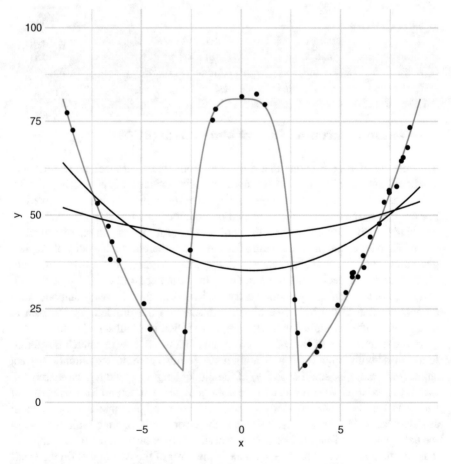

Fig. 5 Illustration of the bias-variance tradeoff. The x-axis shows models' input values and the y-axis is the response. The training data observations are the black points, and the true data generating function is depicted in blue. The two black curves represent two models

represent the observed data points and the blue line f depicts the true generating function, which in this example is:

$$f(x) = \begin{cases} x^2 & when\, x < -3 \\ 81 - x^2 & when -3 \le x \le 3 \\ x^2 & when\, x > 3 \end{cases}$$

The black lines represent quadratic models fit to random samples from this data.

Consider the expected generalization error from this procedure when predicting the point at (say) $x = 0$. The error has three components. First, the observed dependent variable can differ from the true value of the generating function, that is measurement **noise**. Visually, noise is the difference between the black points and the blue line. The second component, **variance**, is the variability of the model due to the specific sample, which is visually represented by the spread of the predictions from the different models (black lines) at x = 0. In this example, with only two models, this ranges from 35 to 45. Finally, the third component is **bias**, which is the difference between the expectation of the prediction (expectation is taken over the different models built on the different samples) and the true value of the dependent variable (the blue line at x = 0). In this example, the expectation of the prediction from different models appears to be approximately 40, while the true value is 81.

The generalization error expressed as MSE at any x can be written as:

$$\mathbf{E}\left[\left(y - \hat{f}(x)\right)^2\right] = \mathbf{E}\left[\left(y - f(x)\right)^2\right] + \mathbf{E}\left[\left(f - E\hat{f}(x)\right)^2\right] + \mathbf{E}\left[\left(\hat{f}(x) - E\hat{f}(x)\right)^2\right]$$

The three terms correspond to noise, bias and variance of $\hat{f}$.

Figure 6 shows the bias (orange), variance (blue) and mean squared error (MSE) (gray) of models of increasing complexity on a test set. Model complexity is controlled by the degree of x the model is allowed to use and how far the optimizer can optimize the training MSE. Complexity increases from left to right. As the model complexity increases, variance increases while bias decreases. For improved readability, bias, variance and MSE are scaled to the same range in the figure. MSE is thus a weighted sum of bias (squared) and variance. The optimal fit is achieved where MSE is minimal (in the middle of the complexity range). Lower complexity leads to underfitting, which is characterized by lower variance and higher bias, while increased complexity leads to overfitting, which is characterized by higher variance and lower bias (compared to the bias and variance at the optimal complexity).

These concepts are critical in helping analysts create models with maximum predictivity (see chapter "Overfitting, Underfitting and General Model Overconfidence and Under-Performance Pitfalls and Best Practices in Machine Learning and AI").

Essential Concepts of Mathematical Statistics Applicable to ML

Mathematical Statistics is the subfield of Statistics that studies the theoretical foundations of statistics. At the same time, many of the concepts and tools of

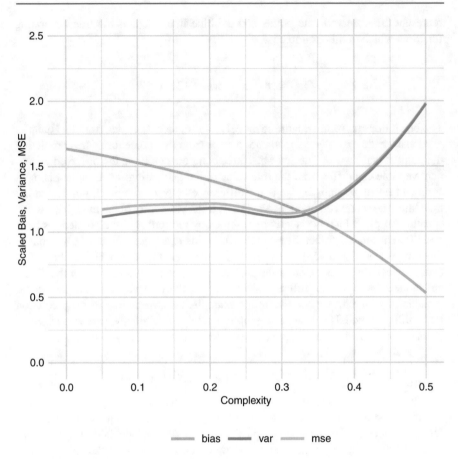

Fig. 6 The relationship between the bias-variance components and complexity in the example (fixed noise is considered). The horizontal axis is complexity (of quadratic models) and the vertical axis is the various bias/variance components scaled to the same range. Orange corresponds to bias, blue to variance and gray is total MSE

mathematical statistics are useful across data science broadly and for ML more specifically. Table 9 provides examples of important areas and analytical tools developed within this field that have value for understanding, advancing, and practicing ML [58].

Techniques and results from mathematical statistics (and its applications) are present throughput the chapters of the present volume.

Table 9 Key concepts and areas of mathematical statistics useful for ML

Area	Subject matter and importance for ML
Special probability distributions and density functions	E.g., Uniform, Bernoulli, Binomial, Hypergeometric, Poisson, Multinomial, etc. distributions; Uniform, Normal, Exponential, Chi-Square, Beta, etc. density functions Uses: • Design and analysis of modeling methods by tailoring them to data characteristics • Instrumental in inference by describing sampling distributions • Also valuable in understanding model errors and other aspects of modeling
Sampling distributions	E.g., Distribution of the mean, Chi-square, t distribution, F distribution Uses: • Measuring the uncertainty of parameters of models, model predictions • Hypothesis testing of whether a sample or model statistic value comes by sampling from a null hypothesis distribution • Estimating the uncertainty of model parameters, structure, and predictions
Estimation and estimators	E.g., Properties of estimators such as unbiasedness, efficiency, consistency, robustness Uses: • Estimators for model construction • Estimators for model error and other properties • Embedding estimators in model selection and construction
Hypothesis testing	E.g., Losses and risk for testing statistical hypotheses. Neyman-Pearson Lemma. Power functions of tests. Control of false positives and false negatives in statistical hypothesis testing decisions Uses: • Deciding whether model properties and function are due to random sampling variation or reliable and generalizable • Deciding on minimum data sample size needed for analysis • Reducing errors when large number of hypotheses are tested when data mining and conducting hypothesis-free discovery

Conclusions

The successful design of problem-solving AI/ML models and systems can be guided by and evaluated according to well specified technical properties. Systems that lack properties are pre-scientific and used heuristically, whereas systems with well-established properties and guarantees provide more solid ground for reliably solving health science and healthcare problems. The nature of the properties listed matches well the practical applications of AI/ML. Properties disconnected from practical implications are not subject of study in the present volume.

AI has both symbolic and non-symbolic methods as well as hybrid variants. Foundational methods in the symbolic category are logics and logic-based systems such as rule based systems, semantic networks, planning systems, NLP parsers and certain AI programming languages. In the non-symbolic category, ML, probabilistic, connectionist, decision-theoretic formalisms, systems and languages dominate.

Among health AI methods capable of reasoning with uncertainty, Bayes Nets and Decision Analysis stand out for their ability to address a variety of uses cases and problem classes.

A major distinction is between shallow systems that essentially are equivalent to function relating outputs to inputs (e.g., most of ML predictive modeling), and systems with rich ontologies and elaborate models of the physical world in the application domain. Non-symbolic AI systems tend to fall in the former category, whereas symbolic ones, in the latter.

The framework of AI search is especially powerful both as a problem-solving technology but also as an analytical tool that helps us understand and architect successful methods and systems. AI search cuts across the symbolic vs. non-symbolic, shallow vs. rich, and the data-driven (Ml) vs. knowledge driven distinctions.

ML has solid and extensive theoretical foundations that include: Computational Learning Theory, ML as AI search, ML as geometrical construction and function optimization, COLT (PAC learning, VC dimension), Theory of feature selection, Theory of causal discovery, Optimal Bayes Classifier, No Free Lunch Theorems, Universal Function Approximation, Generative vs. Discriminative models; Bias-Variance Decomposition of error, and an extensive set of tools borrowed from the field of mathematical statistics.

Key Concepts and Messages Chapter "Foundations and Properties of AI/ML Systems"
- The critical importance of knowing or deriving the properties of AI/ML models and systems.
- The main technical properties of AI/ML systems.
- Tractable vs. intractable problems and computer solutions to them.
- The various forms of Logic-based (symbolic) AI.
- Non-symbolic AI, reasoning under uncertainty and its primary formalisms.
- AI search.
- Foundations of Machine Learning Theory

Pitfalls and Best Practices Chapter "Foundations and Properties of AI/ML Systems"

Pitfall 2.1. From a rigorous science point of view an AI/ML algorithm, program or system with intractable complexity does not constitute a viable solution to the corresponding problem.

Pitfall 2.2. Parallelization cannot make an intractable problem, algorithm or program practical.

Pitfall 2.3. Moore's law improvements to computing power cannot make an intractable problem algorithm or hard program practical.

Pitfall 2.4. Believing that heuristic systems can give "something for nothing" and that have capabilities that surpass those of formal systems. In reality heuristic systems are pre-scientific or in early development stages.

Pitfall 2.5 in Decision Analysis (DA) and Maximum Expected Utility (MEU)-based reasoning

1. Errors in the estimation of probabilities for various events.
2. Errors in eliciting utility estimates in a way that captures patients' true preferences (including using the care providers' utilities rather than the patients').
3. The structure or complexity of the problem setting defies analyst's ability to completely/accurately describe it.
4. Developing a DA for one population and applying in another with different structure of the problem, different probabilities for action-dependent and action-independent events, or with different preferences.

Pitfall 2.6. Using the wrong inductive bias for the ML solution to the problem at hand.

Pitfall 2.7. Ignoring the fit of the data generating procedure with the ML solution to the problem at hand.

Pitfall 2.8. Probably more than other theoretical results, the NFLT for ML has the largest risk to be misunderstood and misapplied.

Pitfall 2.9. If a ML algorithm cannot represent a function class, this outright shows the inability or sub- optimality of this algorithm to solve problems that depend on modeling a data generating function that is not expressible in that algorithm's modeling language.

Pitfall 2.10. UAF theorems should not be over-interpreted. While it is comforting that e.g., algorithm A can represent *any function in the function family* F (i.e., the model space and corresponding inductive bias are expressive enough), learning also requires effective (space and time-tractable, sample efficient, non-overfitting etc.) model search and evaluation in that space.

Best Practices Discussed in Chapter "Foundations and Properties of AI/ML Systems"

Best Practice 2.1. Pursue development of AI/ML algorithm, program or systems that have tractable complexity.

Best Practice 2.2. Do not rely on parallelization to make intractable problems tractable. Pursue tractable algorithms and factor in the tractability analysis any parallelization.

Best Practice 2.3. Do not rely on Moore's law improvements to make an intractable problem algorithm or hard program practical. Pursue tractable algorithms and factor in the tractability analysis any gains from Moore's law.

Best Practice 2.4. When faced with intractable problems, consider using strategies for mitigating the computational intractability by trading off with less important characteristics of the desired solution.

Best Practice 2.5. As much as possible, use models and systems with formal and established properties (theoretical + empirical). Work within the maturation process starting from systems with unknown behaviors and no guarantees, to systems with guaranteed properties.

Best Practice 2.6. Decision Analysis (DA) and Maximum Expected Utility (MEU)-based reasoning

1. Ensure that the structure of the problem setting is sufficiently/accurately described by the DA tree. Omit known or obvious irrelevant factors.
2. Elicit utility estimates in a way that captures patients' true preferences using established utility-elicitation methods.
3. Accurately estimate probabilities of action-dependent events and action-independent events.
4. In most conditions, and whenever applicable, data-driven approaches should be preferred to subjective probability estimates. Use probability-consistent statistical or ML algorithms to estimate the probabilities.
5. Ensure that the decision analysis is applied to the correct population.
6. Conduct sensitivity analyses that reveal how much the estimated optimal decision is influenced by uncertainty in the specification of the model.
7. Whenever possible, produce credible intervals/posterior probability distributions for the utility expectations of decisions.

Best Practice 2.7. Pursue ML solutions with the right inductive bias for the problem at hand.

Best Practice 2.8. Create a data generating or design procedure that matches well the requirements of the problem at hand and works with the inductive bias to achieve strong results.

Best Practice 2.9. Cross validation and independent data validation, as well as their cousin reproducibility, are robust pillars of good science and good ML practice and are not in reality challenged by the NFLT.

Best Practice 2.10. Clustering should not be used for predictive modeling.

Best Practice 2.11. A very useful form of clustering is post-hoc extraction of subtypes from accurate predictor models.

Best Practice 2.12. The choice of generative vs. discriminative modeling affects quality of modeling results and has to be carefully tied to the problem domain characteristics. All else being equal discriminative models confer efficiency (computational and sample) advantages.

Discussion Topics and Assignments, Chapter "Foundations and Properties of AI/ML Systems"

1. Revisit questions (10–13) of chapter "Artificial Intelligence (AI) and Machine Learning (ML) for Healthcare and Health Sciences: the Need for Best Practices Enabling Trust in AI and ML" from the perspective of which properties of the proposed systems are known.

2. Use Table 3 to classify the proposed systems in questions (10–13) of chapter "Artificial Intelligence (AI) and Machine Learning (ML) for Healthcare and Health Sciences: the Need for Best Practices Enabling Trust in AI and ML"

3. Which of the following are heuristic systems (and in what category of the classification of Table 3 in this chapter:
   (a) INTERNIST-I
   (b) MYCIN
   (c) QMR-BN
   (d) A classical regression model for which we do not know if data is normally distributed. Compare to a classical regression model for which we know that data is not normally distributed.
   (e) A Large Language Model implementing an EHR "ChatBot" tool answering queries about the patients' medical history.
   (f) IBM Watson Health

4. Based on your findings in question 3, how would you go about next steps toward putting these systems into practice from a perspective of accuracy and safety?
5. Discuss: are BNs deep or shallow representations?
6. Consider a population with age distribution as in the table below:

Age →	0–10	11–20	21–30	31–40	41–50	51–60	61–70	>70
% →	20	20	10	10	10	15	10	5

   (a) What would be a good 2-way clustering (grouping) of individuals in this population?
   (b) For a pediatrician: what would be a good 2-way clustering (grouping) of individuals in this population?
   (c) For a gerontologist: what would be a good 2-way clustering (grouping) of individuals in this population?
   (d) For an obstetrician: what would be a good 2-way clustering (grouping) of individuals in this population?
   (e) What can you conclude about the value of a priori clustering without any reference to use of the produced groups?

7. Occam's Razor is the epistemological principle that says that given two explanations that fit the data equally well, we should choose the simplest one. Analyze this proposition from a BVDE viewpoint.

References

1. Russell SJ. Artificial intelligence a modern approach. Pearson Education, Inc; 2010.
2. Cook S. The complexity of theorem proving procedures. In: Proceedings of the Third Annual ACM Symposium on Theory of Computing; 1971. p. 151–8.
3. Karp RM. Reducibility among combinatorial problems. In: Miller RE, Thatcher JW, editors. Complexity of computer computations. New York: Plenum; 1972. p. 85–103.
4. Miller RA. A history of the INTERNIST-1 and quick medical reference (QMR) computer-assisted diagnosis projects, with lessons learned. Yearb Med Inform. 2010;19(01):121–36.
5. Aliferis CF, Miller RA. On the heuristic nature of medical decision-support systems. Methods Inf Med. 1995;34(1–2):5–14.
6. Rich, E. and Knight, K., Artificial Intelligence. 1991. Ed.
7. Nilsson NJ. Principles of artificial intelligence. Springer Science & Business Media; 1982.
8. Buchanan BG, Shortliffe EH. Rule based expert systems: the mycin experiments of the Stanford heuristic programming project (the Addison-Wesley series in artificial intelligence). Addison-Wesley Longman Publishing Co., Inc.; 1984.
9. Buchanan BG, Feigenbaum EA. DENDRAL and meta-DENDRAL: their applications dimension. Artif Intell. 1978;11(1–2):5–24.
10. Clocksin WF, Mellish CS. Programming in PROLOG. Springer Science & Business Media; 2003.
11. Hripcsak G, Clayton P, Pryor T, Haug P, Wigertz O, Van der Lei J. The Arden syntax for medical logic modules. In proceedings. Symposium on computer applications in medical care; 1990. p. 200–4.
12. Machado CM, Rebholz-Schuhmann D, Freitas AT, Couto FM. The semantic web in translational medicine: current applications and future directions. Brief Bioinform. 2015;16(1):89–103.
13. McCray A. The UMLS semantic network. In: Proceedings. Symposium on computer applications in medical care; 1989, November. p. 503–7.

14. Shmulevich I, Dougherty ER. Probabilistic Boolean networks: the modeling and control of gene regulatory networks. Society for Industrial and Applied Mathematics; 2010.
15. Noy NF, Shah NH, Whetzel PL, Dai B, Dorf M, Griffith N, Jonquet C, Rubin DL, Storey MA, Chute CG, Musen MA. BioPortal: ontologies and integrated data resources at the click of a mouse. Nucleic Acids Res. 2009;37(suppl_2):W170–3.
16. Torres A, Nieto JJ. Fuzzy logic in medicine and bioinformatics. J Biomed Biotechnol. 2006;2006:1–7.
17. McDermott D, Doyle J. Non-monotonic logic I. Artif Intell. 1980;13(1–2):41–72.
18. Haddawy P. A logic of time, chance, and action for representing plans. Artif Intell. 1996;80(2):243–308.
19. Langlotz CP, Fagan LM, Tu SW, Sikic BI, Shortliffe EH. A therapy planning architecture that combines decision theory and artificial intelligence techniques. Comput Biomed Res. 1987;20(3):279–303.
20. Pauker SG, Kassirer JP. Decision analysis. In: Medical uses of statistics. CRC Press; 2019. p. 159–79.
21. Sox HC, Blatt MA, Marton KI, Higgins MC. Medical decision making. ACP Press; 2007.
22. Pearl J. Probabilistic reasoning in intelligent systems: networks of plausible inference. Morgan kaufmann; 1988.
23. Neapolitan RE. Probabilistic reasoning in expert systems: theory and algorithms. John Wiley & Sons, Inc; 1990.
24. Tsamardinos I, Aliferis CF. Towards principled feature selection: relevancy, filters and wrappers. In: International workshop on artificial intelligence and statistics. PMLR; 2003. p. 300–7.
25. Cooper GF. The computational complexity of probabilistic inference using Bayesian belief networks. Artif Intell. 1990;42(2–3):393–405.
26. Boyd S, Boyd SP, Vandenberghe L. Convex optimization. Cambridge university press; 2004.
27. Rutenbar RA. Simulated annealing algorithms: an overview. IEEE Circuit Devices Magazine. 1989;5(1):19–26.
28. Katoch S, Chauhan SS, Kumar V. A review on genetic algorithm: past, present, and future. Multimed Tools Appl. 2021;80:8091–126.
29. Mitchell TM. Machine learning, vol. 1, No. 9. New York: McGraw-hill; 1997.
30. Dorigo M, Birattari M, Stutzle T. Ant colony optimization. IEEE Comput Intell Mag. 2006;1(4):28–39.
31. Audi R. Epistemology: a contemporary introduction to the theory of knowledge. Routledge; 2010.
32. Duda RO, Hart PE, Stork DG. Pattern classification. New York: John Wiley & Sons. Inc.; 2000. p. 5.
33. Weiss SM, Kulikowski CA. Computer systems that learn: classification and prediction methods from statistics, neural nets, machine learning, and expert systems. Morgan Kaufmann Publishers Inc.; 1991.
34. Anthony M, Biggs NL. Computational learning theory: an introduction. Cambridge University Press; 1992.
35. Kearns MJ, Vazirani U. An introduction to computational learning theory. MIT press; 1994.
36. Langford J. Tutorial on practical prediction theory for classification. J Mach Learn Res. 2005;6(Mar):273–306.
37. Schölkopf C, Burges JC, Smola AJ. Advances in kernel methods—support vector learning. Cambridge, MA: MIT Press; 1999.
38. Herbrich R. Learning kernel classifiers: theory and algorithms, (2002). Cambridge: MA, USA MIT Press; 2002.
39. Kohavi R, John GH. Wrappers for feature subset selection. Artif Intell. 1997;97(1-2):273–324. Prediction (Vol. 2, pp. 1-758). New York: springer.
40. Guyon I, Elisseeff A. An introduction to variable and feature selection. J Mach Learn Res. 2003;3(Mar):1157–82.
41. Guyon I, Aliferis C. Causal feature selection. In: Computational methods of feature selection. Chapman and Hall/CRC; 2007. p. 79–102.

42. Wolpert DH. What the no free lunch theorems really mean; how to improve search algorithms, vol. 7. Santa Fe Institute; 2012. p. 1–13.
43. Hardin D, Tsamardinos I, Aliferis CF. A theoretical characterization of linear SVM-based feature selection. In: Proceedings of the twenty-first international conference on machine learning; 2004. p. 48.
44. Statnikov A, Hardin D, Aliferis C. Using SVM weight-based methods to identify causally relevant and non-causally relevant variables. Signs. 2006;1(4):474–84.
45. Zou H. The adaptive lasso and its oracle properties. J Am Stat Assoc. 2006;101(476):1418–29.
46. Statnikov A, Lemeir J, Aliferis CF. Algorithms for discovery of multiple Markov boundaries. J Mach Learn Res. 2013;14(1):499–566.
47. Statnikov A, Ma S, Henaff M, Lytkin N, Efstathiadis E, Peskin ER, Aliferis CF. Ultra-scalable and efficient methods for hybrid observational and experimental local causal pathway discovery. J Mach Learn Res. 2015;16(1):3219–67.
48. Statnikov A, Aliferis CF. Analysis and computational dissection of molecular signature multiplicity. PLoS Comput Biol. 2010;6(5):e1000790.
49. Pearl J. Causality. Cambridge university press; 2009.
50. Spirtes P, Glymour CN, Scheines R, Heckerman D. Causation, prediction, and search. MIT press; 2000.
51. Eberhardt F, Glymour C, Scheines R. On the number of experiments sufficient and in the worst case necessary to identify all causal relations among N variables. In: Bacchus F, Jaakkola T, editors. Proceedings of the 21st conference on uncertainty in artificial intelligence (UAI); 2005. p. 178–84.
52. Eberhardt F, Glymour C, Scheines R. N-1 experiments suffice to determine the causal relations among N variables. In: Holmes D, Jain L, editors. Innovations in machine learning, theory and applications series: studies in fuzziness and soft computing, vol. 194. Springer-Verlag; 2006. See also Technical Report CMU-PHIL-161 (2005).
53. Mayo-Wilson C. The problem of piecemeal induction. Philos Sci. 2011;78(5):864–74.
54. Mayo-Wilson C. The Limits of Piecemeal Causal Inference. Br J Philos Sci. 2014;65(2):213–49.
55. Dupuy A, Simon RM. Critical review of published microarray studies for cancer outcome and guidelines on statistical analysis and reporting. J Natl Cancer Inst. 2007;99(2):147–57.
56. Hastie T, Tibshirani R, Friedman JH, Friedman JH. The elements of statistical learning: data mining, inference, and prediction, vol. 2. New York: springer; 2009. p. 1–758.
57. Von Neumann J. and Morgenstern O. 2007. Theory of games and economic behavior. In: Theory of games and economic behavior. Princeton university press. Original in Wald, A., 1947. Theory of games and economic behavior.
58. Wackerly D. Mendenhall W. and Scheaffer, RL. 2014. Mathematical statistics with applications. Cengage Learning.

An Appraisal and Operating Characteristics of Major ML Methods Applicable in Healthcare and Health Science

Gyorgy Simon and Constantin Aliferis

Abstract

This chapter provides an outline of most major biomedical ML methods in a manner suitable for both readers who have not delved into ML before, and readers who may already know about some or all of these methods. The former will find here a useful introduction and review. The latter will find additional insights as we critically revisit the key concepts and add summary guidance on whether and when each technique is applicable (or not) in healthcare and health science problem solving. Toward that end, for each technique, we introduce a "Method Label", akin to a drug label, which provides distilled information about the techniques at a glance. The method labels present the primary and secondary uses of each technique, provide context of use, describe the principles of operation, and summarize important theoretical and empirical properties.

Keywords

Method label · Predictive modeling · Feature selection · Exploratory analysis

G. Simon · C. Aliferis (✉)
Institute for Health Informatics, University of Minnesota, Minneapolis, MN, USA
e-mail: constantinaibestpractices@gmail.com

G. J. Simon, C. Aliferis (eds.), *Artificial Intelligence and Machine Learning in Health Care and Medical Sciences*, Health Informatics,
https://doi.org/10.1007/978-3-031-39355-6_3

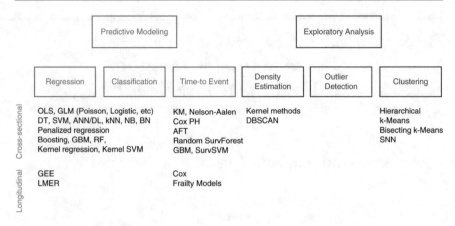

Fig. 1 Lay of the land of biomedical ML. Tabular categorization of major machine learning methods based on modeling task (columns) and predictor type (rows). See the text for abbreviations and details

Introduction

A vast number of machine learning techniques has been proposed for solving a rich set of problems. As we discussed in the Introduction, many of the clinical problems fall into a few categories, some of which are more heavily researched than others. We call these categories **analytic tasks** and, in this chapter, we consider six tasks, which fall into two broader categories: predictive modeling and exploratory analysis.

Figure 1 depicts the lay of the land for predictive and exploratory analysis tabulating the most common techniques. We will address causal modeling separately in chapter "Foundations of Causal ML".

In **predictive modeling**, the goal is to assign values to one or more variables, called outcomes (aka response, or dependent variables), using the known values of other variables (aka predictor variables, independent variables, or features). Somewhat abusing ordinary language, "predictive" in the context of "ML predictive modeling", does not necessarily imply forecasting future events. Any pattern recognition falls under the category including future forecasting, prognosis, diagnosis and recognizing past events (e.g., retroactive diagnosis). Also, "predictor" and "predictor variable" are often used interchangeably although from context it may be clear whether a predictor refers to a variable (feature) or a full model.

In contrast, **exploratory analysis** aims to model the relationships among many variables, none of which is designated as an outcome or predictor variable. For example, predicting patients' risk of mortality (outcome) based on current diagnoses and laboratory results (predictor variables) is a predictive modeling task because variables corresponding to mortality are designated as outcome, variables corresponding to diagnoses and laboratory results are designated as predictors, and we predict the future unknown value of an outcome using known values of the predictor variables. Conversely, understanding a patient population in terms of common comorbidities that co-occur with diabetes is an exploratory analysis task, because there is no particular outcome to predict.

Predictive Modeling Tasks

Within predictive modeling, we distinguish between several tasks based on the outcome type. In the rest of this chapter, we focus on three of them: classification, regression and time-to-event modeling. These are the outcome types and corresponding tasks most frequently encountered in biomedical ML.

Continuous outcomes. Continuous outcomes are measured on a continuous scale. Continuous variables can be **ratio**s (variables that do not have a well-defined 0 point) or **interval**s (which have a well-defined 0 point). For example, lengths are intervals and a length of zero indicates that the object does not have length. Whether we measure length in inches, centimeters, or miles, 0 length is the same. Conversely, temperature is a ratio, because 0 °F or 0 °C does not mean that the object has no temperature. Furthermore, 0 temperature depends on the scale we use: 0°F and 0°C do not designate the same temperature.

Another relevant distinction from a modeling perspective is the distribution of the continuous variable. Commonly used distributions include Gaussian, Poisson, exponential, negative binomial, etc. Prediction problems with a continuous outcome are referred to as **regression** problems.

Categorical variables take a value from a set of finite distinct values. For example, color (red, amber, green), grade (A, B, C, F), or risk category (low, medium, high) are categorical variables. **Binary** (also known as **binomial**) variables are categorical variables that have exactly two levels (they can take one of two values); while **multinomial** variables have more than two levels.

Categorical variables with multiple levels can be further classified as nominal or ordinal variables. In case of **ordinal** variables, the levels are ordered (e.g. good, better, best), while for **nominal** variables, the levels are not ordered (e.g. colors). Prediction problems with categorical outcomes are referred to as **classification** problems. If the outcome is binary, we have **binary classification**; if the outcome is multinomial, we have **multi-class classification** (aka n-ary or polychotomous classification).

Time-to-event outcomes. The measurement of interest is the time between a particular time point (known as **index date or index time**) and an event of interest. The quintessential example is survival, where the measure of interest is the time between the start of the study (index date) and death (the event of interest). The predictive modeling task that predicts time-to-event outcomes is referred to as *time-to-event modeling* or **survival analysis** (when the outcome is survival).

Sequence outcomes. Sequences are ordered sets of observations and when the outcome of interest is a sequence, we have a **sequence prediction** problem. Examples include genomic sequence (ordered set of nucleotides) prediction, *text synthesis or translation* (predicting an ordered set of words), or **trajectory mining** (predicting future sequences of e.g., disease states).

Structured outcomes. The outcome of the predictive model can also be a complex structure such as a graph or the actual structure of an entity (e.g. protein structure prediction). For techniques to discover *causal* structure, see the chapter "Foundations of Causal ML".

Exploratory Analysis Tasks

Density estimation. The goal of density estimation (also encompassing discrete probability functions) is to infer the (often multi-dimensional) probability distribution underlying observed data. The simplest form of density estimation is unidimensional scaled histograms. For example, one might be interested in describing the probability distribution of blood glucose in a population. Density estimation can also be performed on multi-dimensional data and techniques exist for both low and high-dimensional data. Density estimation has several natural uses, including discovery of multiple modes of data, clustering and outlier detection.

Clustering. Clustering creates a grouping of the observations in a data set such that observations that belong to the same group (cluster) are more similar to each other than to observations that belong to a different group. Clustering can be used, for example, for subpopulation discovery, where well-separated groups of observations can represent subpopulations at different states of health or groups of patients with different disease etiology.

Clustering can be achieved based on many principles, one of which is based on data density. In that case, clusters are high-density regions in the data, separated from each other by low-density regions.

Outlier detection. Outliers are observations that are dissimilar to most other observations. Outliers may either fall into low-density regions, or they may behave very differently from model-based expectations (model-based outlier). For example, in a hospitalized population, outliers can be patients who have an unusually long hospital length of stay (LoS), say, above 9 days; or alternatively, they may have a LoS of less than 9 days, but unusually long for the disease that they got admitted for. The first example is clearly patients who fall into a low-density region (very few patients in a patient population stay hospitalized for more than 9 days), while the latter patients are in a low-density region among patients who got admitted with the same disease.

Temporal Characteristics of the Data

A further categorization of methods is based on the temporal characteristics of the data. It is very common for healthcare data to be temporal, thus several AI/ML as well as classical statistical techniques have been developed specifically to take advantage of various temporal characteristics.

Cross-sectional data. This data captures the state of a sample from a population at a specific point in time. The state information often contains temporal information about the past implicitly in the definitions of variables - but not explicitly modeled. The implicit temporal information is typically abstracted to different time scales and granularities. The vast majority of the machine learning techniques expect cross-sectional data.

Cross-sectional data can also be used for predictive modeling in which the outcome occurs at a future time relative to the the index date of the predictor variables. For example, when modeling the 7-year risk of diabetes, the outcome, diabetes, must occur or not within 7 years, but the predictor variables they have been evaluated at a particular point in time (the index date) and changes to them over the 7 years are not of interest.

Longitudinal data. Measurements for a patient population is taken repeatedly over time. Measurements are not necessarily taken at the same time for everyone and not all measurements are taken each time. Routinely collected clinical test data, falls into this category. At most encounters with the health system, some aspect of a patient's health is measured and recorded. Most patients have more than one encounter and at each encounter, different measurements (e.g., lab tests) can be taken.

Time-series data. Similarly to longitudinal data, in time series data, several measurements are taken over time, but unlike longitudinal data, time-series data focuses on a single sampling unit. If we aim to model the glucose trajectory of a single individual over a long period of time, then we are solving a time-series modeling problem; if we aim to model the glucose control of a population of patients over time, then we have a longitudinal data modeling problem.

Figure 1 tabulates some of the techniques from this chapter. The columns correspond to the various analytic tasks, while the rows correspond to the temporal characteristics of the methods. Naturally, several methods can be used for multiple tasks (with appropriate modifications) and with data sets having multiple temporal characteristics. We either put the methods into the categories where they are most prominent (e.g. SVM into classification), or into shared categories (e.g. many techniques that are used for classification can also be used for regression).

Method Labels

In the following sections, we are going to describe the major machine learning methods in terms of their primary use, additional secondary uses, key operating principles, operating characteristics and properties, and provide a context for their use that helps assess their appropriateness for different modeling tasks. We also mention when and why the use of a method is not recommended.

For each method (or family of methods), we are going to present highly digested and operationally-oriented information in what we call a *Method Label*. A Method Label is similar to a drug label, presenting the most vital information about a method at-a-glance.

Format of method labels	
Main Use	This entry describes the main purpose of the model. What kind of tasks can it solve? Within that task, are there specific problems that this method is best suited for? For example, linear regression solves predictive analytic problems with continuous outcomes.
Context of use	In practice, when is this method used? This can be a subset of the intended use or a superset of the intended use. For example, ordinary least square regression is designed for Gaussian outcomes, but is often used for a wide range of continuous outcomes.
Secondary use	This entry describes potential situations where the method can also be used. This may not be the primary intended use of the methods; or this may not be the model that is most appropriate for the use case. For example, SVM can be used for regression, although its primary use is classification.
Pitfalls	**Pitfall 3.1.4.1.** This entry lists negative consequences of using this method under certain conditions. For example, SVM when used for causal problems, leads to wrong causal effect estimates.
Principle of operation	A short description of how the method works. For example, linear regression is approximating a regression using maximum likelihood estimates of the regression parameters.
Theoretical properties and Empirical evidence	This entry describes any known theoretical properties the method may have and the assumptions linked to them, as well as empirical evidence for the method performance.
Best practices	**Best practice 3.1.4.1.** This entry provides prescriptive practice recommendations about when and how to use or not the method.
References	Key literature related to the above.

Readers that cannot delve into technical details can still benefit greatly by the information provided in the Method Labels.

Chapter Layout

We begin (in section "Foundational Methods") with describing the foundational methods for predictive modeling of cross-sectional data. Section "Ensemble Methods" is devoted to ensemble methods which use foundational techniques from "Foundational Methods" to addresses issues related to model stability and performance; and section "Regularization" is devoted to regularization, which addresses high dimensionality, or more broadly, constrains the model complexity. The subsequent three sections address feature selection and dimensionality reduction, time-to-event outcomes, and longitudinal data, respectively. We close the chapter with a brief mention of a few more methods that the reader should be aware of. As the reader will observe we weave classical and modern statistical methods with mainstream ML methods since this reflects modern ML practice and there are significant mathematical, conceptual and computational commonalities between the fields.

Foundational Methods

Foundational methods in the chapter will refer to first-order methods that:
(a) Are of high theoretical and/or practical value on their own, or
(b) Are of high theoretical and/or practical value in conjunction with other higher-order methods.

Ordinary Least Square (OLS) Regression

OLS regression was invented by Sir Francis Galton in 1875 as he described the relationship of the weight of sweet pea seeds and the weight of the seeds from their mother plants. This experiment also gave rise to the correlation coefficient: Karl Pearson, Galton's biographer, developed the mathematical formulation for the Pearson correlation coefficient in 1896 [1].

Given a matrix X of predictor variables (independent variables) and outcome (dependent) variable y, the ordinary linear regression model is

$$y \sim Normal\left(X\beta, \sigma^2\right)$$

where β is a vector of **coefficients**. The outcome is assumed to be normally distributed with mean $X\beta$ and variance σ^2. In other words, the outcome has a deterministic component $X_i\beta$ for the ith observation, and a random component, which is Gaussian noise with mean 0 and variance σ^2. The objective is to find the coefficient vector β, which makes the observations y the most likely, that is to maximize the Gaussian log likelihood

$$\ell\left(\beta\right) = \text{const} - \Sigma_i \frac{\left(y_i - X_i\beta\right)^2}{2\sigma^2},$$

where i iterates over the observations. The coefficient vector β that maximizes the log likelihood is the same vector that minimizes the least square error $\Sigma_i(y_i - X_i\beta)^2$, hence the name Ordinary Least Square regression.

As a least square estimator, OLS is "BLUE" (best linear unbiased estimator) [2]. The coefficient estimates are normally distributed, allowing for a Wald-type test for their significance. The least square problem is convex, thus when a solution exists, it is the global solution.

Assumptions. The assumptions follow from the model: (1) for all observations, the noise component has constant variance (σ^2). Having uniform variance across the observations is referred to as homoscedasticity. (2) The errors of the observations are independent. (3) Observations are identically distributed. (4) The mean of the observations is a linear combination of the predictor variables. The effect of the predictors on the outcome is thus linear and additive.

Expressive capability. OLS, in its native form, is only able to express linear and additive effects. By explicitly including transformations of the original variables, the linear effect assumption can be relaxed. Explicitly including interactions terms of the predictor variables can relax the additivity assumption. OLS has no ability to automatically discover interactions or nonlinearities, so these need be hand-crafted by the data scientist.

Dependent and outcome variable types. Ordinary linear regression assumes that the observations (rows of X) are independently sampled and thus it is more appropriate for dependent variables that can be represented as regular tabular data and a continuous outcome variable that follows a Gaussian distribution.

Sample size requirement. Ordinary linear regression is not appropriate for high-dimensional data, where the number of predictor variables is similar to the number of observations or exceeds them. As a rule of thumb, 10 observations per predictor variable is recommended. This is one of the least sample-intensive techniques, thus when the number of observations is low and the number of predictor variables is low, ordinary linear regression may be the most appropriate modeling technique.

Main use and its context. OLS is intended to solve regression problems with Gaussian outcomes. Guarantees about the solution hold true only for this use case.

Intepretability. For a covariate (predictor variables) X_i with coefficient β_i, every unit increase in X_i is associated with an increase of β_i in the outcome, if all other predictor variables are fixed.

As a result, OLS is highly interpretable, and also fit for use with causal estimation once the causal structure is known (see chapter "Foundations of Causal ML").

We recommend using OLS as a "default" algorithm in low dimensional data unless a generalized linear regression model with a different linkage is more appropriate (see GLM). Building an OLS model, even if its performance is expected to be inferior to more advanced regression techniques, is recommended, because the cost of building an OLS model is minimal, the model is highly interpretable, and it can reveal data problems, biases, design problems and potentially other issues. As we will see the potentially higher predictive performance from other methods needs to be evaluated from the perspective of trading interpretability for performance, and in some applications, higher interpretability can balance out some performance deficit.

Optimality. The coefficients found by maximizing the likelihood are unbiased. Also the log likelihood function is convex, thus the global maximum is easy to find.

Method label: ordinary least squares regression	
Main Use	• Regression problems • Continuous, preferably Gaussian outcomes • Cross-sectional data
Context of use	• First choice, most common regression method in low dimensional data • When highly interpretable model is required
Secondary use	• May achieve acceptable performance for some non-Gaussian continuous outcomes
Pitfalls	**Pitfall 3.2.1.1.** In high-dimensional data, coefficients may be biased or cannot be estimated **Pitfall 3.2.1.2.** OLS is negatively affected by high collinearity
Principle of operation	• Least square estimation (or equivalently, maximizing the Gaussian log likelihood)

Method label: ordinary least squares regression	
Theoretical properties and empirical evidence	• OLS is a consistent, efficient estimator of the coefficients • The coefficients are asymptotically normally distributed • Minimizing the least squares is a convex optimization problem. If a solution exists, numerical solvers will find the global solution. • Highly interpretable and causally consistent models • Vast literature in health sciences documenting successful applications • Because it is a simple model, risk of overfitting in low sample is lower than complex models • By the same token it can fail to capture highly non-linear data generating functions
Best practices	**Best practice 3.2.1.1.** Unless a generalized linear model is more appropriate, OLS is a good default technique. **Best practice 3.2.1.2.** Building an OLS, even if it is known not to produce optimal predictive performance, can reveal data problems, biases, etc.
References	• Numerous good textbooks describe OLS regression. Below is one example. Tabachnick & Fidell. Using Multivariate Statistics. Pearson, 2019

Generalized Linear Models (GLM)

Generalized linear models (GLM) were first introduced by Nelder and Wedderburn in 1972. GLM was born out of the desire to model a broader range of outcome types than Gaussian outcomes and was enabled by advancements in statistical computing [3]. The defining characteristic of GLMs is that the data generating functions is not linear and a **link function** linearizes the relationship between an outcome and the predictor variables, where the outcome is distributed by an exponential family distribution. A fully specified GLM has the following components:

1. The distribution of y
2. A linear predictor $\eta = X\beta$
3. The link function $g(\mu)$ that links the expectation of $E(y) = \mu$ to the linear predictor: $\eta = g(\mu)$; or equivalently, $\mu = g^{-1}(\eta)$.

As an example, let us consider logistic regression, linear regression for outcomes with binomial distribution. The distribution of y_i is Bernoulli with parameter η_i, and the link function is

$$\text{logit}(y_i) = \log\frac{\Pr(y_i)}{1 - \Pr(y_i)} = X_i\beta.$$

The objective is to find the coefficient vector β that maximizes the likelihood of observing y, which in case of the logistic regression is the binomial likelihood.

GLMs are frequently used for modeling outcomes that follow other exponential family distributions, including multinomial, Poisson, and negative binomial [4].

Expressive capability. The link function does not change the model's expressive capability; the relationship between η and the predictor variables is linear, the only difference from OLS is that the linear predictor is transformed through the link function so that GLM can model specific families of non-linear functions.

Dependent and outcome variable types. GLM are best suited for cross-sectional data (with independent and identically distributed observations), but the outcome types have to be distributed in accordance with the link function.

Prediction task. GLM can solve classification problems (logistic and multinomial link) and regression problems where the continuous outcome can be distributed following any of the exponential family distributions.

Theoretical properties. The GLM is a maximum likelihood estimator for the exponential family distributions. Some instances of GLM, such as an overdispersed GLM, does not correspond to an actual exponential family distribution. In such cases, a variance function can be specified and GLM becomes a quasi-likelihood estimator [5]. Both estimators (maximum likelihood and quasi-likelihood) are consistent and efficient. They yield coefficient estimates that are normally distributed and thus the Wald test can be used for testing their significance. Both the likelihood and quasi-likelihood are convex, thus when a solution exists, it is a global solution and solvers can typically find it efficiently.

Method label: generalized linear models	
Main Use	• Predictive modeling with outcomes that follow a distribution from the exponential family (i.e., relationship of outcome and predictor variables can be non-linear) • Most common applications are classification (logistic regression), estimating count outcomes (Poisson regression) and exponential outcomes • Cross-sectional data
Context of use	• First-pass/comparator classifier in low dimensional problems with limited need for input interaction modeling • Highly interpretable model
Secondary use	• Applicable also to deviations from the exponential family, most typically where the sample variance is higher than theoretically expected under the corresponding exponential family distribution (over-dispersion) • Logistic regression may offer acceptable performance in classification problems, where the linear additive assumption is mildly violated
Pitfalls	**Pitfall 3.2.2.1.** In high-dimensional data, coefficients may not be estimatable **Pitfall 3.2.2.2.** Tendency to overfit in the presence of high collinearity
Principle of operation	• When the outcome follows an exponential family distribution, GLM is a maximum likelihood estimator • When the outcome does not follow an exponential family distribution, GLM can be a quasi-likelihood estimator

Method label: generalized linear models	
Theoretical properties and empirical evidence	• GLM provides consistent, efficient estimates of coefficients • The coefficients are asymptotically normally distributed • Minimizing the likelihood or quasi-likelihood is a convex optimization problem. If a solution exists, numerical solvers will find the global solution efficiently. • Highly interpretable models • GLM can have high performance even when the assumptions are violated. Chapter "Lessons Learned from Historical Failures, Limitations and Successes of AI/ML in Healthcare and the Health Sciences. Enduring Problems, and the Role of BPs" discusses comparisons between logistic regression and more modern ML techniques
Best practices	**Best practice 3.2.2.1.** Use GLM as first pass, or main comparator classifier **Best practice 3.2.2.2.** Building a GLM, even if it is known not to produce optimal predictive performance, can reveal data problems, biases, etc.
References	• Walter Stroup. Generalized Mixed Linear Models, CRC Press, 2003 • P. McCullagh, JA Nelder. Generalized Linear Models, CRC Press, 1989

Ordinal Regression Models

There are two main strategies for modeling ordinal outcomes using GLMs. The first one is cumulative logits and the second one is proportional odds [6].

Consider an ordinal outcome variable with J levels, $1 < 2 < \ldots < J$. Under the **cumulative logits** strategy, J-1 logistic regression models are fit. The jth model is a classifier distinguishing $y \leq j$ verus $y > j$. Under the **proportional odds** strategy, again, J-1 models are built, but these models share all coefficients except for the intercept. The jth model is

$$\text{logit}(y \leq j) = \alpha_j + X\beta,$$

where α_j is the level-specific intercept and β are the slopes shared across the J-1 models.

Notice, that the cumulative logits model can use any binary component classifier; while the proportional odds GLM is a special case of multi-task learning.

Key reference: Agresti A. Categorical Data Anlaysis, second edition. Chapter 7.2. Wiley Interscience, 2002.

Artificial Neural Networks (ANNs)

For main milestones in the development of ANNs see chapter "Lessons Learned from Historical Failures, Limitations and Successes of AI/ML in Healthcare and the Health Sciences. Enduring Problems, and the Role of BPs". In this section, we focus on the general form of ANNs for cross-sectional data. Image and language model applications are discussed in Chapters "Considerations for Specialized Health AI and ML Modelling and Applications: NLP" and "Considerations for Specialized Health AI and ML Modelling and Applications: Imaging—Through the perspective of Dermatology".

Artificial neural networks (or neural networks, NN, for short) can be thought of as regression models stacked on top of each other, and each regression model is thus called a **layer**. Each of these layers are *multiple regression models*, meaning they have potentially multivariate inputs as well as multivariate outputs. The outputs from each layer, are transformed using nonlinear functions, called the **activation functions**, and then passed to the subsequent layer as their input. The final layer (aka the output layer) provides the network's output(s).

Figure 2 shows an example NN with two hidden (aka encoding) and an output layer. The output from this network is

$$\hat{y} = f_3\left(b_3 + W_3 f_2\left(b_2 + W_2 f_1\left(b_1 + W_1 X\right)\right)\right),$$

where the $f_i(\cdot)$ is the activation function, b_i are the biases (or bias vectors) and W_i are the weights (weight matrices) of connections coming into layer i. In layer i, the input is multiplied by W_i, the biases b_i are added and the result is passed through the activation function $f_i()$, producing the output from layer i. The input to the first layer is X, and the output from the topmost layer, the third layer in this example, is the outcome $\hat{y}$. Common activation functions include the sigmoid function (logit function), ReLU (rectified linear unit), and softmax.

Expressive power. NNs are universal function approximators, they can express any relationship between the predictors and the output without distributional restrictions. This includes non-linear relationships as well as interactions.

Predictor and outcome types. The basic form of NNs introduced here is most appropriate for cross-sectional data without any special structure. However, when the data has special structure, corresponding network architectures have been proposed for many of them. For example, Convolutional Neural Networks (CNN) [7] have been proposed for image data, Recurrent Neural Networks (RNN) [8] and Long Short-Term Memory (LSTM) [9] for sequence data, Transformers [10] for language models, Graph Neural Networks [11] for graph data, etc. We discuss some of these architectures in chapters "Considerations for Specialized Health AI and ML Modelling and

Fig. 2 An example NN with three layers

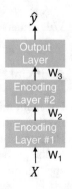

Applications: NLP" and "Considerations for Specialized Health AI and ML Modelling and Applications: Imaging—Through the perspective of Dermatology".

Sample size. The sample size required for NNs can be very large. The deeper the network (the more layers it has), the more parameters it has and the larger the required sample size. Many practical applications of deep learning use millions of parameters. Although the traditional statistical rule of the thumb, that the number of required observations is approximately 10 times the number of parameters, does not hold for deep learning—they can operate on data with fewer samples—the required sample size is still very large.

The largest GPT-3 language model, which has 175 billion parameters, was trained on 45 TB of text data taking 355 GPU-years [12]. Certain structures (most notably convolution) and regularization can alleviate the sample size requirement to some degree.

Interpretability. The key to NNs is to automatically transform the original data space into a new representation that is more amenable to the predictive modeling task at hand. A side effect of this automatic transformation is that the meaning of the original space is lost and the meaning of the resulting variables are often unknown. Thus, NNs are considered black-box (uninterpretable). One way to interpret them is by "local approximation" of the NN using an interpretable model, such as a multi-variate regression model, fitted over input-output pairs sampled from the NN model.

NNs in Less Data-Rich Environments

Two significant shortcomings of NN is the sample size requirement and the training cost. Several strategies exist aiming to alleviate these shortcomings.

Transfer learning. Training neural networks, especially highly performant, large networks, is very expensive not only in terms of CPU time but also in terms of required sample. Large pre-trained *generic* models (so-called *foundational* models) are available in many application areas, including language processing and computer vision. These generic models transform the input space (say written English text) into a representation that is more amenable to carrying out language modeling tasks than the original representation. To solve a *specific* language-related task, such as distinguishing patients with and without dementia, a foundational language model (with many pre-trained encoding layers) can become extended by a task-specific layer so that the new model performs the actual classification task. Only the task-specific layer needs to be trained.

Incorporating domain knowledge. Another avenue to reduce training cost is to incorporate domain knowledge as follows: when synthetic data for a domain can be generated, NNs can be pre-trained using synthetic data to learn a representation of the application. Then this pre-trained model can be further refined using real data to solve specific problems in that domain. Beside pre-training, several other methods exist, which include augmenting the input space of a NN with output from physical models (e.g. climate models) or ascribing meaning to hidden nodes and constraining the connections among such hidden nodes based on what is possible in the real world. See [13] for a survey of incorporating domain knowledge into machine learning models.

Method label: artificial neural networks (including deep learning)	
Main Use	• Solving predictive modeling problems. Classification, including classification with very many classes, is most common, but it can also solve regression and time-to-event problems • In data-rich environments, ANNs can produce highly performant models
Context of use	• ANNs are recommended when sample size is very high and a very complex function needs be modeled • Neural networks work best for specific applications, with network architectures specifically designed for that application. Such applications include image analysis, text and audio modeling, text synthesis, etc.
Secondary use	• Modeling distributions using GANs and auto-encoder variants
Pitfalls	**Pitfall 3.2.4.1.** ANNs can fail when sample size is not large
	Pitfall 3.2.4.2. ANNs are innately black-box models. Their use in applications where transparency is important may be problematic
	Pitfall 3.2.4.3. ANNs do not reduce the number of features needed for prediction and this may be an important requirement in many biomedical problems. However, using strong feature selectors before running the ANN modeling may be a good combination for some problems (but can be detrimental in others)
	Pitfall 3.2.4.4. Training cost is high due to (a) large cost of training a single model, and (b) large number of models that need be trained to explore the immense hyperparameter space
	Pitfall 3.2.4.5. ANNs do not have either formal or empirically competitive causal structure discovery capabilities
	Pitfall 3.2.4.6. Even when a causal structure is known, estimating causal effects with ANNs leads to biased results because the ANN is not designed to condition on known confounders and may introduce other effect estimation biases (e.g., due to blocking mediator paths and opening M-structure paths)
Principle of operation	• Minimizing a penalized loss • Linear combinations of inputs transformed through a non-linear activation function layer-by-layer yields a non-linear model
Theoretical properties and empirical evidence	• ANNs with at least two hidden (encoding) layer and unbounded number of units, can be universal function approximators • NNs are most commonly solved using gradient optimizers. Because the objective function of NNs can be arbitrarily complex with multiple local optima, the optimizers may fail to reach the globally optimal solution • In several biomedical problems deep learning and other ANN learners have exhibited superior accuracy (especially in image recognition). There is also significant evidence that in several clinical domains not involving images they do not outperform vanilla logistic regression (see Chapter "Lessons Learned from Historical Failures, Limitations and Successes of AI/ML in Healthcare and the Health Sciences. Enduring Problems, and the Role of BPs")
Best practices	**Best practice 3.2.4.1.** Deep learning is most recommended for predictive modeling in large imaging datasets. Other domains may also be good candidates. In all cases additional (alternative and comparator) methods should be explored at this time within the same error estimation protocols (see chapter "The Development Process and Lifecycle of Clinical Grade and Other Safety and Performance-Sensitive AI/ML Models")
	Best practice 3.2.4.2. At this time ANNs are not suitable for causal discovery and modeling. Formal causal methods should be preferred (chapter "Foundations of Causal ML")
	Best practice 3.2.4.3. ANNs are not suitable for problems where explainability and transparency are required, or when large reduction of the feature space is important to model application

Method label: artificial neural networks (including deep learning)

References	• Goodfellow I, Bengio Y, Courville A. Deep Learning. MIT Press, 2016 • Discussion and references in Chapter "Lessons Learned from Historical Failures, Limitations and Successes of AI/ML in Healthcare and the Health Sciences. Enduring Problems, and the Role of BPs"

Support Vector Machines

Support Vector Machines (SVMs) is a family of methods that can be used for classification, regression, outlier detection, clustering, feature selection and a special form of learning called transductive learning [14–16]. SVMs use two key principles (1) regularization and (2) kernel projection.

SVM regularization: SVMs cast the classification or regression problems as a non-linear quadratic optimization problem where the solution to predictive modeling is formed as a "*data fit loss + parameter penalty*" mathematical objective function. Intuitively and as depicted in Fig. 3, each object used for training and subsequent model application is represented as a vector of measurements in a space of relevant dimensions (variable inputs). We will discuss regularization in the general (non-SVM) setting in section "Regularization".

Binary classification is formulated in SVMs as a geometrical problem of finding a hyperplane (i.e., the generalization of a straight line from 2 dimensions to n dimensions) such that all the instances above the hyperplane belong to one class and all subjects below the hyperplane to the other. Translating this geometrical problem into

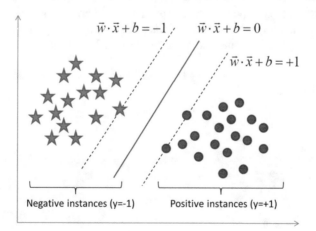

Fig. 3 SVMs and the classification problem as geometrical separation. In the top panel, a geometrical representation of a 2-class predictive modeling (classification problem) with 2 input dimensions (x_1, x_2) is depicted. Each subject is represented by a dot (i.e., a 2-dimensional vector). Blue dots are negative instances and red dots are positive ones. The line that separates negatives from positives—while maximizing the distance between classes—is the solution to the SVM problem. The instances at the border of each class are the "support vectors". In the figure we also see the mathematical expression of the classifier hyperplane and its instantiation for the three support vecotrs of the example. Such problems are easily solved by modern software

linear algebra constraints is a straightforward algebraic exercise. Every variable has a weight and collectively these weights determine the hyperplane decision function.

To ensure a model with good generalization performance and resistance to over fitting, the SVM learning procedure requires two elements: (a) That the hyperplane must be such that the number of misclassified instances is minimized (the "data fit loss" part of the objective function to be minimized). (b) A generalization-enforcing constraint, the so-called "**regularizer**", that is the total sum of squared weights of all variables, must also be minimized. Specifically, the regularizer must be minimized subject to the locations and labels of training data fed into the algorithm. This is an instance of **quadratic program** non-linear optimization function that can be solved exactly and very fast.

$$Minimize \ \frac{1}{2}\sum_{i=1}^{n} w_i^2 \ \text{subject to} \ \ y_i\left(\vec{w}\vec{x}_i + b\right) - 1 \geq 0 \quad \text{for } i = 1, \dots, N$$

A "soft margin" formulation of the learning problem in SVMs allows for handling noisy data (and to some degree non-linearities). The primary method for modeling non-linear decision functions is **kernel projection** which works pictorially as follows (Fig. 4).

In a non-linearly separable problem, there is no straight line (hyperplane) that accurately separates the two classes. The SVM (and other kernel techniques) use a mapping function that transforms the original variables (x_1, x_2 in Fig. 4) into SVM-constructed features, such that there exists a straight line (hyperplane) that separates the data in the new space. Once the solution is found in the mapped space, it is reverse-transformed to the original input variable space. Once projected back to the original input space the solution is a non-linear decision surface. Because the mapping function is very expensive to compute, special kernel functions are used that allow solving the SVM optimization *without incurring the expense of calculating the full mapping*. In mathematical terms the above take the following form:

$$f(x) = sign\left(\vec{w}\vec{x} + b\right)$$

$$\vec{w} = \sum_{i=1}^{N} \alpha_i y_i \vec{x}_i.$$

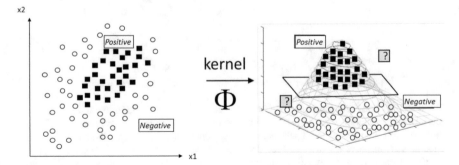

Fig. 4 Non-linearly separable classification by mapping from an original space (x_1, x_2) to a different space (with commonly higher number of dimensions) by using kernel functions

When data is mapped into higher-dimensional features space $\Phi(\vec{x})$,

$$f(x) = sign\left(\vec{w}\Phi(\vec{x}) + b\right)$$

$$\vec{w} = \sum_{i=1}^{N} \alpha_i y_i \Phi\left(\vec{x_i}\right)$$

Combining them into a classifier yields

$$f(x) = sign\left(\sum_{i=1}^{N} \alpha_i y_i \Phi\left(\vec{x_i}\right) \circ \Phi(\vec{x}) + b\right) = sign\left(\sum_{i=1}^{N} \alpha_i y_i K\left(\vec{x_i}, \vec{x}\right) + b\right).$$

The above computations are extremely quick to execute and are solved effectively allowing the SVM to explore an astronomical-size space of non-linear interaction effects in quadratic running time and without over-fitting. Let's demonstrate the remarkable computational and sample efficiency that the kernel projection affords using an example where we will compare the number of parameters that need to be estimated and the sample size needed for a relatively simple non-linear SVM with polynomial kernel degrees of 3 or 5 and number of variables to be modeled ranging from 2 to 100. We will compare with the sample needed and interactions effects that need be constructed and estimated by the corresponding regression model under a conservative requirement of 5 sample instances per parameter.

As can be seen from Table 1. (adapted from [15] for a dataset with 100 variables with up to fifth degree polynomial interaction effects, classical regression would need >96 million parameters to be explicitly constructed and > 482 million sample size in order to estimate the model's parameters. By comparison the SVM algorithm explores the same space in time quadratic to the number of variables (i.e., in practice in seconds in a regular personal computer). Moreover, the SVM generalization error is independent of the number of variables and is bounded by a function of the number of support vectors which is smaller or equal to the available sample size (see chapter "Foundations and Properties of AI/ML Systems" for more details).

One way to think of the effects of regularization is that by forcing weights to be as small as possible, all variables that *are not relevant or are superfluous* to the predictive modeling will tend to have zero or near zero weights and are effectively "filtered" out of the model. Equivalently, the minimization of weights entails that the separation between classes is geometrically maximized and statistical machine learning theory

Table 1 Comparison of non-linear SVM vs classical regression in terms of number of parameters. N denotes the (often very small) sample size available in practice

Number of variables	Polynomial degree	Number of parameters in the SVM model	Number of parameters in the Regression model	Required sample by Regression
2	3	≤N	10	50
10	3		286	1430
10	5		3003	15,015
100	3		176,851	884,255
100	5		96,560,646	482,803,230

shows that this often leads to more generalizable models. In yet another view, regularization entails that the target function is smooth, in the sense that small differences in the input variables result in small changes to the response variable's values.

Additional aspects of SVMs include: **primary and dual formulations** of the learning problem (suitable for low dimensionality/high sample, or high dimensionality/small sample situations respectively), **using only dot product representations of the data**, **Structural Risk Minimization** (i.e., the model complexity classes are neatly organized in embedding classes so that model selection can be orderly and efficient), and **known bounds of error**. These bounds are not dependent on the number of input variables but only on the support vectors (which are at most equal to the sample size N) thus demonstrating the power of SVMs to self-regulate their complexity and avoid overfitting (see also chapter "Overfitting, Underfitting and General Model Overconfidence and Under-Performance Pitfalls and Best Practices in Machine Learning and AI" for comprehensive discussion of overfitting and underfitting). SVM **scores can be converted to probabilities** in a post-hoc manner and can also be used to **perform feature selection for other classifiers.** While SVMs output scores and not probabilities, these scores can be converted to calibrated probabilities [15].

Method label: support vector machines	
Main Use	• Solving classification and feature selection problems • SVMs can produce highly performant models in low sample size/large dimensionality settings • Dominant performance in certain domains (e.g., gene expression and other omics and multi-modal based classifiers, text classification)
Context of use	• SVMs are suitable for clinical data, omic data, text and other unstructured data as well as combinations • Especially suited to non-linear, noisy and small sample data. • Can be combined with other classifiers and feature selectors to form strong analysis stacks and protocols • Are very fast to train and to run model inferences
Secondary use	• Applicable, but not as first choice, to regression, clustering, and outlier detection
Pitfalls	**Pitfall 3.2.5.1.** SVMs are unsuitable for causal discovery. The features they select are not interpretable causally. SVM variable weights are not causally valid even if true causal features only are included in the model **Pitfall 3.2.5.2.** Linear SVMs are easily interpretable. Non-linear SVMs require additional steps for explanation and are innately "black box" models **Pitfall 3.2.5.3.** Error bounds are loose and typically cannot be used to guide model selection
Principle of operation	• Maximum margin (gap) classifiers with hard or soft margins. • Regularization • Quadratic Programming formulation of learning problem guarantees optimal solution in tractable time • Kernel projection enables fast exploration of immense spaces of non-linearities • Structured risk minimization ensures that kernel hyper-parameters relate monotonically to error

Method label: support vector machines	
Theoretical properties and empirical evidence	• Can model practically any function • Known error bounds • Extremely sample and computationally efficient • Overfitting resistant • Best of class performance in several domains
Best practices	**Best practice 3.2.5.1.** Primary choice for omics, text classification, and combined clinical/molecular/text tasks
	Best practice 3.2.5.2. Secondary choice for feature selection (with Markov boundary methods being first choice). In very small sample situations where Markov boundary methods may suffer, SVM feature selection can be first choice
	Best practice 3.2.5.3. SVM weights features or models should not be interpreted causally
	Best practice 3.2.5.4. Explain SVMs by converting them to interpretable models via meta-learning or other approaches; and convert scores to probabilities when needed
References	• Statnikov A, Aliferis CF, Hardin DP, Guyon I. A gentle introduction to support vector machines. In: Biomedicine: Theory and methods (Vol. 1). World scientific. 2011 • Statnikov,A, Aliferis, CF, Hardin DP, Guyon I. A gentle introduction to support vector machines.In: Biomedicine: Case studies and benchmarks (Vol. 2). World scientific. 2012 • Vapnik V. the nature of statistical learning theory. SpringerScience & Business Media. 2013 • Aphinyanaphongs, Y., Tsamardinos, I., Statnikov, A., Hardin, D. and Aliferis, C.F., 2005. Text categorization models for high-quality article retrieval in internal medicine. Journal of the American medical informatics association, 12(2), pp.207–216 • Statnikov, A., Aliferis, C.F., Tsamardinos, I., Hardin, D. and levy, S., 2005. A comprehensive evaluation of multicategory classification methods for microarray gene expression cancer diagnosis. *Bioinformatics, 21*(5), pp.631–643

Naïve Bayesian Classifier (NBC) and Bayesian Networks (BNs)

BNs and the theoretical Optimal Bayes Classifier (OBC) are covered in the AI reasoning under uncertainty, and in the machine leaning theory sections of chapter "Foundations and Properties of AI/ML Systems". Causal BNs are instrumental for causal discovery and modeling. They are covered in Chapter "Foundations of Causal ML". The Markov Boundary feature selection methods have their origins in BN theory and are covered in the previous chapters and in feature selection section "Feature Selection and Dimensionality Reduction" of the present chapter. We thus defined here the Naïve Bayes (NB) classifier and then provide a unified method label that spans NB and BN classification techniques.

Naïve Bayes (NB)

NB is a highly restricted simplification of the complete (brute force) application of Bayes' Theorem in classification.

For an observation vector x_i and corresponding outcome y_i, which takes values from one of the values c_1, c_2, ..., c_m, the predicted probability that the outcome has value c_j can be computed through the Bayes formula

$$\Pr\left(y_i = c_j \mid x_i\right) = \frac{\Pr\left(x_i \mid y_i = c_j\right)\Pr\left(y_i = c_j\right)}{\Pr\left(x_i\right)}.$$

where $\Pr(x_i) = \sum_j \Pr(x_i \mid y_i = c_j) \Pr(y_i = c_j)$. Suppose we constructed a probability table for $\Pr(x_i \mid y_i)$, for binary x_i it would be a table of size exponential to the number of predictor variables. This would also lead to difficulties in estimating the large sample probabilities from a small sample dataset, because the dataset size would have to be large enough to contain sufficient number of observations to estimate every single x_i combination, however low the probability. To reduce this burden, Naïve Bayes classifier makes the assumption that the predictor variables are conditionally independent of each other given the outcome value. This simplifies the computation of $\Pr(x_i \mid y_i)$ to

$$\Pr\left(x_i \mid y_i\right) = \prod_k \Pr\left(x_{ik} \mid y_i\right)$$

where x_{ik} is the kth element (component) of the vector x_i. Under the Naïve Bayes assumption, we only need to estimate $\Pr(x_{ik} \mid y_i)$ for each each variable x_k, which reduces the sample size and compute time required for the estimation from exponential to linear in the number of variables.

The problem with NB is that by adopting unrealistic assumptions of conditional independence, it introduces serious errors in distributions where features are not independent given the target class.

Also, if we allow outcomes to not be mutually exclusive (e.g. a patient may have serval diseases simultaneously), then we need to incorporate $2^{|m|}$ values in the outcome variable which exponentially increases (to the number m of outcome values, e.g., diagnostic categories) the number of probabilities that need be estimated and stored. Hence it is common to see the added NB assumption of mutually exclusive and exhaustive values of the target variable. Of course in medical domains this assumption is very commonly violated as well.

In summary, the problems with brute force Bayes is that of intractability, and of high error in the estimates of joint instantiation (because invariably the real-life sample size is never enough to estimate an exponential number of parameters). The problems with NB is that assumptions rarely hold in numerous biomedical domains.

In early years of AI/ML and before the advent of BNs (that can decompose the joint distribution and store only the smallest number of probabilities needed to accurately represent it), NB was used widely. All modern benchmarks suggest however that NB is no longer a competitive classifier (unless we can tolerate large departures from predictive optimality in order to save storage space). Finally, it is worth noting the work of [17] that show that under specific target functions and loss functions, NB can perform well even though its nominal assumptions are violated. These types of distributions are rare in biomedicine however, and better alternatives exist.

Method label: Naïve Bayes (NB), Bayesian Networks (BNs), causal BNs (CBNs) and Markov Boundary methods	
Main Use	• Classification, causal structure discovery, feature selection
Context of use	• Classification under a range of sufficient assumptions that guarantee asymptotic correctness: Naïve Bayes (NB) have highly restrictive assumptions, while BNs (see chapter "Foundations and Properties of AI/ML Systems") have no restrictions on functions and distributions they can model
	• Flexible classification (chapter "Foundations and Properties of AI/ML Systems") where at model deployment time the inputs can be any subset of variables and the output can also be any subset of variables (while the rest are unobserved)
	• Causal structure discovery (under specific broad assumptions—chapter "Foundations of Causal ML")
	• Causal effect estimation (under specific broad assumptions—chapter "Foundations of Causal ML")
	• Modeling equivalence classes of full or local models (see chapter "Foundations of Causal ML" and "Foundations and Properties of AI/ML Systems")
	• Closely related to Markov boundary feature selection algorithms (see section on "Feature Selection and Dimensionality Reduction")
Secondary use	• Optimal Bayes classifier (OBC) (see chapter "Foundations and Properties of AI/ML Systems"): can be used for theoretical analysis of optimality of the large-sample error of any classifier
	• NB is often used as a minimum baseline comparator in benchmark studies
	• Modeling the full joint distribution of data with BNs (e.g., for simulation or re-simulation purposes)
	• Guiding experiments with hybrid causal discovery and active experimentation
Pitfalls	**Pitfall 3.2.6.1.** Using NB simply because it is computationally fast and has small storage requirements without paying attention to whether data properties match assumptions may lead to high error
	Pitfall 3.2.6.2. Not every probabilistic graphical model is a BN (see chapter "Foundations and Properties of AI/ML Systems")
	Pitfall 3.2.6.3. Not every BN is causal and not every BN learning algorithm guarantees valid causal discovery
	Pitfall 3.2.6.4. Bad or uninformed assignment of priors may lead Bayesian algorithms astray
	Pitfall 3.2.6.5. Discovery algorithms for BNs and CBNs vary widely in output quality and efficiency
	Pitfall 3.2.6.6. BNs and CBNs properties hold in the large sample. In small samples results may be suboptimal
	Pitfall 3.2.6.7. Approximating OBC with Bayesian model averaging with a small number of models, maybe far from the theoretically ideal OBC performance
	Pitfall 3.2.6.8. BN predictive inference with unconstrained models is computationally intractable in the worst case although average case algorithms exist with good performance chapter "Lessons Learned from Historical Failures, Limitations and Successes of AI/ML in Healthcare and the Health Sciences. Enduring Problems, and the Role of BPs")
	Pitfall 3.2.6.9. Discrete BNs are better developed in practice than continuous-function BNs

Method label: Naïve Bayes (NB), Bayesian Networks (BNs), causal BNs (CBNs) and Markov Boundary methods	
Principle of operation	• Application of Bayes' theorem combined with various assumptions about the data, heuristic model search procedures, and algorithms designed to infer from data the most likely model that generated it or estimate model-averaged predictions over a set of models • Causal discovery in addition relies on distributional assumptions such as the causal Markov condition (CMC), the faithfulness condition (FC) and causal sufficiency (CS) • Newer algorithms can discover local or partial models, and overcome violations of CS and FC and worst case complexity
Theoretical properties and empirical evidence	• All Bayesian classifiers have well understood properties ensuring valid predictions, reliable causal structure discovery and unbiased causal effect estimation when the assumptions hold • Closely tied to Markov boundary and causal feature selection • CBNs are the backbone of learning causal models in a sound and scalable manner (see chapter "Foundations of Causal ML") • Large body of validation in causal discovery. Large body of applications and benchmarks for classification and feature selection
Best practices	**Best practice 3.2.6.1.** NB has limited utility in modern health applications and is not a recommended method in usual circumstances
	Best practice 3.2.6.2. Use BNs when flexible classification is needed
	Best practice 3.2.6.3. Use CBNs when causal structure discovery and causal effect estimation are needed
	Best practice 3.2.6.4. Use when modeling equivalence classes of full or local causal or Markov boundary models is needed
	Best practice 3.2.6.5. Markov boundary (identified via specialized algorithms) is typically the feature selection method of choice
	Best practice 3.2.6.6. Use for modeling full joint distributions (e.g., for simulation or re-simulation purposes) while also preserving causal structure
	Best practice 3.2.6.7. Use for guiding experiments in the presence of information equivalences
References	• See references (and discussions thereof) in chapters "Foundations and Properties of AI/ML Systems," "Foundations of Causal ML," "Principles of Rigorous Development and of Appraisal of ML and AI Methods and Systems," "The Development Process and Lifecycle of Clinical Grade and Other Safety and Performance-Sensitive AI/ML Models," and "Lessons Learned from Historical Failures, Limitations and Successes of AI/ML in Healthcare and the Health Sciences. Enduring Problems, and the Role of BPs"

K-Nearest Neighbor

The k nearest neighbor (k-NN) classifier and regression was introduced in 1951 [18]. K-NN is categorized as a "lazy" classifier/regressor, in the sense that it does not actually construct an explicit model from the data. Decisions are made based on the training data set rather than by a model trained on the data set. Specifically, the class of an instance is the (weighted) majority class of its k nearest neighbors, where k is a user-supplied hyperparameter. In case of k-NN regression, the estimated value of an instance is the (possibly weighted) average of the values of the k nearest neighbors.

The critical component of the k-NN classifier/regressor is the similarity function used to determine the k nearest neighbors. Defining an appropriate similarity functions is non-trivial, and is particularly difficult when (i) the data is high-dimensional or (ii) the importance of the variables varies greatly. The similarity function can be often learned from data. The problem of learning a similarity function from data is known as the *distance metric learning*.

When we consider the applicability of a method, we usually think about sample size or the form of the decision boundary between the positive and negative classes in a classification problem. In the case of k-NN, we may need to consider the local density of positive and negative instances. If a clear (low-density) separation exists between the positive and negative classes, kNN can be successful, regardless of the shape of the decision boundary; if a clear separation does not exist, kNN will likely not perform well (Fig. 5).

As we said earlier, kNN classifiers do not build an explicit model, instead, they have to determine the k nearest neighbors at classification time. This makes "training" the model cheap (there is no training), but the actual model application can become expensive. Additionally, this makes the classification less robust, as the classification of a new instance depends on the training sample, especially for small k. Increasing k can reduce the dependence on the specific training sample and can also improve robustness in the presence of noise, however, it makes the classification less local, which is the essence of kNN modeling.

The success of kNN classification depends on the amount of noise in the training sample, the choice of k (which again depends on the noise in the training sample), and a distance function that defines the neighborhood of the instances to be classified. Large-sample analysis of k-NN shows that in the sample limit with k=1 the error is at most double that of the optimal Bayes Classifier, whereas with larger k it can approximate the optimal Bayes Classifier [19].

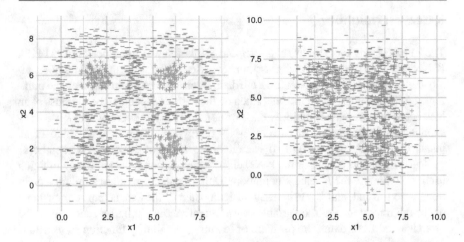

Fig. 5 Two hypothetical two-dimensional problems that can be solved using k-NN classification. Blue '-' signs indicate instances of the negative class; orange '+' the positive class. In the left pane, the positive clusters have a much higher density of positive instances than negative instances, making this an easy problem. In the right pane, there are three positive clusters, and the density of positive (orange) instances in each cluster is similar to that of the negative instances, which makes the problem more difficult

Method label: k-Nearest Neighbor (kNN)	
Main Use	• Classification and regression problems
Context of use	• Classification or regression based on similarity between instances. Its use is most appropriate when a similarity function can be easily constructed
Secondary use	• Density estimation
Pitfalls	**Pitfall 3.2.7.1** kNN asymptotic error is strongly influenced by the choice of k
	Pitfall 3.2.7.2 kNN error convergence to the large sample error as a function of sample size is not well characterized [19]
	Pitfall 3.2.7.3 in high dimensional problems the distance metric values become similar for all instance pairs and this affects accuracy
	Pitfall 3.2.7.4 kNN application is computationally intensive unless special data structures are used
	Pitfall 3.2.7.5 needs to store the entire training data set
	Pitfall 3.2.7.6 kNN will produce poor results when the wrong similarity function is used.
Principle of operation	• Prediction is based on the local density of the k nearest neighbors of the problem instance
Theoretical properties and empirical evidence	• kNN is non-parametric • It can handle arbitrary decision boundaries • In the sample limit, the error of the 1-NN classifier (k = 1), is no more than twice the error of the Optimal Bayes Classifier [18] • Typical similarity functions used in kNN do not perform well in high-dimensional problems • Usually underperforms most modern classifiers in most applications

Method label: k-Nearest Neighbor (kNN)	
Best practices	**Best practice 3.2.7.1.** Use as comparator not as primary classifier.
	Best practice 3.2.7.2. Optimize k with model selection.
	Best practice 3.2.7.3. Use adaptive kNN for high dimensional data.
	Best practice 3.2.7.4. Explore via model selection the right distance metric for the data at hand
References	• Several textbooks, including [19–21]
	• Cover, T. and Hart, P., 1967. Nearest neighbor pattern classification. *IEEE transactions on information theory*, *13*(1), pp.21–27

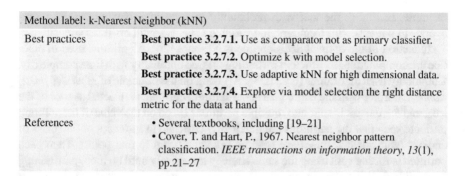

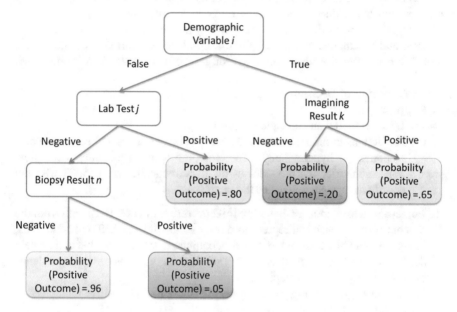

Fig. 6 Illustration of a decision tree classifying patients as having a positive outcome (e.g., successful treatment) depicted as green, or negative outcome (red). Nodes depicted with blue outline are **internal nodes** corresponding to observable variables (e.g., demographic, lab test, biopsy, or imaging test results). **Branches** correspond to the values of each variable. Nodes without children are called "**leaves**" and correspond to DT classifier decisions. Each decision has an associated probability for the values of the response (here, positive patient outcome)

Decision Tree Learning

A decision tree is a predictive model that can be used for classification or regression. Figure 6 depicts an example decision tree for classification built over discrete variables.

Learning a decision tree from data is called *decision tree induction*. Induction algorithms partition the input space into a number of hyperrectangles such that the hyperrectangles are statistically homogeneous for one or the other target class. For example, in Fig. 6, the leaf with probability of a positive outcome =0.80 corresponds to patients with Demographic variable i = False and Lab Test j = Positive.

Induction of the optimal decision tree is NP-hard [20]. Algorithms used in practice are computationally efficient by trading off tree optimality with time complexity. Commonly used algorithms (e.g., ID3 [21]) work on the principle of *recursive partitioning*. Starting with the entire data set, a splitting attribute is selected as root of the tree, and the dataset is split into multiple partitions based on the value of the splitting attribute such that the partitions are maximally enriched in instances of one class or another (equivalently, they have optimal predictivity up to that point). Then each partition is further split using the same strategy recursively until no more partitioning is possible (i.e., the algorithm runs out of sample or informative features). The various decision tree induction algorithms differ in the way the splitting criterion is selected, the stopping criterion, and the way they handle categorical, multi-level categorical and continuous attributes. Often, DT induction algorithms do not have a global objective function, they operate greedily and offer no guarantees of optimality.

Main Properties of Decision Trees
1. **Expressive power**:
   (a) DTs can model any discrete function.
   (b) Predictions in discrete space are made at the leaf nodes and each node corresponds to a hyperrectangle. Therefore, the decision boundary is complex, non-parametric, and the sides of the hyperrectangles are parallel with the coordinate system that spans the input space.

2. **Logic-based and concept-learning interpretation of DTs**. Each path from the root of the tree to each leaf represents a conjunction (logical AND) of conditions. A tree thus can be translated into a set of conjunctive sentences, that collectively define the target as a logical concept. Therefore there is a close correspondence of DTs with logic and concept learning.

   E.g., in the tree of Fig. 6 the Concept "(most likely) Positive Outcome" is defined by the DT as:
   (Positive Outcome = True) iff:
   (((Demographic variable i = False) AND (Lab Test j = Positive)) OR
   ((Demographic variable i = False) AND (Lab Test j = Negative) AND (Biopsy Result n = Negative)) OR
   ((Demographic variable i = True) AND (Imaging Result k = Positive)))

3. **Rule set interpretation of DTs**. A DT can also be thought of as a collection of rules of the type: "if the variables on a path have the observed instantiations depicted by the tree, then the decision is determined by the corresponding leaf's probability". Hence a DT is a system of rules, each one sufficient (when applicable) to establish a decision.

   E.g., in the tree of Fig. 6 the Concept "Positive Outcome" is defined by the DT as:

   RULE 1
   IF ((Demographic variable i = False) AND (Lab Test j = Positive)) THEN

Outcome = Positive with probability 0.80

RULE 2

IF ((Demographic variable i = False) AND (Lab Test j = Negative) AND (Biopsy Result n = Negative)) THEN Outcome = Positive with probability 0.96

RULE 3

IF ((Demographic variable i = True) AND (Imaging Result k = Positive)) THEN Outcome = Positive with probability 0.65

RULE 4

IF ((Demographic variable i = False) AND (Lab Test j = Negative) AND (Biopsy Result n = Positive)) THEN Outcome = Positive with probability 0.05

RULE 5

IF ((Demographic variable i = True) AND (Imaging Result k = Negative)) THEN Outcome = Positive with probability 0.20.

- The rules corresponding to a decision tree, **are individually correct** when they match problem instances, hence fully modular (i.e., one rules does not affect the other and *can be applied in isolation*).
- Moreover the rules **do not need be chained**: each inference made by the tree on a patient is the result of applying the applicable rule.
- The rules are **mutually exclusive**.
- Finally **the order of the variables in each path/rule, does not matter** *after* the tree is constructed, and can be applied in any order. The order of variables during the DT construction from data, however, is very important for the quality of the DT induced.

Notice that such rule sets are trivial to understand. By comparison rule-based systems where the rules have to be chained in complex forward/backward sequences have logic that cannot be understood easily by examining individual rules.

4. **Subpopulation discovery/clustering interpretation of DTs**. Each path of a DT describes a subpopulation that has a defined probability for the target variables and the group members are homogeneous in their probability for the target and in their values for the features along the path. Thus a DT provides a grouping/clustering of the feature space/individual observations that is tied to the outcome. In our running example:

GROUP 1: everyone who has:

((Demographic variable i = False) AND (Lab Test j = Positive))

GROUP 2: everyone who has:

((Demographic variable i = False) AND (Lab Test j = Negative) AND (Biopsy Result n = Negative))

Etc. for the other paths.

From the tree:

Group1 will have 0.80 probability of Outcome = Positive

Group2 will have 0.96 probability of Outcome = Positive

Etc. for the other groups.

Because DTs can be understood in several ways (rules, concepts, groups) and in a modular manner they are an exemplary model of interpretable and explainable ML (as long as DTs are of modest size).

5. A key problem with interpretability is *subtree replication*. Especially in the presence of noise, the exact same subtrees can appear under multiple nodes across the tree, which creates redundancy, hindering interpretation.
6. Decision trees are susceptible to overfitting. During tree induction, some method of protection against overfitting needs to be applied. Such methods include empirical testing on a validation set, regularizers (e.g., maximum allowed number of instances in a leaf, or maximum allowed tree depth, maximum allowed model complexity as part of the stopping criterion). Some of these can be enforced during learning, or after a tree is created.

Method label: Decision Trees	
Main Use	• Classification with maximum interpretability • As component of ensemble and boosted algorithms
Context of use	• DTs are highly interpretable: a decision tree can be translated into a set of rules. Interpretation is the main reason to use a decision tree • DTs are non-parametric, non-additive models that can represent linear and nonlinear relationships. • DTs are commonly used as a base learner in an ensemble • Baseline comparator
Secondary use	• Regression problems (regression trees) • Explaining black box ML models by converting them to functionally equivalent DTs
Pitfalls	**Pitfall 3.2.8.1.** A single DT on its own typically does not have very high performance **Pitfall 3.2.8.2.** DTs depending on how they are used can be unstable (which makes them a good choice for bagging) **Pitfall 3.2.8.3.** DTs if not regularized have a tendency for overfitting **Pitfall 3.2.8.4.** High dimensionality is a problem when feature selection has not been pre-applied
Principle of operation	• Recursive partitioning of the data. The inductive algorithm may build a DT following a partitioning strategy, or may follow other procedures (e.g. genetic algorithms or other search). Once a DT is built, however, it encodes a partitioning of the data
Theoretical properties and empirical evidence	• DT induction is NP-hard. Greedy algorithms are used, which provide no guarantees of optimality • Unless regularization and feature selection are applied, they have a tendency to overfit • DTs are highly interpretable • In an ensemble learning context, DTs can handle very high dimensionality, noise, and can identify interaction terms

Method label: Decision Trees	
Best practices	**Best practice 3.2.8.1.** Use DT for interpretable modeling alone or in conjunction with other methods
	Best practice 3.2.8.2. Use for target variable-specific subpopulation discovery
	Best practice 3.2.8.3. Use as baseline comparator method
	Best practice 3.2.8.4. Use in ensembling (boosting or bagging (Random Forest)) algorithms
References	Quinlan, J. R. C4.5: *Programs for Machine Learning*. Morgan Kaufmann Publishers, 1993
	Several textbooks e.g. [19–21]

Clustering

The family of clustering techniques deals with grouping objects into meaningful categories (e.g., subjects into disease groups or treatment-response groups). Typically, the produced clusters contain objects that are similar to one another but dissimilar to objects in other clusters [19, 20]. As has been shown mathematically, there is no single measure of similarity that is suitable for all types of analyses nor is clustering the most powerful method for all types of analysis even when applicable. Thus this generally useful set of methods is known to be often abused or misused [22]. We demonstrate these dangers with the following two figures.

Figures 7 and 8 show that *it is not possible for a clustering algorithm to anticipate predictive use of the clusters if the clustering algorithm does not have information about the labels (or other assumptions that amount to such information).*

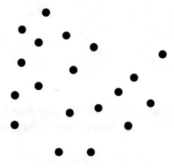

Fig. 7 Demonstration of the fallacy of using unsupervised clustering for predictive modeling. Question: what is a good clustering of the above data?

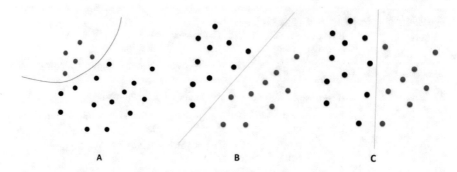

Fig. 8 Demonstration of the fallacy of using unsupervised clustering for predictive modeling, continued. Effect of the target function that generates data labels. As shown, identifying "good" (in the predictive sense) clusters of the above (and any) data, absolutely depends on the values of the target function. Case (**a**) left, case (**b**) middle, and case (**c**), right, involve exactly the same data in terms of input space but with different target functions defined over the input data (positive class depicted in red, negative in black). As a result, classifiers (blue lines) have to the class labels take into account in order to be accurate. The resulting classifiers are radically different and cannot be identified without reference to the target function that generates the class assignments

Pitfall 3.2.9

Use of clustering for predictive modeling will lead to under-performing models.

Best Practice 3.2.9

Do not use unsupervised clustering to produce groups that you intend to use predictively. Use predictive modeling, instead. Once accurate and interpretable classifiers have been built, subpopulations or other useful clusters can be extracted (see section on Decision Trees for a detailed example).

Clarifying Misconceptions About Unsupervised/Supervised Learning, Similarity/Distance-Based Learning, and Clustering

(a) As explained in chapter "Overfitting, Underfitting and General Model Overconfidence and Under-Performance Pitfalls and Best Practices in Machine Learning and AI" a common way that unsupervised clustering apparently yields decent predictive performance (e.g., in some parts of the high-throughput based genomics literature), is because a pre-selection of features was performed on the data based on how strongly the features correlated with the outcome. The analysts in these cases *inductively biased* the clustering toward classification of the desired response variable. This inductive bias is not enough to lead a clustering algorithm to optimal accuracy levels, however. Moreover, if such feature pre-selection is not done in a nested cross-validated manner (see chapter "Overfitting, Underfitting and General Model Overconfidence and Under-Performance Pitfalls and Best Practices in Machine Learning and AI") the resulting classification accuracy estimates will be highly biased (in the error estimation sense) and generalization will suffer.

(b) Because clustering is often defined in terms of *similarity*, it may be tempting to think that all similarity-based classification is predictively flawed. In reality, powerful classifiers exist that use distance and similarity functions (e.g., KNN, SVMs, etc. see section in the present chapter) however they are *supervised* (i.e., they approximate a particular target function that generates the data) which allows them (along with the rest of their design) to be capable of accurate predictive modeling.

(c) Conversely, and to re-iterate the point previously made, because good similarity-based predictive modeling exists, that does not mean that an unsupervised method, such as clustering, can be successful for predictive modeling.

(d) Finally, users of learning methods such as BNs and Causal Probabilistic Graphical Models (CPGMs) do not specify a target response variable and some may confuse them with unsupervised methods. In reality, because they model the joint probability distribution (and underlying causal generating function for CPGMs) they are *supervised learners for all variables* which can then be used as potential target responses at model execution time (see also chapter "Foundations and Properties of AI/ML Systems", section on flexible modeling with BNs).

Importance of Feature Selection for Similarity-Based Classification

If the features *containing all information about the response variable* are not included in the training data, then the predictive accuracy of similarity-based (*and any other sufficiently powerful classifier* family) will be compromised relative to the best classifier that can be built with this data. Compromised performance may also happen because of using feature selectors that allow large numbers of redundant or irrelevant features. This can overwhelm classifiers that, for example, lack sufficiently strong regularization or other anti-overfitting measures. In high dimensional spaces it is critical to apply sound feature selection algorithms so that choice of features enhances rather than hinders classification.

The following table summarizes essential properties of clustering algorithms.

Method label: clustering	
Main Use	• Group data for exploratory analysis, summarization and visualization purposes
Context of use	• Summarize, visualize and explore data (e.g., outliers, apparent distribution mixtures, etc.)
Secondary use	• Often used *inappropriately* for causal discovery and classification purposes
Non-recommended Uses and Pitfalls	**Pitfall 3.2.9.1.** Clustering variables should not be used to infer that they are causally related (a common mistake in genomics literature) **Pitfall 3.2.9.2.** Clustering individuals should not be used to build classifiers (also a common mistake in genomics literature) **Pitfall 3.2.9.3.** Choice of similarity metric, algorithm, and parameters inductively biases results toward specific groupings. There is no such thing as "unbiased" clustering analysis
Principle of operation	• Typically unsupervised method (i.e., clustering algorithms do not have access to response variable values) • Group together data instances that are similar and apart dissimilar instances • In other versions, cluster variables or cluster *simultaneously* variables and instances • Use similarity metrics and algorithms that employ those to create clusters • Clusters can be overlapping or mutually exclusive (soft vs hard clustering) • Clusters can be hierarchically organized or distinct
Theoretical properties and Empirical evidence	• Across all possible uses all clustering algorithms are on average equivalent ("Ugly Duck Theorem") • Clustering lucks the inductive bias, information capacity and the computational complexity to be compatible with causal discovery
Best practices	**Best practice 3.2.9.1.** Do no use clustering to discover causal structure **Best practice 3.2.9.2.** Do not use clustering to create accurate classifiers **Best practice 3.2.9.3.** Tailor the use of clustering algorithm and metric to the problem at hand **Best practice 3.2.9.4.** Derive predictive subgroups from properly-built and validated classifiers (Decision Trees are particularly good candidates—See "Decision Tree Learning") **Best practice 3.2.9.5.** Perform sensitivity analysis to study the impact of the choice of parameters, metrics and algorithms **Best practice 3.2.9.6.** Repeat and summarize multiple runs of randomized clustering algorithms **Best practice 3.2.9.7.** Either start from causal and predictive algorithms and use clustering to summarize, visualize, etc. their results, or start from clustering analysis in preliminary data to inform the design and analysis with focused techniques

Method label: clustering	
References	• Dupuy, A. and Simon, R.M., 2007. Critical review of published microarray studies for cancer outcome and guidelines on statistical analysis and reporting. *Journal of the National Cancer Institute*, *99*(2), pp.147–157. • Several textbooks [19–21]

Ensemble Methods

So far, a single predictive model has been trained on a training data set and the prediction from this model is the final prediction. In **ensemble learning**, an ensemble, i.e., a set of models, is trained on the training data and their output is combined into a final prediction. Figure 9. illustrates the ensemble learning process. A set of m models, called **base learners**, $L_1, \ldots, L_m$ are trained on their corresponding data sets $X_1, \ldots, X_m$. The data set X_i can be the data set X itself or a sample from it. Predictions from the m base learners are combined using the **meta learner** L^*. The meta learner can be as simple as majority voting or as complex as a neural network. The different ensemble learning methods depend on (i) how they generate the data set X_i from X, (ii) the base learners they use and (iii) the meta learner.

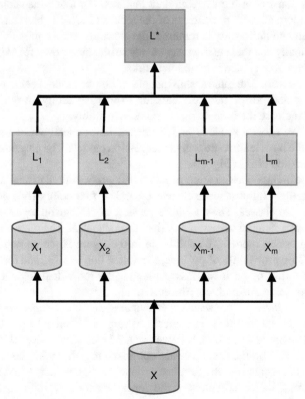

Fig. 9 Generic form of Ensemble Learning

The key motivation for using ensembles is improving predictive performance. This is achieved in four possibly overlapping ways. First, if we assume that the base learners make mistakes independently, as long as the base learners achieve better (lower) than random error rate, the ensemble will have a lower error rate than the individual base learners. In practice, the base learners do not make errors independently, but the ensemble still tends to achieve better performance than the base learners. Second, the ensemble learning framework allows us to combine models of different characteristics, potentially allowing for compensating for biases inherent in some of the methods. Third, ensembles of various types of base learners can expand the base learners' expressive capabilities: the ensemble can express much more complex relationships than base learners. Fourth, the ensemble may reduce the variance of a collection of models built on small samples.

Model Stacking

Model stacking is essentially the generic form of ensemble learning. The data sets X_i can be the original data set (X), a bootstrap resample of X, or a subsample of X. For high-dimensional data sets, X_i can be a random projection of X, which helps most when X consists of highly redundant features. For low dimensional X, X_i can consist of random linear combinations of the features in X. The base learners can be of any type and no uniformity is required: the ensemble can contain different types of models. Finally, the meta learner can be any sufficiently powerful ML algorithm; as of late, a common choice is neural networks.

Expressive ability. The relationship that ensembles can model between the inputs and the output depends on the base learners' expressive ability. In practice, model stacking can increase the base learners' expressive ability.

Example. We show a stack of logistic regression models, where both the base learners and the meta learner are logistic regression models. The ensemble is applied to the problem depicted in Fig. 10.

This is a two-class classification problem using a two-dimensional data set with strong interactions (almost an exclusive OR). The two colors (orange and blue) represent the two classes. The ensemble consists of 10 logistic regression models, each trained on a random subsample of the original data X. The meta learner is also a logistic regression model. The solid line in the figure is the contour line corresponding to 20% probability of positive, the dotted line to 50%, and the dashed line to 80% probability of positive class. Although the individual logistic regression models cannot solve this problem, the ensemble can.

Note on the difference between stacked linear regression and neural networks. This example of stacked logistic regressions appears similar to a 2-layer neural network with sigmoid activation, however, in a 2-layer neural network the "logistic regression models" on the first layer are optimized together with the second layer, while in stacked regression, the first layer models are constructed first (on random subsamples) with the actual output as the dependent variable, their coefficients are

Fig. 10 Illustration of an ensemble of 10 logistic regression models with a logistic regression meta learner on a two-dimensional classification problem

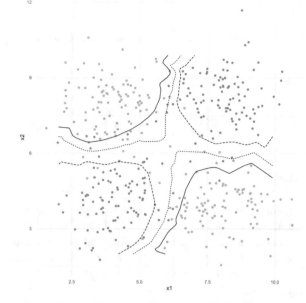

fixed, and only then is the second layer model (the meta learner) constructed. While the second layer logistic regression is being fitted, the coefficients of the first layer are not modified.

Method label: model stacking	
Main Use	• Classification or regression

Context of use	• This is a generic form of ensemble learning
	• There are four main reasons for using ensemble learning:
	   – Ensembling can reduce error by taking advantage of independent errors of the base learners
	   – Base learners have different inductive biases
	   – The ensemble can expand the base learners' hypothesis spaces by combining their spaces
	   – The ensemble may reduce variance of base learners

Secondary use	• Other types of learning (not only classification or regression) can be ensembled
Pitfalls	**Pitfall 3.3.1.1.** Interpretability suffers **Pitfall 3.3.1.2.** Increased computational cost **Pitfall 3.3.1.3.** Potentially additional data may be needed for training the ensemble
Principle of operation	• Multiple base learners are built and then a meta learner is trained on the output of the base learners and the actual outcome. The prediction from the meta learner is the prediction of the ensemble
Theoretical properties and empirical evidence	• Stacking draws its formal foundations from fundamentals of ML theory plus the theory of weak learner boosting and bagging • Several stacking algorithms exhibit best of class performance in various domains. [23, 24] individual algorithms (e.g., Adaboost, random forests) have distinct characteristics (described below)

Method label: model stacking	
Best practices	**Best practice 3.3.1.1.** Consider stacking as a high priority choice of algorithm when high performance is needed, base algorithms do not perform well, and interpretability is not a strong requirement
References	• Wolpert (1992). "Stacked Generalization". Neural Networks. 5 (2): 241–259 • Breiman, Leo (1996). "Stacked regressions". *Machine Learning*. **24**: 49–64. • Textbooks [20]

Bagging

Bagging, also known as *bootstrap aggregation*, forms the data sets for the base learners as a bootstrap resample (i.e., sample with replacement) of the original dataset. The base learner can be any learning algorithm and the "meta learner" is simply majority voting (or average in the continuous outcome case).

The key benefit of bagging is reducing the variance of the base learner. If a classifier's predictions are sensitive to minor perturbations in the data, this means that the generalization error is negatively affected by the variance of the base learning. Bagging can help reduce random fluctuations across possible training samples. If the base learner is robust to small perturbations, then the generalization error is caused mainly by bias in the base learner, and bagging cannot help. Thus, bagging is most useful in conjunction with base learners that have high variance (such as decision trees).

Figure 11 illustrates bagging. The left panel shows a one-dimensional data set, where the horizontal axis shows the data ("x") and the vertical axis is simply a

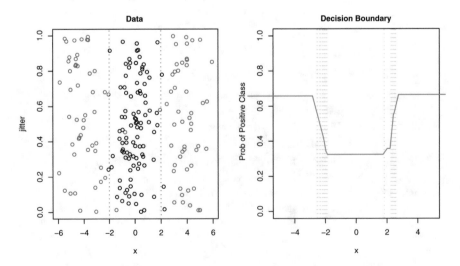

Fig. 11 Illustration of bagging

jitter-plot visualization (i.e., the y axis spreads randomly the corresponding x points so that data points on the x axis are not plotted on top of each other). Red points represent the positive class and black points the negative class. The true decision boundary for the positive class is x < = −2 or x > 2; this is shown as two dashed lines. We constructed 200 decision stumps (decision tree with depth 1, with a single binary split of the input dimension) on bootstrap samples of this data set. Such stumps can accurately learn the target function in x ≥ 2 or in x ≤ −2. The right panel shows 200 decision boundaries from these 200 decision trees as dotted gray lines. The horizontal axis is the data dimension ("x") and the vertical axis is the probability (from the trees) of an instance with the corresponding x value belonging to the positive class. The blue line corresponds to **the bagged prediction** using the previously constructed 200 trees.

Bagging can also help increase the expressive capability of the base learner. Fig. 11 demonstrates that by bagging weak learners, improved accuracy can be achieved in a simple example. Bagging decision stumps, for example can form a decision boundary that can only be achieved by deeper (more than one-level) trees without bagging. Also it can be seen in Fig. 11 that the bagged classifier smooths the decision surface.

Bagging a set of models is more resilient to overfitting than overfitting any single model. Overfitting that arises as a result of a predictor aligning with an outcome randomly (i.e. in a specific sample), is not likely to happen in a different sample. Therefore, only one (or very few) trees are affected by this particular random alignment. Other random alignments can also occur in other samples, and they will tend to average out. Thus overfitting is still much possible on the individual model level, but less so at the level of bag of models.

Random Forests

A Random Forest (RF) is an ensemble classification method using decision trees as the base learning algorithm combining the following four ideas: (a) bagging decision trees, (b) random feature projection, (c) off training sample error estimation, and (d) model complexity restrictions.

The RF generates X_i, the data set on which the ith tree is grown by bootstrapping once at the start of modeling. The features are randomized at each tree's node expansion step. Feature randomization increases the independence among the trees in the forest, while bagging aims to reduce the variance of the predictions by each tree. The predictions from the tree in the forest are combined using majority voting or averaging (for continuous outcomes).

Method label: fandom forest	
Main Use	• Classification
Context of use	• RFs achieve high predictive performance
Secondary use	• Regression, time-to-Event (Random Survival Forest)

Method label: fandom forest	
Pitfalls	**Pitfall 3.3.3.1.** As with all ensemble techniques interpretability suffers **Pitfall 3.3.3.2.** If not restricting the size of trees RFs can overfit
Principle of operation	• Bagging trees • Random projection of the features • Off-training sample error estimation • Model complexity restrictions
Theoretical properties and Empirical evidence	• Overfitting is controlled • In practice, RFs can handle very high dimensional problems • Excellent empirical performance observed in benchmarks across biomedical domains [25]
Best practices	**Best practice 3.3.3.1.** Use as primary or high priority choice when high predictivity is required and interpretability is not of high importance **Best practice 3.3.3.2.** Do not rely on internal error estimation but use an independent unbiased error estimator **Best practice 3.3.3.3.** When feature selection is important, combine with an external feature selection algorithm **Best practice 3.3.3.4.** Control DT size using as starting point the recommendations of the inventor in original publication [24]
References	• Breiman L (2001). "Random Forests". Machine Learning. 45 (1): 5–32 • Hastie, Friedman, Tibshirani. Elements of statistical learning second edition, Chpater 15. 2009, springer • Tan, Steinbach, Karpatne, Kumar. Introduction to data mining, second edition. Chapter 4.10.6., 2018, Pearson

Boosting

Boosting creates an ensemble of base models sequentially, where the ith base model is aimed at correcting errors made by the ensemble of the previous i-1 base models. The resulting ensemble is an additive model, where the final prediction is the sum of the predictions from the base models. The data set X_i for the ith model can be the data set X itself, a bootstrap resampled version of X, or a weighted version of X to emphasize difficult-to-classify instances.

Consider a boosted ensemble of m models. The prediction for an instance X_i is

$$y_i = f\left(\sum_{j=1}^{m} m_j\left(X_i\right)\right)$$

where $f(\cdot)$ is the link function and $m_j(\cdot)$ is jth model. Similarly to GLM, $f()$ is identity for gaussian outcomes, logit/expit for binomial outcomes, exp for counts and survival outcomes, etc. The ensemble is built up iteratively, following a gradient descent procedure

$$M_{j+1} = M_j + \gamma \frac{\partial l}{\partial M_j},$$

where M_j is the ensemble after the jth iteration, l is the log likelihood of M_j, and γ is the learning rate. For the exponential family of distributions, including the Gaussian, binomial (and multinomial) and Poisson (survival) outcomes, the derivative of the log likelihood is the residual. Thus the $(j + 1)^{st}$ model is the model fitted to the residual of the ensemble M_j. This leads to a very straightforward interpretation that the subsequent model is built to the errors (residual) of the ensemble M_j thus the $(j + 1)^{st}$ base model aims to correct the mistakes made by the previous j base models.

Gradient boosting can overfit, but typically only slowly to the number of modeling iterations. The number of base models in a boosted model (the number of iterations to perform) is a hyperparameter h. It has been observed that models consisting of substantially more base models than optimal still overfit only minimally. A potential reason for this is that when a model reaches overfitting, adding further base models has very minimal impact. However, boosting will eventually overfit, so overfitting should be controlled by h.

Gradient Boosting Machines (GBM) are a special case of boosting, where the base learners are decision trees, often decision stumps (1 level-deep trees). Similar to bagging, boosting can also expand the base model's expressive capability.

AdaBoost is another special case of boosting which relates to the generic gradient boosting the same way as Fisher scoring (or Newton Raphson) optimization algorithm relate to gradient descent. AdaBoost is specifically designed for binomial (multinomial) outcomes.

The $(j + 1)^{st}$ model is added to the ensemble using

$$M_{j+1} = M_j + \gamma \left(\frac{\partial^2 l}{\partial M_j^2} \right)^{-1} \frac{\partial l}{\partial M_j},$$

where $\frac{\partial^2 l}{\partial M_j^2}$ is a diagonal matrix containing the second derivatives of the log likelihood l. For binomial outcomes, the second derivative is $p(1-p)$, where $p_i = expit\left(M_j\left(X_i\right)\right) = \dfrac{\exp\left(M_j\left(X_i\right)\right)}{1 + \exp\left(M_j\left(X_i\right)\right)}$.

AdaBoost is implemented by weighing the ith training instance by $(p_i(1 - p_i))^{-1}$ and using the residuals $r_i = y_i - p_i$ as the dependent variable.

Method label: gradient boosting machines (GBM)	
Main Use	• Classification
Context of se	• GBMs offer high predictive performance • Interpretability is limited to variable importance
Secondary use	• Exponential family distributions, including time-to-event
Pitfalls	**Pitfal 3.3.4.1.** As with all ensemble techniques interpretability suffers
	Pitfal 3.3.4.2 If not controlling the complexity parameter it can overfit

Method label: gradient boosting machines (GBM)	
Principle of operation	• Gradient Boosting with decision stumps as base learners • Gradient descent (GBM) or Fisher-scoring (AdaBoost) in model space • Can be thought of as successively reducing the residual errors from previous cycles of modeling.
Theoretical properties and empirical evidence	• Very expressive • Overfitting can be controlled • Can handle very high dimensional data • For AdaBoost, theoretical (but loose) error bounds are proven. • Certain boosting algorithms (e.g., Adaboost) have sensitivity to noise • Top performer in several types problems/data
Best practices	**Best practices 3.3.4.1.** Use as primary or high priority choice when high predictivity is required and interpretability is not of high importance **Best practices 3.3.4.2.** When feature selection is important, combine with an external feature selection algorithm **Best practices 3.3.4.3.** Control overfitting by restricting number of iterations (number of trees) **Best practices 3.3.4.4.** If data is noisy, prefer noise-robust variants. **Best practices 3.3.4.5.** Select appropriate link function for exponential family outcomes
References	• Schapire, R.E., 1990. The strength of weak learnability. *Machine learning*, 5, pp.197–227 • Freund, Y., 1999, July. An adaptive version of the boost by majority algorithm. In *proceedings of the twelfth annual conference on computational learning theory* (pp. 102–113) • G. Ridgeway (1999). "The state of boosting," Computing Science and Statistics 31:172–181 • Long, P.M. and Servedio, R.A., 2008, July. Random classification noise defeats all convex potential boosters. In *proceedings of the 25th international conference on machine learning* (pp. 608–615)

Regularization

A problem is considered high-dimensional when the number of predictors is comparable to or exceeds the number of observations. When the number of predictors equals the number of observations, an OLS regression fit can be an exact fit, with 0 training error. Such a model will be most likely overfitted. When we consider other types of models, with the number of predictors very close to or exceeding the number of observations, overfitting becomes highly likely. We start our discussion with an explanation of regularization, a general solution to the high-dimensionality problem, and next, we discuss ways in which regularization can be added to various modeling techniques.

Regularization from a Bias/Variance Perspective

The material builds on the BVDE in chapter "Foundations and Properties of AI/ML Systems". When a model is overfitting and has high variance and low bias, it can be advantageous to increase bias provided that it reduces variance. One way to achieve this is to reduce complexity and another way, the subject of this section, is regularization [26].

We previously saw how SVMs perform regularization and that the resulting RFE-SVM feature selector is one of the strongest feature selectors (second in performance to Markov Boundary methods in empirical performance across various domains). See section "Support Vector Machines" for SVM regularization, and section "Feature Selection and Dimensionality Reduction" for feature selectors. See also chapter "Lessons Learned from Historical Failures, Limitations and Successes of AI/ML In Healthcare and the Health Sciences. Enduring Problems, and the Role of Best Practices" when feature should be interpreted causally or not.

Next we examine the Elastic net family of regularizers which we will call Maximum Likelihood (ML) Regularizers.

Let $l(\beta)$ denote the log likelihood function, with β representing the model parameters. Model fitting without regularization solves

$$\max_\beta l(\beta).$$

ML regularization adds a penalty term $P(\beta)$

$$\max_\beta l(\beta) - \lambda P(\beta),$$

where λ controls the amount of regularization. Different ML regularization methods differ in the form of $P()$. Table 2. shows the most common regularization terms.

L1 regularization modifies the coefficients by pulling them away from maximum likelihood estimate. The maximum likelihood estimate is unbiased, thus regularization introduces bias, in hope of reducing variance. The various ML regularization methods differ in the way they modify the coefficients. Lasso is shrinking the coefficients towards 0 and it has the ability to set some of the coefficients exactly to 0. This allows Lasso to be used as a feature selector. Therefore, Lasso penalty is in principle most useful when some of the features are not truly related to the outcome.

Table 2. Common penalty (regularization) terms

Name	Penalty term	Remark
Lasso	$\|\beta\|_1 = \sum_j \| \beta_j \|$	Can set the coefficient β_j to exactly 0
Ridge	$\|\beta\|_2^2 = \sum_j \beta_j^2$	
Elastic net	$(1-\alpha)\|\beta\|_2^2 + \alpha\|\beta\|_1$	Balance between Ridge and Lasso
Adaptive Lasso	$\sum_j w_j \| \beta_j \|$	w_j reduces the penalty on important variables. A common choice is $\frac{1}{\beta_j^*}$, , where β_j^* is the OLS estimate.

In contrast, Ridge penalty simply shrinks coefficients towards zero without actually setting them to 0. Elastic net allows to blend these two penalties together.

Adaptive lasso [27] also addresses the situation where some of the variables are not related to the outcome. However, by weighing the penalty on the individual coefficients, it aims to shrink important variables less and eliminate variables that are not related to the outcome (shrink their coefficients all the way to 0). The property that the adaptive lasso can set non-zero coefficients to variables that are relevant with probability approaching one is called the *oracle property*. Feature selection is discussed in more detail in the section "Feature Selection".

The procedure for the adaptive lasso proceeds in two steps. First, a regular lasso model is constructed. In the second step, an adaptive lasso model is constructed, with the weights being the inverse of the coefficients from the first lasso.

We will discuss overfitting in chapter "Overfitting, Underfitting and General Model Overconfidence and Under-Performance Pitfalls and Best Practices in Machine Learning and AI". There are many reasons for overfitting, including high dimensionality, with many irrelevant features and highly correlated features in a problem with moderate dimensionality. In the former case, lasso or adaptive lasso is most appropriate: lasso will discard some of the features. In the latter case, Lasso and Ridge will have different effect. When overfitting occurs as a result of high collinearity, the OLS estimator tends to set the coefficients of collinear variables to very high positive and similarly high negative values. Lasso will select one of the correlated features and set the coefficients of the others to zero, while Ridge will set the coefficients to similar values across the correlated features. Ridge prevents the coefficient from taking the extremely high values.

Bias and correctness. Since the penalties aim to trade bias for variance, the estimates are likely biased. Lasso has feature selection ability, however, it is not guaranteed to find the correct support (the exact set of variables that are predictive of the outcome). Adaptive lasso in theory finds the correct support and may help reduce or even eliminate the bias.

Method label: penalized regression	
Main Use	• Predictive modeling with exponential family outcomes
Context of use	• High-dimensional data
	• Data with collinear variables
Secondary use	• Lasso can be used for variable selection
Pitfalls	**Pitfall 3.4.1.1.** The models assume linearity and additivity. They are not appropriate if these assumptions are violated
	Pitfall 3.4.1.2. Does not have the same interpretability as unregularized regression models. Specifically cannot be used to estimate effects of an exposure on outcomes controlling for confounders given to the model
	Pitfall 3.4.1.3. The theory of optimality of the ML regularized regression does not address the selection of strongly vs weakly relevant vs irrelevant features which is essential to feature selection
	Pitfall 3.4.1.4. Extensive benchmark results show weak empirical feature selection performance across many datasets, loss functions and comparator algorithms
Principle of operation	• Regression models
	• Biases the coefficient estimates to reduce variance (bias-variance tradeoff)

Method label: penalized regression	
Theoretical Properties and empirical evidence	• They tend to give biased estimates (on purpose) • BVDE give theoretical support to the means of operation • "Oracle property" (as defined by [27])
Best practices	**Best practice 3.4.1.1.** Penalized regression can operate in high dimensional datasets that classic regression cannot handle at all
	Best practice 3.4.1.2. Use as comparator method along with others as appropriate for the application domain
	Best practice 3.4.1.3. May be useful for feature selection, but not as first-choice methods
	Best practice 3.4.1.4. When non-linear regularized models are needed, consider link functions that model the non-linearity as well as kernel SVMs, kernel regression
References	Hastie, T., Tibshirani, R., Friedman, J.H. and Friedman, J.H., 2009. *The elements of statistical learning: Data mining, inference, and prediction* (Vol. 2, pp. 1–758). New York: Springer

Regularizing Groups of Variables

In the previous section, Lasso was used for variable selection, primarily in the context when many variables could be assumed irrelevant to the outcome. Variables may be related to each other and form groups. It may be useful to select variables on a per-group basis [28].

Assume that variables form K groups with p_k variables in the kth group. Let $\beta^{(k)}$ denote the coefficients of the variables in group k. With l denoting the log likelihood function, the group lasso is formulated as

$$\max_\beta l(\beta) - \lambda \sum_{k=1}^{K} \sqrt{p_k} \left\| \beta^{(k)} \right\|_2.$$

The sparse group lasso [29] formulation

$$\max_\beta l(\beta) - \lambda \alpha \|\beta\|_1 - \lambda(1-\alpha) \sum_{k=1}^{K} \sqrt{p_k} \left\| \beta^{(k)} \right\|_2$$

also has a (regular) lasso penalty, allowing for selecting variables on a per-group basis and further selecting variables within the groups.

Regularizing Partial Correlations

The precision matrix, that is the inverse of the variance-covariance matrix, is a key parameter of a multivariate normal distribution. Regularization is necessary to estimate the precision matrix when sufficient observations are not available.

Let Θ denote the precision matrix and S the sample covariance matrix. The regularized estimate of Θ is computed as

$$\max_{\theta \geq 0} \log \det \Theta - tr(S\Theta) - \lambda \sum_{j \neq k} \Theta_{jk}.$$

The inverse covariance matrix contains the partial correlations. Two random variables X_i and X_j are independent if their covariance is 0; and they are *conditionally* independent (conditioned on all other variables) if the ijth element of the inverse covariance matrix is 0 [30].

Regularization to Constrain the Search Space of Models

So far, we have shown examples of regularization to avoid overfitting, either by computing a sparse solution (some parameters/coefficients are set to exactly 0) or by introducing bias to reduce variance. We have done so mostly in the context of regression.

Regularization is more general. It can be broadly viewed as a means to constrain the search space of models to confer some desirable property on the model. It is not limited to regression, but it is often used in conjunction with likelihoods. This is not a requirement, it can be used with any kind of quasi-likelihood or arbitrary loss functions. Constraining the search space of models through regularization is arguably the most common use and providing an exhaustive overview is impractical as new applications are continuously developed. In this section, we simply show some examples.

Knowledge distillation. Deep learning models are regarded complex highly performing models. Very complex DL models have been trained in many areas that can be further modified for particular applications (See chapters "Considerations for Specialized Health AI and ML Modelling and Applications: NLP," "Considerations for Specialized Health AI and ML Modelling and Applications: Imaging—Through the perspective of Dermatology"). These modified models are still very large, and deploying such models into resource-limited environment is difficult. The teacher-student paradigm, consist of a large teacher model used to train a small student model. Knowledge distillation is the process of generating smaller student models (models with fewer parameters), deployable in limited-resource environment, that are trained based on the more complex teacher models. Knowledge distillation is often implemented using regularization: the student model is regularized so that it resembles the teacher model in various aspects [31].

Learning DAGs. Traditionally, learning DAGs is a combinatorial optimization problem. However, the NOTEARS method introduced a penalty term, applicable to weight matrices, that enforces DAG-ness when this weight matrix is used as an adjacency matrix [32].

Dropout (Neural Networks)

Dropout layers in Neural Networks aim to reduce overfitting due to noise. In dropout, a pre-defined (as hyperparameter) proportion (**dropout portion**) of nodes are dropped from the hidden layers and possibly from the input layers. "Dropping from the network" means that the inputs and outputs of these nodes are severed and thus these nodes no longer influence the prediction. The set of nodes to be dropped is selected at random in each epoch. After the epoch, the nodes are restored [33].

Dropout layers have properties both from regularization as well as from ensemble learning. Clearly, they are similar to regularization, because they constrain the network architecture by dropping some nodes.

The ensemble perspective can be explained as follows. One way to reduce the risk of overfitting in a neural network would be to build an ensemble of neural networks, i.e. multiple neural network models with different parameterizations. Given the high cost of training neural networks, this approach is impractical. Instead, dropout re-configures the network temporarily, which means that the network being trained in each epoch has a (slightly) different architecture. Over the training epochs, a range of different network architectures are explored.

An alternative explanation of the dropout layers is, that the potentially high number of parameters a network has over possibly many layers, makes the network susceptible to **co-adaptation**, where multiple parts (sets of nodes) of the network get optimized so that some parts can correct for errors made by other parts. This co-correction allows for easely fitting noise, which is undesirable. Dropping nodes out of the network at random, breaks these co-adaptation patterns.

Dropouts can be defined on the input layer, as well. In this case, the network temporarily ignores some of the input features. This is similar to introducing noise into the data to make the model more robust.

When a neural network model is used to make predictions, all nodes are used for the prediction, i.e. no dropout is used for prediction. Since the nodes were trained with some of the nodes missing, the weights of the nodes may be too high. To correct for this, the weights are scaled down by the dropout portion at prediction time.

Why Regularized Models and Other Predictive Modeling Should Not Be Used For Reliable Causal Modeling

Regularization, with the exception of penalizing the precision (partial correlation matrix), has profound impact on a modeling technique's ability to condition on variables.

Figure 12 depicts a dataset with two variables A and B and an outcome (target) T. The target T is binary, points in red correspond to positive outcome and the points in black to negative. The data generating causal relationships are $A{\rightarrow}T$ and $A{\rightarrow}B$. This means that B is independent of T given A; or in other words, A alone is sufficient to classify the instances, B contains no additional information. From a causal perspective, the association of B with the target is confounded by A (their

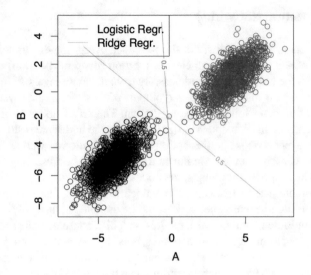

Fig. 12 Illustration of the ability and inability to condition on a variable

common cause). Any valid causal method must be able to differentiate correlation from causation, i.e., determine which correlations are causal and which are confounded. This is not happening in the example since the decision surface (orange line) of the (logistic) ridge regression gives the same weights to both A and B. Ridge regression is not designed to realize that B and T are conditionally independent given (conditioned on) A. Contrast this with the decision surface (blue line) produced by unpenalized Logistic Regression, which assigns almost zero weight to the confounded variable (B) and nearly all the weight to the true cause (A) since LR is capable of correctly conditioning on any set of confounders (thus correctly estimating direct causal effects).

Ridge regression is not the only method that has this problem. The maximal margin decision boundary that SVMs would select, is similar to the orange line; and most classifiers including modern regularized regression methods, principal component and other classical dimensionality reduction methods, as well as all predictive modeling without causal properties, will make similar errors.

Figure 13 illustrates another example where Lasso penalized regression (and other non-causal techniques) will fail to correctly condition on variables. In this example, we have 7 variables, $A, B, …, E, S$ and the target variable T. $A, B, …, E$ are direct causes of T. Variable S which is not causal for T (but confounded with it via $A,….E$) synthesizes information from causal variables $A, B, …, E$. In this setup, S and T are independent conditioned on $A, B, …, E$. However, since S synthesizes information from $A, B, …, E$, it can contain more information about T than any subset of $A, B, …,$ or E. Thus, when building a predictive model for T, a penalized model, like Lasso, can prefer a set of predictor variables that contains S over the correct set of $A, B, …, E$. In contrast, unpenalized logistic regression (and any sound

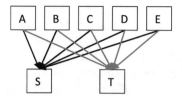

Fig. 13 Simple example where a confounded correlate synthesizes information from multiple true causes

causal algorithm) will correctly identify that S is independent of T given the other variables and will assign a zero coefficient to S given the true causes.

For large scale benchmark studies comparing all modern predictive modeling algorithms with causal algorithms see refs. [34, 35]. In these references, it is explained why various additional non-causal methods fail to model causality.

Implications for interpreting models. Not being able to condition on variables has two important model interpretation implications. The interpretability of the penalized models differs from unpenalized models. (a) In an (unpenalized) regression model, if a variable has non-zero coefficient, it is not conditionally independent of the target. However, in a regularized model, in general, having non-zero coefficient does not imply that the variable is not conditionally independent of the target.

(b) The broader implication is that because discovering causal structure and estimating effects require sound conditional independence tests and conditional association estimation, regularized regression and other purely predictive methods cannot be used for causal structure discovery or causal effect estimation even for simple questions (e.g. direct causal effect estimation) and even when the complete set of confounders is measured and are included in the model. Although unpenalized regression can be used for causal effect estimation, note that this has to be guided by knowledge of the causal structure (or elicitation of it using complex causal modeling algorithms).

See chapter "Foundations of Causal AI/ML" for more details and best practices.

Feature Selection and Dimensionality Reduction

Variable selection (aka feature selection) for predictive modeling has received considerable attention during the last three decades in a variety of data science fields [36, 37]. Feature selection and dimensionality reduction are techniques of choice to tame high dimensionalities in diverse big data applications. Intuitively, **feature**

selection for prediction aims to select a subset of variables for constructing a diagnostic or predictive model for a given classification or regression task. Ideally this selected set should include all variables with unique information and discard variables the information of which is subsumed by the selected set (since they add no information to the classifier). **Dimensionality reduction** maps the original data on a smaller number of dimensions so that fitting models is faster, less prone to overfitting and less sample intensive (all problems created by the high dimensionality and collectively known as "**Curse of Dimensionality**").

Feature Selection

Key concepts of the theory of feature selection were introduced in chapter "Foundations and Properties of AI/ML Systems". Here we will extend that material with a refinement of the types of feature selection problems typically addressed in practice, their relative complexity, examples, and algorithms that are used for feature selection.

Motivation and *Standard Feature Selection Problem*

In practice, reducing the number of features in clinical predictor models can reduce costs, and increase ease of deployment. Second, a more parsimonious model can be easier to interpret. Third, sometimes, identifying the most impactful features helps gain an understanding of the underlying process that generated the data. Finally, many classifiers do not perform well with very high dimensional data: they may overfit, exhibit too long compute times, or even fail to fit models.

Feature selection can be approached from three high-level theoretical perspectives. (1) The first one is that of overfitting/underfitting. In high-dimensional data sets, feature selection can reduce overfitting, but in lower dimensions if not conducted properly it can introduce both overfitting and underfitting (not both at the same time). It can underfit relative to a model that has more features (i.e., resulting model does not have enough capacity); and it can overfit if it is overly influenced by random variations in the data; a model with the same number of features could perform worse on the training set but perform better on a test set. (2) Feature selection in moderate or low dimensions can be used specifically to produce a parsimonious (and thus potentially more interpretable and practical) model, but this may induce underfitting if feature selection is not optimal. (3) Suboptimal feature selection can introduce instability when it selection of features is influenced by random perturbations in the data. To what extent such instability affects predictivity depends on whether the unstable features share the same information for the target or not. It is therefore important to deploy feature selection methods which are both theoretically sound and empirically strong.

The *standard feature selection problem* (chapter "Foundations and Properties of AI/ML Systems") is typically defined as:

Find the smallest set of variables St in the training data such that the predictive accuracy of the best classifier than can be fit for response T from the data is maximized

A commonly used classification of feature selection considers three primary categories of methods: wrapper methods, filter methods and embedded methods [36]. We will further elaborate this taxonomy by considering whether the feature selection methods have a strong theoretical framework and properties (formal) vs not (heuristic).

Heuristic Algorithms

Wrapper methods. These methods conduct a heuristic search in the space of all subsets of the variables to assess each subset's predictive information with respect to the selected predictive model. Wrapper methods treat the classifier as a black box, fit a model to that data with a particular feature set and evaluate the model. Then they build a model with a different feature set and re-evaluate the new model. This process continues until some stopping criterion is met. This approach is computationally expensive, often overfits and underperforms, and also has great variation in performance depending on methods.

a. *Stepwise Regression.* Historically it has been used broadly for statistical regression modeling but its use is reduced because (a) standard implementations have been shown to overfit and are unstable [38] and (b) regularized regression has alleviated the need to use them substantially.

These methods can start from an empty model and use a forward single variable inclusion step, iterated with a backward single variable elimination step method until no improvement can be made. Backward elimination starts with a full model (a model contains all predictor variables) and eliminates one feature at a time. It eliminates the feature with least statistical significance (or equivalently, the one that improves the objective criterion the least). Stepwise feature selection stops when all features in the model achieve a certain level of significance (e.g. p-value of 0.05) and no other significant feature can be added. Alternatively, a penalized objective criterion (e.g. AIC—described later) can be used and the stepwise feature selection process terminates when this penalized objective is maximized.

b. *SVM-RFE* (recursive feature elimination) is an example of a more recent (and surprisingly powerful) wrapper method. SVM-RFE builds an SVM model and examines the contribution of features in the model. In each iteration, 50% of features with the lowest importance are eliminated, a model is re-fit and its accuracy evaluated in a test set. The process iterates recursively until predictivity drops. Due to SVM's resilience to high dimensions, SVM-RFE can produce a stable, highly accurate and non-overfitted set of features. What it typically lacks is minimality (although in practice it often selects parsimonious models).

c. *Bagging for feature selection.* In an attempt to improve the stability of feature selection methods and reduce their bias, bagging can be used. Models are constructed on bootstrapped versions of the training data using a base feature selection technique. Features that appear in some percentage (e.g. 50%) of the models are selected. The tendency of the feature selection method to select a feature because it randomly appears better than another can be mitigated by using multiple samples.

Univariate Selection Filtering. Filter methods select (or pre-select) features before the learning algorithm is applied to the data. Unlike wrapper methods, filter methods do not use a predictive model for evaluating the features, but rather use statistical criteria to select features. The advantage of this approach is that it is agnostic of the learning algorithm and can be much more computationally efficient than fitting the model to the data.

Univariate variable screening (aka Univariate Association Screening, UAS or univariate association filtering, UAF) is the most commonly-used filter method for pre-selecting a set of variables that have significant association with the outcome at a predefined significance level; or in the case of UAF, variables are ranked based on their univariate association with the outcome and the top k variables are selected. Any common measure of association (e.g. correlation, signal-to-noise, G2, etc.) can be used. The rationale for univariate variable screening is that variables without a univariate association with the outcome are (often) not relevant to the outcome. A key advantage of variable screening is saving computational effort since the dimensionality of problems can be reduced early in the analysis.

Embedded methods. In embedded methods, the modeling technique itself incorporates a method to reduce the influence of irrelevant variables. Examples of this approach are regularization techniques such as SVMs, LASSO and similar methods. These methods and the mechanism by which they eliminate features is described in section "Regularization".

Feature Selector Algorithms Based on Formal Theories of Relevancy

The previously described feature selection methods are essentially heuristic because they do not utilize a principled framework for optimal feature selection. In the remainder we will discuss formal feature selection frameworks (i.e., Kohavi-John and Markov Boundary) and will describe algorithms that conduct provably optimal feature selection.

Kohavi-John and Markov Boundary framework for Standard predictive feature selection problem. Kohavi and John [37] decompose the standard feature selection problem as follows:

- A feature X is **strongly relevant** if removal of X alone will result in performance deterioration of an optimal Bayes classifier built on all data.
- A feature X is **weakly relevant** if it is not strongly relevant and there exists a subset of features, S, such that the performance of the Optimal Bayes Classifier fit with S is worse than the performance using S U {X}.
- A feature is **irrelevant** if it is not strongly or weakly relevant.

Intuitively, choosing the strongly relevant features provides the minimal set of features with maximum information content and thus solves the standard feature selection problem (since a powerful classifier in the small sample or the Optimal Bayes Classifier in the large sample) will achieve maximum predictivity.

Recall from chapter "Foundations and Properties of AI/ML Systems" that a set S is the Markov Boundary of variable T (S = MB(T)), if S renders T independent on every other subset of the remaining variables, given S, and S is minimal (cannot be reduced without losing its conditional independence property). This is the MB(T) in the probabilistic sense.

Tsamardinos and Aliferis connected the Kohavi-John relevancy concepts with BNs and Markov Boundaries as follows: In faithful distributions (see chapter "Foundations and Properties of AI/ML Systems," "Foundations of Causal ML") there is a BN representing the distribution and mapping the dependencies and independencies so that:

We will further elaborate on the nature of these problem types by explaining subtypes 3 and 10 in the next two figures. These explanations along with the material of chapter "Foundations and Properties of AI/ML Systems" and especially the

1. The strongly relevant features to T are the members of the MB(T).
2. Weakly relevant features are variables, not in MB(T), that have a path to T.
3. Irrelevant features are not in MB(T) and do not have a path to T.

Thus in faithful distributions: the Markov boundary MB(T) = solution to the standard feature selection problem.

Local causally augmented feature selection problem and Causal Markov Boundary. In faithful distributions with causal sufficiency (see chapter "Foundations of Causal ML") there is a causal BN that is consistent with the data generating process and can be inferred from data in which: strongly relevant features = members of MB(T) and comprise the solution to the local causally augmented feature selection problem of finding:

1. The direct causes of T
2. The direct effects of T
3. The direct causes of direct effects of T

Thus in faithful distributions with causal sufficiency the causal graphical MB(T) set is connected with the probabilistic MB(T). Inducing the probabilistic MB(T) then:

1. Solves the standard predictive feature selection problem, and
2. Solves the *local causally augmented feature selection problem.*

Equivalency-augmented feature selection problem and Markov Boundary Equivalence Class. In faithful distributions the MB(T) exists and is unique [39]. However, in non-faithful distributions where target information equivalences exist ("TIE distributions") we may have more than one MB(T) [40]. The number of Markov Boundaries can be exponential to the number of variables and in empirical tests Statnikov and Aliferis extracted tens of thousands of Markov boundaries before terminating the experiments [40].

In TIE distributions:

1. The Kohavi John definitions of relevancy break down since there are no Kohavi-John strongly relevant features any more, only weakly relevant and irrelevant ones. This is because if S1, S2 are both in the MB equivalence class {MBi(T)} then: *independent (S1, T | S2) and independent (S2, T | S1).*
2. *The 1-to-1 causal and probabilistic relationship of the probabilistic and graphical MB(T) breaks down.* A variable can be a member in some MBi(T) without having a direct causal or causal spouse relationship with T.
3. The standard predictive feature selection problem is solved by the smallest member in the equivalence class of MBi(T).
4. The *Equivalency-augmented feature selection problem* is to find the equivalence class of all probabilistic MBi(T).

These feature selection problem types can be further subdivided as shown in Fig. 14. The problem types depicted were chosen on the grounds that (a) applied ML papers often aim to solve them, and (b) proofs of feature selection soundness often use these subtypes as the goal. They are organized from simpler/lower complexity or hardness in the bottom, increasing while moving to the top.

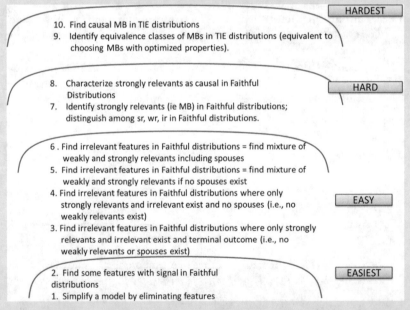

Fig. 14 A taxonomy of progressively harder feature selection problems. *From bottom to top of the figure, ten FS problem types of increasing complexity are depicted. Problems 1–5 are addressed with simple association criteria and can be tackled with regularized algorithms. Problems 6–7 correspond to the Standard Feature Selection Problem and require specialized algorithms. Problem 8 corresponds to the Causally-extended Standard Feature Selection Problem and requires specialized algorithms. Problems 9–10 correspond to the Causally-extended Standard Feature Selection Problem with Equivalence Classes and requires specialized algorithms.*

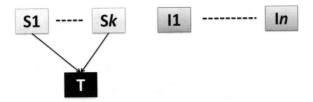

Fig. 15 **Demonstration of FS Problem type 3 in the feature selection complexity taxonomy.**
The response variable is depicted in black. Green variables are the ones we seek to retain and red
the ones to be discarded. Variables starting with *S* depict *strongly relevant* variables (i.e., cannot be
discarded without loss of information—see chapter "Foundations and Properties of AI/ML
Systems"). Variables starting with *I* depict *irrelevant* variables (i.e., can be discarded without loss
of information—see chapter "Foundations and Properties of AI/ML Systems"). In domains with
the data structure depicted and Faithful distributions, this problem is easily solvable by selecting
all and only variables with non-zero marginal (i.e. univariate) association with the response.
Regularized methods typically give zero weights to such irrelevant variables under these conditions

definitions of standard, causal and equivalency class problems, should make obvious their relevance to many real-life tasks (Figs. 15 and 16).

Modern Markov Boundary Algorithms—Faithful Distributions
We do not mention MB algorithms with only historical significance. For a review
see [34]. Modern MB algorithms with guaranteed correctness, sample efficiency,
and excellent empirical performance are instantiations of a broad family called GLL
and include several HITON variants (HITON MB, HITON PC, interleaved or not,
with symmetry correction or not, with additional wrapping or not, etc.), and MMMB
and MMPC algorithms. They can be instantiated for recovery of full Markov boundaries or direct causal edges only. The IAMB family also exhibits sound and computationally efficient behavior in real data but is not as sample efficient.

These algorithms have been extensively tested and compared to all major feature
selectors including wrappers, UAF, SVM-RFE, Lasso, LARS, LARS-EN, etc. See
the benchmarks in [34, 41] for experiments covering in total > 120 algorithms,
>270 dataset/tasks and multiple loss functions and data types. Consistent with the
theory of feature selection the Markov Boundary algorithms in these benchmarks
return the smallest feature sets and lead to classifiers with maximum predictivity.
They also achieve near-perfect empirical discrimination among strongly relevant,
weakly relevant and irrelevant features and are causally consistent.

Modern Markov Boundary Algorithms—TIE Distributions
Statnikov et al. [40, 42] invented the TIE* and iTIE* algorithhm families that can
extract the full equivalence class of Markov Boundaries. The algorithms are correct
and efficient. In typical usage they utilize GLL as subroutines . In [40, 42] extensive
experiments are reported with comparisons to dozens of real and simulated datasets
over multiple domains including comparisons with all availialbel comparators for
feature selection equivalence class discovery. According to these benchmarks, MB

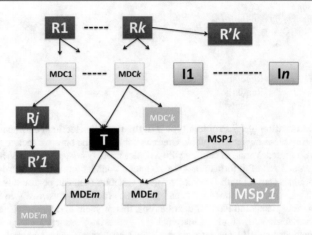

Fig. 16 **Demonstration of feature selection Problem type 10 in the FS complexity taxonomy.**
The response variable is depicted in black. Plain green variables are the ones we seek to retain and
differentiate. Red ones are to be differentiated (deep vs pale red) and discarded from predictive
modeling. Variables starting with M depict Markov Boundary variables (cannot be eliminated
without loss of predictive accuracy). An example MB is {MDC1, ..., MDCk, MDEm, ..., MDEn,
MSP1}. Variables with names starting with MDC are members of the MB and direct causes of
T. Variables with names starting with MDE are members of the MB and direct effects of T. Variables
with names starting with MSP are members of the MB and direct causes of direct effects of T (i.e.,
"spouses" of T). Variables starting with I depict irrelevant variables (i.e., have no information about
T and can be discarded without loss of information). Variables starting with R depict redundant
variables (i.e., have information about T but should be discarded without loss of information if
most compact models are needed). Variables with same name and the corresponding "prime" ones
without prime names are equivalent in information content with respect to the response T (we only
consider for simplicity contect-free equivalence [40]). A variable or variable set can have a large
number of equivalent variables/sets (not depicted here for simplicity). By substituting equivalent
variables, we obtain equivalent Markov Boundaries. For example MB {MDC1, ..., MDCk,
MDEm, ..., MDEn, MSP1} is equivalent to MB {MDC1, ..., MDC'k, MDEm, ..., MDEn,
MSP1}, and to {MDC1, ..., MDCk, MDEm, ..., MDEn, MSP'1}, and {MDC1, ..., MDCk,
MDEm, ..., MDE'n, MSP1}, and so on. An exponentially large number of equivalent MBs can
exist in a distribution. The feature selection/causal FS problem depicted requires highly specialized algorithms and cannot be solved with simple regularization or variable filtering

equivalence classes are common, their sizes varies across domains, and TIE* algorithms recover them with great accuracy.

We next provide a summary table (Table 3.) with properties of widely used feature selection approaches comparing their ability to tackle the feature selection
problems 1–10.

We close this section with the method label of feature selection methods.

Table 3 *Comparative capabilities of current FS strategies and algorithms including simple univariate filtering, regularized regression,* SVM-RFE and Markov Boundary methods across the FS complexity categories of Fig. 10."+" = can solve, "-"cannot solve

	UAF	Regularized Regression Variants (e.g., Lasso, LARS, LARS-EN)	SVM-RFE	Markov boundary induction in faithful distributions (e.g., GLL, IAMB)	Markov boundary induction in tie distributions (e.g., TIE*)	Markov boundary induction and active experimentation in tie distributions (e.g., ODLP)
FS problem type 1	N/A (model-dependent)	+	+	N/A (model-dependent)	N/A (model-dependent)	N/A (model-dependent)
FS problem types 2–5	+	+	+	+	+	+
FS problem type 6	-	-	-	+	+	+
FS problem type 7	-	-	-	+	+	+
FS problem type 8	-	-	-	+	+	+
FS problem type 9	-	-	-	−	+	+
FS problem type 10	-	-	-	−	+	+

Method label: feature selection (FS)	
Main Use	• Finding a small set of variables that has all information about the response (FS)

Context of use	• Can be used to reduce the number of inputs to a classifier or regressor model so that:
	  – Over fitting is avoided
	  – Learning is faster
	  – Deployment of a model is easier, faster, cheaper
	  – The ML models are more understandable
	• Causal FS methods also reveal local causal structure around the response variable
	• Some learning algorithms have embedded FS (for example Decision Tree learning and Random Forests). In such cases adding formal FS algorithms often further enhances their performance

Secondary use	• Data simplification, compression and visualization • Clustering and subgrouping based on FS transforms of the data

Method label: feature selection (FS)	
Pitfalls	**Pitfall 3.5.1.2.** FS methods that are not designed for causal discovery cannot be interpreted causally and any estimates of causal effects will be biased
	Pitfall 3.5.1.3. FS itself can be over fitted to the data if model selection protocols used are not well-designed (see chapter on overfitting)
	Pitfall 3.5.1.4. FS like any other component of analysis needs be tailored to the data and problem. Using a default FS everywhere may lead to suboptimal results
	Pittfall 3.5.1.5. If a classifier has embedded FS, DR, or regularization does not mean that it cannot benefit from FS
Principle of operation	Highly-dependent on the specific FS method
	• Markov boundary FS is based on Bayesian Network theory and is additionally concordant with Kohavi-John FS theory in faithful distributions. In non-faithful distributions MB FS has strong advantages over Kohavi-John FS
	• RFE-SVM is based on fitting SVM models and performing wrapping over models with progressively smaller feature sets chosen based on the SVM weights
	• Univariate association filtering (UAF) rank-orders variables according to association with the response and chooses the top *k variables*
	• Wrapping is heuristic search over the space of all possible subsets, each one evaluated for a specific classifier and loss function of interest
	• Stepwise regression procedures originated in statistics and examine a series of regression models by iteratively including and discarding variables according to inclusion and exclusion criteria while conducting tests of statistical significance of model improvement at each step
Theoretical properties and empirical evidence	• Markov boundary FS accurately solves the standard FS problem by finding the smallest subset of variables that has all the information in the data about the response. Worst case computational complexity for inferring the MB is exponential to the number of variables but real-life complexity of best-of-class algorithms on common data is very efficient. In faithful distributions with causal sufficiency the Markov boundary solves a causal version of the standard FS problem: It finds the direct causes, directs effects and direct causes of direct effects of the response. Equivalence class MB induction recovers the whole set of MBs in the data. Excellent empirical performance in most domains
	• RFE-SVM is not guaranteed to find the optimal FS solution and is not causally valid. Computational complexity is low order polynomial. It is very robust to small sample size and has very good performance in many domains
	• Univariate filter selection (UAF) is not guaranteed to give the smallest set of variables with all information about the response. The top-ranked UAF variables do not need to be causally related to the response. Computational complexity is very small and sample efficiency is high
	• Wrapping is learner-specific, computationally intensive and tends to overfit. Not suitable for causal discovery, typically
	• Stepwise regression procedures are relatively fast but do not guarantee correct results and tend to overfit

Method label: feature selection (FS)	
Best practices	**Best practice 3.5.1.1.** Markov boundary procedures are first choice for FS when modest sample size (or more) is available and regardless of how high is the dimensionality. They are particularly appropriate when causal interpretation of findings is desired and when we wish to have consistent and coherent predictive and valid causal models. Also when we wish to find equivalence classes of optimal feature sets or optimal classifiers
	Best practice 3.5.1.2. SVM-RFE is a first choice in very small sample size and high dimensional/small sample when causal conclusions are not sought
	Best practice 3.5.1.3. UAF is common in genomics. Contrary to common over-interpretation by some researchers, the top ranked variables are not strongly suggestive of biologically/mechanistically/causally important or even valid factors. UAF has a place however when sample sizes are extremely small
	Best practice 3.5.1.4. Generic wrapping and stepwise procedures should be (and are increasingly) retired from practice
References	[36–42]

Dimensionality Reduction

As we mentioned earlier, the main objective of dimensionality reduction is to transform a high-dimensional space into a lower-dimensional representation. While feature selection achieves a lower dimensional space by keeping a subset of the original features without modifying the actual features, dimensionality reduction combines several of the original features into new features.

Dimensionality reduction techniques can be categorized as supervised vs unsupervised and linear vs nonlinear.

1. *Supervised versus unsupervised*: supervised techniques can use supervising information (such as outcome) to guide the dimensionality reduction. For example, linear discriminant analysis uses the class label to help project a multi-dimensional feature space into a lower-dimensional representation that maximally distinguishes among the classes. Unsupervised dimensionality reduction does not use outcome information. In this section, we focus on unsupervised dimensionality reduction; high-dimensional classification or regression are handled in other parts of this chapter.
2. *Linear vs nonlinear*. The transformation that reduces a high-dimensional space into a the lower-dimensional representation can be linear or non-linear. New features created by linear dimensionality reduction techniques are linear combinations of the original features, while non-linear dimensionality reduction uses nonlinear combinations. For example, autoencoders are arbitrarily complex non-linear transformations (they may increase or reduce the dimensionality), while classic Principal Component Analysis PCA is linear. Nonlinear dimensionality reduction is also known as manifold learning ([43], Chapter 20). Unsupervised dimensionality reduction has a vast literature; here, we focus on two classical approaches. For other popular dimensionality reduction techniques, the reader is referred to [44].

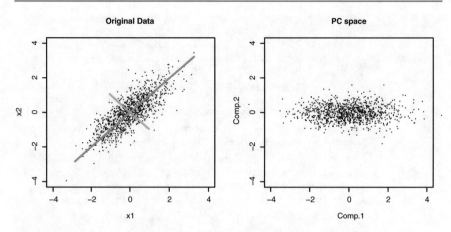

Fig. 17 Illustration of PCA. The left pane depicts a two-dimensional synthetic dataset. The blue and orange lines are the axes of the transformed space. The right pane depicts the same data set in the principal component space. The horizontal axis is the first and the vertical axis is the second principal component. The variance of the data is much higher along the first principal component than along the second

Principal Component Analysis (PCA)

Given a data matrix X, with columns as variables and rows as observations, find a matrix $U = [u_1, u_2, ..., u_p]$, such that (i) the u_i 's are orthogonal to each other and (ii) each subsequent **principal component** (or component for short) u_i, captures a maximal portion of the remaining variance.

Figure 17 depicts an illustration of PCA. The left pane shows the original Gaussian data. The variance of the data along both dimensions is approximately equal. PCA transforms this space into a new representation, the principal component (PC) space. Data in the PC space is depicted in the right pane. The horizontal axis corresponds to the first PC and the vertical axis to the second. As we can see, the variance (and thus information content) of the data along the first PC is much larger than along the 2nd. If we had to create a lower dimensional (i.e. one-dimensional) representation of the original data, we could choose the first PC as this new dimension, as it would capture much more variability than any of the original variables. In fact, among all linear combinations of the original variables, the first PC captures the highest amount of variance (under the constraint the total variances of the original and transformed space must equal).

Properties of PCA

1. The components computed by PCA are linear combinations of the original features. Thus PCA is a linear dimensionality reduction method.
2. Each vector u_i is an eigenvector of $X^T X$ for centered X.
3. The ith PC has variance λ_i, where λ_i is the eigenvalue corresponding to the ith eigenvector.
4. $\sum \lambda_i$ is the total variance.

Exploratory Factor Analysis

The motivation behind factor analysis is that a (relatively) small number of unobservable **factors** can explain the observed variables. For example, "intelligence" is a quantity that is directly unobservable, thus it is measured through a battery of tests that is believed to be related to intelligence. In this example, the test results are the observations and intelligence is the latent factor.

Given an $m \times n$ observation matrix X consisting of n observations (columns) and m features (rows), we wish to explain these observations by p factors, then a factor model is of form

$$X - M = \Lambda F + \varepsilon$$

where M is the mean matrix containing the row means of X in its rows, Λ is the $(m \times p)$ **loadings** matrix, F is the $(p \times n)$ **factor** matrix, and ε is the error matrix $(m \times n)$ with mean 0 and finite variance.

Assumptions. We assume that

1. F and ε are independent
2. The factors in F are independent of each other
3. F is centered.

PCA can be viewed as a special case of factor analysis where Λ is orthogonal.

Method label: dimensionality reduction (DR)	
Main Use	• Computes a lower dimensional representation of a high-dimensional features space
Context of use	• Lower dimensional mapping can help with visualization • Can be used to reduce the number of inputs to a classifier or regressor model so that: – Overfitting is avoided – Learning is faster • May reveal structure properties of the domain • Some learning algorithms have embedded DR (for example deep learning and other ANNs) • Factor analysis: Estimate the values of unobserved factors through multiple observed variables
Secondary use	• Data simplification, compression and visualization • Clustering and subgrouping based on DR transforms of the data
Pitfalls	**Pitfall 3.5.2.1.** Some nonlinear methods can be very computation intensive **Pitfall 3.5.2.2.** DR does not reduce the number of inputs that need to be measured in order to deploy a model. Many expensive, dangerous (to measure) and unnecessary inputs discarded by FS will be needed by DR to be measured for model deployment **Pitfall 3.5.2.3.** DR methods that are not designed for causal discovery cannot be interpreted causally and any estimates of causal effects will be biased **Pitfall 3.5.2.4.** DR itself can be overfitted to the data if model selection protocols using it are not well-designed (see chapter "Evaluation") **Pitfall 3.5.2.5.** DR like any other component of analysis needs be tailored to the data and problem. Using a default DR everywhere may lead to suboptimal results **Pittfall 3.5.2.6.** If a classifier has embedded DR, that does not mean that it cannot benefit from FS or regularization

Method label: dimensionality reduction (DR)	
Principle of operation	• Greatly differs by the method • Generally, variables in the transformed representation are required to have some sort of independence of each other, and they collectively capture maximal amount of information across the full distribution • Embedded DR constructs lower-dimensional transforms of the original data in a way that is consistent with the inductive bias of the embedding learner
Theoretical properties and empirical evidence	PCA: • The number of PCs does not exceed the sample size • PCs are independent of one another • PCs cannot be interpreted as causal factors and loadings cannot be interpreted as causal effect sizes EFA: • It is a probabilistic model • PCA is a special case of EFA when loadings vectors are orthogonal • Causal interpretation of hidden factor effects on measured variables under strong assumptions
Best practices	**Best practice 3.5.2.1.** When eliminating expensive, dangerous and unnecessary inputs by predictor models is beneficial, then use FS instead of DR **Best practice 3.5.2.2.** For prediction of specific outcomes, FS targeting these outcomes should be the methods of choice **Best practice 3.5.2.3.** Using a top-2 PC data transform is a staple of data visualization for exploratory purposes **Best practice 3.5.2.4.** Both PCA and EFA should not be over interpreted causally, predictively or otherwise **Best practice 3.5.2.5.** PCA for classification can be overfitted, so it needs to be treated like any other data operation by the model selection and error estimation protocol
References	• For an overview, see chapter 20 in Murphy KP. Probabilistic Machine Learning: An Introduction. MIT Press, 2022 • Hinton, G.E. and Roweis, S., 2002. Stochastic neighbor embedding. *Advances in neural information processing systems, 15*

Time-to-Event Outcomes

Survival data, (aka **time-to-event data**), describes the distribution of time until an event occurs. This **event** can be the failure of a device, incidence of a disease, a recurrence of a disease, an adverse event, or death. **Time** is the number of days, weeks, months, years, etc. from the beginning of follow-up until the event. Alternatively, it can also be calendar time such as the subject's age at the time of the event. We tend to think of events as negative, such as death (after all the field of survival analysis is named after studying survival time, the time to death), but it can also be a positive event, such as discharge from hospital. In the following, we use the terms "survival" and "time-to-event" interchangeably as long as context clarifies the use, and we also use the terms "event", "failure" and "death" interchangeably, unless this causes confusion.

Analytic tasks involving a time-to-event outcome are analogous to most other outcome distributions. The main tasks are (1) estimating the time-to-event (or the survival probability distribution S(t)); (2) testing whether two time-to-event distributions are statistically different; and (3) assessing whether one or more covariates (e.g. exposures) significantly affect the survival distribution.

The need for survival analysis. At first glance, time-to-event could be viewed as a continuous quantity and be modeled as one of the many known non-negative distributions, however, this approach breaks down for the following reasons. First, some subjects never experience the event of interest within the practical time frame of the study. Discarding these patients (with unknown time-to-event) leads to loss of information, because we know that these patients did not experience an event until the end of the study. In other words, time-to-event is not missing completely, it has been bounded. Second, some subjects are lost to follow-up before the study ends. Again, discarding such patients because their time-to-event is missing, discards useful information (i.e., that they had not experienced an event until the time they were lost to follow-up). Both of these situations are referred to as *right censoring* (see terminology section below). Third, in a study where the outcome is not death, many enrollees may have already experienced the event before enrollment. If this is allowed, cases with time-to-event = 0 can have high probability. Moreover, parametric distributions handle the general properties of time-to-event modeling poorly. As an example, fourth, outliers (extreme survivors) are common, and they have potential to become an *influential point* for some distributions. Also, fifth, many parametric distributions have parameters that mathematically relate to their moments (mean, variance). Censored data can make the estimation of moments on which model parameters depend, difficult, thus compromising the model.

Pitfall 3.6.1
In most practical settings, it is a significant pitfall to model time-to-event/ survival using ordinary predictive modeling classification or regression.

Best Practice 3.6.1
When modeling time-to-event outcomes, specialized methods, such as the ones described in this section, should be used, at minimum as comparators with conventional techniques.

Terminology

Let T be a random variable with T_i denoting the time at which an event happened to subject i. Let $f(t)$ denote the density of T and let $F(t)$ denote the cumulative density of T. The cumulative density is referred to as the **failure** function and is defined as

$$F(t) = \Pr(T \le t) = \int_0^t f(\tau)d\tau.$$

The **survival** (or survivor) function is the complement of the failure function and is defined as the probability that a subject survives beyond a particular time t

$$S(t) = \Pr(T > t) = \int_t^\infty f(\tau)d\tau = 1 - F(t).$$

Properties of the survival function. The survival function is monotonic, non-increasing, equals 1 at time 0 and decreases to 0 as time approaches infinity. [45].

Often, instead of the survival function, we model the instantaneous "probability" of an event. The **hazard** function is the instantaneous "probability" per unit time that an event occurs exactly at time t given that the patient has survived at least until time t,

$$h(t) = \lim_{\Delta T \to 0} \Pr\left(T \le t \le T + \Delta T \,|\, T > t\right)$$

Properties of the hazard function. The hazard function can be thought of as the "velocity" of the failure function or the rate of change in the failure function. Since the survival function is non-increasing, the failure function is non-decreasing and $h(t)$ is non-negative. The hazard is not a true probability, it is a rate [45].

The **cumulative hazard** is

$$H(t) = \int_0^t h(\tau)d\tau.$$

The hazard and survival functions are linked to each other through the following relationship [46]. By taking the derivative of $\ln S(t)$, we get

$$\frac{d\ln S(t)}{dt} = \frac{dS(t)/dt}{S(t)} = -\frac{f(t)}{S(t)} = -h(t),$$

which leads to

$$S(t) = \exp\left(-H(t)\right)$$

Figure 18. shows the survival (left) and the hazard (right) functions for the diabetes dataset in [47]. The horizontal axis corresponds to the follow-up time (in years). For visualization purposes we show points (in grey color) on the actual hazard "curve". There is one point every follow-up day. The hazard estimates can change frequently in any direction as long as they remain non-negative. To further improve interpretability, a smoothed version of the hazard curve is also presented in black. The survival curve is a non-increasing step function starting at 1 at time 0 and ending at 0 at time infinity. It appears smooth in this figure because of the high resolution (daily) and large sample size, but it is nonetheless a step function. Note that the survival

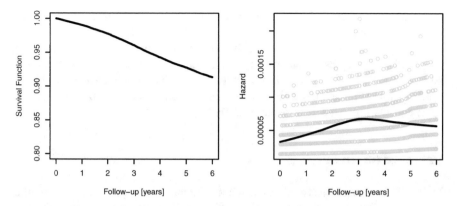

Fig. 18 Illustration of the Survival and Hazard functions. The left panel shows the survival function, while the right panel shows the smoothed hazard function for the diabetes data set in [47]

function relates to the *lack of* event (probability of *not having* an event), while the hazard function relates to experiencing an event (the rate of *having* an event).

Censoring

When a patient is lost to follow-up and is no longer observable, the time-to-event beyond the time of the patient dropping out cannot be observed. This is not a typical missing data problem as it first appears, because we have partial observations: the event did not occur while the subject was under observation. This partial observability is called **censoring**.

Left censoring happens, when the event takes place before the subject enters observation. We know that the event has already occurred at time 0, but we do not know when. **Right censoring** happens when the event takes place after the subject is no longer observed. We know that the event did not take place during the observation period but we do not know when/whether it occurred afterwards. Common reasons for right censoring are that the study ended, the subject is lost to follow-up or the subject withdrew from the study. Finally, **interval censoring** brackets the time of the event between two time points. We know that the event did not take place before the first time point and that it already occurred by the second time point.

Let C denote the time to censoring with density $g()$ and cumulative density $G()$. With $\tilde{T}$ denoting the true time-to-event, the subject's **follow-up time** T is $T = \min\left(C, \tilde{T}\right)$. Let δ denote the event type: $\delta = 1$ if an event took place ($\tilde{T} \, " \, C$); and $\delta = 0$ if the subject got censored ($\tilde{T} > C$).

Censoring is **random**, if $\tilde{T}_i$ is independent of C_i given X_i, where X_i is the covariate vector of observation i. Random censoring assumes that subjects who are censored at time t are similar in terms of their survival experience to the subjects remaining in the study. **Independent censoring** is a related concept. When a study has subgroups of interest, **independent censoring** is satisfied if censoring is random in all subgroups. **Uninformative censoring** happens when the distribution of C_i and $\tilde{T}_i$ do not share parameters [46, 48].

Competing risks arises when we have multiple outcomes of interest and the occurrence of one outcome prevents us from observing another outcome. As an example, consider heart disease and mortality as two outcomes of interest. If a patient dies (from a cause other than heart disease) we can no longer observe the patient's time to heart disease. In this case, we may have complete observation of the time-to-death, but we only have partial information about the time to heart disease: we only know that it is greater than the time-to-death.

Inference About Survival

In this section, we discuss methods to summarize the time-to-event distribution of a population. First, the time-to-event distribution can be summarized into a statistic (a single number) much in the same way as the mean or median summarizes aspects of a typical distribution. The fundamental difference is censoring: some subjects may not experience an event and thus their exact time-to-event is unknown. Next, we describe the time-to-event distribution as a function of time. We show methods to estimate the survival function and equivalently the cumulative hazard function. Finally, we present methods of constructing confidence intervals around the survival and cumulative hazard functions.

Summary Statistics of Survival

A concise way of describing the survival distribution is by presenting summary statistics. Often used summary statistics of common statistical distributions include the mean, the standard deviation, and the median. However in survival analysis, in the presence of censoring, it is desirable to account for the follow-up times when we compute summary statistics. Below, in Table 4, we describe some of the commonly used survival statistics [45].

Estimating the Survival Function

We present two estimators of the survival function: the Kaplan-Meier and the Nelson-Aalen estimator. They yield very similar results.

Table 4 Common statistics to summarize survival time distributions

Statistic	Definition	Remark
Average survival time	$\bar{T} = 1/N \sum_i T_i$.	Ignores censoring
Average hazard rate	$\bar{h} = \dfrac{\sum_i \delta_i}{\sum_i T_i}$	Uses hazard instead of survival to account for censoring
Median survival time	Survival time t, where $S(t) = 0.5$	Lessens the impact of outliers
k-year survival rate	Percentage of patients surviving k-years after their diagnosis [49]	Common choices for k include 5, 7, 10

The Kaplan-Meier estimator is more commonly used for estimating survival itself, and this is the preferred method for exploring and visualizing time-to-event data.

The Nelson-Aalen estimator, on the other hand, estimates the cumulative hazard function, and is mostly utilized by other methods, such as the Cox Proportional Hazards model.

Kaplan-Meier (Product Limit) Estimator

Let the index j iterate over the distinct time points t_j when an event took place. Let us assume that there are J such time points. The product limit formula is

$$
\begin{aligned}
\hat{S}(t_j) = P(T > t_j) &= P(T > t_j | t > t_{j-1}) P(T > t_{j-1}) \\
&= \left[1 - P(T = t_j | T > t_{j-1}) \right] P(T > t_{j-1}) \\
&= \quad (1 - h_j) S(t_{j-1}),
\end{aligned}
$$

where h_j is the hazard at time t_j. Expanding this formula yields the Kaplan-Meier estimate

$$
\hat{S}(t_j) = \Pi_j (1 - \hat{h}_j) = \Pi_j \left(1 - \frac{d_j}{n_j} \right),
$$

where d_j is the number of events and n_j is the number of patients at risk at time t_j.

Nelson-Aalen Estimator

The Nelson-Aalen estimator estimates the cumulative hazard as

$$
\hat{H}(t) = \Sigma_{j:t_j \le t} \frac{d_j}{n_j}.
$$

The relationship between the cumulative hazard and the survival function can be used to estimate survival, yielding the **Breslow formula**

$$
\hat{S}(t_j) = \exp\left(-\hat{H}(t)\right) = \Pi_{j:t_j \le t} \exp\left(-\frac{d_j}{n_j} \right)
$$

Comparison of the Kaplan-Meier and the Breslow (Nelson-Aalen) estimators (Fig. 19). Since $exp(-h_j) \sim 1 - h_j$ for small h_j, the Kaplan-Meier and the Breslow estimates are very similar and asymptotically equal. The Breslow estimate has uniformly lower variance but is upwards biased [46]. When ties are present in the data, the Kaplan-Meier estimate is more accurate. **Fleming and Harrington** proposed a

Fig. 19 The Kaplan-Meier and the Nelson-Aalen survival curves for the diabetes data set [47]. The two curves are so close that they are virtually indistinguishable

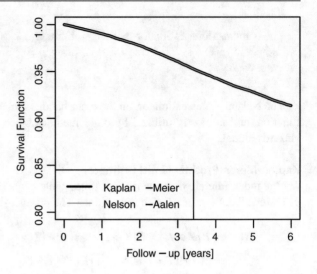

modification to the Breslow estimate by introducing a small jitter to break the ties in the follow-up times.

Confidence Intervals for the Survival Curves

Whenever conducting a survival analysis it is imperative to present confidence intervals (CIs). Statistical packages routinely offer such estimates. However when survival analysis is conducted with less conventional time-to-event modeling methods, often packages that implement these methods offer no facilities for CI estimation. We thus present here the fundamentals of estimating CIs for survival curves and hazard curves.

There are two fundamentally different approaches to constructing the confidence intervals and for each approach there are numerous variants. For brevity, in this section, we focus on one common method for directly estimating the confidence interval of the survival function. The interested reader is referred to Appendix 1 for the other methods.

Greenwood's formula. We consider constructing the confidence interval in survival space (as opposed to log survival or hazard space). The variance of the log survival function can be estimated using Greenwood's formula

$$\mathrm{Var}\left(\log \hat{S}(t)\right) = \sum_{j:t_j \le t} \frac{d_j}{n_j\left(n_j - d_j\right)},$$

where d_j and n_j are defined previously as the number of events at t_j and the number of patients at risk at time t_j, respectively. The *delta method* can be used to derive the variance of the (non-log) survival function, which yields the **plain-scale** confidence interval

$$\hat{S}(t) \pm z \sqrt{\hat{S}(t)^2 \sum_{j:t_j \le t} \frac{d_j}{n_j(n_j - d_j)}},$$

where z is the normal quantile corresponding to the confidence level [46].

Method label: Kaplan-Meier (KM) estimator of survival curves	
Main Use	• Estimate survival curves • Visualize the survival curves
Context of use	• Non-parametric modeling • Predict survival probability at time t • The data does not meet the assumptions of more sophisticated (e.g., cox regression) survival modeling
Secondary use	• Checking the proportional hazards assumptions
Pitfalls	**Pitfall 3.6.1.1.** Estimating the effect of covariates is difficult. A separate curve is computed for each covariate combination. Does not scale to more than a very small number of covariates
Principle of operation	• Non-parametric estimator
Theoretical properties and empirical evidence	• In biomedicine it is practically expected and used in every publication involving survival
Best practices	**Best practice 3.6.1.1.** Plotting the KM curve can reveal data problems. Consider the complementary log-log plot of the KM curve
References	Recommended textbooks include [45, 46, 48]

Comparing Survival Curves

Comparing the estimated survival curves from two or more populations. Two survival curves are considered statistically equivalent when the data supports the hypothesis that these two curves are identical and any apparent difference between them is due merely to random variations in the samples that were used to estimate the curves.

In this section, we focus on the **log rank test**. Extensions of the log rank test are described in Appendix 1. Consider a group variable, which divides the population into G groups. At each unique event time, $j = 1,...,J$, the association between grouping and survival can be assessed. The null hypothesis is that the hazard at time t_j is the same across all groups for all j. The alternative hypothesis is that the hazard differs between the groups at at least one j.

Let n_{gj} denote the number of subjects at risk in group g at time t_j and let d_{gj} denote the number of failures in group g at time t_j. For simplicity, we concentrate on the two-sample test, where $G = 2$. The expected number of failures in group 1 at time t_j is

$$e_{1j} = \frac{n_{1j}}{n_{1j} + n_{2j}} \left(d_{1j} + d_{2j} \right)$$

The observed number of failures across time in group g is $O_g = \sum_j d_{gj}$ and the expected number of failures is $E_g = \sum_j e_{gj}$. The **log-rank statistic** becomes

$$Z = \frac{\left(O_g - E_g \right)^2}{\mathrm{Var}\left(O_g - E_g \right)},$$

and the variance can be estimated from the hypergeometric distribution. Z follows a X^2 distribution with 1 degree of freedom and can be used as test of curve equivalence [48].

Cox Proportional Hazards Regression

Two important uses of regression models is to assess the effect of covariates on the hazard and to make predictions. Regression models we consider fall into two categories: semi-parametric and parametric models. **Semi-parametric** models, the Cox proportional hazards regression in particular, models the hazard as a product of a non-parametric **baseline hazard** function (which is a function of time) and (the time-invariant) **multiplicative effect** of the covariates. The covariates thus have a proportional (multiplicative) effect on the baseline hazard. **Fully parametric** models make a distributional assumption about the cumulative hazard (as a function of time) and model the parameter of this distribution as a linear additive function of the covariates. In this section, we focus on the Cox proportional hazard model (aka Cox model, Cox PH); fully parametric models will be discussed in the section "Parametric Survival Models".

The proportional hazards assumption. Fig. 20 illustrates the proportional hazards assumption using the diabetes example from [47]. The left panel shows the cumulative hazard of diabetes as a function of years of follow-up time. The orange curve in the plot corresponds to patients with impaired fasting glucose (IFG) and the blue line corresponds to patients with healthy glucose. At all time points, the ratio of cumulative hazard along the orange line versus the blue line is constant, 6.37. In other words, having IFG (versus not having IFG) confers a proportional, 6.37-fold, increase of diabetes risk upon the patients, and it remains constant across time. To translate this into the terminology of Cox models, the **baseline hazard** corresponds to patients without IFG (the corresponding covariate $x = 0$) and they have a time-dependent risk of diabetes depicted by the blue curve. Patients with IFG ($x = 1$), experience a risk (hazard) that is proportionally (6.37 times) higher across the entire timeline (orange curve).

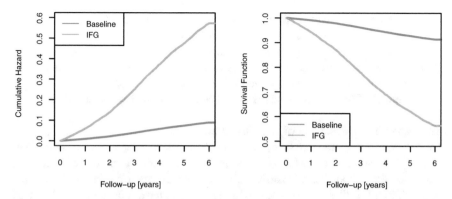

Fig. 20 Proportional Hazards Assumption. The left panel shows the cumulative hazard of patients with normal glucose (in blue) and impaired fasting glucose (IFG) (in orange) as a function of follow-up time (in years). The ratio of the underlying hazards of the orange line to the blue line is constant: the hazard along the orange line versus the blue line has the same proportion. The right panel transforms the cumulative hazard into survival probability

The Cox model. Let X be the covariate matrix, and let X_i denote the covariate vector for subject i. The hazard at time t is modeled as

$$h_i(t) = h_0(t)\exp(X_i\beta) \tag{1}$$

where $h_i(t)$ is the hazard of the ith subject at time t, $h_0(t)$ is the baseline hazard (common across all subjects) at time t, and β are regression coefficients. The cumulative hazards can be expressed as

$$H_i(t) = H_0(t)\exp(X_i\beta) = \exp(X_i\beta)\int_0^t h_0(\tau)d\tau$$

showing that the covariates increase (or decrease) the cumulative hazard proportionally relative to the baseline cumulative hazard. For additional details about the model (e.g. the partial likelihood function), see Appendix 1.

Assumptions.
1. The proportional hazards assumption: the covariates have a proportional (multiplicative) effect on the hazard relative to the baseline hazard.

    Consider two subjects, i and j, with covariate vectors X_i and X_j, respectively. The **hazard ratio** of these two subjects is

$$\frac{H_i(t)}{H_j(t)} = \frac{H_0(t)\exp(X_i\beta)}{H_0(t)\exp(X_j\beta)} = \frac{\exp(X_i\beta)}{\exp(X_j\beta)}$$

and is constant with respect to time (the $\dfrac{(\exp(X_i\beta))}{(\exp(X_j\beta))}$ ratio does not depend on time). The name proportional hazards reflects the fact that the hazards of two patients are proportional to each other.

Continuing with the diabetes example, if patient i has IFG ($X_i = 1$) and patient j does not ($X_j = 0$), with $\beta = 1.85$, the hazard ratio is exp.$(1.85) = 6.37$. Therefore, the ratio of the hazards between the orange and the blue curves in Fig. 20 is 6.37.

2. Independence. Observations with an event are independent of each other. Only observations with an event are multiplied in the partial likelihood.
3. The effect of the covariates is linear and additive on the log-log survival.

Testing the Significance of the Covariates

Generally, in regression, we have two ways to test the significance of a coefficient. The first method is the **likelihood ratio test** and the second one is the **Wald test**. Although the proportional hazards regression maximizes a partial likelihood (as opposed to a full likelihood) as it leaves the baseline hazard unspecified, this does not affect the likelihood ratio test and both methods remain applicable.

Estimating the Baseline Hazard

Fitting a Cox proportional hazards model does not require the estimation of the baseline hazard. After the model has been fitted, the baseline hazardfunction is estimated using a variant of the Nelson-Aalen estimator that incorporates effects of covariates

$$\hat{H}_0(t) = \sum_{j:t_j \le t} \frac{\delta_j}{\sum_k R_k(t_j) \exp(X_k \beta)}.$$

where $R_k(t)$ indicates whether subject k is in the risk set at time t_j. Notice, that when $\beta = 0$, this reduces to the Nelson-Aalen estimatorfrom the "Terminology" section.

The variance of the baseline hazard is also based on the Nelson-Aalen estimator $\mathrm{Var}(\hat{H}_0(t)) = \sum_{j:t_j \le t} \frac{d_j}{\left(\sum_k R_k(t_j) \exp(X_k \beta)\right)^2}.$

Making Predictions

For an individual i, hazard can be estimated as

$$\hat{H}_i(t) = \hat{H}_0(t) \exp(X_i \beta)$$

and the corresponding survival can be computed using the Breslow estimator (see section "Estimating the Survival Function".)

$$\hat{S}_i(t) = \exp(-\hat{H}_i(t))$$

Testing the Proportional Hazards Assumption

There are three methods for testing the proportional hazards assumption: (1) visual inspection, (2) formal statistical testing with time-dependent covariates, and (3) Schoenfeld residuals. We describe the first two methods and refer the interested reader to Appendix 1 for a more thorough discussion of the Schoenfeld residuals.

Visual Inspection

The first method is visual inspection of the log-log survival plot. Since under the proportional hazards assumption,

$$\hat{S}_i(t) = \exp\left(-\hat{H}_0(t)\exp\left(X_i\beta\right)\right),$$

its log-log transform is

$$\log\left(-\log\hat{S}_i(t)\right) = \left(\log\hat{H}_0(t)\right) + X_i\beta.$$

The log-log transform of two survival curves, corresponding to two different values of X_i, (say) x_1 and x_2, only differ in the $X_i\beta$ term, which is not a function of time t, thus the two curves should be parallel with a distance of $(x_2 - x_1)\beta$ between them.

To check the validity of the proportional hazards assumption, we plot the log-log transform of the Kaplan-Meier survival curves for two different values of X_i and expect these curves to be parallel.

A benefit of visual inspection is that we can see where (at what t) the violation of the proportional hazards assumptions happens and we may also see patterns that suggest the functional forms to correct the violation. *However, the decision whether the proportional hazards assumption is violated is subjective, no formal test is applied and hence no test statistic or p-value is obtained to guide the decision as to whether the proportional hazards assumption is violated.*

Figure 21 shows the complementary log-log plot of the diabetes data set. The two curves correspond to two levels of the covariate glucose status: the blue line shows

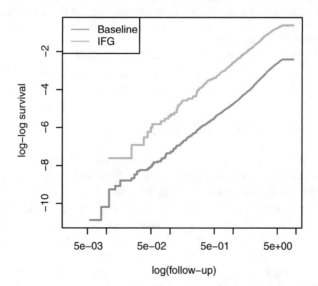

Fig. 21 Log-log survival plot of the diabetes dataset. The blue line corresponds to patients with healthy glucose levels, and the orange line to patients with impaired glucose levels. The log-log plots for the two levels of glucose status (normal versus impaired glucose) are parallel, suggesting that the proportional hazards assumption is acceptable

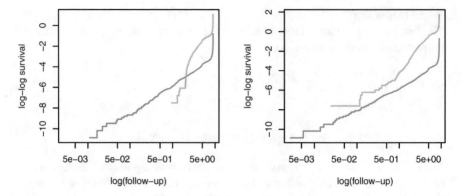

Fig. 22 *Violations of the proportional hazardassumption. The blue line is the baseline hazard,* while the orange line corresponds to some treatment. The left panel shows a violation where the treatment effect "switches over": while it is beneficial initially, it becomes harmful after some time. The right panel shows a violation, where the treatment line is a function of time. The curve suggests a function form (quadratic)

patients without impaired fasting glucose (IFG) while the orange line shows patients with IFG. Since the two curves are parallel, the proportional hazards assumption appears to hold for glucose status.

Figure 22 shows two synthetic examples where the proportional hazards assumption is violated. In both examples, the blue line represents the baseline hazardand the orange line corresponds to some exposure. In the left panel, the effect of the exposure changes from beneficial to harmful at about 2 years. In the right panel, the effect of the exposure (orange line) is quadratically related to (log) time.

Time-Dependent Covariates

The second method is based on time-dependent covariates. Under the proportional hazards assumption, adding regression terms involving interactions between the covariates and functions of time should not improve the fit. To check the validity of the proportional hazards assumption, we fit models of the form

$$h(t) = h_0(t)\exp\left(X\beta + \left(X \times g(t)\right)\gamma\right),$$

where $g(t)$ are vectors of function of time, $X \times g(t)$ are covariate-time interactions and γ is the coefficient vector of the covariate-time interaction terms. Under the proportional hazards assumption, we expect $\gamma = 0$.

A benefit of this method is that a statistical test is performed, a p-value is obtained, and thus the decision is objective. A weakness is the need for choosing an appropriate function $g(t)$. Different choices of $g()$ can lead to different conclusions. Common choices include the identity: $g(t) = t$; the log transform of time: $g(t) = log\ t$; and the heaviside function, where $g(t) = 1$ if t exceeds a threshold τ and $g(t) = 0$ otherwise.

> In practice different functions of t are tested. The complementary log-log plot can provide hints as to the functional form of the violation.

Addressing the Violations of the Proportional Hazards Assumption

The consequences of violating the proportional hazards assumption are usually not dire. Violations do not usually affect the predictions, they mostly affect the error estimates.

Workarounds for the violations exist, however, they end up answering a question that is different from the original research question.

When the data set is large, violations are almost unavoidable. Thus depending on the extent of the violation and purpose of the study, we may opt to ignore the violation.

Suppose a test reports a proportional hazards violation, we start by verifying that the non-proportionality is substantial. Not all non-proportionalities are substantial. Statistically significant non-proportionality can arise from large sample sizes, where even small deviations from proportionality can become significant; or violation can arise also from influential points. The former can be ignored, the latter can be removed. To assess whether a non-proportionality is substantial, the key method is visualization. Not only can visualization show whether the non-proportionality is substantial, but it can also suggest a functional form to correct it.

For example, a formal test reports violations for the diabetes data set. However, inspecting the complementary log-log plot (Fig. 21) shows no violation of concern; the statistically significant violation is simply a result of the large sample size (54,700 patients) and is inconsequential to the analysis results.

Once we verified that the violation is substantial and decided to address it, we have several options.

1. The first option is **stratified Cox models**. If the covariate with the non-proportionality is a factor with relatively few levels, it can be used as a stratification factor in a stratified Cox model. The non-proportional effect now becomes part of the baseline hazard. If the covariate is a quantitative (continuous valued) variable, stratified Cox models can still be constructed, but the variable needs to be categorized (into a few categories) before it can be used as a stratification factor.

2. If the non-proportionality is present in a relatively short timeframe and not in the entire timeline, the **timeline can be partitioned into segments** in which the proportional hazards assumption holds and separate Cox models can be constructed in each time segment.

3. Finally, if the non-proportionality was detected through methods (2) or (3—see Appendix 1), using time or a **transformation of time**, $g(t)$, adding an interaction term with the appropriate time-transformation can resolve the non-proportionality.

Method label: Cox proportional hazards regression	
Main Use	• Regression models for time-to-event outcomes
Context of use	• Right-censored data • Interest is the effect of covariates and making predictions • Same interpretability as classical regression models for other outcome types
Secondary use	N/A
Pitfalls	**Pitfall 3.6.3.1.** The key assumption is the proportional hazards assumption. Often, violation of the proportional hazards assumption is a non-issue, occasionally it can lead to problems **Pitfall 3.6.3.2.** The models assume linearity and additivity. Not appropriate if these assumptions are violated **Pitfall 3.6.3.3.** High dimensionality is a problem for the unregularized model
Principle of operation	• It is a semi-parametric regression model • The effect of covariates is a proportional (multiplicative) increase/decrease relative to a time-dependent baseline hazard • Coefficient estimates are obtained from maximizing a partial likelihood
Theoretical properties and empirical evidence	• Although a partial likelihood is maximized, the favorable properties of maximum likelihood estimation are preserved: Estimates are consistent, efficient and asymptotically normally distributed • Partial likelihood is convex and thus easy to solve
Best practices	**Best practice 3.6.3.1.** First-choice model for time-to-event data **Best practice 3.6.3.2.** Consider, additionally, whether the problem can be solved as a classification problem, or using survival modeling versions of ML predictive models **Best practice 3.6.3.3.** In the presence of substantial violations, different models, including extensions of the cox PH, may be more appropriate **Best practice 3.6.3.4.** Consider the Markov boundary feature selector for survival analysis that results from using cox proportional hazards models as conditional independence testing within the Markov boundary algorithm **Best practice 3.6.3.5.** For high-dimensional data, consider regularized cox proportional hazards models. Also consider the cox Markov boundary method described above **Best practice 3.6.3.6.** If age is included in the model and is nonlinear, consider an age-scale Cox PH model
References	Kleinbaum DG, Klein M. survival Analysis. A self-learning text. 2020, springer Therneau T, Grambsch P. modeling survival data. Extending the cox model. 2000, springer

Extensions of the Cox Proportional Hazards Regression

Several extensions to the Cox PH model have been proposed. In this section, we review some of them.

Stratified Cox Model

Stratified Cox models allow the population to be divided into different non-overlapping groups, called "strata". Each stratum has its own baseline hazard and each group may also have its own coefficient vector. The standard form of a stratified Cox models is

$$h_i(t) = h_{0k}(t) \exp(X_i \beta)$$

which assumes a common covariate effect across all strata that is proportional to the stratum-specific baseline hazard, $h_{0k}(t)$ for the kth stratum. The coefficients represent an "average" hazard ratio across the population (regardless of strata). This is the most flexible way of incorporating effects that violate the proportional hazards assumption, but stratified cox models offer no direct way of assessing the significance of the stratifying factor. An alternative form of the stratified Cox models considers the possibility of some covariates in a stratum (or some of the strata) having an effect that differs from its effect in other strata. Such effects are incorporated as interaction effects between the covariate and the stratum. If all covariates have interactions with the strata, then the resulting Cox model is the same as fitting separate Cox models for each stratum. Naturally, having to estimate separate baseline hazards and interaction terms requires sufficient sample size.

Recurring Events and Counting Process Cox Model

So far, time-to-event data was described by the triplet $\{T_i, \delta_i, X_i\}$, where T_i denotes the time to event, δ_i the event type (event or censoring), and X_i is the covariate vector. Alternatively, each subject's timeline can be divided into multiple segments and each segment can be described by a quartet $\{start_i, end_i, \delta_i, X_i\}$, where $start_i$ and end_i are the two end points of the time segment, δ_i denotes whether an event occured in the time segment, and X_i is the covariate vector. This format is called the **counting process format**. Many applications of the counting process format exist, here we highlight a few.

The first application is the change of the time scale. The term time scale refers to the way time is measured. The triplet format measures time on the *study scale*, and, specifically, time 0 is when subjects entered the study. The counting process format allows for different time scales. For example, time can be measured as patients' age, where $start_i$ is the age when they entered the study and end_i is the age when they experienced an event. We discuss different time scales later in more detail.

Another commonly used application of the counting process format is **time-dependent covariate Cox models**. Time-dependent covariate Cox models allow for modeling under the assumption that the covariates can change over time. The time scale is divided into multiple segments and each segment can have its own covariate vector. As long as the subjects experience at most one event, the time-dependent covariate Cox model does not cause any complications, even though each subject can contribute multiple observations (rows). This stands in contrast to longitudinal data analysis (section "Longitudinal Data Analysis"), where observations from the same subject are correlated and this causes estimation issues. The key assumption to avoid such estimation problems is that the subjects have at most one event.

A third application of the counting process format is when subjects can experience multiple events. The timeline can be divided into multiple segments when subjects experience an event: resulting in a separate timeline for the first, second, etc. event. Now, each subject can enter the partial likelihood function multiple times. Several remedies exist. First, we can consider only the first event of all patients. Second, we can use longitudinal data analysis techniques. Analogues of both GEEs and mixed effect models exist for time to event outcomes. A third, commonly used option is to initially fit a model ignoring the correlation due to the possibly multiple observations per subject (with event) and then re-computing the error estimates, taking the correlation into account. Chapter 8.2.2 of [19, 46] describes three popular variations of this option in detail.

Age-Scale Models

The term **time scale** refers to the way time is measured for a time-to-event outcome. Typically, time is measured from a particular event, e.g. enrollment into the study, to the end of study. This is the **study time scale**. An alternative is **calendar scale**, where time is measured based on a calendar, e.g. the age of the participant.

Changing the time scale has two important effects. First, the risk sets are different. At first sight it may appear that age scale can be easily converted into a study-scale by $T_i = end_i - start_i$, however, the risk sets are different. Consider two patients. The first one enters the study at the age of 40 and suffers a heart attack (event of interest) at the age of 51. The second one enters the study at 55 and suffers a heart attack 5 years later at the age of 50. On the study-time scale, we have two events, one at 5 and one at 11 years. At the time of the first event, at year 5, we have a risk set of two patients. In contrast, on the age scale, we have two events, one at 51 and one at 60. At both events, the risk set contains only one patient. Since the risk sets are different, the survival estimates (or equivalently the hazard estimates) are different, as well. These two time-scales yield different results and admit different interpretations.

The second effect of age-scale relates to how age is entered into the model. One option is to use study-scale and add a covariate that represents age; and the other option is to use age-scale. In case of using age scale, age is modeled completely non-parametrically; the baseline hazard is a function of age. As such, the statistical significance of the age effect is difficult to assess. Conversely, when age is added as a covariate, the usual assumptions (linear, additive effect) apply and the baseline hazard is based on time in the study. Whether we use age-scale or study-time scale can also be determined based on whether the model assumptions about age as a covariate are reasonable.

Parametric Survival Models

The Cox proportional hazards model estimates the effects of the covariates first and then estimates the baseline hazard in a non-parametric manner. Non-parametric estimation typically requires more samples than parametric estimation.

Parametric models that model the time-dependent hazard (or equivalently, the survivor) curves in a fully parametric manner, can be more sample efficient if their assumptions are met.

In this section, we model the time-to-event variable T using parametric distributions. Consider X, a covariate matrix, β the regression coefficients and W is the error term. Rather than modeling T directly, we model its natural logarithm as

$$\log T = \mu + X\beta + \sigma W$$

In this model, μ is called a **location parameter**, σ is called the **scale parameter** and W is the error term. Similarly to linear regression, in parametric survival models, the coefficients have a linear effect on the location parameter of the distribution of $\log T$.

Principle of operation. Recall from section "Predictive Modeling Tasks", that in OLS regression with covariates X, outcome y, and error term ε, the model can be written as $y = X\beta + \varepsilon$. The error term is assumed to follow a normal (Gaussian) distribution, with location parameter (mean) $\mu = 0$ and scale parameter (standard deviation) σ. The covariates linearly affect the location parameter and the outcome thus have the same distribution as the noise, i.e. Gaussian, but with location parameter $\mu = X\beta$ and scale parameter σ (which remained unchanged).

Parametric survival models work analogously. The error term W is assumed to have a particular distribution with location and scale parameters μ and σ, respectively. The outcome $\log T$ then follows the same distribution as W, with location parameter $\mu + X\beta$. The model assumes that the covariates effect the location parameter linearly. The various parametric survival models differ in their choice of the distribution of W. We refer the reader to Appendix 1, which discusses several such distributions and the corresponding parametric survival model.

Property [Accelerated Failure Time (AFT)]. The covariates shift the location μ, which accelerates or decelerates the passing of time. This class of models is referred to as **accelerated failure time (AFT)** models. Let $S_0(t)$ denote the survival time distribution when all covariates are 0. The survival time distribution for a subject with covariates X is

$$\begin{aligned}
S(t) &= \Pr(T > t) = \Pr(\log T > \log t) \\
&= \Pr(\mu + X\beta + \sigma W > \log t) \\
&= \Pr(\mu + \sigma W > \log t - X\beta) \\
&= \Pr\left(\exp(\mu + \sigma W) > t \exp(-X\beta)\right) \\
&= S_0\left(t \exp(X\beta)\right)
\end{aligned}$$

The covariates, depending on the sign of $X\beta$, accelerate or decelerate the passing of time by a factor of $\exp(-X\beta)$.

Figure 23 shows an AFT model fitted to the diabetes dataset. The outcome is diabetes-free survival, the horizontal axis is follow-up years. The orange line

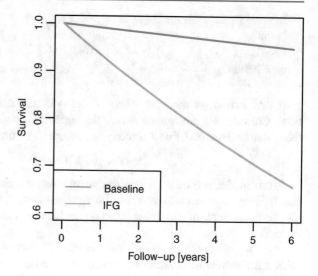

Fig. 23 Illustration of an accelerated failure time model on the diabetes data set

represents patients with impaired fasting glucose (IFG) and the blue represents patients with normal fasting glucose. Patients with normal fasting glucose have higher diabetes-free survival probability. If we draw a horizontal line at a particular (diabetes-free) survival probability, and compute the ratio of the time it takes to get to that probability along the blue line versus the orange line, we would find that this ratio is constant, exp.(−2.08) = 0.12 in this example. In other words, the time it takes for the diabetes-free survival to drop to a probability P is much shorter (takes 0.12 times as long) for patients with IFG than without.

Method label: accelerated failure time (AFT) models	
Main Use	• Regression models for time-to-event outcomes
Context of use	• Right-censored data • Interest is the effect of covariates and making predictions • Same interpretability as regression models for other outcome types
Secondary use	
Non-recommended Uses and Pitfalls	**Pitfall 3.6.4.1.** The key assumption is the accelerated failure time (AFT) assumption. Not appropriate if this assumption is violated
	Pitfall 3.6.4.2. The models assume linearity and additivity (location shift). Not appropriate if these assumptions are violated
	Pitfall 3.6.4.3. High dimensionality is a problem
Principle of operation	• Fully parametric model that specifies the full likelihood • The error term is assumed to have a location-scale distribution. This ensures that the log survival time has the same distribution. Covariates change the location parameter, accelerating/decelerating the passing of time

Method label: accelerated failure time (AFT) models	
Theoretical Properties and empirical evidence	• Parameter estimates are obtained using maximum likelihood estimation. They are consistent, unbiased, efficient and asymptotically normally distributed • AFT is a family of distribution with different properties Exponential survival model—Constant hazard assumption Weibull survival model—AFT and PH Log-logistic survival model—AFT and proportional odds assumption
Best practices	**Best practice 3.6.4.1.** Use AFT if the assumptions are met **Best practice 3.6.4.2.** Use cox PH if only the PH assumption is met
References	KleinJP, Moeschberger ML. SURVIVAL ANALYSIS techniques for censored and truncated data. 2003, springer Kleinbaum DG, Klein M. survival Analysis. A self-learning text. 2020, springer

Parametric Survival Models Versus Cox PH Models

If the model assumptions of the parametric models are met, the parametric models are more sample efficient. If the assumptions are not met or if we are in doubt, the semi-parametric model is more robust to model misspecification and only requires the proportional hazards assumption.

Appendix 1 describes method to check the appropriateness of various parametric survival models. In this section, we show one example, comparing the fit from a Weibull model (a particular type of parametric survival model) with Cox PH model.

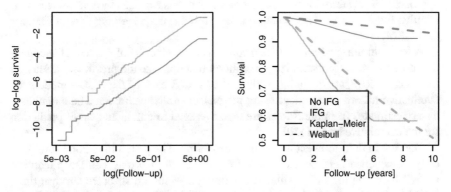

Fig. 24 Weibull survival model on the diabetes data set. The right panel shows the complementary log-log survival curve. The orange line corresponds to patients with IFG and the blue line without. The right panel shows the survival curves. The solid lines are estimated using the Kaplan-Meier estimator, while the dashed lines are computed from a Weibull model (see Appendix 1 for details). Orange corresponds to patients with IFG, while blue corresponds to patient with healthy fasting glucose

The left panel in Fig. 24 shows the complementary log-log plot of the diabetes data set. We continue to use impaired fasting glucose (IFG) as the sole covariate and the two survival curves were computed using the Kaplan-Meier estimator. The two lines corresponding to the two values of this covariate, IFG in orange and non-IFG in blue, are reasonably straight and parallel for the first 6 years. As shown in Appendix 1, the curves being parallel indicates that the proportional hazards assumption holds. If the curves are straight the AFT assumption holds. Beyond 6 years, the curves turn and become horizontal. They remain parallel but they no longer continue to have a constant slope. The turn signals a violation of the AFT assumption, however, they remain parallel, indicating that the PH assumption is still met. This appears to be a small violation, however, a large portion of the population have a follow-up time in excess of 6 years.

The right panel in Fig. 24 shows the Weibull fit (in dashed lines) and the Kaplan-Meier survival curve (in solid line) for the IFG patients (orange) and non-IFG patients (blue). We can see that the lack of events beyond 6 years caused a substantial bias in the Weibull estimates. We expected this bias based on the violation of the AFT assumption. Since the PH assumption is still met, a Cox model would be a better fit for this data.

Non-Linear Survival Models

The regression models in the previous sections all assume that the covariates have a linear (additive and proportional) relationship with the log hazard or log survival time. To overcome this limitation, the original features X can be transformed through a non-linear non-additive transformation to serve as the input to the partial or full likelihood function of the above models. Deep-learning based survival models and the Gradient Boosting Machine (GBM) for time-to-event outcome have taken this approach. The $X\beta$ term in the Cox partial likelihood is replaced by a non-linear non-additive function $f(X)$. This function is an ANN for deep learning and a GBM for Cox GBM.

A Random Survival Forest (RSF) consists of a collection of B trees. This collection does not directly maximize a likelihood function like the previously discussed methods, so RSF works slightly differently. In RSF, each of the B trees models the cumulative hazard of a patient using the Nelson-Aalen estimator. The cumulative hazard estimates from the B trees are then averaged to obtain an overall prediction for the cumulative hazard [50].

One key in time-to-event modeling is censoring. The partial likelihood automatically takes censoring into account, but the full likelihood may not. Deep learning models based on the full likelihood, assuming a Weibull distributed survival time, have been proposed. An alternative to the partial likelihood in the presence of censoring is the censoring unbiased loss (CUL), which is a general method for bias-correcting the unobservable loss. Censoring unbiased deep learning (CUDL) follows this strategy [51, 52].

High-dimensional data. Similar to non-survival regression models, high dimensionality, when the number of predictor variables is large relative to the number of observations, poses a challenge. In non-survival regression, regularizing the likelihood function was one of the solutions. Analogous solutions by regularizing the partial likelihood function of the survival models has been proposed in the form of an elastic-net style Cox model.

Survival models for longitudinal data. When we have longitudinal data, the covariates and the outcome can change over time. We have already discussed extensions to the Cox model that allow for changing predictors (time-dependent covariates) and recurring events. In the general regression setting, longitudinal data is handled through marginal models or through mixed effect models, because the observations become correlated. We have also discussed that in the Cox model, as long as we only have one event per patient, marginal or mixed effect models are not required [46].

Apart from providing the correct error estimates in the longitudinal setting, mixed effect models are also used for separating subject-specific and population effects. Frailty models are the time-to-event outcome analogues of the mixed effect regression models and allow for separating subject-specific effects and population effects.

Longitudinal Data Analysis

Longitudinal data is generated when measurements are taken for the same subjects on multiple occasions. For example, EHR data of patients is longitudinal as the same measurements, e.g. vitals, are taken at multiple encounters. Longitudinal data stands in contrast with single cross-sectional data, where measurements are taken (or aggregated) at a single particular time point. It also contrasts with **time series** data, where measurements are taken for a single subject (or for few subjects) for a long period of time and inference is conducted within the subject.

Using longitudinal data offers several advantages. (1) It can provide more information about each subject than data from a single cross-section since we observe the subject over a time span. (2) It also allows for a crossover study design, where a patient can be a control patient for himself: When a subject experiences an exposure during the study period, he/she is a "control" subject before the exposure and is an "exposed" patient after the exposure. (3) it also allows for separating aging effects from intervention effects. Finally, (4) it allows for separating subject-specific effects from population effects [5, 53].

Figure 25 shows an illustrative synthetic data set. Five subjects are followed over 10 time periods and a measurement is taken in each time period. The left panel shows a plot of the data set. The horizontal axis represents time, and the vertical axis is the measurement. We can see an overall upward trend: as time increases the measured values increase. We fitted a linear regression model to the entire data, which is shown as the bold black line. This model is a **population-level** model and it confirms this increasing trend. We also fitted a regression line, shown as dashed gray

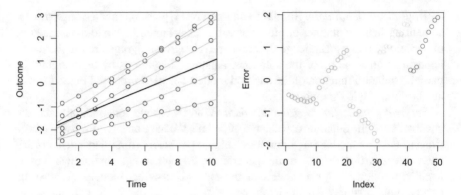

Fig. 25 Longitudinal Data Illustration. Five subjects are followed over 10 time periods and a measurement is taken in each time period. The left panel shows a plot of the data set. The horizontal axis represents time and the vertical axis is the measurement. The bold black line depicts an overall trend (population trend) and the 5 dashed lines represent the (individual) trends of the five subjects. The right panel shows the error relative to the population trend. The horizontal axis is an index, grouped by subject. Different colors represent different subjects

lines, to each individual subject. These are called **individual-level** lines. We can see that most (all five in this sample) subjects also exhibit an increasing trend, but their initial points (y-intercepts) vary, and their slopes also vary. Some methods allow for modeling individual effects such as the per-subject intercept and per-subject slope.

These advantages of longitudinal data analysis, however, come at a price. The multiple observations of the same patients are correlated with each other, which violates the i.i.d. (independent, identically distributed) assumption that most analytic methods make.

The right panel in Fig. 25 shows the error relative to the population-level regression model (the bold black line in the left panel). The horizontal axis is simply an observation index and the vertical axis is the (signed) error (residual). Observations from the five subjects are grouped together along the horizontal axis in increasing order of time: index 1–10 corresponds to the 10 time points of the first subjects, etc. Different subjects are depicted in different colors. We can see that the errors of each subject (errors depicted in the same color) tend to form clusters. Within a subject, once we know the error of one observation, errors of the other observations will typically not differ as much as errors from a different subject. This means that *errors of the same subject are correlated with each other*. There is also a trend within each subject: as time increases, the errors tend to increase or decrease. This is due to the differences in the growth rates of the different subjects (the differences across the slopes of the gray lines in the left panel).

When we assume that the errors in the right panel are generated from 50 independent observations, we would estimate the variance of the outcome to be about 1 (ranging between −2 and 2). Once we account for the fact that the observations came from 5 different subjects, the spread of the error becomes the range covered by the same color, and the variance becomes approximately 0.57; and after accounting for the differences in individual growth rates, the error variance drops to (approx.) 0.1. Such reduction in the noise variance leads to much improved estimates and is very beneficial for detecting significant effects from exposures.

> The data is **balanced** when measurements for all subjects are taken at the same time points.

When the data is balanced, coefficient estimates, whether they are computed using methods for longitudinal data or for cross-sectional data, will be similar albeit with substantially different errors. If the purpose of the analysis is prediction for previously unseen subjects, no individual effect estimates will be available, thus the results obtained from the regular regression models will be very similar to those obtained from the longitudinal models.

> Conversely, when the design is not balanced, methods specifically designed for longitudinal data should be used. Also, when the significance of the coefficients needs to be estimated, or estimating errors is important, or individual (within-subject) effects are of interest, or if predictions are to be made for previously seen patients (whose individual effect sizes are already estimated), methods specifically designed for longitudinal data should be used (regardless of whether the design is balanced or not).

As we mentioned earlier, the key drawback of using longitudinal data is the correlation among the observations of the same subject. All methods in this section address this correlation. Moreover, linear mixed models (LMMs) can additionally model within-subject variability, while generalized estimating equations (GEE) offer improved coefficient estimates at lower computation cost relative to LMMs. Both of these techniques are described in later sections.

Terminology and Notation

The sampling unit of the analysis is a subject or a patient and we index the sampling units $i = 1, .., N$. The analytic units are observations. Each patient can have multiple observations, indexed by $j = 1, ..., n_i$, taken at n_i different occasions (time points). The time of these occasions are denoted by t_{ij}, the time of the jth occasion for the ith patient.

The design is **balanced**, if all subjects share the same time points.

Let y_{ij} denote the response variable (of patient i at occasion j) and let X be covariates. The covariates for subject i can be time-invariant (constant across time) or they can vary across time (a situation referred to as **time-varying covariates**). The vector of time-invariant covariates for subject i is denoted by X_i and the vector of time-varying covariates from subject i at occasion j is denoted by X_{ij}.

Random effects are effect estimates that are computed for observation units that are thought of as a random sample from a population. In contrast, **fixed effects** are effect estimates computed for specific observation units. The within-subject effects are random effects, because the corresponding units, namely the subjects, are thought of as a (hopefully) representative random sample (the discovery cohort) from a population of patients. We could have conducted our study with a different random sample from the same population and we would expect similar results. Conversely, the time effects are fixed effects, because we wish to know the effect of a specific time period j on the outcome. The time points are not a representative random sample from a population of time points, they represent periods of exposure to the intervention. If we conducted our study using different time periods, say 2 months exposures as opposed to 2 days, we would certainly expect to get different results.

The questions we ask about longitudinal data are similar to and are a superset of the questions we ask about cross-sectional data. These questions include:

1. Are two sets of observations (y_{i1}, y_{i2}, ..., y_{in} and y_{k1}, y_{k2}, ..., y_{kn}), one for patient i and the other one for patient k, different?
2. Are observations at different time points j and k different ($y_{.j} =^? y_{.k}$)? Or more broadly, describe the changes in observations over time.
3. Making predictions. We may wish to predict the value of the observation at a particular time point for a subject we have observed before; or we may want to predict the value of an observation for a subject that we have not seen before.
4. Estimate the effect of exposures.
5. Estimate subject-specific effects.

ANOVA and MANOVA for Repeated Measures

Before the advent of more advanced and flexible analysis methods, repeated ANOVA and MANOVA were the first-choice methods for analyzing repeated measures data. In this chapter, we focus on the more advanced methods (which subsume ANOVA and MANOVA), and detailed discussion of ANOVA and MANOVA are presented in Appendix 2. Given their historic importance and hence presence in the health sciences literature, we still provide method labels for them below.

Method Label: Repeated Measures ANOVA	
Main Use	• ANOVA for repeated measures data
Context of use	• Single-sample or multiple-sample ANOVA
	• Assumes the data to be in the PP (person-period) format
	• Assessing the significance of time effects and treatment effects
Secondary use	
Pitfalls	**Pitfall 3.7.2.1.** Repeated measures ANOVA is not a predictive model
	Pitfall 3.7.2.2. Repeated measures ANOVA assumes compound symmetry; not appropriate when this assumption is violated
Principle of operation	• Operates on the same principle as most ANOVA methods
	• See Appendix 2 for detailed models

Method Label: Repeated Measures ANOVA	
Theoretical properties and empirical evidence	• Requires balanced design • Assumes the compound symmetry • Performs statistical tests of time effect and treatment effects • Contrasts can be used to perform specific tests (e.g. difference between two treatment levels)
Best practices	**Best practice 3.7.2.1.** Also consider the random intercept LMM. The LMM is more flexible and contains the ANOVA specification as a special case
References	• Hedeker D, Gibbons RD. Longitudinal Data Analsyis. Wiley, 2006. Chapter 2

Method label: repeated measures MANOVA	
Main Use Context of use	• MANOVA for repeated measures data • Single-sample or multiple-sample MANOVA • Assumes the data to be in the PL (person-level) format • Assessing the significance of time effects and treatment effects
Secondary use Pitfalls	**Pitfall 3.7.2.3.** Repeated measures MANOVA is not a predictive model **Pitfall 3.7.2.3.** Repeated measures MANOVA in its original form, does not allow for missing observations
Principle of operation	• Operates on the same principle as most ANOVA /MANOVA methods • See Appendix 2 for detailed models
Theoretical properties and Empirical evidence	• Requires balanced design • In contrast to ANOVA, it does not make the compound symmetry assumption, but it does not allow missing values • Performs statistical tests of time effect and treatment effects • Contrasts can be used to perform specific tests (e.g. difference between two treatment levels)
Best practices References	**Best practice 3.7.2.2.** Also consider LMMs • Hedeker D, Gibbons RD. Longitudinal Data Analsyis. Wiley, 2006. Chapter 3

Linear Mixed Effect Models

The key difference between methods developed for longitudinal data and for cross-sectional data lies in their ability to take within-subject correlations into account. Linear Mixed Effect Models (LMM), the subject of the present section, aim to partition the variance-covariance matrix into within-subject and between-subject variances.

If differentiating and estimating within-subject versus between-subject variance is of interest, then Linear Mixed Effect Models should be used.

Model Specification and Principle of Operation. Regular regression models model the outcome as a combination of deterministic "fixed" effects and a random noise

$$y_i = \beta_0 + X_i\beta + \varepsilon_i,$$

where β_0 is an intercept, β is a vector of coefficients for the fixed effects imparted by the covariates X_i and ε is a normally distributed noise term with mean 0 and variance σ^2.

Mixed effects regression models, similarly to regular regression models, allow for fixed effects, but they further partition the "noise" into different anticipated random effects. Different types of LMM models differ in the random effects they anticipate, which in turn, confers different structures on the variance-covariance matrix.

Let the subscript i correspond to the subject and j to the (index of) the occasion when the subject was observed. Let X_{ij} denote the covariate vector and y_{ij} the response of subject i at occasion j. The time point of this occasion is t_{ij}.

Mixed effect models are often expressed in the hierarchical format. The **first-level model** is on the *level of the population*

$$y_{ij} = \beta_{0i} + X_{ij}\beta + t_{ij}\beta_{ti} + \varepsilon_{ij}$$

and the **second-level** (*subject-level*) models define the models for the (subject-specific) intercept β_{0i} and (time) trend β_{ti} for subject i. Mixed effect models are a family of models that chiefly differ in the way β_{0i} and β_{ti} are defined.

Assumptions. Different definitions lead to different variance-covariance matrices based on different assumptions, however, all mixed effect models share some common assumptions.

1. As in all linear models, the fixed effects, X_{ij}, are assumed to have a linear (additive and proportional) relationship with y_{ij}. This assumption can be relaxed by including a priori known interactions and nonlinearities.
2. Time enters the mixed effect models explicitly (t_{ij}). This allows for observation times to vary across subjects. In many models, time has a linear additive effect on the response, however, models with curvilinear relationships will be discussed later.
3. The structure of the variance-covariance matrix is specified through a random intercept and/or trend. This allows for the dimension of the variance-covariance matrix to vary across patients, which in turn, allows for a differing number of observations across subjects. The second and third properties combined make mixed effect models appropriate for the analysis of longitudinal data that is not of repeated measures design (observation times vary) or for repeated measures design with missing observations.
4. Models in this chapter assume an outcome with Gaussian distribution, but mixed effect models have been extended to the exponential family outcomes through a linkage function that linearizes these outcomes. These models, Generalized Mixed Effect Models, are the mixed-effect analogues of GLMs.

In the following sections, we describe specific mixed effect models, their assumptions, relationships between covariates, time and outcome they can represent, and the variance-covariance matrix forms these assumptions yield.

Random Intercept Models

Random intercept models are mixed effect models with a subject-specific random intercept effect but only with a population average trend effect. The second level models are thus

$$\beta_{0i} = \beta_0 + \upsilon_i$$

$$\beta_{ti} = \beta_t$$

The subject-specific intercept β_{0i} is decomposed into a population average effect β_0 and a subject-specific random effect υ_i. The time effect β_{ti} is simply the population average trend (slope) β_t (without a subject-specific random effect). Thus, the random intercept model decomposes the "noise" into a subject-specific random effect υ_i and the actual noise at the jth occasion ε_{ij}.

It is further assumed that

$$\upsilon_i \sim N\left(0, \sigma_\upsilon^2\right)$$

$$\varepsilon_i \sim N\left(0, \sigma_e^2\right)$$

This yields a block-diagonal variance-covariance matrix. Each block corresponds to a subject and is of the form

$$\Sigma_i = \begin{bmatrix} \sigma_\upsilon^2 + \sigma_e^2 & \sigma_\upsilon^2 & \sigma_\upsilon^2 & \cdots & \sigma_\upsilon^2 \\ \sigma_\upsilon^2 & \sigma_\upsilon^2 + \sigma_e^2 & \sigma_\upsilon^2 & \cdots & \sigma_\upsilon^2 \\ \sigma_\upsilon^2 & \sigma_\upsilon^2 & \sigma_\upsilon^2 + \sigma_e^2 & \cdots & \sigma_\upsilon^2 \\ \vdots & \vdots & \vdots & \ddots & \vdots \\ \sigma_\upsilon^2 & \sigma_\upsilon^2 & \sigma_\upsilon^2 & \cdots & \sigma_\upsilon^2 + \sigma_e^2 \end{bmatrix}$$

This form of variance-covariance matrix is referred to as **compound symmetry**. It assumes that the covariance between observations of the same subject are constant over time. This is often unrealistic: observations closer to each other in time are typically more correlated than observations further away in time.

Random Growth Models

Random growth models, in addition to the subject-specific random intercept, also have a random slope for time. This allows (i) for changes (slopes) to vary across subjects and (ii) for time to enter the variance-covariance matrix. The second-level model is

$$\beta_{0i} = \beta_0 + \upsilon_{0i}$$

$$\beta_{ti} = \beta_t + \upsilon_{ti}$$

Similarly to the way the intercept was decomposed into a subject-specific effect υ_{0i} and a population-level effect β_0 in the random intercept model, in the random growth model the time effect is also decomposed into a subject-specific effect υ_{ti} and a population-level time effect β_t. It is assumed that

$$\upsilon_{0i} \sim N\left(0, \sigma_{\upsilon_0}^2\right), \upsilon_{ti} \sim N\left(0, \sigma_{\upsilon_t}^2\right)$$

$$\varepsilon_i \sim N\left(0, \sigma_e^2\right)$$

With subjects i and k being independent, the variance-covariance matrix is block-diagonal, with each block representing a patient and taking a form of

$$\Sigma_i = \sigma_e^2 I + T_i \Sigma_\upsilon T_i^T$$

where

$$T_i^T = \begin{bmatrix} 1 & 1 & \cdots & 1 \\ t_1 & t_2 & \cdots & t_{n_i} \end{bmatrix}$$

and

$$\Sigma_i = \begin{bmatrix} \sigma_{\upsilon_0}^2 & \sigma_{\upsilon_0 \upsilon_t} \\ \sigma_{\upsilon_0 \upsilon_t} & \sigma_{\upsilon_t}^2 \end{bmatrix}.$$

With time entering the covariance matrix, the covariance among the observations of the same patient can change over time.

Polynomial Growth Model

To model non-linear time effects, the level-1 model can be extended with polynomials of time.

Specifically, in vector notation, it becomes

$$y_i = \beta_{0i} + X_i \beta + T_i \upsilon_i + \varepsilon_i.$$

where T_i contains polynomial of t_i. To be able to model a quadratic time effect, T_i would be

$$T_i = \begin{bmatrix} 1 & t_1 & t_1^2 \\ 1 & t_2 & t_2^2 \\ 1 & \vdots & \vdots \\ 1 & t_{n_i} & t_{n_i}^2 \end{bmatrix}.$$

Comparison of the Various Model Assumptions

Figure 26 illustrates the difference among the three model types. Four synthetic data sets were generated using four different assumptions. In all four data sets, five subjects were observed at 10 time points. The four data sets are plotted in the four panels. For all four panels, the horizontal axis is the index j of the observations, grouped by subject. Since the key issue in longitudinal data is partitioning the errors (based on these four assumptions), the vertical axis corresponds to the error relative to a population-level model.

The first assumption is the *random intercept*. This causes errors to cluster by subject. The mean of the error in each subject is the subject's random intercept β_{oi}. No other structure can be observed: the scale of the errors remains the same over time.

The second assumption corresponds to the *growth model*. In addition to clustering due to the random intercept, the plot also shows that the errors consistently increase over time, at a rate that differs across patients. This growth rate is the random slope v_{it}. Observations of the same subject closer together in time have more similar errors (and thus observations) than observations of the same subject further apart in time. This is a violation of the compound symmetry structure, but the random growth model can handle this situation correctly.

The third assumption is *quadratic time, random intercept*. The data has both linear and quadratic population-level time effect but only a random intercept. We

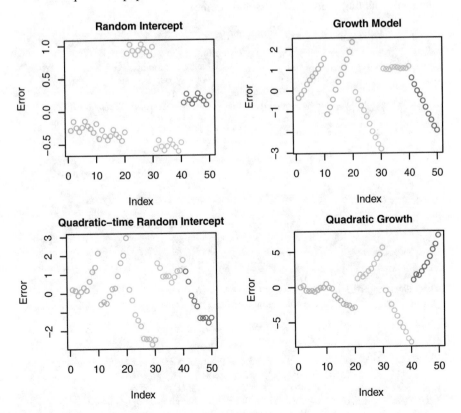

Fig. 26 Comparison of the various model assumptions

only removed the linear time effect, thus the errors (residuals) form a per-subject parabola, indicative of a quadratic effect. The parabolas have similar shape across patients (although different parts of the same parabola are visible), which suggests that this is a (quadratic) population-level effect, but the parabolas have different foci along the y axis, suggesting a subject-level random intercept.

Finally, the *quadratic growth model* has both population-level as well as a subject-level quadratic time effect. The quadratic structure is apparent in the parabolic shapes of the within-subject errors, however, the shape of the parabolas change across the patients, suggesting a subject-level effect. Because of the strong population-level quadratic time-effect, it is difficult to see whether the subject-level time effect is only linear or quadratic. The parabolas are located at different positions along the vertical axis, which indicates a subject-level random intercept.

Generalized Linear Mixed Effect Models (GLMM)

Generalized Linear Mixed Effect Models relate to LMMs the same way as Generalized Linear Models (GLMs) relate to linear regression models. GLMMs allow for a link function to link the expectation of the outcome with the linear predictor. Similarly to GLMs, GLMMs can thus be used to solve regression problems with non-Gaussian dependent variables, such as classification problems (logistic outcome), counting problems (Poisson outcome), etc.

Method label: linear mixed effect models (LMM)	
Main Use	• Regression models for longitudinal data
Context of use	• Longitudinal data with balanced or unbalanced design
	• Separates subject-level effects from population-level effects
	• Predictive modeling with within-subject predictions
	• Accurate error estimates are required or the interest is the statistical significance of covariates
Secondary use	• Generalized LMM has been developed for non-Gaussian response variables
Pitfalls	**Pitfall 3.7.3.2.** GEEs can be computationally more efficient and may produce better predictive models. Use LMM when the goal is to identify subject-level effects
Principle of operation	• Partitions the error into subject-level and population-level components
	• Random intercept model: Assumes a subject-specific intercept
	• Random growth model: Assumes a subject-specific intercept and time-trend
	• Polynomial growth model: Assumes a subject-specific curvilinear time effect
Theoretical properties and empirical evidence	• See the text for the detailed assumptions
	• ML estimator. Coefficient estimates are consistent, asymptotically normal
Best practices	**Best practice 3.7.3.1.** Use LMM when the goal is to identify subject-level effects
	Best practice 3.7.3.2. If the main purpose is estimating the effect size of covariates or making predictions for previously unseen subjects, GEE can be more computationally effective
References	• Hedeker D, Gibbons RD. Longitudinal Data Analsyis. Wiley, 2006. Chapter 4

Generalized Estimating Equations

As discussed earlier, the key statistical challenge with longitudinal data is the correlation among the observations of the same subject. This challenge is addressed by assuming a variance-covariance matrix for the error when the regression parameters are estimated. In the previous section ("Linear Mixed Effect Models"), we described a method for constructing such a matrix by separating the error variation into a set of subject-specific and a set of population-level effects. These effects define the form of the variance-covariance matrix. An alternative strategy is to assume a functional form for the variance-covariance matrix. This second strategy is the subject of the current section.

In this approach, the parameters that define the variance-covariance matrix are treated as nuisance parameters and the main interest is the coefficients of the covariates, including time. The variance-covariance parameters are marginalized (integrated out) and hence this type of models are referred to as **marginal models**.

Model Specification. The specification of the generalized estimating equations models proceeds similarly to that of generalized linear models (see section "Foundational Methods"). Given a covariate matrix X, the following components are defined.

1. Linear predictor: $\eta_{ij} = X_{ij}\beta$;
2. Linkage function that links the mean of the linear predictor to the expectation of the outcome $g(E(Y_{ij})) = \mu_{ij}$;
3. A variance function relating the mean of the outcome to its variance: $\text{Var}(y_{ij}) = \phi V(\mu_{ij})$;
4. A working variance-covariance matrix parameterized by a: $R(a)$

The first three components are shared with the generalized linear models; GEEs add the fourth component.

Several variance-covariance matrix forms are implemented by statistical software packages and the most common matrices are described below.

1. **Identity**: $R(a) = I$. This assumes that the observations of a subject are independent of each other and thus it reduces a GEE to a regular GLM.
2. **Exchangeable**: $R(a) = \rho$. Observations of the same subject have constant covariance ρ, which does not depend on time. This matrix form is the same as the compound symmetry in the random intercept models.
3. **Autoregressive**: $R(a) = \rho^{|j-j'|}$. With j and j' denoting two time steps, the covariance among observations of the same subject depends on time. If $\rho < 1$, then the further away the observations are in time, the smaller the covariance.
4. **Unstructured**. Each element of the matrix is estimated from data.

Among the four matrices, we have already seen the identity and the exchangeable structures and the unstructured matrix is straightforward to imagine. The autoregressive matrix will take the following form

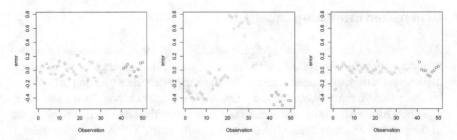

Fig. 27 Illustration of the error distributions corresponding to the Independent, Exchangeable and autocorrelated variance/covariance structures

$$R(\rho) = \begin{bmatrix} 1 & \rho & \rho^2 & \rho^3 & \cdots \\ \rho & 1 & \rho & \rho^2 & \cdots \\ \rho^2 & \rho & 1 & \rho & \cdots \\ \vdots & \vdots & \vdots & 1 & \ddots \end{bmatrix}.$$

When $|\rho| < 1$, increasing powers of ρ become smaller, thus the more distant two observations are in time, the smaller their covariance.

Figure 27 shows three types of error distributions. For 5 subjects, 10 observations were generated using independent error (left panel), exchangeable error (middle panel) and autocorrelated error (right panel). The 5 subjects are shown in different colors and their 10 observations are ordered by time along the horizontal axis. The noise has standard normal distribution with $\sigma = .1$ in all three cases. The error in the left panel is noise and all errors, regardless of which subject they came from, are independent: knowing the error of an observation for a patient does not provide any information about the error of another observation of the same patient or about any observation of any other subject. In the middle panel, the error has a noise component and a random intercept component. Errors are correlated within each subject and subjects are independent of each other. We have seen this correlation structure earlier. Finally, in the right panel, we have autocorrelated errors. Two errors of the same subject are more similar to each other the closer they are to each other in time

Method label: generalized estimating equations (GEE)	
Main Use	• Regression models for longitudinal data • A linkage function can be specified
Context of use	• Longitudinal data with unbalanced design • Most used when the focus is on coefficient estimates and making predictions for previously unseen patients

Method label: generalized estimating equations (GEE)	
Secondary use	
Pitfalls	**Pitfall 3.7.4.1.** No individualized effects are estimated. Consider the LMM if separation of the individual effects from the population effect is desired
Principle of operation	• Uses estimating equations • It is a marginal model. Assumes a parametric form for the working variance/covariance matrix and marginalizes it out
Theoretical properties and empirical evidence	• Uses M estimation. Specification of the likelihood is not required • Solving estimating equations is very computationally efficient • Even if the structure of the variance/covariance matrix is misspecified, it yields good results
Best practices	**Best practice 3.7.4.1.** Use GEE when predictions for previously unseen subjects is needed **Best practice 3.7.4.2.** Use LMM when subject-specific effects are of interest **Best practice 3.7.4.3.** GEE can be more computationally efficient than LMM
References	• Hardin, J.W. and Hilbe, J.M., 2002. *Generalized estimating equations*. Chapman and hall/CRC • Hedeker D, Gibbons RD. Longitudinal Data Analsyis. Wiley, 2006. Chapter 3

Brief Summary of Other Techniques of Interest

Network science. The field of network science [54] offers a completely different approach to conventional predictive modeling and causal discovery methods. Network Science leverages the remarkable consistency in the properties of a broad array of systems that are adaptive and robust. Systems that exhibit these measurable properties are called *Complex Adaptive Systems* (CAS) [55]. The application of Network Science to problems of health and disease is called *Network Medicine* [56] and its main idea follows: a disease represents a pathologic biological process that emerges, and is sustained over time, because it is embedded in a transformed biologic system that acquires adaptive properties. Accordingly, if such an adaptive system related to a given disease is identified, the capacity to determine its areas of vulnerability may reveal promising targets or new approaches for treatment. A typical network science analysis proceeds by building network representations of complex systems and then calculating a number of metrics on the network model. Such metrics include: Network Diameter, Characteristic Path Length, Shortest Path Distribution, Degree Distribution, and Clustering Coefficient. The specific structure and properties of the network model help the analyst identify drug or other intervention targets and other important system properties.

Active learning. The field of Active Learning studies methods for the iterative collection of data and corresponding refinement of models until an accurate enough model is built or other termination criteria are met. Active Learning methods address both predictive modeling and causal discovery tasks [57–61].

Outlier detection. Outlier (or novelty) detection methods seek to find extreme or otherwise atypical observations among data. "Super utilizer" patients is a prototypical example of outliers that has great importance for healthcare. Numerous methods have been invented for outlier detection over the years in many fields including statistics, engineering, computer science, applied mathematics etc. and they are based on multivariate statistics, density estimation, "1-class" SVMs, clustering, and other approaches [15, 62].

Genetic Algorithms (GAs). Genetic Algorithms are heuristic search procedures in the space of models that the analyst wishes to consider. For example, the analyst may use GAs to find a good linear regression, a good SVM, a good Decision Tree or other model of choice. The search resembles the process of genetic evolution and can be shown to advance rapidly to better models [21]. On the other hand, GAs are computationally very expensive and prone to get trapped in local optima (i.e., solutions that cannot be improved in the next reachable steps in any direction in the model search space, although a better solution does exist several steps away). GAs also are used when the analyst does not have a good insight about the process that generates the data, or about which method may perform well for the task at hand. When such insight exists, it is typically better to use methods that have known properties that guarantee high performance for the desired analysis [63, 64].

Visualization. Visualization methods rely on the capability of the human visual apparatus to decode complex patterns when these patterns have been represented in convenient visual forms. Another use of visualization serves explanatory purposes; that is, presenting and explaining results that were obtained via computational means. Interactive data visualizations, where users are allowed to manipulate their views of the data to obtain more information, have been found to be rapid and efficacious in identifying early infection and rejection events in lung transplant patients [65]. Data visualization can also be useful in displaying health care data, such as that coded with the Omaha System; and intraoperative anesthesia data, such as maintenance of blood pressure [66]. Evaluation techniques have been developed to gauge visualization effectiveness in clinical care [67]. Significant challenges exist, however, in implementing visualization more widely in electronic health records, many of them resulting from the highly multivariable nature of case-oriented medical data which can lead to misleading results. In biological research, heatmaps, clustering, PCA-based visualization and lately t-SNE are very widely used [68].

Recommended Level of Understanding for Professional Data Scientists

The information provided in chapters "Foundations and Properties of AI/ML Systems," "An Appraisal and Operating Characteristics of Major ML Methods Applicable in Healthcare and Health Science," and "Foundations of Causal ML" describing fundamental techniques and their properties aims to provide on one hand a **big picture description** of methods, and a **concise summary of their relative and absolute strengths and weaknesses and types of outputs (e.g., models) produced by each method**.

We recommend that the reader commits to memory the methods information in the above chapters to the extent feasible, and especially for the application domain(s) of interest to them. This will help them evaluate, choose and appropriately apply the right methods, a skill set that eventually, with time and practice will become second nature.

The professional data scientist however should have a much deeper level of understanding that in addition to the information here includes knowing the key algorithms of each method family and possess the ability[1] for each algorithm to:

(a) Describe it in pseudocode from memory;
(b) code it in a programming language of choice;
(c) trace the algorithm on paper for small but representative example problems;
(d) describe the algorithm's function to an expert, a novice, or a lay person at the appropriate level of nuance/simplification;
(e) recite its key theoretical properties;
(f) prove the properties or at least outline the essence of the proofs; and
(g) interpret the algorithms' output.

These skills are typically developed with a combination of formal training, and hands-on experience. The many technical references provided throughout this volume provide a core knowledge base for the technically-oriented reader.

[1] "Possessing the ability" should not be interpreted that the professional data scientists should code all the programs personally, but rather know how it should be done correctly so that they can manage programmers, or evaluate third party codes.

Classroom Assignments and Discussion Topics Chapter "An Appraisal and Operating Characteristics of Major ML Methods Applicable in Healthcare and Health Science"

1. What kind of ML tasks are implied by the following questions? (There could be more than one correct answers.)

    (a) What is a particular patient's risk of type-2 diabetes mellitus (T2DM) in 7 years?
    (b) How many years will it take for a particular patient to develop T2DM?
    (c) What is the likely next diseases a particular patient with T2DM will develop?
    (d) What diseases do patients with T2DM typically develop?
    (e) In patients with T2DM, what other diseases are commonly present?
    (f) What is the average age at which patients develop T2DM?
    (g) At what age is a particular patient going to develop T2DM?
    (h) What is the expected cost of medications (per annum) for an average T2DM patient?
    (i) What is the expected cost of medications (per annum) for a particular patient (given other diseases the patient may suffer from)?

2. What kind of modeling tasks are described by the following questions? Also, name the outcome type. There can be more than one solution; give as many answers as you can.

    (a) Predicting the length-of-stay for hospitalized patients.
    (b) Predicting whether the length-of-stay of hospitalized patients will exceed 9 days.
    (c) Predicting the risk of developing diabetes (in patients who are not known to have diabetes currently).

        • We wish to know the probability that the patient develops diabetes within 7 years from now.
        • We wish to know the probability that the patient develops diabetes on any day between now and 7 years from now.
        • We wish to know how many days (from now) it will take for a patient to develop diabetes.

    (d) Predicting the type of cancer (e.g. small-cell, non-small-cell, large-cell, squamous cell).
    (e) Given a sequence of diseases a patient has already developed, predict the most likely next disease.
    (f) What kind of diseases do hospitalized patients with a length-of-stay in excess of 4 days suffer from?
    (g) What are the most common reasons (e.g. admitting diagnoses) for receiving opioids?
    (h) Identify distinct patient groups, based on their lab results, in a cohort of pre-operative patients.

3. What are the most appropriate modelling methods in the following scenarios? Assume you are tasked with building a diabetes risk prediction model that estimates the probability that a patient develops diabetes in 7 years given the patients' health records.

   (a) Suppose you have 20 different predictor variables, which are reasonably informative and uncorrelated, have 100 patients in your training sample, and each patient has one observation vector (for all 20 predictor variables).
   (b) Suppose you have the same 20 predictor variables as in (a), but now you have 10,000 patients, each contributing one observation vector.
   (c) Suppose you have 200 predictor variables that form highly correlated blocks. Each variable is important and has its own unique effect despite the high correlation. Further, you only have 200 patients, one observation vector per patient.
   (d) Suppose you have 2000 predictor variables, most of which are irrelevant to the task at hand. Unfortunately, you do not know a priori which variables are irrelevant. You have 200 patients, one observation vector per patient.
   (e) Suppose you have 20 different predictor variables, which are reasonably informative and uncorrelated, 1000 patients, and you have 10 observation vectors per patient. These 10 observations were collected at equally spaced time intervals for all patients.
   (f) Suppose you have 20 different predictor variables, which are reasonably informative and uncorrelated, 1000 patients, and you have 10 observation vectors per patient. These 10 observations were collected at exactly the same time for all patients.
   (g) Suppose you have 20 different predictor variables, which are reasonably informative and uncorrelated, 1000 patients, and you have 10 observation vectors per patient. These 10 observations were collected at different times for each patient and the collection time is known.
   (h) Suppose you have 20 different predictor variables, which are reasonably informative and uncorrelated, 1000 patients, and you have varying number of observations per patient.

4. You are tasked with building a survival (time-to-event) model that estimates patients' risk of developing diabetes at any time within the next 7 years. What kind of model would you use in the same scenarios as in question 3?

5. You have decided to build classifiers for a classification task. You are given the predictor variables, the outcome and a training data set. What models would be appropriate under the following scenarios?

   (a) The predictor variables are not highly correlated, all have approximately linear effects, and your training data set contains 10 observations per predictor variable.
   (b) The predictor variables are not highly correlated, all have approximately linear effects, and you have several million observations per predictor variable. Which algorithms are most likely to run into computational problems?

(c) The predictor variables are not highly correlated, but they may have unknown non-linear effects. You have sufficient amount of data, but not to the extent where you would expect computational issues.

(d) The predictor variables are not highly correlated, but they may have unknown non-linear effects. You have only 1 observation per predictor variable.

(e) The predictor variables are correlated and may have unknown non-linear effects. You have sufficient amount of data for any algorithm.

(f) The predictor variables are not highly correlated, all have approximately linear effects, and the clinical expects are asking for an "interpretable model". Select a model type and explain why (or how) it is "interpretable".

(g) The predictor variables are correlated and may have unknown non-linear effects. You need to build an "interpretable" model. The predictive performance "is not the primary concern".

(h) The clinical experts are asking for a model that is highly interpretable and has the best possible predictive performance. What do you tell the experts?

6. A data representation is a collection of features (variables) obtained by transforming the original variables. For example, a variable set obtained through dimensionality reduction is a (lower-dimensional) data representation. In this question, your goal is to create a data representation, appropriate under the following conditions.

(a) Predictor variables are reasonably linear, have no interactions, and sufficient observations exist. We want the resulting variables to be orthogonal to each other.

(b) Predictor variables are reasonably linear, have no interactions, and sufficient observations exist. We want the resulting variables to be "independent" of each other in some sense. Select a method and explain what "independent" means for that method.

(c) Predictor variables are reasonably linear, have no interactions, and we wish to have a low-dimensional representation to visualize the data.

(d) Predictor variables may have nonlinear effects, interactions and we wish to build a survival model or a classifier (we do not know yet) using the new representation.

References

1. Stanton, J.M., 2001. Galton, Pearson, and the peas: a brief history of linear regression for statistics instructors. J Stat Educ, 9(3).
2. Taboga M. "Gauss Markov theorem", Lectures on probability theory and mathematical statistics. Kindle Direct Publishing; 2021. Online appendix. https://www.statlect.com/fundamentals-of-statistics/Gauss-Markov-theorem.
3. Hilbe JM. Generalized linear models. Encyclopedia of mathematics. http://encyclopediaofmath.org/index.php?title=Generalized_linear_models&oldid=38890.
4. GLM N, McCullagh P, Nelder JA. Generalized linear models. CRC Press; 1989.
5. Stroup WW. Generalized linear mixed models. Modern Concepts: Methods and Applications. CRC Press; 2013.

6. Agresti A. Categorical data anlaysis. 2nd ed. Chapter 7.2. Wiley Interscience; 2002.
7. Zhang, Wei. Shift-invariant pattern recognition neural network and its optical architecture. Proceedings of Annual Conference of the Japan Society of Applied Physics.1988.
8. Rumelhart DE, Hinton GE, Williams RJ. Learning internal representations by error propagation. Tech. rep. ICS 8504. San Diego, California: Institute for Cognitive Science, University of California; 1985.
9. Hochreiter S, Schmidhuber J. Long short-term memory. Neural Comput. 1997;9(8):1735–80. https://doi.org/10.1162/neco.1997.9.8.1735.
10. Attention is all you need. NIPS'17: Proceedings of the 31st International Conference on Neural Information Processing Systems. 2017 P. 6000–6010.
11. Scarselli F, Gori M, Tsoi AC, Hagenbuchner M, Monfardini G. The graph neural network model. IEEE Trans Neural Netw. 2009 Jan;20(1):61–80. https://doi.org/10.1109/TNN.2008.2005605.
12. Zhang M, Li J. A commentary of GPT-3 in MIT technology review 2021. Fundament Res. 2021;1(6):831–3.
13. Jia X, Willard J, Karpatne A, Read JS, Zwart JA, Steinbach M, Kumar V. Physics-guided machine learning for scientific discovery: an application in simulating lake temperature profiles. ACM/IMS Transactions on Data Science. 2021;2(3):1–26.
14. Vapnik V. The nature of statistical learning theory. Springer Science & Business Media; 2013.
15. Statnikov A, Aliferis CF, Hardin DP, Guyon I. A gentle introduction to support vector machines. In: Biomedicine: theory and methods, vol. 1. World Scientific; 2011.
16. Statnikov,A, Aliferis, CF, Hardin DP, Guyon I. A gentle introduction to support vector machines. In: Biomedicine: case studies and benchmarks (Vol. 2). World Scientific. 2012.
17. Domingos P, Pazzani M. On the optimality of the simple Bayesian classifier under zero-one loss. Mach Learn. 1997;29:103–30.
18. Cover T, Hart P. Nearest neighbor pattern classification. IEEE Trans Inf Theory. 1967;13(1):21–7.
19. Hart PE, Stork DG, Duda RO. Pattern classification. Hoboken: Wiley; 2000.
20. Tan PN, Steinbach M, Kumar V. Introduction to data mining. Pearson Education; 2018.
21. Mitchell, T.M., 1997. Machine learning (Vol. 1, 9). New York: McGraw.
22. Dupuy A, Simon RM. Critical review of published microarray studies for cancer outcome and guidelines on statistical analysis and reporting. J Natl Cancer Inst. 2007;99(2):147–57.
23. Wolpert DH. Stacked generalization. Neural Netw. 1992;5(2):241–59. https://doi.org/10.1016/s0893-6080(05)80023-1.
24. Breiman L. Stacked regressions. Mach Learn. 1996;24:49–64. https://doi.org/10.1007/BF00117832.
25. Couronné R, Probst P, Boulesteix AL. Random forest versus logistic regression: a large-scale benchmark experiment. BMC Bioinformatics. 2018;19:270. https://doi.org/10.1186/s12859-018-2264-5.
26. Hastie T, Tibshirani R, Friedman JH, Friedman JH. The elements of statistical learning: data mining, inference, and prediction, vol. 2. New York: springer; 2009. p. 1–758.
27. Zou H. The adaptive lasso and its oracle properties. J Am Stat Assoc. 2006;101(476):1418–29.
28. Yuan M, Lin Y. Model selection and estimation in regression with grouped variables. J R Stat Soc Ser B. 2007;68(1):49–67.
29. Simon N, Friedman J, Hastie T, Tibshirani R. A sparse-group lasso. J Comput Graphical Stat. 2013;22(2)
30. Friedman J, Hastie T, Tibshirani R. Sparse inverse covariance estimation with the graphical lasso. Biostatistics. 2008;9(3):432–41.
31. You J, Yu B, Maybank SJ, Tao D. Knowledge distillation: a survey. 2021. https://arxiv.org/abs/2006.05525.
32. Zheng X, Aragam B, Ravikumar P, Xing EP. DAGs with no tears: continuous optimization for structure learning. 2018.
33. Goodfellow I, Bengio Y, Courville A. Deep learning. MIT Press; 2016.

34. Aliferis CF, Statnikov A, Tsamardinos I, Mani S, Koutsoukos XD. Local causal and Markov blanket induction for causal discovery and feature selection for classification part I: algorithms and empirical evaluation. J Mach Learn Res. 2010;11(1):171–234.

35. Aliferis, CF, Statnikov, A, Tsamardinos, I, Mani, S and Koutsoukos, XD, 2010. Local causal and Markov blanket induction for causal discovery and feature selection for classification part II: analysis and extensions. Journal of Machine Learning Research, 11(1).

36. Guyon I, Elisseeff A. An introduction to variable and feature selection. J Mach Learn Res. 2003;3(Mar):1157–82.

37. Kohavi R, John GH. Wrappers for feature subset selection. Artif Intell. 1997;97(1–2):273–324.

38. Harrell FE. Regression modeling strategies: with applications to linear models, logistic regression, and survival analysis, vol. 608. New York: springer; 2001.

39. Pearl J. Causality. Cambridge university press; 2009.

40. Statnikov A, Lemeir J, Aliferis CF. Algorithms for discovery of multiple Markov boundaries. J Mach Learn Res. 2013;14(1):499–566.

41. Aphinyanaphongs Y, Tsamardinos I, Statnikov A, Hardin D, Aliferis CF. Text categorization models for high-quality article retrieval in internal medicine. J Am Med Inform Assoc. 2005;12(2):207–16.

42. Statnikov A, Aliferis CF. Analysis and computational dissection of molecular signature multiplicity. PLoS Comput Biol. 2010;6(5):e1000790.

43. Murphy KP. Manifold learning. In: Probabilistic machine learning: an introduction, chapter 20. MIT Press; 2022.

44. Murphy KP. Probabilistic machine learning: an introduction. MIT Press; 2022.

45. Kleinbaum DG, Klein M. Survival Analysis. A self-learning text. Springer; 2020.

46. Therneau T, Grambsch P. Modeling Survival Data: extending the Cox Model. Springer; 2000.

47. Castro MR, Simon G, Cha SS, Yawn BP, Melton LJ, Caraballo PJ. Statin use, diabetes incidence and overall mortality in normoglycemic and impaired fasting glucose patients. J Gen Intern Med. 2016;31:502–8.

48. KleinJP MML. Survival Analysis techniques for censored and truncated data. Springer; 2003.

49. National Cancer Institute. Five-year survival rate. https://www.cancer.gov/publications/dictionaries/cancer-terms/def/five-year-survival-rate

50. Ishwaran, H., Kogalur, U.B., Blackstone, E.H. and Lauer, M.S., 2008. Random survival forests.

51. Wang P, Li Y, Reddy CK. Machine learning for survival analysis: a survey. ACM Comput Surv. 2019;51(6):1–36.

52. Buckley J, James I. Linear regression with censored data. Biometrika. 1979;66:429–36.

53. Hedeker D, Gibbons RD. Longitudinal Data Analsyis. Wiley; 2006.

54. Barabási AL. Network science. Philos Trans R Soc A Math Phys Eng Sci. 2013;371(1987):20120375.

55. Holland JH. Complex adaptive systems. Daedalus. 1992;121(1):17–30.

56. Barabási AL, Gulbahce N, Loscalzo J. Network medicine: a network-based approach to human disease. Nat Rev Genet. 2011;12(1):56–68.

57. Tong S, Koller D. Support vector machine active learning with applications to text classification. J Mach Learn Res. 2001;2(Nov):45–66.

58. Meganck S, Leray P, Manderick B. modeling decisions for artificial intelligence 58–69. Springer; 2006.

59. Settles, B., 2009. Active learning literature survey.

60. Ren P, Xiao Y, Chang X, Huang PY, Li Z, Gupta BB, Chen X, Wang X. A survey of deep active learning. ACM computing surveys (CSUR). 2021;54(9):1–40.

61. Olsson, F., 2009. A literature survey of active machine learning in the context of natural language processing.

62. Zimek A, Schubert E, Kriegel HP. A survey on unsupervised outlier detection in high-dimensional numerical data. Stat Anal Data Min: ASA Data Sci J. 2012;5(5):363–87.

63. Katoch S, Chauhan SS, Kumar V. A review on genetic algorithm: past, present, and future. Multimed Tools Appl. 2021;80:8091–126.

64. Srinivas M, Patnaik LM. Genetic algorithms: A survey. Computer. 1994;27(6):17–26.

65. Pieczkiewicz DS, Finkelstein SM, Hertz MI. Design and evaluation of a web-based interactive visualization system for lung transplant home monitoring data. AMIA Annu Symp Proc. 2007;2007:598–602.
66. Lee S, Kim E, Monsen KA. Public health nurse perceptions of Omaha system data visualization. Int J Med Inform. 2015;84(10):826–34. https://doi.org/10.1016/j.ijmedinf.2015.06.010.
67. Pieczkiewicz DS, Finkelstein SM. Evaluating the decision accuracy and speed of clinical data visualizations. J Am Med Inform Assoc. 2010;17(2):178–81. https://doi.org/10.1136/jamia.2009.001651.
68. Van der Maaten L, Hinton G. Visualizing data using t-SNE. J Mach Learn Res. 2008;9(11):2579–605.
69. Hardin JW, Hilbe JM. Generalized estimating equations. Chapman and hall/CRC; 2002.

Foundations of Causal ML

Erich Kummerfeld, Bryan Andrews, and Sisi Ma

Abstract

The present chapter covers the important dimension of causality in ML both in terms of causal structure discovery and causal inference. The vast majority of biomedical ML focuses on predictive modeling and does not address causal methods, their requirements and properties. Yet these are essential for determining and assisting patient-level or healthcare-level interventions toward improving a set of outcomes of interest. Moreover causal ML techniques can be instrumental for health science discovery.

Introduction

Previous chapters have discussed methods for using ML to predict outcomes. We will start by illustrating the concepts of causal ML techniques using a hypothetical vignette. Imagine a scenario where we have used predictive methods that estimate that a particular patient, Amy Anonymous, who has been diagnosed with alcohol use disorder (AUD) but is currently abstaining, has a high probability of relapsing. The next step would naturally be to perform interventions with the goal of preventing the relapse. Can ML help identify the best interventions for preventing Amy's relapse? Causal ML methods can help solve such problems, specifically addressing questions like:

1. How much would Amy's chance of relapsing be reduced if Amy receives a specific therapy?

E. Kummerfeld (✉) · B. Andrews · S. Ma
Institute for Health Informatics, University of Minnesota, Minneapolis, MN, USA
e-mail: erichk@umn.edu

© The Author(s) 2024

G. J. Simon, C. Aliferis (eds.), *Artificial Intelligence and Machine Learning in Health Care and Medical Sciences*, Health Informatics,
https://doi.org/10.1007/978-3-031-39355-6_4

2. What factors other than therapy, if any, might also help prevent relapse?
3. What additional complications might ensue if Amy receives a specific therapy?

These are all fundamentally causal questions because they refer to actions that change the usual function of the modeled system, whereas predictive modeling applies only when we model the system's (the human organism or a healthcare system) behavior in its natural state (without any interventions). Using data to answer them requires causal ML. Using data to answer the first of these questions is a **causal inference** problem, [1] while using data to answer the second and third questions are **causal structure discovery** problems [2].

> **Causal inference** is the problem of quantifying the effect of specific interventions on specific outcomes.
>
> **Causal structure discovery** is the problem of identifying the causal relationships among a set of variables.
>
> Like regression and classification, these are very broad problems. Numerous solutions within AI/ML and outside these disciplines have been developed for each. Both of these problems can further be complicated by the presence of unmeasured (aka "hidden" or "latent") variables. Specialized algorithms exist to address such settings [1–4]. For pedagogical simplicity we focus in the present chapter mostly on situations where all relevant factors have been measured.

We will next review the core concepts of causal modeling. As we saw in chapter "Foundations and Properties of AI/ML Systems" any ML method can be conceptualized as search in the space of models appropriate for the problem domain. Causal ML therefore deals with the space of causal models.

Causal Models Versus Predictive Models

Predictive knowledge is associative, capturing co-variation between two or more phenomena. In contrast, causal knowledge is etiological, and captures whether and to what degree the manipulation of one phenomenon results in changes in another. For example, to reduce Amy's risk for relapse, one needs to manipulate, (aka intervene on, or treat), its causes. In contrast, while being in a rehab facility is strongly associated with experiencing the symptoms of a relapse, preventing Amy from entering the rehab will not prevent or treat a relapse, since presence in the rehab facility is not a cause of relapse but an effect. These forms of knowledge are distinct, and distinct methods are required to model them.

Causal models must therefore be able to (a) represent cause-effect relationships; (b) answer questions of the type "what will be the effects of manipulating factor X" and "which factors should one manipulate in order to affect X"; (c) generate data from the model for simulation purposes. In addition, causal models can answer also the usual predictive queries, e.g.: if we observe X what is the probability of Y?"

The **fundamental distinction between predictive and causal ML models** is that predictive models inform us about the **unperturbed distribution** over a set of variables (i.e., patterns that occur "normally", without any intervention on the factors); whereas causal models inform on what modified patterns and distributions one will obtain when interfering and altering the underlying process that generates the data.

Pitfall 4.1
Popular and successful predictive ML methods are not designed and equipped to satisfy the essential requirements of causal modeling.

While causal ML methods are capable of being used for prediction under no interventions as well under interventions, predictive ML methods have several practical advantages over causal ML ones when used for prediction under no intervention. Therefore:

Best Practice 4.1
For predictive tasks (i.e., without interventions contemplated) use of Predictive ML should be first priority. For causal tasks (i.e., with interventions contemplated) use of Causal ML should be first priority.

Also as discussed in chapter "Foundations and Properties of AI/ML Systems", in some cases we need to construct **flexible predictive models** that can accept queries designating any subset of variables as evidence and other subsets as outcomes of interest, while leaving the remaining variables unspecified. We saw in chapter "Foundations and Properties of AI/ML Systems" how BNs can attain this goal without building a new model for every new query (as the majority of predictive modeling algorithms do; see chapter "An Appraisal and Operating Characteristics of Major ML Methods Applicable in Healthcare and Health Science"). The same is true when a mixture of observational and manipulation evidence variables are part of the query (i.e., **flexible causal/predictive modeling**). Causal Probabilistic Graphs (e.g., Causal BNs) can handle such flexible reasoning.

Properties of Well-Constructed Causal Models[1]

First and Foremost Causal Models Must Be Able to Represent the Cause-and-Effect Relationships Among Variables

For causal discovery, this is necessary for answering questions about which variables cause which other variables. For causal inference, this is necessary for removing bias due to confounding. For example, consider a study (Fig. 1) on diet and alcohol abuse, that finds that people who eat fast food regularly are more likely to abuse alcohol. This does not mean that preventing a fast food diet will decrease the chance of Amy's alcohol abuse relapse. Other factors, for example motivation and stress may lead a person to eat more fast food and may also lead a person to abuse alcohol (thus the relationship between fast food and alcohol abuse is confounded by motivation and stress in the Fig. 1 hypothetical example). Causal models can represent complex systems of relationships involving up to hundreds of thousands of variables with clear distinction between confounded vs causal associations.

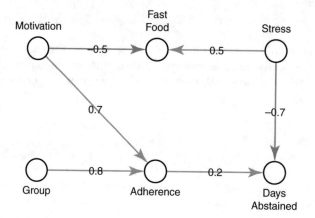

Fig. 1. *A highly simplified example of a clinical trial for a hypothetical drug for treating alcohol use disorder (AUD). Group (Treatment) indicates whether participants receive a placebo or the tested treatment, Adherence indicates how often the participant takes the assigned treatment pills, Motivation indicates a measure of the participant's motivation to have a healthy lifestyle, Fast Food indicates the amount of fast food the participant eats, Stress indicates the stress levels that the participant experiences, and Days Abstained indicates primary outcome, of number of days the person is able to go without relapsing into problematic alcohol use behaviors.* Note: causal ML does not require experimentation in the form of randomized clinical trials (RCTs) or otherwise to infer causal relationships, although it can as in this example be combined with such data to uncover more fine grain information about the causal process than a simple average treatment effect that a RCT provides.

---

[1] So that the present chapter is self-contained some of the BN definitions and properties of chapter "Foundations and Properties of AI/ML Systems" are re-visited in "Properties of Causal Models" and "Structural Equation Models (SEMs)". Readers can skip previously encountered material.

Second, Causal Models are Markovian

That is, **from the perspective of what are the effects of causal manipulations**, the distribution of every variable can be entirely determined by its immediate causes [1]. If Variable T has direct causes A and B and we manipulate A and B this will have the maximum possible effect on T. No other simultaneous manipulation of variables in the system will have an effect on T once we manipulate A and B. Stated differently, T is "shielded" causally by all variables once we manipulate its direct causes.

From an information transfer (and thus predictive) perspective, however, every variable is independent of every non-descendant variable given its immediate causes (a condition known as the Markov Condition [1]). In other words, non-direct causes of T will have no information about what happened to T after we manipulated A and B. Downstream effects of T *and spouses of T* (i.e., direct causes of the direct effects of T) *will have additional information* about what happened to T after we manipulated A and B.

It is widely accepted that causation itself is Markovian (in the macroscopic world, whereas exceptions happen in the quantum world [2], luckily with no relevance to health science and care). This is reflected by common practice in medical science, epidemiology, biology etc., where causation is studied in two fundamental ways:

(a) Causal chains of the type A → B → C
(b) Causal chains of the type A ← C → B

In the chain (a) common health science and health care intuitions are that manipulating A will affect B and thru B will affect C; A, B and C all correlated with one another; once we fix B then manipulation of A will stop affecting C; the correlation of A and C will vanish if we observe or fix B; and the correlation of A and B and of B and C will not ever vanish regardless of observing any other variable.

In the chain (b) common health science and health care intuitions are that manipulating A will not affect B and manipulating B will not affect A; A, B and C all correlated with one another; once we fix C or observe C then the correlation of A and B will vanish; and the correlation of A with C and of C with B will not ever vanish regardless of observing or fixing any other variable.

Third, Causal Models are Modular [1]

Being Markovian leads to the models being decomposable into smaller parts, where we can study these local regions and their function without reference to remote areas in the causal process.

Fourth, Causal Models Are Manipulatable and Generative

Manipulatable refers to capturing in the model the changes that a physical manipulation makes in the actual part of the world that the model represents. A way to represent a physical world manipulation in the model is to assign the corresponding value to the manipulated variable and eliminate all causal edges to it (i.e., because physical manipulations neutralize all other possible causes).

A generative model is one that encodes the full distribution of variables at hand so that every probabilistic calculation can be made with the model. This is sharp distinction with discriminative predictive models that only seek to encode a small fragment of the full distribution, typically the conditional probability of a response given a fixed set of inputs (and in many cases less than that, for example decision surfaces that encode even less information but manage to predict the response to arbitrary accuracy).

In the next sections, we review the predominant class of causal models.

Causal Probabilistic Graphical Models (CPGMs) Based on Directed Acyclic Graphs (DAGs)

A CPGM comprises (1) a DAG; (2) a joint probability distribution (JPD) over variable set V such that each variable corresponds to a node in the DAG; and (3) a restriction of how the JPD relates to the DAG, known as the Causal Markov Condition (CMC).

1. A directed graph is a tuple $<V,E>$, where V is a set of nodes representing variables 1-to-1, and E is a set of directed edges, or arrows, each one of which connects a pair of members of V. A *path* is any set of adjacent edges. A directed path is a path where all edges are pointing in the same direction. A directed graph is a DAG if it has no cycles in it, that is, if there is no directed path that contains the same node more than once. Fig. 1 is an example of a DAG.
2. The JPD over V is any proper probability distribution (i.e., every possible joint instantiation of variables has a probability associated with it and the sum of those is 1).
3. The CMC states that every variable V is independent of all variables that are non-descendants (i.e., not downstream effects) of V given its direct causes.

Causal ML Models Have Well-Defined Formal Causal Semantics

They typically take the form:

1. Parent set (direct causes) $Pa(Vi)$ of variable V_i, $Pa(Vi) = \{Pa(V_i)_1, Pa(V_i)_2, \ldots\}$ is defined over all V_i; and
2. Probability $\Pr(V_i = j | Pa(V_i)_1 = k, Pa(V_i)_2 = l, \ldots)$ is defined over all variables V_i for all value combinations of V_i and its direct causes.

1. Describes the direct causal relationships among all variables
2. Describes the conditional probability distribution of every variable given its direct causes.

If V_i has Parent $Pa(V_i)_j$ that means that in a randomized experiment where one would manipulate $Pa(V_i)_j$, changes would be observed in the distributions of V_i relative to the distribution when $Pa(V_i)_j$ is not manipulated and these changes are entailed by the conditional probability distribution of the variable given its parents.

Unique and Full Joint Distribution Specification in GCPMs

If the fundamental property of the Causal Markov Condition (CMC) holds, then (1) and (2) (parents set, and conditional probabilities of each variable given its parents, respectively) together specify a full and unique joint distribution over variables set V.

Joint Distribution of GCPMs Can Be Factorized Based on Local Causes

This joint distribution is factorized as a product of the conditional probability distribution of every V_i given its direct causes $Pa(Vi)$:

$$\Pr\left(\{V_1,V_2,\dots,V_n\}\right)=\prod_i \Pr\left(V_i\Big|,Pa\left(V_i\right)_1\Big|,Pa\left(V_i\right)_2\Big|,\dots\Big|,Pa\left(V_i\right)_{m_i}\right),\qquad(3)$$

where V_i has m_i parents.

Inspection of the Causal Graph of a GPCM Informs About Conditional Independencies in the Data

By inspection of the causal graph (and application of an interpretive rule following from the CMC, called *d-separation*) we can infer a set of conditional independencies in the data, *without statistically analyzing the data.*

If furthermore, *all dependencies and independencies* in the data are the ones following from the CMC, then we speak of **Faithful distributions** encoded by such GCPMs.

A CPGM encoding a faithful distribution entails that all dependencies and independencies in the JPD can be inferred from the DAG. Therefore the DAG becomes a map (so-called i-map) of dependencies and independencies in the data JPD. Conversely by inferring dependencies and indecencies in the data we can construct the CPGM's DAG and parameterize the CPDs of every variable given its parents effectively recovering the causal process that generates the data. This is the **fundamental principle of operation of causal ML methods.**

Additional Notes

Two nodes are **adjacent** if they are connected by an edge. Two edges are **adjacent** if they share a node.

Parents, children, ancestors, and descendants: In a directed graph, if variables X, Y share an edge X → Y then X is called the parent of Y, and Y is called the child of X. In Fig. 1, Motivation is a parent of Adherence, and Adherence is a child of Motivation. If there is a directed path from X to Y then X is an ancestor of Y and Y is a descendant of X.

Degree: The degree of a node is the number of edges connected to it. In a directed graph, this can be further divided into in-degree and out-degree, corresponding to the number of parents (connected edges oriented towards the node) and children (connected edges oriented away from the node) that the node has. For example, in Fig. 1, Group has degree 1, in-degree 0, and out-degree 1. In the same figure, Adherence has degree 3, in-degree 2 and out-degree 1. A node with degree 0 is said to be "disconnected".

Collider: A collider is a variable receiving incoming edges from two variables. For example in: X → Y ← Z, Y is the collider. A collider is either "shielded" or "unshielded" iff the corresponding parents of the collider are connected by an edge or not, respectively. Unshielded colliders give form to the so-called "v-structure". In Fig. 1, Fast Food is a collider of stress, and motivation.

Trek: A trek is a path that contains no colliders. In Fig. 1, the path from Motivation to Days Abstinent through Adherence is a trek; also the path connecting Fast Food and Days Abstinent through Stress is also a trek. However, the path connecting Motivation and Group through Adherence is not a trek, since it contains the collider Adherence.

D-Separation

1. Two variables X, Y connected by a path are d-separated (aka the path is "blocked") given a set of variables **S**, if and only if on this path, there is (1) a non-collider variable contained in **S**, or (2) a collider such that neither it nor any of its descendants are contained in **S**.
2. Two variables, X and Y, connected by several paths are d-separated given a set of variables **S**, if and only if for all paths connecting X to Y, they are d-separated by **S**.
3. Two disjoint variable sets **X** and **Y** are d-separated by variable set **S** iff every pair <X_i, Y_j> are d-separated by **S**, where X_i and Y_j are members of **X, Y** respectively.

Structural Equation Models (SEMs)

SEMs are causal inference models that can be used after causal relationships have been discovered or when they are known a priori. Left panel of Fig. 2 shows an example causal graph with three variables X, Y, and Z. The three SEM equations show the quantitative functions for each variable given its parents.

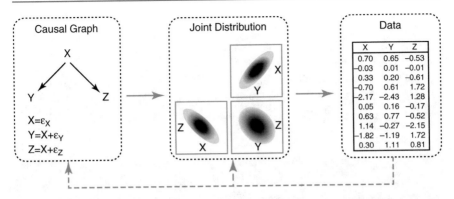

Fig. 2 Correspondence of causal models (left), distribution properties (middle) and data sample (right)

Note that these equations are termed structural equations to emphasize the causal/generative nature of the relationship. SEMs can be continuous, discrete, or mixed, thus extending the definitions of discrete causal models we have seen so far.

The general form of a structural equation for modeling variable x is $x = f(Parent(x), \varepsilon)$, where $Parent(x)$ represents the parents of x, and ε is a noise term representing the unexplained variance in x. The variables on the right hand side of the causal structural equations are causes of the variables on the left hand side. This information mirrors the causal graph, where directed edges (−>) represent direct causal relationships. The quantitative aspect of the causal relationship (e.g. how much change in Y is expected if X is manipulated from 0 to 1) is represented by function f. For example, in the structural equation for Y in Fig. 2, Y is a linear function of X with additive noise ε_Y.

In the same example the expected effect of changing X from 0 to 1 via manipulation of X, on Y is 1 (measured in units of Y), which can be computed by $E(Y|do(X = 1))-E(Y|do(X = 0)) = E(1 + e\_Y)-E(0 + e\_Y) = 1$. The $do(.)$ notation in the equation represents a manipulation involving the assignment of a value that is enacted regardless of other factors in the model that appear as parents of the manipulated variable. To further clarify the causal vs. associational relationship, consider variables Y and Z. The expected effect of changing Z from 0 to 1 on Y is 0, which can be computed by $E(Y|do(Z = 1))-E(Y|do(Z = 0)) = E(X + e\_Y)-E(X + e\_Y) = 0$. Y is not affected by manipulating Z, since Z is not a cause of Y. This is also obvious from the causal graph, since there is no directed path (sequence of variables connected by directed edges pointing to the same direction) leading from Z to Y. However, the values of Y are associated with values of Z since they are both caused by X.

In summary, when Z is manipulated from value 0 to value 1, Y does not change, even though Y and Z are correlated in observational data without manipulations. The correct causal model explains the observed statistical association between Y and Z as confounded by X and indicates that if we wish to change (e.g., treat) Y, we should manipulate X rather than Z.

The above could be inferred using a CPGM with equivalent results (albeit using probabilities and probabilistic inference rather than structural equations and expectations).

The fundamental difference however is that for a SEM model to be useful we need to first infer the causal relationships via an external mechanism. By contrast many algorithms exist that infer a CPGM from data automatically.

Pitfall 4.2
Using SEMs to estimate causal effects with the wrong causal structure.

Going back to Fig. 1 assume that this model represents the causal process correctly and further that motivation and stress were not measured in this RCT. Also assume that a data analyst is interested in how diet affects relapse rates in patients with AUD, and has access to the trial data, which includes how much the participants eat fast food. The analyst regresses Days Abstinent on Fast Food, and finds that eating more fast food is negatively associated with days abstinent. With the goal of ensuring that this association is not related to the RCT design itself, the analyst also regresses Days Abstinent against both Fast Food and Group, and again finds that there is a negative association between fast food consumption and days abstinent. Excitedly, the analyst goes forth to publicize the findings, and recommends that perhaps limiting the consumption of fast food will reduce relapse rates for AUD patients. Based on these findings, other researchers carry out an RCT to test this theory, but find that (as expected by the true causal model) restricting fast food consumption has no effect on relapse.

The analyst has fallen into a common pitfall when they performed regression analyses without any knowledge of the structure of the underlying causal process, and inappropriately interpreted confounded associations as causal. Even if the analyst reports that an association was found, and does not make claims of causal effects, such associations carry a promise of possible valuable causal relationships.

The same problem is encountered when applying any predictive ML method. It is a grave error to apply such non causal methods when causal results are sought.

Consider the following variant of the above scenario where Group (treatment) is not manipulated but observed. Furthermore consider that the analyst, in an effort to eliminate confounding bias, models Adherence as a confounder (on the grounds that it correlates with both group and days abstained). In such a scenario the estimated causal effect of Group will be falsely zero because the plausible confounder, in reality, is on the causal path between group and the outcome.

> **Pitfall 4.3**
> Using regression to estimate causal effects without knowing the true causal structure (and making assumptions about which are the true measured confounders).

Causal Effect Estimation[2]

Further elaborating on causal inference, often we wish to estimate the quantitative causal influence that a variable C has on variable T for a manipulation that causes a 1 unit change of C. The key to obtaining unbiased causal effect estimates from observational data is to partition the total (bivariate, i.e., marginal) statistical association between pairs of variables into the components of that total association due to causal vs. confounded relationships across all connecting paths. In principle, this is relatively straightforward if we know the true causal structure governing the variables we observe. For example, consider estimating the causal effect of C on T using data generated from the causal system depicted in Fig. 3.

In the true causal graph, there are two paths contributing to the overall observed association between C and T. path 1: $C \rightarrow T$, and path 2: $C \leftarrow A \rightarrow D \rightarrow T$[3]. The first path is a causal path, and when one changes the value of C, the value of T will change as a result through this path. The second path is a confounding path, since the change in C cannot causally propagate through this path to affect T. In other

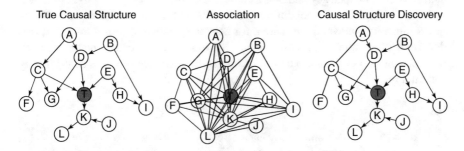

Fig. 3 Illustration of the local causal structure around a variable T

---

[2] In this section we make extensive use of d-separation to infer whether variables are dependent or independent given other variables (also assuming a faithful distribution encoded by the CPGM). Readers not proficient in application of d-separation in faithful DAGs are advised to simply use the provided dependence/independence statements.

[3] There are other connecting paths between C and T, but they do not contribute to the observed bivariate association between C and T because for the information to travel across them, we need condition on collider nodes. For example $C \rightarrow G \leftarrow D \rightarrow T$ does not contribute to the association between C and T, unless G is observed, since G is a collider (i.e. both edges involving G have arrow head pointing to G).

words, when we compute the total marginal (aka univariate) association between C and T, the resulting value reflects the combined contributions from the causal effect $C \to T$ and the confounding $C \leftarrow A \to D \to T$.

In order to estimate the causal effect of C on T, we need to eliminate the component of association due to the confounding path. This can be easily achieved by estimating the relationship between T and C, using A as a covariate in a regression model, or more generally controlling for the associational effect of A. Assuming for example linear functions with Gaussian noise, the causal effect of C on T can be estimated by fitting the linear regression $T = \beta_c * C + \beta_A * A + \varepsilon$.

The estimated coefficient for C then will be the unbiased causal effect estimate of the causal influence of C on T. The reason that this regression model can result in unbiased estimates of causal effects is because adding A to the regression model (i.e. conditioning on A) blocks the confounding path $C \leftarrow A \to D \to T$ and therefore removes the association component between C and T due to the confounding (path 2).

Conditioning on the wrong variables will likely result in biased effect estimation. For example, conditioning on G by fitting the regression model $T = \beta_c * C + \beta_g * G + \varepsilon$ results in biased effect estimation, since conditioning on G, which is a collider on the $C \to G \leftarrow D \to T$ opens the path and introduces additional association between C and T due to this non-causal path (plus the confounding thru A is not controlled).

In practice there are numerous choices for variables to condition on, especially in high dimensional data and in domains with poor prior knowledge. For example, as an alternative to A, conditioning on D by fitting the regression $T = \beta_c * C + \beta_d * D + \varepsilon$ will also result in unbiased effect estimation, since it also blocks the $C \leftarrow A \to D \to T$ path and does not open any additional paths (the $C \leftarrow A \to D \leftarrow B \to I \leftarrow H \leftarrow E \to T$ path is still blocked when conditioning on D, due to the presence of I as a collider).

As illustrated above, the principle for achieving unbiased causal effect estimation from observation data is to ensure that only the true causal paths are open (between the pair of variables under consideration) given the variables controlled by conditioning.

Best Practice 4.2
In order to estimate unbiased causal effects, control variables that are sufficient to block all confounding paths. These variables can be identified by causal structure ML algorithms.

Best Practice 4.3
Often there is a choice of multiple alternative variable sets that block confounding paths. An applicable choice is to control/condition on the set Pa(A) in order to block all confounding paths connecting A and T. However this sufficient confounding blocking variable set is not the minimal one and it is recommended to use the minimal blocking variable set in order to maximize statistical power and minimize uncertainty in the estimation of the causal effect.

> **Pitfall 4.4**
> Discovering the correct variables to condition on can be hard or even impossible in the presence of hidden variables. Discovering the minimal blocking variable set may be computationally hard or intractable when the causal structure is large and complex.

It is also possible that the causal effect for a specific variable cannot be estimated from observational data for some causal data generating functions. In these cases experiments are needed. For those cases that causal effect estimation is feasible from experimental data, Pearl's Do-Calculus procedure will return the right set of conditioning variables. Do-calculus specifies a systematic procedure to determine if a causal effect is estimable and sequences of operations to compute the causal effect when possible [1].

Also in some distributions, discovery of a causal edge may require conditioning on all variables (which is statistically not feasible).

The Do-Calculus is critically different from conventional methods for causal structural learning and causal inference, e.g. structural equation modeling [5], path analysis [6], matching [7], propensity scoring [8]. The conventional methods of the structural equation family are generally hypothesis-driven and only examine a small fraction of possible causal structures governing the data, which make them likely to miss the true causal structure and result in biased estimates of causal effects. Moreover, even without any hidden variables present, the number of possible models is astronomical for even a few dozen variables, making specification of a good model like winning the lottery. Causal structure discovery algorithms together with Do-calculus circumvent these difficulties in many practical settings.

Causal Structure Discovery ML Algorithms

Given that the definition of causes involves manipulation, experimentation is by default one way to discover causal knowledge. However, in domains where experiments are unethical, technically not feasible, or resource prohibitive, or when we want to construct system-level causal models with numerous variables and all their interactions, it is inefficient, impractical and occasionally impossible to derive causation strictly with experimentation. When combining experimentation with observational causal algortihms (and simultaneous measurement of all variables) however, in the worst case, N-1 experiments are needed to derive all causal relationships in a non-cyclic causal system with N variables, given that one variable can be randomized per experiment [9].

Instead, investigating the statistical relationships among variables in observational data and using the result to guide experimentation can be more efficient. In fact, in many scientific domains, in order to discover causal factors, investigators often first examine observational data for variables that are associated with their outcome of interest and then conduct experiments on a subset of the associated factors to determine the causes. This common practice reflects the attempt to use observational data to improve the efficiency of experimental causal discovery. However, as we will illustrate, association is a poor heuristic for causation. In some cases, it provides very little guidance to which experiments need to be performed.

The right panel of Fig. 3 illustrates the local causal structure around a variable T of interest. Based on this causal structure, association will be identified among most variables, indicated by lines connecting most pairs of variables shown in the middle panel (this is referred to as the *correlation network* in some literature). Specifically, other than variable J, all measured variables would be univariately associated with T. Therefore, statistical association is not a good strategy for identifying causes of T. Furthermore, the strength of the association is also not a good indicator of causality, since given the true causal structure, there exist distributions where non-causal variables (e.g. G, K, L) can have stronger associations with T than that of the causes of T. Chapter "Foundations and Properties of AI/ML Systems" provides additional theoretical results about causal ML.

Different from association based methods, causal structure discovery methods are designed to discover causal relationships given observational data up to statistical equivalency [2]. Domain knowledge and knowledge regarding the data collection process can be readily incorporated to facilitate the discovery process [1, 2]. Different algorithms for causal structure discovery leverage different statistical relationships. For example, **constraint-based algorithms** infer causal relationships using conditional independence relationships, whereas **score-based algorithms** search for the causal structure that maximizes likelihood-based scores given data. Further, algorithms such as the IC* [1] and FCI[3] [2] can identify hidden confounding variables, which is very helpful when we are not certain if we have measured all possible entities that participate in the causal process.

When the Causal Markov Condition and Faithfulness Condition hold, statistical associations that are non-causal can be identified by examining statistical properties such as conditional independence. For example, the association between A and T is deemed not directly causal, since A and T are independent given variables C and D (denoted as $A \perp T \mid C, D$ where $\perp$ denotes conditional independence, and | denotes conditioning. Conditional dependence is denoted with $\not\perp$. Also, determination of the direction of causal relation can be resolved due to the collider relations (i.e., in "Y structures" such as $T \rightarrow C \leftarrow A$, where C is a variable known as an "unshielded collider"). Importantly, the presence of hidden variables can also be identified by examining conditional independence. It is worth noting that even in systems with a moderate number of variables (e.g. > a few dozen), it is computationally impossible and sample inefficient, to examine all conditional independence relationships, since the number of all possible conditional independence tests grows exponentially with the number of variables. Therefore, modern causal discovery ML algorithms implement efficient search strategies to ensure that the discovered causal structure is correct and the procedure is scalable to millions of variables in many real-life settings (see Chapter "Principles of Rigorous Development and of Appraisal of ML and AI Methods and Systems" for detailed description of development and validation of such methods). Table 1. below lists several classic causal structure discovery

Table 1 Summary of classic causal discovery algorithms

Method	Assumptions	Statistics	Search strategy
PC [2, 10]	CMC, faithfulness, causal sufficiency, acyclic	Conditional Independence	Start from full graph, eliminate indicated by CI tests
FCI [2, 11]	CMC, faithfulness, acyclic	Conditional Independence	Same as PC in the first phase. Potential hidden variables are identified by examining conditional independences in a second phase
GES [12]	CMC, faithfulness, causal sufficiency, acyclic	Likelihood of model equivalence class given data	Start from empty graph, greedy edge addition and greedy edge elimination operating on the model equivalence class
GFCI [13]	CMC, faithfulness, acyclic	Likelihood of model given data for skeleton discovery and causal orientation, conditional independence for hidden variable identification.	Same as GES in the first phase. Potential hidden variables identified by examining conditional independence in the second phase
MMHC [14]	CMC, faithfulness, causal sufficiency, acyclic	Conditional Independence; likelihood of model given data	Identify local graph of each variable by conditional independence tests, connect local graphs to global graph, greedy edge addition, elimination, and reversal according to likelihood
LGL-GLL [15, 16]	CMC, faithfulness, causal sufficiency, acyclic	Conditional Independence	Flexible algorithm families. Generalized local learning (GLL) identifies local graph of each variable by conditional independence tests, local to global learning (LGL) constructs the global graph by stitching the local neighborhood of variables together. Maybe combined with additional algorithms, e.g., post-process results with equivalence class and hidden variable algorithms
LiNGAM [17]	CMC, faithfulness, causal sufficiency, acyclic, non-Gaussianity	ICA; Wald test; chi-square test; difference test	A combination of ICA, causal-order permutations, and edge pruning tests

algorithms, their assumptions, the statistical relationships they examine, and the search strategies they employ.

It is worth noting that models that rely solely on conditional independence cannot fully resolve the orientation of all edges in the causal system in general. Since the same conditional independence relationships can correspond to multiple causal structures (i.e., belonging to the same so-called Markov Equivalence Class). For example, the conditional independence relationships corresponding to the following causal three structures $X \rightarrow Y \rightarrow Z$, $X \leftarrow Y \rightarrow Z$, and $X \leftarrow Y \leftarrow Z$, are identical (i.e. X, Y, and Z are pairwise dependent, but $X \perp Z \mid Y$, $X \not\perp Y \mid Z$, $Y \not\perp Z \mid X$), i.e. they are Markov equivalent. Markov equivalent causal structures may still be distinguishable by statistical properties other than conditional independence. Methods that aim to tackle this problem are generally referred to as pairwise edge orientation methods, since they explore the statistical asymmetry between pairs of variables to determine causal direction. These methods, originally pioneered by D. Janzing et al. [42] typically require non-linear generating function and/or non-Gaussian noise terms to break the symmetry in causal direction [18].

Trace of PC on Alcohol Abstinence Example

The PC algorithm is an early algorithm in the field that is no longer used in practice (because of low efficiency and high error) but is useful pedagogically to explain how causal discovery may take place. PC begins by forming a completely connected graph of undirected edges, representing no conditional independence anywhere. The algorithm proceeds by iteratively testing for conditional independence between pairs of (currently) adjacent variables conditioned on sets of increasing size. To begin with, unconditional independence is tested, followed by conditional independence with conditioning sets of cardinality one, then of cardinality two, then of cardinality three, and so forth. The members of these conditioning sets are pulled from the variables adjacent to either member of the current pair being tested. After completing all such conditional independence tests (which thins out the graph), the PC algorithm orients the undirected edges by referencing which conditioning sets were used to separate the independent pairs. For each unshielded triple, if the mediating node was not in the stored conditioning set (aka "sepset"), then it orients the triple as a collider. Lastly, a final set of orientation rules are applied that take advantage of the acyclicity constraint [2].

Let us revisit the AUD example and step through a run of the PC algorithm. First, a completely connected graph of undirected edges is formed in Fig. 4. This represents that we have not yet seen any conditional independences. Next, unconditional independence relations are tested (i.e., conditional sets of size zero). In this case, five independencies are found which results in the removal of five edges as shown in Fig. 5. Next conditional independence relations with conditioning sets of cardinality one are tested. In this case, three conditional independencies are found which results in the removal of three more edges as shown in Fig. 6. Next conditional independence relations with conditioning sets of cardinality two are tested. In this case, one more conditional independence is found which results in the removal or one more edge in Fig. 7. The PC algorithm will go on testing conditional independences (up to the point that the conditioning sets lead to under-powered test), but it will not find any more. Accordingly, the conditional independence phase of the algorithm will result in the undirected graph in Fig. 8.

Fig. 4 PC trace on the AUD example: forming a completely connected graph

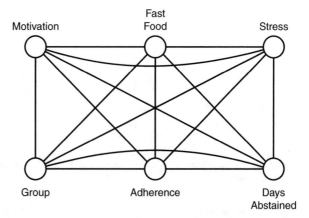

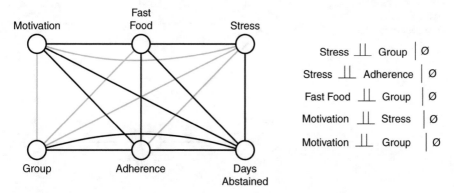

Stress $\perp\!\!\!\perp$ Group | ∅

Stress $\perp\!\!\!\perp$ Adherence | ∅

Fast Food $\perp\!\!\!\perp$ Group | ∅

Motivation $\perp\!\!\!\perp$ Stress | ∅

Motivation $\perp\!\!\!\perp$ Group | ∅

Fig. 5 PC on the AUD example after testing unconditional independence

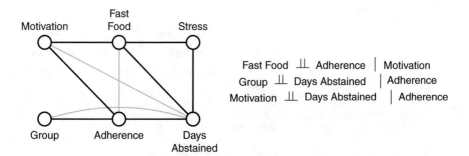

Fast Food $\perp\!\!\!\perp$ Adherence | Motivation

Group $\perp\!\!\!\perp$ Days Abstained | Adherence

Motivation $\perp\!\!\!\perp$ Days Abstained | Adherence

Fig. 6 PC on the AUD example after testing conditional independence with conditioning sets of cardinality one

The edges of the undirected graph in Fig. 8 are oriented by referencing which conditioning sets were used to separate the independent pairs. For each unshielded triplet, if the mediating node was not in the conditioning set, then PC orients the

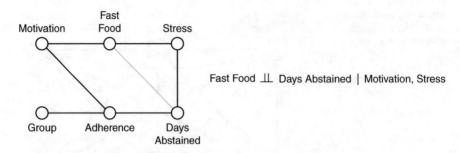

Fast Food ⊥⊥ Days Abstained | Motivation, Stress

Fig. 7 PC on the AUD example after testing conditional independence with conditioning sets of cardinality two

Fig. 8 PC on the AUD example after completing the conditional independence phase

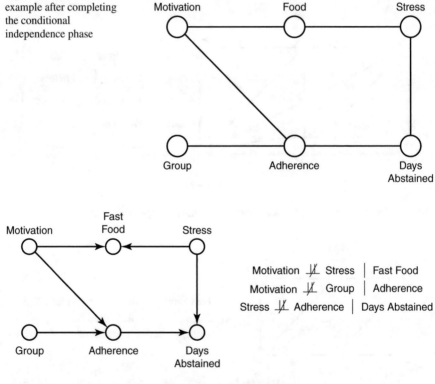

Motivation ⫫̸ Stress | Fast Food
Motivation ⫫̸ Group | Adherence
Stress ⫫̸ Adherence | Days Abstained

Fig. 9 PC on the AUD example after orienting unshielded colliders

edges to make the middle node in the triplet a collider. In the AUD example, the endpoints of the triplets <Motivation, Fast Food, Stress>, <Motivation, Adherence, Group>, and < Stress, Adherence, Days Abstained> were not separated by Fast Food, Adherence, and Days Abstained, respectively. Accordingly, PC orients these triplets as involving colliders in Fig. 9. At this point, the final set of orientation rules would be normally applied, however, the graph has already been fully oriented. Note that in general, there are many cases where the final model produced by PC will have some undirected edges remaining, corresponding to a set of possible graphs that are not fully resolved.

Latent Variables

As depicted in Fig. 10 (left), suppose Motivation and Stress are latent (i.e., unmeasured, aka "hidden"). In this case, if we run PC, the resulting graph would be the one shown in Fig. 10 (right). This graph correctly identifies the causal path from Group to Days Abstained and can be used to correct estimation the effect of Group to adherence. However the graph is misleading in that it suggest that the effect of Adherence to Days Abstained can be estimated by conditioning on Fast Food, when in reality conditioning on Fast Food opens a confounding path and leads to inaccurate causal effect estimate. Such examples showcase the need to use algorithms that reveal latent variables and their confounding on measured ones.

We can think about latent variables as variables that have been marginalized out of a larger, complete, but not fully observed, set of variables. In this paradigm, we assume that the causal model over the complete set of variables is a DAG. Thus, under this assumption, the "margin" of a DAG is a natural choice to represent the model's structure over the observed set of variables.

Intuitively, the "margin" of a DAG should be a graph whose restriction of the model manifests as conditional independence in the marginal probability distribution. More precisely, the conditional independence statements implied by the marginalized graph should be the subset of conditional independence statements implied by the DAG over the remaining variables after marginalization.

Unfortunately, DAGs are not closed under marginalization in this sense. That is, there are DAGs with margins that are not consistent with any DAG. For example, in Fig. 10 (left), Group is independent of Fast Food and independent of Days Abstained

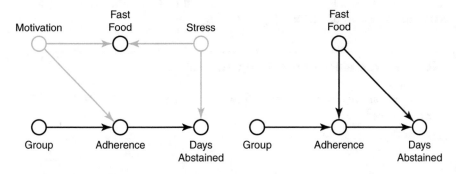

Fig. 10 A DAG with latents and the corresponding PC output

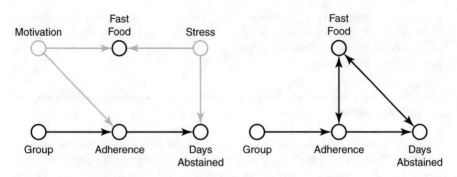

Fig. 11 A DAG with latents and the corresponding ADMG

conditioned on Adherence, however, no DAG represents these exact relations. Accordingly, a richer family of graphs is required to represent margins of DAGs.

Acyclic Directed Mixed Graphs

Acyclic directed mixed graphs (ADMGs) characterize margins of DAGs (Richardson and Spirtes 2002, Richardson 2003). These graphs additionally include bi-directed edges; see Fig. 11 (right) for an illustration. Intuitively, an ADMG can be constructed from a DAG with latent variables by a simple latent projection.
1. For each unshielded non-collider with a latent mediating variable,

   (a) If the triple is directed, add a similarly directed edge between the endpoints,
   (b) Otherwise, add a bi-directed edge.

2. Remove all latent variables.
Importantly, ancestral relationships are invariant under latent projection. For example, in Fig. 11, Group and Adherence are ancestors of Days Abstained while Fast Food is not. These (non-)ancestral relationships are preserved during the marginalization process. Accordingly, it is sufficient to learn an ADMG over the measured subset of variables to infer the presence (or absence) of causal relationships between the measured variables. To this end, the FCI and GFCI algorithms learn Markov equivalence classes of ADMGs [2, 11, 13].

General Practical Approach to Causal ML

In this section, we describe a protocol for conducting causal analysis that involves the following 6 steps:

> **Best Practice 4.4**
> **A Protocol for health science causal ML**
> 1. Define the goal of the analysis.
> 2. Preprocess the data.
> 3. Conduct causal structure discovery.
> 4. Conduct causal effect estimation.
> 5. Assess the quality and reliability of the results.
> 6. Implementation and enhancement of results.

We will next walk the reader through the six step process, pointing also out common pitfalls and how to overcome them.

Evaluate whether the Goals of Modeling Require Causal Analysis

Problem solving that is causal in nature is best addressed by causal modeling. In health-related domains, causal questions generally involve the mechanism and especially the treatment of diseases or interventions on the healthcare system, or discovery of biological causality etc. Some example causal questions in our simple vignette are: (1) what are the *causes* of alcohol abuse? (2) How much improvement in abstinence days can be expected if some motivation enhancer improves it by one standard deviation? (3) What is the best *treatment* for a 35 year-old male with a high stress job that suffers from alcohol abuse?

Questions regarding risk prediction, (e.g. what is the probability of failing 30 days abstinence for a 35 year-old male with a high stress job?), can also be answered with causal discovery analysis. After all, if we have a accurate causal model, we can instantiate the causal model with relevant observational information to deduce a risk prediction. However, the current generation of predictive modeling methods have advantages in answering risk prediction questions not involving manipulations compared to the current generation of causal discovery methods. The main reasons for this are: the current generation of predictive models are discriminant and not generative, can represent more complex mathematical relationships, have built in regularization to avoid overfitting, and most importantly are fitted by analytical protocols such as nested cross validation to maximize their predictive performance via model selection and unbiased performance estimation (whereas causal models seek first and foremost causal validity and have no access to causal error estimators that are available to predictive models). Therefore, we recommend using predictive modeling methods (see chapter "An Appraisal and Operating Characteristics of Major ML Methods Applicable in Healthcare and Health Science") for prediction related tasks.

We also note that Markov Boundary feature selectors **naturally bridge the predictive and causal domains by revealing local causal edges and retaining the maximum predictive information**. They are not however full-fledged causal discovery procedures and need be combined with other causal algorithms for complete causal discovery (chapter "An Appraisal and Operating Characteristics of Major ML Methods Applicable in Healthcare and Health Science").

It is also worth noting that some questions appear to require predictive modeling on the surface, but they actually require casual knowledge to answer correctly. For example, the question "what is the risk of relapse within 30 days for a 35 year-old who suffers from alcohol abuse, if he were treated with naltrexone?" This question can be addressed correctly with predictive modeling if we have observed similar patients taking the medication and others not in a randomized assignment. If, however, observed treatments were not randomized, then we would need causal modeling to answer correctly.

Check If the Data Is Suitable for Causal Discovery Analysis and Preprocess Data Appropriately

Causal discovery analysis can be applied to a wide range of data. To ensure that the discovered causal relationships correspond to the goal of the project and have biological and clinical relevance, special attention needs to be paid to the data design, the data collection process, and the data elements being collected. We point out several common situations where data preprocessing might be needed.

Deterministic relationships: Existing causal discovery algorithms may produce erroneous results when deterministic relationships are present among variables. Examples of deterministic relationships are: item scores for a depression inventory vs. the total score for the same depression inventory; height and weight vs. BMI. How to incorporate this kind of information into causal discovery analysis is an area of active research, but at present our recommendation is to eliminate deterministic relationships by using a subset of the variables that are involved in the deterministic relationships.

Specificity of Measurements: Some measurements/variables can contain information from multiple related variables. This is common in mental health data. For example, the depression inventory also often measures anxiety symptoms, and vice versa. As a result, when causal discovery analysis is conducted on these types of variables, a high amount of interconnectivity is found. High connectivity in a causal graph is not in general problematic. But in this case, it is an artifact of the lack of specificity in the measurements and the findings are hard to interpret causally. One way to improve the measurement specificity is through feature engineering, i.e. instead of directly using the original variables with low specificity, we can construct new variables (e.g. separate out depression specific items from the depression inventory and anxiety inventory, and construct a variable that represents depression more specifically). This can be done by either using prior knowledge, or using data driven methods such as factor analysis [19].

Using EHR Data: Different from observational research and clinical trial data, EHR data are collected at irregular time intervals as part of the patients' clinical care. Using the EHR data for any modeling generally requires the researcher to come up with a study design, construct a specific patient cohort, extract relevant EHR data from it, and preprocess the data according to the goal of the study. These steps should follow the same principles for designing observational studies while considering specific properties of the EHR data [20–23]. For data preprocessing, one needs to consider the nature of various EHR data elements and the nature of diseases. For example, a diagnosis code might appear in the patients' record multiple times. This may be due to multiple episodes of acute disease, or may be due to chronic disease and differentiating between them may be important. Similarly, the timestamps in the EHR reflect the documentation time of an event and often do not coincide with the onset time of the measured event. Further, missing measurements in the EHR data is almost definitely not missing at random, since the care providers decide if a measurement would be taken based on the patients' symptoms. Therefore, using imputation algorithms that assume missing at random would cause errors in the analysis. Some of these challenges in the EHR data can be handled with preprocessing, but others might require adaptations to generic causal discovery algorithms [24, 25].

Causal Structure Discovery

Prior knowledge can be readily incorporated into many causal structure discovery algorithms and can greatly facilitate the structure discovery, especially for edge orientation. Prior knowledge can come from multiple sources. One source is the knowledge of the data collection process. For example, in datasets with longitudinal design, information is collected at multiple time points. This timing information can assist edge orientation since events that happen later cannot be the cause of events that happened earlier. It is worth noting that one needs to distinguish between the time that an event happens vs. the timing that the event was measured or documented. For example, we might have measured a patient's Single-nucleotide polymorphism (SNP) and their depression score at the same clinical encounter, but to study the causes of depression, we would assign the SNP to an earlier time point than the depression score. Further, one needs to consider if the variable contains information over a time span. For example, HbA1C contains information regarding glucose over the past 2 or 3 months, it can be assigned an earlier time point compared to variables that reflect instantaneous information such as the blood oxygen level if these variables were measured at the same time.

Prior knowledge can also come from experimental design. For example, in randomized trials, due to the randomization, the participant's pretreatment measurements should not cause the treatment assignment. This prior knowledge can be encoded by prohibiting edges that emerge from the pretreatment variables to the treatment variable.

A third source of prior knowledge is existing domain knowledge. One can enforce the presence or absence of edges according to existing domain knowledge, but this needs to be done with caution. Since the condition under which the domain knowledge was obtained can be different from the current dataset and its data generating process.

Since incorporating prior knowledge can have a significant effect on the resulting causal structure, we recommend only incorporating the most reliable prior knowledge as input to the causal discovery algorithm. We also encourage performing the causal structure discovery analysis with and without all or a subset of the prior knowledge as sensitivity analysis to investigate the added value of incorporating prior knowledge.

Choice of Algorithms At a high level, the performance of the causal structure discovery largely depends on: (1) if the algorithm used is theoretically guaranteed to produce the correct results under its assumptions, (2) how far does the data deviate from the assumptions of the algorithms, and (3) statistical power. One should always choose algorithms that have solid theoretical properties and clearly defined assumptions (see for example the list of algorithms and assumptions in Table 1). Choice of algorithms can also be informed by benchmark studies applied to data with similar characteristics [15, 26, 27].

One important assumption is causal sufficiency, i.e. the absence of latent common causes. *Latent common cause*, also referred to as *latent variables* are likely present for health data, therefore, it is recommended to apply algorithms that can detect latent variables such as the FCI or GFCI directly to the data for causal discovery, or use FCI and GFCI [2] as a second step for latent variable discovery following the skeleton discovery by another more scalable algorithm.

Another common violation of assumptions of most causal discovery algorithms *is target information equivalence* [28]. In health data, overlapping or redundant information often exists, such as co-occurring symptoms in multiple organs and systems, concurrent abnormal lab values from different lab tests, and simultaneously disturbed molecular pathways. This information redundancy can result in target information equivalence, where multiple variable sets contain statistically equivalent information regarding a target variable of interest. Due to the statistical equivalency, the causal role of these variables cannot be determined from observational data alone. Applying algorithms that are not designed and equipped to handle target information equivalence will likely result in missing important causal information. We recommend to always investigate presence and consequences of target information equivalence when appropriate algorithms are available (e.g., TIE*) [28–31].

Statistical power also influences the choice of algorithm. For smaller sample sizes with large numbers of variables, local causal discovery algorithms have advantages over global causal discovery algorithms due to their sample efficiency [15, 16]. It is also worth noting that the algorithms' parameter setting also impacts statistical power and therefore the algorithms' performance. The choice of the underlying statistical test (for constraint based algorithms) or scores (for score based algorithms) need to correspond to the distribution of data to maximize the statistical power. For example, for constraint based algorithms, Fisher's test is recommended for multivariate Gaussian data, and the G^2 test is recommended for discrete data. Special distributions and data designs (e.g., time-to-event longitudinal designs) might require specially-designed statistical tests. Further, only a subset of algorithms can scale to a very high number of variables without compromising correctness thus being applicable to high dimensional data such as omics data [15].

Causal Effect Estimation

Causal effect estimation should follow the causal structure discovery and be based on the discovered causal structure. Causal effects can be estimated using the Do-calculus principles with SEM as stated in section "Structural Equation Models (SEMs)" above. Note that the SEM model for effect estimation is not restricted to linear regressions. Other mathematical models can be adopted to accommodate non-Gaussian distributions and complex relationships as needed.

It is worth noting that traditional causal effect estimation methods, such as **propensity score-based methods and matching** generally are either based on hypothesized causal graphs, untestable assumptions for correctness (i.e., "strong ignorability") or do not have an explicitly defined causal graph associated with the effect estimation. Given the large space of possible graphs over the set of observed variables, it is highly unlikely that the hypothesized graph would correspond to the true causal structure, therefore these methods can and often lead to biased effect estimation. On the other hand, the lack of an explicitly defined causal graph makes it difficult to interpret the result practically and state the properties of the result of effect estimations [1].

Quality Check and Interpretation of Results

There are several ways to evaluate the discovered causal graphs and estimated causal effects. We recommend several analyses that are suitable for most causal analysis, but problem-specific evaluation should be designed and conducted when appropriate.

Stability of causal discovery. The stability of the causal discovery procedure due to sampling variability can be assessed by bootstrap analysis [32]. In bootstrapping, the same causal discovery procedure (causal structure discovery and causal effect estimation) that was performed on the entire sample can be repeatedly applied to different bootstrap samples. The percentage of time an edge is discovered across all bootstrap samples represents the stability of the causal structure discovery. Edges with percentages closer to 0 or 1 indicate higher stability, representing they are consistently absent or present across all bootstrap samples (i.e., they are more robust to sampling variation). The empirical distribution of the estimated causal effect for manipulating one variable on another variable over all bootstrap samples represents the stability of both the causal structure discovery and the effect estimation. An empirical distribution with smaller variance indicates better stability. Poor stability can indicate issues related to the distribution of the data. For example, it is possible that the identification of a particular edge based on the entire dataset was driven by outliers and such edges would have low stability in bootstrap samples. When poor stability is observed, we recommend careful inspection of the empirical distribution of the data, as well as target information equivalence analysis (that may be driving the instablity).

Fit of the causal model to the data. After the causal structure discovery and parameterization of the causal model (i.e. estimating all parameters for functions $X_i = f(Parent(x))$), one can assess the fit of the causal model to the data. In general, the fit can be assessed with scores like the BIC. If the model parameters are estimated with SEM softwares (e.g. OpenMx, Mplus, Lavaan), one can also examine common metrics for goodness of fit from the SEM literature [33–35].

Generalizability. To test the generalizability of causal discovery results, one can identify a separate dataset that contains the same or similar measurements as the primary dataset, conduct causal analysis and compare the results. For example, comparing the causal discovery results on EHR data collected from different hospital systems to assess the generalizability of causal mechanisms over different patient populations [24]; comparing the causal discovery results in a veteran population with PTSD vs. civilian population with traumatic brain injury tests the generalizability of causal mechanism over different disease populations [36].

It is worth noting that the goal for testing generalizability is not to require that the causal mechanism underlying two datasets must be the same, but rather to assess whether the causal mechanisms are indeed the same in different populations. The discrepancies among causal mechanisms discovered from multiple datasets do not indicate that the discovered causal mechanisms are incorrect. It merely indicates that the discovered causal mechanisms are different (because of population or external factor differences). The differences can be due to a variety of technical factors, such as sample sizes, sampling bias in one or more of the datasets, differences in data collection protocol, and differences in measurements. They can also be due to genuine differences in the causal mechanisms of the two populations. Nevertheless, assessing causal mechanisms in multiple datasets that bear similarity is beneficial, since it helps identify stable causal relationships across different datasets and highlights different causal pathways.

Quality of the local causal neighborhood. The predictive performance for a variable of interest can be used to assess the quality of the local causal structure around the variable. This is related to the concept of Markov boundary (chapter "An Appraisal and Operating Characteristics of Major ML Methods Applicable in Healthcare and Health Science"). Recall that the Markov boundary of a variable of interest is the smallest variable set that contains the maximum amount of (predictive) information about the variable [1]. Under the faithfulness condition, and with no latents, the Markov boundary consists of the direct causes, direct effects and direct causes of the direct effects of the variable of interest [37]. Therefore, one way to assess if our causal structure discovered captures the Markov boundary of the response variable, we can compare the predictive performance of the discovered Markov boundary to the best predictive model (see chapters "The Development Process and Lifecycle of Clinical Grade and Other Safety and Performance-Sensitive AI/ML Models,"

"Overfitting, Underfitting and General Model Overconfidence and Under-Performance Pitfalls and Best Practices in Machine Learning and AI" for more details) we can build for this variable given this dataset. If the predictive performance of the discovered Markov boundary is statistically indistinguishable from that of the best model, we can be assured that the Markov boundary variables contain the true local causes and effects (subject to any confounding due to latents). It is worth noting that, when target information equivalency is present for the response variable of interest (which constitutes a faithfulness violation), there are many variable sets (Multiple Markov Boundaries) that are predictively equivalent and contain the maximum amount of information regarding the variable of interest, and are minimal. In this case, observing statistically indistinguishable predictive performance of one Markov boundary vs. the best model does not guarantee the causal role of that Markov boundary. However one of the multiple Markov boundaries contains exactly the direct causes, direct effects, and direct causes of direct effects of the variable of interest (always subject to latent confounding). Finally, a variable that appears in all members of the Markov boundary equivalence class is guaranteed to be causal subject to confounding. An example of applying this method is [31].

Experimental Validation. Another way to partially assess the validity of the discovered causal relationships and effect sizes is experimental validation. For example, one can select a variable to manipulate, observe its effects on another variable, and compare the experimental result with the effect estimated by the causal model. This form of validation is in general costly and possibly not feasible. Experimental results can also come from prior studies, such as RCTs. An example of this is [38].

Implementation and Enhancement of Results

Causal Discovery Guided Experimentation. In many domains of medicine, it is common practice to observe correlational relationships, hypothesize that they are causal, and then test this hypothesis with experimentation. This procedure is not efficient since numerous correlational relationships are due to confounding and are not causal. A more efficient approach is to use causal structure discovery algorithms to eliminate the majority of correlational relationships that are non-causal and resolve any false positives by experimentation. Hybrid causal ML/experimental algorithms exist that are designed to minimize the number of experiments needed for discovery [39].

Consideration for Clinical Translation. One of the main goals for causal discovery applied to biomedical data is to discover novel treatments that can benefit patients. Molecular and other targets that causally affect patient outcomes are potential treatments. Key considerations for which targets to select for treatment depend on their effectiveness, robustness and safety. Causal modeling can help us evaluate these aspects. For example, a causal factor with large effect size and small variability indicates that a corresponding drug treatment would work well and have consistent performance over the patient population. Also in such cases, this potential treatment could be prescribed to patients regardless of their characteristics. If a putative treatment's effect has large variability, however, this indicates that the response to the treatment could benefit precision medicine administration [40, 41]). Further, with the help of causal analysis, one can also evaluate not only the effect of the treatment on outcomes but also side effects, and select therapeutic targets that maximize patient benefit and minimize side effects.

In summary, the goals for causal ML in health is to discover knowledge that are (1) biologically and clinically relevant, (2) correct and generalizable, and (3) can be translated into clinical application and incorporated into the clinical workflow to benefit patients. A multidisciplinary team consisting of clinical and biological domain experts, health data scientists specialized in causal discovery, clinical informaticists and implementation scientists working closely together is well suited to achieve these goals.

Key Concepts Discussed in Chapter "Foundations of Causal ML"

Causal Inference, Causal Structure Discovery.
Graph, Directed Acyclic Graph (DAG).
Causal Model, Causal Markov Condition, Causal Probabilistic Graphical Model (CPGM), Properties of CPGMs.
Distinction between predictive and causal ML models.
d-separation and Faithfulness.
Structural Equation Models (SEMs).
Causal Effect Estimation and Do-Calculus.
Causal Structure Discovery algorithms.
Acyclic Directed Mixed Graphs (ADMG).
Protocol for health science causal ML.

Pitfalls Discussed in Chapter "Foundations of Causal ML"

Pitfall 4.1. Popular and successful predictive ML methods are not designed and equipped to satisfy the essential requirements of causal modeling.

Pitfall 4.2.: Using SEMs to estimate causal effects with the wrong causal structure.

Pitfall 4.3. Using regression to estimate causal effects without knowing the true causal structure (and making assumptions about which are the true measured confounders).

Pitfall 4.4. Discovering the correct variables to condition on can be hard or even impossible in the presence of hidden variables. Discovering the minimal blocking variable set may be computationally hard in intractable in when the causal structure is large and complex.

Best Practices Discussed in Chapter "Foundations of Causal ML"

Best Practice 4.1. For predictive tasks (i.e., without interventions contemplated) use of Predictive ML should be first priority. For causal tasks (i.e., with interventions contemplated) use of Causal ML should be first priority.

Best Practice 4.2. In order to estimate unbiased causal effects, control variables that are sufficient to block all confounding paths. These variables can be identified by causal structure ML algorithms.

Best Practice 4.3. Often there is a choice of multiple alternative variable sets that block confounding paths. An applicable choice is to control/condition on the set Pa(A) in order to block all confounding paths connecting A and T. However this sufficient confounding blocking variable set is not the minimal one and it is recommended to use the minimal blocking variable set in order to maximize statistical power and minimize uncertainty in the estimation of the causal effect.

Best Practice 4.4. A Protocol for health science causal ML.
1. Define the goal of the analysis.
2. Preprocess the data.
3. Conduct causal structure discovery.
4. Conduct causal effect estimation.
5. Assess the quality and reliability of the results.
6. Implementation and enhancement of results.

Classroom Assignments and Discussion Topics for Chapter "Foundations of Causal ML"
1. Give:

   (a) 2 examples of causal discovery problems and 2 examples of predictive problems in healthcare management.
   (b) 2 examples of causal discovery problems and 2 examples of predictive problems in clinical care.
   (c) 2 examples of causal discovery problems and 2 examples of predictive problems in health sciences research.
   (d) Discuss how predictive modeling that does not take into account causality may lead to flawed decisions in each of the above causal example applications.

2. Someone presented to you a model for predicting the probability of cancer relapse with high predictive performance, derived from observational data using a convolutional neural network. Can you deduce potential relapse prevention strategies from this model?

3. Write a computer program in your favorite programming language to generate data based on the causal graph specified in Fig. 1.

   (a) Based on the data you generated and the causal structure in Fig. 1, estimate the causal effect for each cause-effect pair in Fig. 1 (hint: you should obtain coefficients similar to what is specified in Fig. 1).

   (b) Apply the PC algorithm or the FGES algorithm to the data you generated to discover the causal structure and compare it to the true causal structure specified in the figure.

References

1. Pearl J. Causality. Cambridge University Press; 2009.
2. Spirtes P, Glymour CN, Scheines R. Causation, prediction, and search. MIT Press; 2000.
3. Kummerfeld E, Ramsey J. Causal clustering for 1-factor measurement models. In: Proceedings of the 22nd ACM SIGKDD International Conference on Knowledge Discovery and Data Mining, KDD '16. New York, NY, USA: ACM; 2016. p. 1655–64.
4. Kummerfeld E, Ramsey J, Yang R, Spirtes P, Scheines R. Causal clustering for 2-factor measurement models. In: Calders T, Esposito F, Hullermeier E, Meo R, editors. Machine learning and knowledge discovery in databases, volume 8725 of Lecture notes in computer science. Berlin, Heidelberg: Springer; 2014. p. 34–49.
5. Kaplan D. Structural equation modeling: foundations and extensions, vol. 10. Sage Publications; 2008.
6. Wright S. Correlation and causation. J Agric Res. 1921;20:557–85.
7. Rubin DB. Matching to remove bias in observational studies. Biometrics. 1973;29:159–83.
8. Rosenbaum PR, Rubin DB. The central role of the propensity score in observational studies for causal effects. Biometrika. 1983;70:41–55.
9. Eberhardt, F., Glymour, C. & Scheines, R. On the number of experiments sufficient and in the worst case necessary to identify all causal relations among n variables. arXiv preprint, arXiv:1207.1389 (2012).
10. Colombo D, Maathuis MH. Order-independent constraint-based causal structure learning. J Mach Learn Res. 2014;15:3741–82.
11. Zhang J. On the completeness of orientation rules for causal discovery in the presence of latent confounders and selection bias. Artif Intell. 2008;172:1873–96.
12. Chickering DM. Optimal structure identification with greedy search. J Mach Learn Res. 2002;3:507–54.
13. Ogarrio JM, Spirtes P, Ramsey J. A hybrid causal search algorithm for latent variable models. In: Conference on probabilistic graphical models. PMLR; 2016. p. 368–79.
14. Tsamardinos I, Brown LE, Aliferis CF. The max-min hill-climbing Bayesian network structure learning algorithm. Mach Learn. 2006;65:31–78.
15. Aliferis CF, Statnikov A, Tsamardinos I, Mani S, Koutsoukos XD. Local causal and Markov blanket induction for causal discovery and feature selection for classification part I: algorithms and empirical evaluation. J Mach Learn Res. 2010;11(7):171–234.
16. Aliferis CF, Statnikov A, Tsamardinos I, Mani S, Koutsoukos XD. Local causal and Markov blanket induction for causal discovery and feature selection for classification part II: algorithms and empirical evaluation. J Mach Learn Res. 2010;11(8):235–84.
17. Shimizu S. LiNGAM: non-Gaussian methods for estimating causal structures. Behaviormetrika. 2014;41(1):65–98.

18. Statnikov A, Henaff M, Lytkin NI, Aliferis CF. New methods for separating causes from effects in genomics data. BMC Genomics. 2012;13(8):1–16.
19. Rawls E, Kummerfeld E, Mueller BA, Ma S, Zilverstand A. The resting-state causal human connectome is characterized by hub connectivity of executive and attentional networks. NeuroImage. 2022;255:119211.
20. Rosenbaum PR, Rosenbaum PR, Briskman. Design of observational studies, vol. 10. New York: Springer; 2010.
21. Kramer MS. Clinical epidemiology and biostatistics: a primer for clinical investigators and decision-makers. Springer Science and Business Media; 2012.
22. Botsis T, Hartvigsen G, Chen F, Weng C. Secondary use of EHR: data quality issues and informatics opportunities. Summit Transl Bioinform. 2010;2010:1–5.
23. Weiskopf NG, Bakken S, Hripcsak G, Weng C. A data quality assessment guideline for electronic health record data reuse. Egems. 2017;5(1):14.
24. Shen X, Ma S, Vemuri P, Castro MR, Caraballo PJ, Simon GJ. A novel method for causal structure discovery from EHR data and its application to type-2 diabetes mellitus. Sci Rep. 2021;11(1):1–9.
25. Shen X, Ma S, Caraballo PJ, Vemuri P, Simon GJ. A novel method for handling missing not at random data in the electronic health records. In: 2022 IEEE 10th international conference on healthcare informatics (ICHI). IEEE; 2022. p. 21–6.
26. Sanchez-Romero R, et al. Estimating feedforward and feedback effective connections from fMRI time series: assessments of statistical methods. Netw Neurosci. 2019;3(2):274–306.
27. Ma S, Kemmeren P, Gresham D, Statnikov A. De-Novo learning of genome-scale regulatory networks in S. cerevisiae. PLOS ONE. 2014;9(9):e106479.
28. Statnikov A, Lemeir J, Aliferis CF. Algorithms for discovery of multiple Markov boundaries. J Mach Learn Res. 2013;14(1):499–566.
29. Karstoft KI, Galatzer-Levy IR, Statnikov A, Li Z, Shalev AY. Bridging a translational gap: using machine learning to improve the prediction of PTSD. BMC Psychiatry. 2015;15(1):1–7.
30. Statnikov A, Aliferis CF. Analysis and computational dissection of molecular signature multiplicity. PLoS Comput Biol. 2010;6(5):e1000790.
31. Kraus VB, Ma S, Tourani R, Fillenbaum GG, Burchett BM, Parker DC, Kraus WE, Connelly MA, Otvos JD, Cohen HJ, Orenduff MC. Causal analysis identifies small HDL particles and physical activity as key determinants of longevity of older adults. EBioMedicine. 2022;85:104292.
32. Kummerfeld E, Rix A. Simulations evaluating resampling methods for causal discovery: ensemble performance and calibration. In: 2019 IEEE international conference on bioinformatics and biomedicine (BIBM). IEEE; 2019. p. 2586–93.
33. Fan X, Thompson B, Wang L. Effects of sample size, estimation methods, and model specification on structural equation modeling fit indexes. Struct Equ Model Multidiscip J. 1999;6(1):56–83.
34. Bentler PM. On tests and indices for evaluating structural models. Personal Individ Differ. 2007;42(5):825–9.
35. Barrett P. Structural equation modelling: adjudging model fit. Personal Individ Differ. 2007;42(5):815–24.
36. Pierce B, Kirsh T, Ferguson AR, Neylan T, Ma S, Kummerfeld E, Cohen B, Nielson JL. Causal discovery replicates symptomatic and functional interrelations of posttraumatic stress across five patient populations. Front Psychiatry. 2023;13:1018111.
37. Guyon I, Aliferis C. Causal feature selection. In: Computational methods of feature selection. Chapman and Hall/CRC; 2007. p. 79–102.
38. Maathuis MH, et al. Predicting causal effects in large-scale systems from observational data. Nat Methods. 2010;7(4):247–8.

39. Statnikov A, Ma S, Henaff M, Lytkin N, Efstathiadis E, Peskin ER, Aliferis CF. Ultra-scalable and efficient methods for hybrid observational and experimental local causal pathway discovery. J Mach Learn Res. 2015;16(1):3219–67.
40. Gunlicks-Stoessel M, Klimes-Dougan B, VanZomeren A, Ma S. Developing a data-driven algorithm for guiding selection between cognitive behavioral therapy, fluoxetine, and combination treatment for adolescent depression. Transl Psychiatry. 2020;10(1):1–11.
41. Winterhoff B, Kommoss S, Heitz F, Konecny GE, Dowdy SC, Mullany SA, Park-Simon TW, Baumann K, Hilpert F, Brucker S, du Bois A. Developing a clinico-molecular test for individualized treatment of ovarian cancer: the interplay of precision medicine informatics with clinical and health economics dimensions. In: AMIA annual symposium proceedings, vol. 2018. American Medical Informatics Association; 2018. p. 1093.
42. Janzing D, Mooij J, Zhang K, Lemeire J, Zscheischler J, Daniušis P, Steudel B, Schölkopf B. Information-geometric approach to inferring causal directions. Artif Intell. 2012;182:1–31.

Principles of Rigorous Development and of Appraisal of ML and AI Methods and Systems

Constantin Aliferis and Gyorgy Simon

Abstract

The chapter outlines a comprehensive process, governing all steps from analysis and problem domain needs specification, to creation and validation of AI/ML methods that can address them. The stages are explained and grounded using existing methods examples. The process discussed equates to a generalizable Best Practice guideline applicable across all of AI/ML. An equally important use of this Best Practice is as a guide for understanding and evaluating any ML/AI technology under consideration for adoption for a particular problem domain.

Keywords

Method development and evaluation process · Properties of AI/ML methods (theoretical, empirical) · AI/ML stacks · Protocols · Engines · AI/ML method properties map

Establishing Properties of AI/ML Methods During New Method Development and Evaluating Properties when Choosing the Best Method for the Problem at Hand

In chapters "Foundations and Properties of AI/ML Systems", "An Appraisal and Operating Characteristics of Major ML Methods Applicable in Healthcare and Health Science", and "Foundations of Causal ML" we reviewed major health AI/ML methods in common use in healthcare and the health sciences. We examined

C. Aliferis (✉) · G. Simon
Institute for Health Informatics, University of Minnesota, Minneapolis, MN, USA
e-mail: constantinaibestpractices@gmail.com

© The Author(s) 2024
G. J. Simon, C. Aliferis (eds.), *Artificial Intelligence and Machine Learning in Health Care and Medical Sciences*, Health Informatics,
https://doi.org/10.1007/978-3-031-39355-6_5

how they work and summarized important properties. We especially focused on the following **theoretical properties and corresponding conditions (if known) that guarantee these properties**:

1. Representation power: can the models produced by the method represent all relevant problem instances and their solutions?
2. Transparency: are the models produced by the method easy to understand (i.e., are they "transparent box") and can they be easily understood by human inspection (i.e., are they explainable and human interpretable)?
3. Soundness: When the methods output a solution to a problem instance, is this solution correct? If there is a degree of error (measured in some scale of loss, risk or other scale) how large is the error and its uncertainty?
4. Completeness: Does the method produce correct answers to all problem instances? If only for a fraction of the problem space, how large or important is the fraction?
5. Computational complexity for learning models: what is the exact or asymptotic computational complexity of running the method to produce models as a function of the input size (e.g., number of variables, or sample size)?
6. Computational complexity for using models: what is the exact or asymptotic computational complexity of running the models produced by the method to answer problems as a function of the input size (e.g., number of input variables)?
7. Other cost functions: for example, what is the cost to obtain and store input data and run analyses on a compute environment, either at model discovery or at model deployment time?
8. Space complexity for learning models: what is the exact or asymptotic storage complexity of running the method to produce models as a function of the input size (e.g., number of variables, or sample size)?
9. Space complexity for storing and using models: what is the exact or asymptotic storage complexity of running the models to answer problems as a function of the input size (e.g., number of variables, or sample size)?
10. Sample complexity, learning curves, power-sample requirements: how does the error of the produced models varies as function of sample size of discovery data? How much sample size do we need in order to build models with a specific degree of accuracy and acceptable statistical error uncertainty, and how much sample size is needed to establish statistically superiority to random or specific models and performance levels?
11. Probability and decision theoretic consistency: is the ML/AI method compatible with probability and utility theory?

We also discussed **empirical performance properties which we can differentiate for the purposes of the present chapter into**:

1. **Comparative and absolute empirical performance in simulation studies**: when we give the method discovery data produced by simulations, what is the empirical performance of the method?
2. **Comparative and absolute performance in real data with hard and soft gold standard known answers**: when we give the method discovery data from real world sampling, what is the empirical performance of the method?

Chapters "Foundations and Properties of AI/ML Systems", "An Appraisal and Operating Characteristics of Major ML Methods Applicable in Healthcare and Health Science", and "Foundations of Causal ML" made it abundantly clear to the reader that the majority of widely-used formal methods have known properties along the above dimensions. Ad hoc and heuristic systems and methods do not, however, and thus are viewed in this volume as pre-scientific or early-stage and preliminary, thus carrying great risk of failure (at the present stage of scientific knowledge about them). It also became obvious that knowing the above properties is essential knowledge for determining which among several available methods and corresponding libraries, tools and commercial offerings are the ones that are best suited for a problem we wish to solve using AI/ML.

In general, theoretical properties are stronger than empirical ones in the sense that they describe very large parts of the problem-solving domain more efficiently and with greater clarity than empirical studies. Figure 1 shows the coverage and interpretation of **sufficient conditions**, vs. those provided by **sufficient and necessary conditions and vs. necessary conditions**. Sufficient and necessary criteria describe the whole problem space, whereas sufficient conditions and necessary conditions only part of it, but they are usually more difficult to establish, thus usually theoretical analysis for AI/Ml methods is provided in the form of sufficient conditions. It is not uncommon for the set of sufficient conditions to grow over time so that the total problem space is better understood.

Notice that sufficient conditions point to parts of the problem space where desired performance is achieved. So, if we establish that in some domain a set of sufficient conditions hold, we can expect desirable performance. In other words, *sufficient conditions are constructive*. Necessary conditions point to parts of the problem space where undesired performance will occur. They provide warnings against pitfalls, but do not tell us the complete picture of how to obtain desirable results (other than avoiding the pitfalls, i.e., safeguarding that necessary conditions are not violated).

Even if we do not violate necessary conditions, we are not guaranteed desired performance however (because additional sufficient conditions may not hold). Necessary and sufficient criteria map out precisely the totality of the problem space

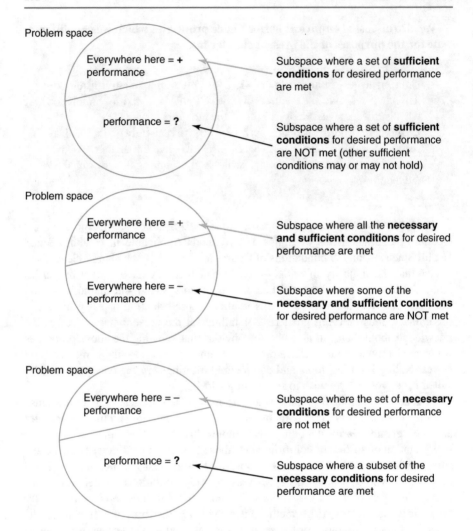

Fig. 1 Conditions for desirable performance of AI/ML methods. Sufficient vs. sufficient and necessary, vs. necessary conditions

in which we will obtain desirable performance and the space that we will not. Again, it is much harder in practice to derive necessary and sufficient conditions.

By comparison to the above, empirical studies provide *limited coverage* of the problem space as shown in Fig. 2. In the absence of theory it would take an astronomical number of empirical studies to cover the space that a single theorem can (assuming that the combinatorial space of factors involved is non-trivial).

One caveat of applying theoretical analysis is that we may not know with absolute certainty if sufficient, necessary, or sufficient and necessary conditions are met in some problem domain. It is very important for **theoretical conditions to be testable**. For example, we can easily test whether the data is multivariate normal and thus we can know whether in some domain we satisfy the relevant sufficient

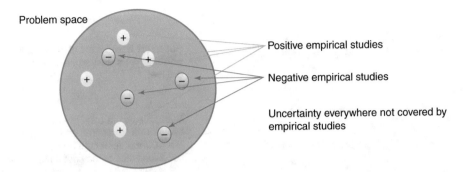

Fig. 2 Empirical studies. Empirical studies showing positive (green) and negative (red) performance results, can sample the problem space and collect evidence about the applicability of method (s) of interest (extrapolated, inductively, to similar populations). The vast majority of the space (grey) has unknown performance however since it has properties that may affect performance, and which properties are not covered by the empirical studies. Empirical studies are vastly less efficient than theoretical analysis

condition of OLS regression (chapter "An Appraisal and Operating Characteristics of Major ML Methods Applicable in Healthcare and Health Science"). By comparison, within classical statistics frameworks we do not know in general, and cannot test practically, whether the strong ignorability sufficient condition of propensity scoring method holds (chapter "Lessons Learned from Historical Failures, Limitations and Successes of AI/ML In Healthcare and the Health Sciences. Enduring problems, and the role of Best Practicess"). The existence of such a condition then just says that it is *theoretically possible* for the method to work in some real or hypothetical distribution (but we cannot tell whether it will work in any real life data of interest with certainty).

In some situations it is also possible to fix violations of conditions. For example, we can transform (some) non normal distributions so that they become normal. Sometimes, violating sufficient conditions for desired performance is mistaken to imply guranteed undesired perfromance. This is not the case, always, since not meeting a set of suffiecient conditions may still be followed by good performance (i.e., if other sufficient conditions exist and are met, aka "mitigation factors" [1]).

There is a clear relevance of pitfalls and guidelines for best practices, to the above concepts. These must describe sufficient, necessary or sufficient and necessary conditions for desired or undesired performance, and these conditions must be testable or identifiable.

In Fig. 3 we demonstrate the importance of **combining theoretical analysis with empirical testing**. If theory predicts that in some identifiable part of the problem space - described in the example of the figure by the subspace where sufficient conditions hold - we expect there desirable behavior. But we may still be unsure about whether these conditions were tested accurately. Or if no testing of conditions was conducted, whether the theory applies to this particular problem space and data sampled from it, that we are facing. By 'sampling" this part of the problem space we can obtain evidence strengthening or refuting the appropriateness of the applicability of the methods in question.

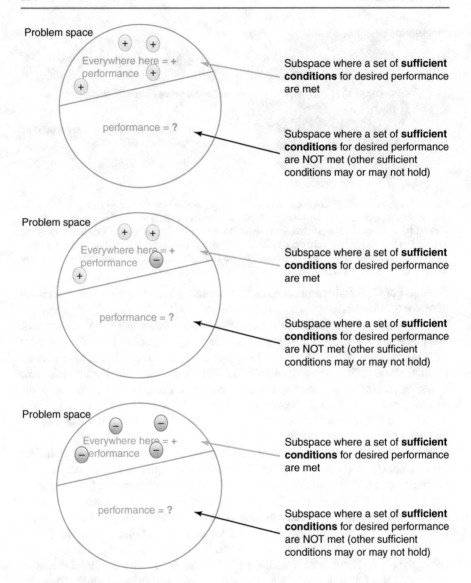

Fig. 3 Combining theoretical analysis' expectations with empirical studies (green = empirical studies showing desired performance, red = empirical studies with undesired performance). Top: empirical studies (verify that our problem space is well aligned with theoretical expectations of AI/ML method performance. Middle: some studies show misalignment with theoretical expectations. Possibly, criteria used to test whether assumptions hold may be inaccurate, or the empirical studies were flawed, or both. Bottom: many studies show misalignment of our domain with theoretical expectations. Either criteria used to test whether assumptions hold are wrong or assumptions were never tested (and the problem domain does not oblige)

To elaborate, if we obtain positive empirical verification of theoretical expectations, we can be sure that the theoretical roadmap is aligned with our practical problem solving setting. If, however we see empirical results that violate the theoretical expectations, this is evidence that we did not sufficiently test the preconditions for method success, or that the means in our disposal for testing the preconditions of the theoretical properties are not accurate and we need better ways to test the suitability of our methods to the real-life problem.

Going back to Fig. 2, the reader may wonder: why don't we dispense with theory and treat the characterization of the problem space with regards to performance of any set of methods, as an empirical ML problem itself? For example, dispel with theory and base acceptance of, e.g., clinical AI models by doing Clinical Trials? With enough methods and enough trials/datasets over enough problem spaces we can circumvent the need to derive complex theoretical analyses. The answer is three-fold:

1. As indicated earlier, the number of empirical studies needed would be astronomical, as the number of studies needed grows combinatorially to the number of factors involved.

2. In the absence of theory we do not even known which factors affect performance and thus lack the knowledge necessary to design a set of empirical studies that can cover the space of interest. This is a *Theory Ladeness* problem (i.e., scientific conclusions are affected by the framework determining what to study, how to measure it etc. [2, 3].

3. This practice may jeopardize human subjects or waste valuable resources, and is thus unethical in such cases. Moreover, as the field of ML matured, it has become evident that even thousands of datasets used for a variety of benchmarks across domains cannot cover the full space of possibilities of evaluating a single method. At most we can divide and conquer the full ML problem space into application areas and conduct large benchmark studies there. However for this endeavor in order to be efficient and practical, the specific choices of focused areas and datasets must be constrained and guided by a robust theoretical understanding of the factors affecting successful modeling.

In summary, theory and empirical study work synergistically together and provide a concrete roadmap of which methods are suitable for what task, by establishing the properties of AI/ML methods. The same is true for individual models produced by such methods as detailed in the next chapter on developing and validating AI/ML models. Knowing AI/ML properties (theoretical and empirical) provides crucial information that allows one to make informed decisions about the **Performance, Safety and Cost-effectiveness requirements and potential** of corresponding AI/ML approaches, methods and systems (and the decision models produced by them). Successfully meeting requirements that ensure desirable AI/ML behavior can then lead to building trust in the AI/ML solution (as discussed in chapter "Artificial Intelligence (AI) and Machine Learning (ML) for Healthcare and Health Sciences: the Need for Best Practices Enabling Trust in AI and ML") which encompasses: *Scientific and Technical Trust; Institutional Trust; System-of-science Trust; Beneficiary Trust; Delivery Trust; Regulatory Trust; and Ethical Trust.* We can codify the above as 4 best practices:

Best Practice 5.1
Methods developers should strive to characterize the new methods according to the dimensions of theoretical and empirical properties.

Best Practice 5.2
Methods developers should carefully disclose the known and unknown properties of new methods at each stage of their development and provide full evidence for how these properties were established.

Best Practice 5.3
Methods adopters and evaluators (users, funding agencies, editorial boards etc.) should seek to obtain valid information according to the dimensions of theoretical and empirical properties for every method, tool, and system under consideration.

Best Practice 5.4
Methods adopters and evaluators should map the dimensions of theoretical and empirical properties for every method, tool, and system under consideration to the problem at hand and select methods based on best matching of method properties to problem needs.

Major pitfalls can and do ensue when the above best practices are not followed. In chapter "Lessons Learned from Historical Failures, Limitations and Successes of AI/ML In Healthcare and the Health Sciences. Enduring problems, and the role of Best Practices" we will discuss many case studies of real-life dire consequences of failing to follow these best practices.

Pitfall 5.1
Developing methods with theoretical and empirical properties that are:
(a) Unknown, or
(b) Poorly characterized in disclosures and technical, scientific or commercial communications and publications, or
(c) Clearly stated (disclosed) properties but not proven, or
(d) Not matching the characteristics of the problem to be solved at the level of performance and trust needed opens the possibility for major errors, under-performance, poor safety, unacceptable cost-effectiveness, and lack of trust in AI.

Best Practice Workflow to Establish the Properties of any New or Pre-Existing Method, Tool or System

In the remainder of the present chapter we will outline a best practice workflow, shown in Figs. 4, and 5 that can be used to create new (Fig. 4) or establish the properties of any pre-existing (Fig. 5) method, tool or system, so that a rational, effective and efficient solution to the problem at hand can be identified as per the guidelines 5.1–5.4.

Throughout the description of the process details that follow, we will highlight how the steps apply to several well-known methods (which are detailed in chapters "Foundations and Properties of AI/ML Systems", "An Appraisal and Operating Characteristics of Major ML Methods Applicable in Healthcare and Health Science", and "Foundations of Causal ML") and furthermore interleave a running in-depth example of putting these principles to practice in a real-life method development context (new method development for biomarker, signatures and biomedical pathway discovery).

Step 1. Rigorous problem definition (in precise mathematical terms, and with precise correspondence to health care or health science objectives)

It is always worthwhile to invest time to define the problem addressed by new methods we plan to develop or evaluate, in very precise terms. This enables an

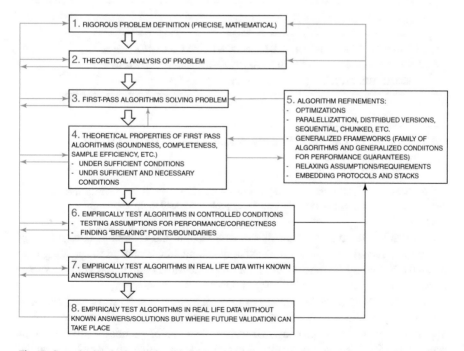

Fig. 4 Steps in developing and validating new AI/ML methods. Details in text. Notice the highly non-linear flow that describes the frequent need to go back and revise earlier steps if they do not lead to desired performance

1. APPRAISAL OF OPERATING PROBLEM DOMAIN SPECIFICATION PRECISION

2. APPRAISAL OF THEORETICAL ANALYSIS OF OPERATING DOMAIN

3. APPRAISAL OF THEORETICAL PROPERTIES OF METHOD/SYSTEM
(SOUNDNESS, COMPLETENESS, SAMPLE EFFICIENCY, ETC.)
- UNDER SUFFICIENT CONDITIONS
- UNDR SUFFICIENT AND NECESSARY CONDITIONS

4. APPRAISAL OF OTHER CAPABILITIES, EXTENSIONS AND DERIVATIVES:
- OPTIMIZATIONS
- PARALELLIZATTION, DISTRIBUED VERSIONS, SEQUENTIAL, CHUNKED, ETC.
- GENERALIZED FRAMEWORKS
- RELAXING ASSUMPTIONS/REQUIREMENTS
- EMBEDDING PROTOCOLS AND STACKS

5. APPRAISAL OF EMPIRICAL TESTS IN CONTROLLED CONDITIONS
- TESTING ASSUMPTIONS FOR PERFORMANCE/CORRECTNESS
- FINDING "BREAKING" POINTS/BOUNDARIES

6. APPRAISAL OF EMPIRICALL TESTS IN REAL LIFE DATA WITH KNOWN
ANSWERS/SOLUTIONS

Fig. 5 Steps in evaluating existing AI/ML methods. Details in text. This process is linear since the evaluators do not concern themselves with fixing problems found in the appraisal

accurate and effective mapping of the data design and modeling onto the most appropriate AI/ML methods if they exist, or establishing the need for creating new methods (if methods do not exist or their properties are not up to par with the specifications of the problem solving effort at hand).

A mathematical-level description of the problem we wish to solve enables theoretical (mathematical, algorithmic, information theoretic, statistical, or other) appropriate analysis and proving that the problem can or cannot be solved, within specific performance requirements. This includes whether the problem can be solved in acceptably small time, storage, or sample size and input costs. Or, if it cannot, whether, the development effort needs to focus on subclasses of the broad problem space that are solvable efficiently.

Unfortunately it is often the case that AI/ML is used by applying on data and expecting that "useful" patterns will be revealed, or "insights" will be generated without a precise description of what constitutes a desired solution.

Real-life relevance. Characteristic examples of this pitfall in healthcare AI/ML applications is seeking "useful patterns", "anomalies", "practice variation", "actionable insights", "subpopulations", or any number of other fuzzy goals that are hard to critically and conclusively evaluate in terms of meaningfully meeting the goals of the project. Another common pitfall is in the risk and predictive modeling domains where "accurate" algorithms (or models) are being sought without reference to the degree of accuracy expressed in some evaluation scale, that is required to advance the goals of the project at hand.

In the health sciences, a characteristic example of this pitfall is in bioinformatics analyses of high-dimensional omic molecular data where application of AI/ML methods is used to reveal "biological insights", "structure in data", "shape of the data", "clusters", "pathways", "signatures", "gene lists", often with very imprecise or inconsistent language about what exactly each one of these entities is meant to encompass, or about how discovering them will enable a specific scientific investigation, answer a concrete hypothesis, or generate results with practical clinical, scientific or technological value. Often such fuzzy goals and results are combined with ex post facto narratives by the authors of the study that overlay meaning and significance to the findings although they may inherently lack such meaning.

The ability of experts to create explanations in their field is an important component of their professional success [4]. A serious possibility exists that the domain expert investigators may be prone to creating (on the surface) convincing narratives around any set of results, even random ones, however. The term *Scientific Apophenia* describes the tendency to find evidence of order where none exists in scientific results [5]. The human mind is a powerful recognizer of patterns but is also subject to seeing patterns over random sequences and conversely, believing that non-random patterns are random [6].

Moreover some pattern may emerge out of random structures as a result of mathematical necessity as studied by Ramsey Theory [7]. For example, in any group of 6 people, by mathematical necessity, either at least three of them are (pairwise) mutual strangers or at least three of them are (pairwise) mutual acquaintances. The reader can see the relevance of this theorem to, e.g., interpreting bioinformatics analyses describing clusters among genes or other molecules. Such clusters even, if randomly generated, will contain structured patterns of known relationships and in turn will give credence to the (false) validity of previously unknown relationships.

The requirement for rigorous problem definitions prevents such problems early in the discovery process, at a stage where the very methods used for discovery are formulated and validated.

Another common pitfall of new method development related to defining the goals of methods is to define them in mathematical terms but without establishing how the mathematical goal maps to the health science discovery goals, or clinical value, or how it addresses known limitations of existing methods. For example, the problem of topological clustering can be very precisely defined (and is a worthwhile and non-trivial mathematical theoretical endeavor), however it is not clear how solving this class of problems overcomes practical limitations of existing methods for concrete health problems.

A related pitfall to imprecise problem definitions is that of "re-inventing the wheel", that is creating an unnecessary new solution to a problem for which equally good or better solutions exist. In the history and practice of AI/ML re-invention of solutions to problems with established solutions is unfortunately rampant. For example, numerous pathway reverse engineering methods have been proposed in bioinformatics without leveraging or acknowledging the mathematically and algorithmically robust literature on causal discovery or improving upon their performance. Similarly the kernel regression method has been re-discovered several times in recent decades. In yet another example, numerous heuristic feature selection algorithms with "non-redundancy" properties have been proposed well after several sound, complete and efficient Markov Boundary algorithms (that solve this class of problem optimally) had been previously introduced, validated and successfully applied.

> **Pitfall 5.2**
> Evaluating the success of methods with poorly defined objectives, by employing ex post facto expert narratives as a proxy of "validity".

> **Pitfall 5.3**
> Defining the goals of methods in mathematical terms but without establishing how the mathematical goals map to the healthcare or health science discovery goals.

> **Pitfall 5.4**
> Reinventing the wheel: whereby a new method is introduced but it has been previously discovered yet ignored (willfully or not) by the "new" method developers.

> **Pitfall 5.5**
> Reinventing a method but make it worse to established methods (…"reinventing the wheel and making it square"!).

In-depth real-life example for step 1 (Rigorous problem definition): Development and evaluation of scalable discovery methods of biomarkers and molecular pathways from high dimensional biomedical data.

Investigators started by asking: how can we make this problem concrete? Biomarkers are a diverse group of conceptual entities which across the literature includes the following: (1) substitutes (proxy outcomes) for outcomes in clinical trials; (2) downstream effects of interventions that are indicative of toxicity and adverse events; (3) complex computable models (aka "signatures") that can be used to diagnose, prognosticate or precision-treat patients; Pathways, on the other hand, are causal subsystems in bigger healthcare or biological systems with defined functions and modularity. Pathways can be instrumental in revealing drug targets for new therapeutics. Biomarkers are involved in one or more drug target pathways [8–10].

One can see that the general concepts of biomarkers and related disease or drug pathways includes, therefore, both predictive and causal modeling which indicates that one would need to develop methods that seamlessly support both types of reasoning. In addition, such development is sensitive to the need for discovery and modeling with very high dimensional and often low sample size datasets.

One natural way to frame the predictive/prognostic/outcome surrogate biomarker discovery aspect is as a feature selection problem, and the causal aspect as a causal induction problem. Recall from chapters "Foundations and Properties of AI/ML Systems", "An Appraisal and Operating Characteristics of Major ML Methods Applicable in Healthcare and Health Science", and "Foundations of Causal ML" that the feature selection problem in its simplest standard form can be stated as: *given a distribution P, with variable set V including a response variable ("target") T, and data sampled iid from P, find the smallest set of variables S in V such that S contains all predictive information about T in P.* The observational causal induction problem can be stated as: *given a distribution P, generated by a causal process C comprising a variable set V including a response variable ("target") T, and data sampled iid from P, without interventions on V, find the set of ordered relations (Vi,Vj) such that Vi directly causes Vj, whereby the causal semantics are as follows: Vi, temporally precedes Vj and a randomized experiment determining values of Vi yields changes in the distribution of Vj (compared to not manipulating Vi).*

These definitions directly point to three computational and mathematical frameworks for AI/ML modeling addressing the problem definitions: first, theory of relevancy; second, theory of causal graph induction; and third, theory of Bayesian Networks and in particular Markov Boundaries [11–14].

Step 2. Theoretical analysis of problem (complexity, problem space characteristics etc.)

The second step, after the method goals are precisely defined, is to conduct theoretical analysis that shows the characteristics *of the problem, across all possible AI/ML methods* that could be employed. This at first glance may seem to the non-expert exceedingly hard, or even impossible, since there is an infinity of possible AI/ML algorithms that one can devise. In practice, a precise and thoughtful problem definition in step 1 of the development process presented, often makes it feasible or even easy to derive properties by mapping the problem considered (i.e., by establishing its correspondence) to known problems which themselves have established properties.

For example, recall from chapter "Foundations and Properties of AI/ML Systems" one of the foundational achievements of computer science is the theoretical toolkit to prove that a problem class has a certain computational complexity. Similarly, the whole practice of Operations Research relies on having a catalog of prototypical problems with efficient solution algorithms such that practitioners can solve infinite problems just by mapping them to the smaller set of pre-established archetypal problem solutions [15].

If such mapping is not possible, the methods developers or evaluators can apply other established more granular and general-purpose techniques from the field of design and analysis of algorithms to understand the feasibility and hardness of the problem space [16].

Real-life example for step 2 (Theoretical analysis of problem). Development or evaluation of scalable discovery methods of biomarkers and molecular pathways from high dimensional biomedical data, CONTINUED.

How one would go about characterizing the theoretical properties of the problem as formally defined in step1? Recall from chapters "Foundations and Properties of AI/ML Systems", "An Appraisal and Operating Characteristics of Major ML Methods Applicable in Healthcare and Health Science" that existing theory of relevancy includes the Kohavi-John framework (K-J) which differentiates between *strongly relevant, weakly relevant and irrelevant features*. Strongly relevant features in K-J theory are features that have unique information and can never be dropped by feature selection without loss of predictive signal. Weakly relevant features are predictive but lack unique signal, thus can be dropped by feature selection without loss of predictivity. Irrelevant features carry no signal so they are effectively noise (for the target T) and can be dismissed by feature selection. So there is a theory guiding the discovery of predictive biomarkers. What about the causal aspect?

As we saw, the connective tissue between causation, feature selection and causal discovery is given, locally around a target variable T, by the Markov Boundary (MB) of T. Specifically, a Markov Blanket of T is any set of variables that renders all other variables in the data independent of T, once we know the Markov Blanket variables. A Markov Boundary is a minimal

Markov Blanket which means that we cannot discard any member of the Markov Boundary without losing its Markov Blanket property. Moreover in a vast family of distributions (the majority of all possible distributions including all distributions modeled by classical statistics), called Faithful Distributions, and when no latent variables are present,: (a) there is always a single Markov Boundary and (b) the Markov Boundary comprises the direct causes, plus direct effects plus direct causes of the direct effects of T (so-called "spouses" of T). Thus, the Markov Boundary contains the local causal pathway around T (minus those spouses that lack causal edges to T). Moreover because BNs are probability and decision theoretically sound, MBs are also consistent with probability and decision theory. Finally, the Markov Boundary feature selection is connected with K-J relevancy since in Faithful distributions the strongly relevant features are the members of the Markov Boundary [11–14].

So far the problem space was well-characterized, looked feasible and the natural next question was what are algorithms that solve it?

Step 3. First-pass algorithms solving problem

The third stage of new AI/ML method development is a first attempt at identifying or (if none exists) creating an algorithmic method that solves the problem as previously defined and analyzed. If the problem has been precisely defined and its properties established in steps 1 and 2, then it is often easy to modify existing methods or put together a first algorithm that solves the problem. Typically this first-pass solution is not meant to be optimally efficient, as such optimization is attempted in subsequent steps. Existing method evaluation may also apply here if the existing method is an early-stage one.

Real-life example for step 3 (First-pass algorithms solving the problem). Development or evaluation of scalable discovery methods of biomarkers and molecular pathways from high dimensional biomedical data, CONTINUED.

In our running example, the theoretical specifications and analysis described above provide solid footing for moving to first-pass algorithm development. Algorithms that solve the example problem do exist (chapters "Foundations and Properties of AI/ML Systems", "An Appraisal and Operating Characteristics of Major ML Methods Applicable in Healthcare and Health Science") and have solid properties, however for illustrative and pedagogical purposes we will consider their development at the time that they did not exist and had to be invented.

Developing new such algorithms was a necessity in the early 00s because at the time there was no sound and scalable algorithms for discovery of Markov

Boundaries from data. In principle, one could use existing causal graph induction algorithms to discover the whole graph and then extract the Markov Boundaries from it. However the algorithms were not scalable beyond approx. 100 variables in practice, and it had been shown that learning the causal graph with Bayesian search and score algorithms was NP-Hard, whereas the Conditional Independence and constraint-based algorithm family was worst case exponential (chapter "Foundations of Causal ML"). Heuristic algorithms introduced by Kohler and Sahami in 1996 and by Cooper et al. in 1997 were informative first attempts but not sound. In the Kohler-Sahami case they were also poor empirical performers, whereas the Cooper et al. algorithm was better performer in small data but was not scalable in compute time or sample size. Another recent (at the time) algorithm by Margaritis and Thrun was sound but not scalable and also not sample efficient. With these necessities in mind Tsamardinos and Aliferis invented a novel sound and scalable algorithm IAMB, and variants, that could be instantiated in a variety of ways (e.g. by combining it with full-graph algorithms for intermediate results pruning or post-processing) [18–21].

Step 4. Theoretical properties of first pass algorithms: focus on representation power, soundness and completeness.

Once a first algorithm that *prima facie* solves the problem has been created, its key theoretical properties should ideally be established, typically under (a) sufficient or necessary conditions, or (b) sufficient and necessary conditions. If analysis shows that no such conditions exist, or that they are too narrow and unworkable in real life conditions, then revisiting step 3 is mandated and steps 3 and 4 are iterated until a method has been identified that guarantees soundness and completeness (or reasonable approximations thereof) under real-life realistic conditions.

Real-life example for step 4 (Theoretical properties of first pass algorithms: focus on representation power, soundness and completeness). Development or evaluation of scalable discovery methods of biomarkers and molecular pathways from high dimensional biomedical data, CONTINUED.

In our running example and from the viewpoint of when the corresponding development steps were conducted, the IAMB algorithm family was theoretically sound and complete. In preliminary empirical analyses its inventors established that it is both sound and scalable. IAMB was however a *definitional* Markov Boundary algorithm meaning it would apply the definition of the Markov Boundary in each step of its operation. This entailed that it would conduct conditional independence tests with large sets of variables which increased its sample size needs to exponentially large to the number of conditioning variables. So, refinements and optimizations were needed which led to a second (more refined) family of algorithms (see below).

Step 5. Algorithm refinements, extensions and derivatives

Step 5 is a multi-faceted and critical step in the sense that its success will determine the practical utility of the new method. This is the step where various optimizations and adaptations to real life performance requirements will take place. This step has several sub-steps that may require many years' worth of incremental improvements. Hardly ever the full range of optimizations is accomplished close to the first time a method appears in the literature. It is not uncommon for such efforts to constitute a career-long research program of the method innovators and their teams, as well as independent researchers. The refinement sub-steps comprise:

Step 5.a. Performance Optimizations that cover achieving high computational efficiency for learning and for using models; optimizations for other costs (for example cost to obtain and store input data and run analyses on a compute environment, either at model discovery or at model deployment time); efficient space complexity for learning, storing and using models; efficient sample complexity and establishing learning curves and broad power-sample requirements.

Real-life example for step 5.a. (Performance Optimizations - Sample efficient algorithms and going beyond local pathways). Development or evaluation of scalable discovery methods of biomarkers and molecular pathways from high dimensional biomedical data, CONTINUED.

In our running example, the second-pass algorithms designed to overcome IAMB's sample size inefficiency described earlier was HITON and MMMB. These were *compositional* algorithms, that is, instead of applying the definition of Markov Boundary, they composed it edge-by-edge (exploiting the link between graphical and probabilistic Markov Boundaries and causality).

At the core of the causal discovery problem from observational data there is a foundational theorem (chapter "Foundations of Causal ML") that states that to establish a direct edge between variables Vi and Vj one must establish the conditional dependence of these variables given every subset of the remainder of the variables in the data [13]. This is clearly an exponential cost operation in both compute time and sample, which becomes super-astronomical in datasets with more than a few dozen variables. Thus smart algorithms are needed to exploit the sparsity of causal processes and identify quickly a single subset that shows independence so that the vast majority of tests can be omitted from computations.

With this asymmetry in mind, the designers of HITON and MMMB sought to apply informed search functions that would identify quickly a single subset needed to establish that variable Vi was not directly linked to T, for every Vi in the data. Whereas the algorithms are still worst-case exponential (because the problem is itself worst-case exponential regardless of algorithm), their exponentiality is directly linked to the connectivity of the underlying causal structure. For sparse or predominantly sparse causal data generating processes (as most biological networks are, for example), the majority of the causal process can be identified fast if **the algorithms' time complexity is adaptive to the connectivity**. Both HITON and MMMB are locally adaptive to the hardness of the causal problem at hand. Additional variants return direct causes and effects only (HITON-PC, MMPC) and Markov Boundaries (HITON-MB, MMMB).

Because of the compositional nature of this second generation of algorithms these investigators and their collaborators were able to introduce algorithm variants that discover not just the Markov Boundary for T, but also *the local causal pathways (causal neighborhood) only* around T (i.e. without need to find spouses and remove them with post processing), also *local causal regions* of depth *k* (depth specified by the user), and *the full causal graph* by inducing all local causal edges around every variable in the data (algorithm MMHC and it generalized family LGL) [22–24].

Step 5.b. Parallelization, distributed/federated, sequential, chunked, versions [25–27]. These are derivative and enhanced forms of the main algorithmic solution with the following properties:

Parallel algorithms: can be run in parallel computing architectures and environments whereby the computational steps are divided among many processors. The parallelization can be *coarse, intermediate, or fine grain*, depending on how large and complicated are the unit computations divided among the parallel processors.

Distributed/federated algorithms: operate across federated and distributed databases which exist in diverse locations without the need to bring all data into a centralized database and computing environment.

Sequential algorithms operate in steps corresponding to incremental availability of input data, for example with increasing sample size over time, or with increasing sets of variables over time. At each processing step, a different set of results is obtained that over time increases in quality (i.e., converges to the right solution or approximation thereof).

Chunked algorithms address the situation where data is so large that overwhelms the memory limits of the computing environment. The data is divided then in chunks, each one of which fits in memory, and analysis proceeds across all chunks until all data is analyzed and final results obtained.

Real-life example for step 5.b. (Performance Optimizations - Parallelization, distributed/federated, sequential, chunked, versions). Development or evaluation of scalable discovery methods of biomarkers and molecular pathways from high dimensional biomedical data, CONTINUED.

In our running example, and motivated by the need to process datasets with vast numbers of variables not fitting in single-computer memories of the time, the investigator team was also forced to invent a chunked version of IAMB and HITON. Because of the nature of these algorithms it was immediately obvious that they can also be modified to obtain parallel, distributed, and sequential versions as well. Over the years, the investigator team conducted massive experiments in parallel compute clusters taking advantage of these algorithms. These algorithms also gave important insights on the feasibility and requirements for **sound federated** Markov Boundary and causal discovery. For example, it was established that for sound federated/distributed Markov Boundary discovery exactly two passes of local processing was required plus one global step with the results from the first two passes, and a subset of variables had to be shared among all nodes depending on intermediate results [1, 28].

Step 5.c. Relaxing assumptions/requirements. This step corresponds to efforts to relax the assumptions guaranteeing its properties and broaden the space of conditions under which the new or existing method will have the desired guaranteed properties.

Real-life relevance. For example, extending Bayesian classifiers from restricted distributions with Naive Bayes, to algorithms that can operate on all discrete distributions. Other examples include: extending from discrete to continuous decision trees, extending single tree models to ensembles of trees (e.g., Random Forests) that are more robust to sampling variance, extending artificial neural networks from linearly separable functions to non linearly-separable ones, extending SVM binary classification to multi-class classification, extending SVMs from noiseless data to noisy data, extending linear to non-linear SVMs, extending standard Cox Proportional Hazards regression to accommodate time-dependent covariate effects, extending causal discovery algorithms that require no hidden (aka latent) variables to ones that can operate in the presence of latents, etc. (see chapters "Foundations and Properties of AI/ML Systems", "An Appraisal and Operating Characteristics of Major ML Methods Applicable in Healthcare and Health Science", and "Foundations of Causal ML" for details and more examples).

In-depth example for step 5.c. (Performance Optimizations: Relaxing assumptions/requirements allowing equivalence classes, latent variables, guided experimentation). Development or evaluation of scalable discovery methods of biomarkers and molecular pathways from high dimensional biomedical data, CONTINUED.

In our running example, the methods outlined so far depended on two fundamental assumptions: one is Faithful distributions and the other is causal sufficiency (i.e., no unmeasured confounders). To address the former, the development team introduced new algorithms addressing distributions with *information equivalences*, i.e., distributions where several variable groups can have the same information regarding the target response. Such situations are very common in omics data, complex survey data, clinical data, and many other types of biomedical data. The result of information equivalency is the existence of multiple (not just one) Markov Boundaries and ambiguity of the causal pathways.

Specifically, in such distributions there is an equivalence class containing multiple statistically indistinguishable MBs and local causal edges and the size of this class can be exponential to the number of variables. Statnikov et al. introduced a family of algorithms called TIE* which extract from data all MBs and local causal neighborhoods. TIE* algorithm family members are sound, complete and adaptable to the distribution at hand by choice of conditional independence tests and component subroutines (used for single Markov Boundary induction).

The second relaxation concerning latent variables was addressed by postprocessing the main algorithms' results with algorithms that can detect presence of hidden variables (e.g., IC* and FCI, see chapter "Foundations of Causal ML"). Such algorithms could not be used for end-to-end analysis because they are not scalable and in most cases they are also error prone empirically.

Another important algorithmic extension addressing both equivalence classes and latent variables was the introduction of algorithms that resolve these ambiguities by limited algorithm-guided experimentation. Specifically the ODLP algorithm family combines using MB and local neighborhood algorithms plus equivalency class algorithms and guides an experimenter to conduct a series of experiments that resolve statistical ambiguity due to latents and equivalence class due to information equivalency. The ODLP algorithm attempts to minimize the number of experiments and has worst-case number of experiments that is at most the total number of variables in the equivalence class of the local pathway [29–31].

Step 5.d. Generalized frameworks (generalized family of algorithms and generalized conditions for performance guarantees).

This step involves extending the new method to a more general family of inter-related similar methods. It also involves establishing testable rules for instantiating the family into specific methods in that class, and testable rules for guaranteeing that the properties of the family will be shared by every method in that family (without further need to prove these properties of empirically test them).

It is not always obvious if such generalizations are possible, and if yes how to accomplish them. Thus it is not always pursued, especially in initial stages of developing a new method. But whenever it is possible, it confers a number of important benefits which we summarize here. Developing a generalization of a fundamental method explains in mathematically precise terms how the core method can be modified so that:

(a) It can address slightly different problem instance classes and situations;

(b) To allow for modifications that do not alter its foundational nature;

(c) It will enable other method developers to create variations without having to undergo the whole development process from scratch and at the same time inherit the main performance and other properties of the core method;

(d) It will help understand other methods and their properties by showing how they relate to the generalized core method;

(e) It will prevent confusion about apparently similar methods with different properties or apparently different methods with same properties; and

(f) It will protect scientific priority claims and commercial intellectual property, by establishing which methods are just variations or derivatives of the original core methods, especially when such variations and derivatives were anticipated by the generalized framework.

Real-life relevance. Examples of generalized families of inter-related algorithms are many and include: the Best-First-Search algorithm family (chapter "Foundations and Properties of AI/ML Systems"), the General Linear Model (GLM) family (chapter "An Appraisal and Operating Characteristics of Major ML Methods Applicable in Healthcare and Health Science"), the penalty+loss regularized classifier family (chapter "An Appraisal and Operating Characteristics of Major ML Methods Applicable in Healthcare and Health Science"), the Generalized Local Learning (GLL) and Local to Global causal discovery (LGL) algorithm families (chapters "Foundations and Properties of AI/ML Systems", "An Appraisal and Operating Characteristics of Major ML Methods Applicable in Healthcare and Health Science", and "Foundations of Causal ML"), and the TIE* family for equivalence class modeling (chapters "Foundations and Properties of AI/ML Systems", "An Appraisal and Operating Characteristics of Major ML Methods Applicable in Healthcare and Health Science").

In-depth example for step 5.d. (Performance Optimizations: Generalized frameworks). Development or evaluation of scalable discovery methods of biomarkers and molecular pathways from high dimensional biomedical data, CONTINUED.

In our running example, of developing principled and scalable biomarker and pathway discovery algorithms, it was realized within the team developing these algorithms, that infinite variations could be had that would preserve the soundness, completeness and other desired properties of the first algorithms introduced. To facilitate the study and further analysis and development of the families of the algorithms in a systematic way and minimizing confusion, Aliferis at al introduced a generalization of HITON-PC/HITON-MB and MMMP/MMMB, and of MMHC.

The former was termed GLL family and the latter LGL. Around the same time Statnikov and Aliferis introduced the generalized TIE family termed TIE*, and later generalized versions of ODLP and of parallel/distributed/sequential and chunked variants. Aliferis et al. introduced the notion of a 2-part **Generative Algorithm Framework** comprising:

1. *A general template* statement of the algorithm family.
2. *Admissibility rules* for instantiation of the template components.

If the admissibility rules are followed when instantiating components, then this guarantees that the instantiated algorithm have guaranteed properties *without the need for de novo theory or proofs*.

Figure 6 illustrates one instantiation of the GLL-PC generative template algorithm (shown in 6.a) by the admissibility rules of the Generative Algorithm Framework (shown in 6.b) to yield an infinity of algortihms with guaranteed properties such as the original MMPC (presented in 6.c). Contrary to the intricacy of the original MMPC, however, the generative framework describes the whole family of algorithms by specification of a few simple components.

Moreover, a Generative Algorithm Framework does not allow just the re-creation and compact representation of pre-existing algorithms, but as shown by these investigators, several new instantiations of the original generalized algorithms were demonstrated and they matched or exceed empirical performance of the original set of algorithms in validation data. One of the new algorithms is shown in part (6.d) of the figure. The new instantiations exhibited different traces of navigating the solution space toward the correct (same) output, demonstrating that they are not just a rehash of known algorithms [1, 29–32].

a

GLL-PC: High-level pseudocode and main components of Generalized Local Learning - Parents and Children. Returns PC(T)

1. U ← GLL-PC-nonsym(T) // first approximate $PC(T)$ without symmetry check

2. For all $X \in U$

3.   If $T \notin$ GLL-PC-nonsym(X) then $U \leftarrow U \setminus \{X\}$ // <u>check for symmetry</u>

4. Return U // true set of parents and children

GLL-PC-nonsym(T) // *return a set which is a subset of EPC(T) and a superset of PC(T)*

1. Initialization

   a. Initialize a set of candidates for the true $PC(T)$ set: $TPC(T) \leftarrow S$, s.t. $S \subseteq V \setminus \{T\}$
   b. Initialize a priority queue of variables to be examined for inclusion in
      $TPC(T)$: OPEN ← $V \setminus \{T \cup TPC(T)\}$

2. Apply <u>inclusion heuristic function</u>

   a. Prioritize variables in OPEN for inclusion in $TPC(T)$;
   b. Throw away non-eligible variables from OPEN;
   c. Insert in $TPC(T)$ the highest-priority variable(s) in OPEN and remove them
      from OPEN

3. Apply <u>elimination strategy</u> to remove variables from $TPC(T)$

4. Apply <u>interleaving strategy</u> by repeating steps #2 and #3 until a termination
   criterion is met

5. Return $TPC(T)$

Fig. 6 Example of Generative Algorithm Framework. GLL-PC shown here and generating two from an infinite number of members of this family of algorithms (pre-existing MMPC algorithm in part (**c**) and new algorithm semi-interleaved HITON-PC with symmetry correction in part **d**), with guaranteed properties, merely by instantiating a simple general template statement (part **a**), following a small set of admissibility rules (part **b**)

b

GLL-PC: Admissibility rules

1. The inclusion heuristic function should respect the following requirement:

    // Admissibility rule #1

    All variables $X \in PC(T)$ are eligible for inclusion in the candidate set $TPC(T)$ and each one is assigned a non-zero value by the ranking function. Variables with zero values are discarded and never considered again.

    Note that variables may be re-ranked after each update of the candidate set, or the original ranking may be used throughout the algorithm's operation.

2. The elimination strategy should satisfy the following requirement:

    // Admissibility rule #2

    All and only variables that become independent of the target variable T given any subset of the candidate set $TPC(T)$ are discarded and never considered again (whether they are inside or outside $TPC(T)$).

3. The interleaving strategy iterates inclusion and elimination any number of times provided that iterating stops when the following criterion is satisfied:

    // Admissibility rule #3

    At termination no variable outside the set $TPC(T)$ is eligible for inclusion and no variable in the candidate set can be removed at termination.

Fig. 6 (continued)

c

Algorithm 1 $\overline{MMPC}$ Algorithm

1: **Procedure** $\overline{MMPC}$ (T,$\mathcal{D}$)

      Input: target variable T; data $\mathcal{D}$

      Output: the parents and children of T in any Bayesian network faithfully representing the data distribution

      %Phase I: Forward

2:      **CPC** $= \emptyset$

3:      **repeat**

4:         $\langle F. \, assocF \rangle = MaxMinHeuristic(T; \textbf{CPC})$

5:         **if** $assocF \neq 0$ **then**

6:            **CPC** = **CPC** $\cup \, F$

7:         **end if**

8:      **until CPC** has not changed

      %Phase II: Backward

9:      **for all** $X \in$ **CPC do**

10:     **if** $\exists \textbf{S} \subseteq$ **CPC**, s.t. Ind $(X; T \mid S)$ **then**

11:         **CPC** = **CPC** $\setminus \{X\}$

12:     **end if**

13:     **end for**

14:     **return CPC**

15: **end procedure**

16: **Procedure** MAXMINHEURISTIC(T,**CPC**)

      Input: target variable T; subset of variables **CPC**

      Output: the maximum over all variables of the minimum association with T relative to **CPC**, and the variable that achieves the maximum

17:     $assocF = \max_{X \in V} MinAssoc(X; T|\textbf{CPC})$

18:     $F = \arg \max_{X \in V} MinAssoc(X;T|\textbf{CPC})$

19:     **return** $\langle F, \, assocF \rangle$

20: **end procedure**

Fig. 6 (continued)

d

Semi-Interleaved HITON-PC with symmetry correction

Derived from GLL-PC with following instantiation specifics:

Initialization

$TPC(T) \leftarrow \emptyset$

Inclusion heuristic function

a. Sort in descending order the variables X in OPEN according to their pairwise association with T, i.e., $Assoc(X, T|\emptyset)$.

b. Remove from OPEN variables with zero association with T, i.e., when $I(X, T|\emptyset)$

c. Insert at end of $TPC(T)$ the first variable in OPEN and remove it from OPEN

Elimination strategy

  If OPEN=$\emptyset$

    For each $X \in TPC(T)$

      If $\exists\, Z \subseteq TPC(T)\backslash\{X\}$, s.t. $I(X, T|Z)$ remove X from $TPC(T)$

  Else

    $X \leftarrow$ last variable added to $TPC(T)$ // in step 2 of GLL-PC-nonsym

    If $\exists\, Z \subseteq TPC(T)\backslash\{X\}$, s.t. $I(X, T|Z)$ remove X from $TPC(T)$

Interleaving strategy

Repeat

  steps #2 and #3 of GLL-PC-nonsym

Until OPEN=$\emptyset$

Fig. 6 (continued)

Step 5.e. Nested algorithms, embedding protocols and stacks, interactions with data design.

Real-life relevance. Per traditional computer science and AI/ML practice, algorithms can be used as subroutines in higher complexity algorithms. For example, decision tree induction algorithms can be used inside Random Forests. Weak learning algorithms can be used as components of boosting algorithms. Algorithms of various kinds can be components of Stacked ML models, and so on.

Generative Algorithm Frameworks can also be used to create more complicated and hierarchically- nested algorithms families, creating **nested systems of generalized algorithms tackling an increasingly complex problem-solving AI/ML construct**. For example the GLL-PC generative family is nested in the GLL_MB family, which is nested in the TIE* family, which is nested in the ODLP* family. The nesting does not force use of the most complex level algorithm. To the contrary, the algorithms with smallest complexity that solve a problem are sufficient for that problem.

Algorithms and their implementations are the conceptual and scientific backbone and "engines" of real-life AI/ML. Complicated tools and systems, designed to solve health science and healthcare problems are almost always organized in complex data science "stacks".

AI/ML (or data science) Stack: a hierarchically-integrated *architecture* for AI/ML software system delivery comprising data input management at the lower level, going upward to model selection, to error estimation, to error management, to decision support delivery and end-user interfacing, to embedding and healthcare integration, to model monitoring and full model lifecycle support (see chapter "The Development Process and Lifecycle of Clinical Grade and Other Safety and Performance-Sensitive AI/ML Models" for details).

At the core of the ML stack is the *ML protocol* (see chapter "Foundations and Properties of AI/ML Systems" and "The development process and lifecycle of clinical grade and other safety and performance-sensitive AI/ML models" for details).

ML Protocol. A ML system *architecture* implements a ML method which can be understood as a combination of data design, algorithm, and model selection procedure that ideally will incorporate an error estimator procedure. The higher-level algorithm that combines the ML algorithms, data processing subroutines, model selection strategies and error estimators used, is the ML protocol.

AI/ML "Pipelines", Automodelers, and Platforms. These represent discrete *software implementation* entities embodying implementation of the chosen algorithms and protocol, plus all other layers of the full AI/ML stack and are designed to be used reproducibly, in either fully automatic mode ("automodeler") or semi-automatically, or as a component of a broader modeling system (a "pipeline"). Platforms refer to even more complex software systems with additional facilities for user experimentation, model sandboxing, training, model development, integration with other enterprise systems, etc.

Best Practice 5.5
The properties of a ML algorithm can be negatively or positively affected by the ML protocol to extreme degrees (see chapter "Lessons Learned from Historical Failures, Limitations and Successes of AI/ML In Healthcare and the Health Sciences. Enduring problems, and the Role of Best Practices" for several important case studies that show the immense and often under-appreciated practical consequences). Similarly the data design can negatively or positively affect the ML protocol and its embedded algorithms to extreme degrees. Therefore, it is imperative to design AI/ML methods taking into account any positive or negative interactions of data design with the protocols and embedded algorithms employed.

In-depth example for step 5.e. (Performance Optimizations: Nested algorithms, embedding protocols and stacks, interactions with data design). Development or evaluation of scalable discovery methods of biomarkers and molecular pathways from high dimensional biomedical data, CONTINUED.

In our running example, of developing principled and scalable biomarker and pathway discovery algorithms, a core choice was made to design the algorithms and ML protocols with a focus on nested balanced cross validation as a "canonical" preferred model selection and error estimation protocol (see chapter "The Development Process and Lifecycle of Clinical Grade and Other Safety and Performance-Sensitive AI/ML Models" for more details). The anticipated data designs were primarily case-control or natural, cross-sectional or longitudinal, i.i.d. sample designs. As long as distributions were faithful or TIE, the algorithms were guaranteed to exhibit well-defined and desirable soundness, completeness, computational and sample efficiency properties. Deviations from these "canonical" designs were also tolerated but would need careful tailoring of the methods to data designs outside these "canonical" specifications.

Many of the produced algorithms were embedded in software with data ingestion/transform, model selection, error estimation and adaptive selection among the core methods and state of the art comparators. Examples include the GEMS auto modeler system for microarray analysis, the FAST-Aims auto modeler system for Mass Spectrometry analysis, and several psychiatry-oriented, as well as bioinformatics, clinical and translational predictive and causal modeling stacks and pipelines. The construction of the auto modelers was further guided by extensive benchmarking of these and comparator methods and cross-referencing to expert analyses in the literature on the same datasets. These empirical performance benchmark studies measured a level of performance that matched or exceeded that of faculty level experts in AI/ML with the added advantage of almost immediate analysis, at no cost other than an inexpensive laptop or desktop [33–36].

Figure 7 shows components of the GEMS auto modeler.

Step 5.f. Explanation, clarity, and transparency
This step addresses the needs for **transparency and clarity in the method's semantics, syntax, inference mechanisms and mode of operation**, and including its transparency, explainability, and ability for humans to inspect and understand the **models produced by the new AI/ML method** and of the operations that led to these models.

We frequently refer to AI/ML methods as being "black box, and "transparent", "explainable", or "open box".

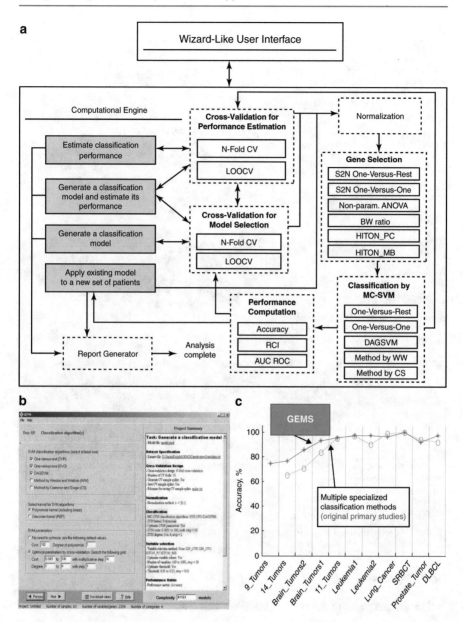

Fig. 7 Example of an auto modeler system. Components of the GEMS auto-modeler shown. (**a**) System architecture. (**b**) "Wizard"-like user interface (the user could enter values for specific parameters, load analysis templates, or run in fully automatic mode). (**c**) Empirical results of GEMS analyzing datasets from the relevant literature and comparison with performance of original studies conducted by experts. (**d**) Algorithms benchmarked to inform the construction of the system [37]. (**e**) Algorithms chosen to be included in the system based on results of the benchmarks

d

Classification algorithms
- K-Nearest Neighbors
- Backpropagation Neural Networks
- Probabilistic Neural Networks
- Multi-Class SVM: one-versus-rest
- Multi-Class SVM: one-versus-one
- Multi-Class SVM: DAGSVM
- Multi-Class SVM by Weston and Watkins
- Multi-Class SVM by Crammer and Singer
- Weighted Voting: one-versus-rest
- Weighted Voting: one-versus-one
- Decision Trees: CART

Ensemble classification algorithms
Based on output of Multi-Class SVM methods
- Majority voting
- Decision Trees: CART
- Multi-Class SVM: DAGSVM
- Multi-Class SVM: one-versus-rest
- Multi-Class SVM: one-versus-one

Based on output of all classifiers
- Majority voting
- Decision Trees: CART

Computational experimental design
- Leave-one-out cross-validation for performance estimation (outer loop) and 10-fold cross-validation for model selection (inner loop)
- 10-fold cross-validation for performance estimation (outer loop) and 9-fold cross-validation for model selection (inner loop)

Gene selection methods
- Signal-to-noise ratio in one-versus-rest fashion
- Signal-to-noise ratio in one-versus-one fashion
- Kruskal-Wallis nonparametric one-way ANOVA
- Ratio of genes between-categories to within-category sum of squares

Performance metrics
- Accurancy
- Relative classifier information (entropy-based performance metric)

Statistical comparison among classifiers
- Custom randomized permutation procedure

e

Classification algorithms
- Multi-Class SVM: one-versus-rest
- Multi-Class SVM: one-versus-one
- Multi-Class SVM: DAGSVM
- Multi-Class SVM by Weston and Watkins
- Multi-Class SVM by Crammer and Singer

Gene selection methods
- Signal-to-noise ratio in one-versus-rest fashion
- Signal-to-noise ratio in one-versus-one fashion
- Kruskal—Wallis nonparametric one-way ANOVA
- Ration of genes between-categores to within-category sum of squares
- HITON_PC
- HITON_MB

Normalization techniques
- For every gene x [a, b]
- For every gene x $[x - \text{mean}(x)]/\text{std.}(x)$
- For every gene x $x/\text{std.}(x)$
- For every gene x $x/\text{mean}(x)$
- For every gene x $x/\text{median}(x)$
- For every gene x $x/\|x\|$
- For every gene x $x - \text{mean}(x)$
- For every gene x $x - \text{median}(x)$
- For every gene x $|x|$
- For every gene x $x + |x|$
- For every gene x $\log(x)$

Computational experimental design
- Leave-one-out cross-validation for performance estimation (outer loop) and N-fold cross-validation for model selection (inner loop)
- N-fold cross-validation for performance estimation (outer loop) and $(N-1)$-fold cross-validation (inner loop)
- Leave-one-out cross-validation for model selection
- N-fold cross-validation for model selection

Performance metrics
- Accuracy
- Relatives classifier information (entropy-based performance metric)
- **Area under ROC curve (AUC)**

Fig. 7 (continued)

For the purposes of the present book we will define:

Black box AI/ML methods and/or models: are methods or models for which the user (and possibly even the developer) know only the inputs and outputs but not the internal operation; or, alternatively, the internal operation is accessible but it is not readily fully interpretable by humans.

Transparent (aka explainable, open, or white, or clear box) are methods or models for which the user and the developer know not only the inputs and outputs but also the internal operation which is readily fully interpretable by humans.

The transparency of the new method and its models are critical for (a) debugging the method and models (see chapter "Characterizing, Diagnosing and Managing the Risk of Error of ML and AI Models in Clinical and Organizational Application"), and (b) managing risks associated with its use and establishing trust in the AI/ML method and its outputs (see chapters "Artificial Intelligence (AI) and Machine Learning (ML) for Healthcare and Health Sciences: the Need for Best Practices Enabling Trust in AI and ML" and "Characterizing, Diagnosing and Managing the Risk of Error of ML and AI Models in Clinical and Organizational Application"), as well as "Regulatory Aspects and Ethical Legal Societal Implications (ELSI)").

When AI/ML methods are transparent we can also explain and justify their results including on a case-by-case, input-output basis. However there is a somewhat subtle but important distinction between explanation by translation and other forms of justification which is germane to the purposes of best practices in AI/ML.

Justification of a method or a model (and their outputs) is any argument that supports the validity of the method, the models produced by it, and the outputs produced by the models.

Explanation of a method or model (and their outputs) by functional translation is a justification of the method or model's logic by fully equivalent translation in humanly-understandable language.

Where:

Human understandable language includes natural language but also other formalisms readily understood by humans such as decision diagrams, decision trees, propositional and first order logic, etc.

A common pitfall in AI/ML is providing peripheral/oblique and thus inadequate justifications of the model and its decisions which may be persuasive in some settings, but do not "open" the black box in the sense of creating a human-understandable and mathematically equivalent model to the black box model. For example, consider a hypothetical similarity-based "explanation" module of a neural network AI/ML model using exemplars. The module attempts to justify model decisions on a case C, by presenting a small number of cases similar to C, with gold standard labels same as the model's prediction for C. Because the neural network does not make decisions based on similarity to exemplars, this whole justification exercise amounts to a "sleight of hand". It can also be argued that local simple (e.g. linear) approximations to a very complex decision functions underlying the black box models, attempt to justify the decisions of the model are generally meaningful and trustworthy by examining a simplified version of the local individual decisions of the neural net but not explaining the global complex inductive logic of the model and its generalization.

We also highlight the distinction between "open source" and "closed source" software implementing AI/ML methods and models.

Open source software is software whose source code is at minimum open for inspection. Depending on the specific licensing terms of open source software, it may or not come with other rights granted, such as the right to modify the source code and release such modifications under same or different licensing terms.

Closed source (or proprietary) software is software with restrictions on code inspection, use, modifications/derivatives creation, sharing derivatives, or sharing the software.

A pitfall in AI/ML is conflating "open source" for open box" and "closed source" for "black box" software.

In reality an open source implementation of a method or model does not entail "open box" status, and a "closed-source" software does not entail "black box status. Artificial neural Network models are notoriously "black box" ones, yet this does not change if we have access to the code implementing them, or the right to modify and re-distribute implementation code. Conversely, a closed source implementation of, for example the ID3 decision tree algorithm, can be transparent in terms of both the algorithm used (which is well understood and openly accessible in the literature, and may also be accessible by licensed users), and the models it produces (i.e., decision trees which are intuitive and readily understood by humans). The latter case requires that the disclosures of the algorithms used by the software are (a) complete and (b) accurate.

Pitfall 5.6
Providing persuasive but peripheral/oblique justifications that lack fidelity to the AI/ML method, the models produced by them and their decisions.

Pitfall 5.7
Confusing "open source" for "transparent" and "closed source" for black box".

In this section we covered only introductory concepts about explainability, since at the method development stage it is typically quite clear whether the method and its models are interpretable. In chapter "The development Process and Lifecycle of Clinical Grade and Other Safety and Performance-Sensitive AI/ML Models" we will delve into the details of explainable AI (XAI) [38], interpretable ML [39] and some of the key techniques and nuances of explaining back box models.

In-depth example for step 5.f. (Performance Optimizations: Explanation, clarity, and transparency). Development or evaluation of scalable discovery methods of biomarkers and molecular pathways from high dimensional biomedical data, CONTINUED.

In our running example, of developing principled and scalable biomarker and pathway discovery algorithms, a core choice was made to design the algorithms and ML protocols within a causal graphical modeling framework. Causal graphs are very intuitive representations of causality, and Markov Boundaries have an intuitive causal and probabilistic meaning and lead to very compact and transparent models as well. Depending on the classifier used (e.g., decision trees, conditional probability tables/heatpmaps, rules, regression) results can be readily reviewed by human non-experts. In addition, the team members devised a more sophisticated method whereby if the MB was used to create black box models (because they were optimally predictive) or for any black box model for that matter, data would be sampled from the black box model and then a meta learning step involving MB induction and learning decision tree models over the MB that were equivalent to the black box, but perfectly transparent to humans. This explanation method was used to understand the black box reasoning of human physicians in the diagnosis of melanoma by Sboner et al. [40, 41]. More details are presented in chapter "The Development Process and Lifecycle of Clinical Grade and Other Safety and Performance-Sensitive AI/ML Models" in the context of general explanation of black box models.

Step 6. Empirically test algorithms in controlled conditions

The next stage in the development of new AI/ML methods is testing them in controlled conditions whereby they are given data that comply with the sufficient or necessary and sufficient conditions for their theoretical performance properties to hold. In these empirical tests, developers also vary parameters such as sample size, variable measurement noise, strength of signal for the functions to be learnt, dimensionality of the data as well as various parameters relevant to the specific characteristics of the learning methods (as dictated by their properties established in previous steps) The methods are also tested with data where assumptions are violated to varying degree and the effect on performance characteristics is studied.

There are four important types of controlled condition data testing:

(a) **Simulated data**: where developers or other evaluators first define a mathematical or computational model representing the data generating function to be learned. Then they sample from this function via simulation, give the data to the AI/ML method and study its performance characteristics.

(b) **Label-reshuffled data**: these are real data where evaluators randomly re-assign the response variable's values (aka "labels") across the dataset (Fig. 8). This has

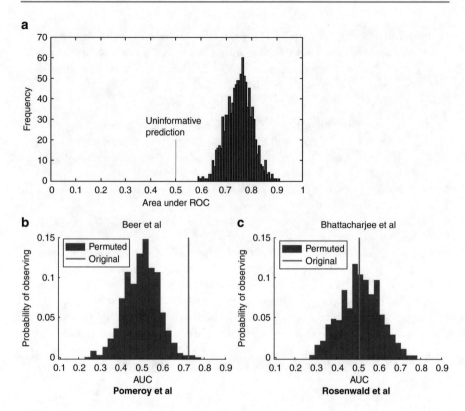

Fig. 8 Label reshuffling and its uses. In the top panel (**a**), the distribution of estimated predictivity for a hypothetical new ML method operating in a dataset that has been label-reshuffled (measured as area under the ROC curve—AUC ROC) is shown in blue. As can be seen, the distribution is not centered at the 0.5 point (the uninformative or no-signal point) in the AUC ROC. This indicates that the new ML method significantly overestimates performance [42]. In the bottom left panel (**b**) from a real data set modeling it can be seen that (1) the modeling protocol does not overestimate the model performance (because the distribution is centered on AUC ROC 0.5) and (2) the actual model obtained (red line) has performance that is statistically significantly different than that of the null hypothesis (i.e., no signal, represented again by the 0.5 point of the AUC ROC distribution of label-reshuffled datasets). By contrast, the analysis of the data depicted in the bottom right panel (**c**), leads to a model devoid of signal. Again the protocol used is unbiased with respect to error estimation [43]

the effect of maintaining the real joint distribution of inputs, as well as the real marginal distribution of response variable, but decoupling the inputs from outputs, so that over multiple such label-reshuffled datasets, on average there is no signal to be learned. This type of simulation is essential for testing ML methods' error estimation procedures. It is also a valuable tool for testing a learnt model against the hull hypothesis of no predictive signal in the data [42, 43]. See also chapter "Overfitting, Underfitting and General Model Overconfidence and Under-Performance Pitfalls and Best Practices in Machine Learning and AI" on model over confidence for more details.

(c) **Re-simulated data**. *Resimulation* attempts to create controlled data simulations that are ideally hi-fidelity approximations of real data distributions of interest. Resimulation works as follows [32, 44]:

- We start with one or more real life datasets D^{real} where all variables (including response variables) have known values.
- Then we use a learning algorithm A to learn one or more models Mi capturing all or at least some desired characteristics of the real-life distribution from which the real data was sampled from.
- Then we sample from the encoded distribution in Mi using simulation ("resimulation" in his context) creating resimulated data D^{resim}.
- Then we test the properties of D^{resim} against the real data D^{real}. A variety of distribution similarity metrics can be used as well as custom predictive modeling, and custom tests of properties can be used for establishing that the resimulated data is a hi-fidelity representation of the real data.
- If adjustments are needed, we can iterate between the second and fourth steps until sufficiently accurate resimulated data is obtained.
- Once we have the hi-fidelity resimulated data we can now feed it in the new method, while varying parameters and obtain performance metrics just like in the case of simple simulation.

A conceptual nuance about resimulation is that if the resimulated data is perfectly indistinguishable from real data *in all modeling aspects of interest to us* (not just modeling the joint distribution), that implies that algorithm A is an optimal algorithm for discovery for the data generating function of the real distribution. Algorithm A would then represent a correct discovery algorithm procedure, rendering further method development effort potentially unnecessary (barring efficiency considerations). In common practice, we rarely have a perfect algorithm A at hand when performing resimulations. Instead we use algorithms that capture simplified and controllable aspects of the real data and therefore the performance of our new method is (loosely) an upper bound on the performance with real data. The rationale being that, if a new method cannot learn the process that creates the simplified version of real data D^{real}, i.e., D^{resim}, then the new method will most likely not be able to learn much more complicated real life data generating functions. If a perfect algortihm A exists in terms of quality of output, then the new algorithms may be more efficient ones.

(d) **Statistical tests for distributional or other conditions for method correctness.** These typically encompass statistical tests that do not test the algorithms but the data per se. For example, if an algorithm is devised to create regression models under multivariate normality of the data, we can test the real data for conformance to this assumption. This type of test is an important supplement to simulation studies and may also serve as a preferred alternative if no credible simulation or resimulation can be designed, and the algorithm's theory of correctness is well established.

In-depth example for step 6 (Empirically test algorithms in controlled conditions). Development or evaluation of scalable discovery methods of biomarkers and molecular pathways from high dimensional biomedical data, CONTINUED.

In our running example, of developing principled and scalable biomarker and pathway discovery algorithms, all of the algorithms discussed in section "Over- and Under-Interpreting Results", were tested extensively with simulated and resimulated data. These experiments revealed a number of important properties including: (1) verifying the MB theoretical expectation of maximum compactness and maximum predicitivity; (2) verified causal consistency; (3) showed high stability; (4) showed large added value over comparators and over random selection; (5) showed the role of various hyperparameters; (6) established the natural false discovery rate control in the GLL algorithm family that protecting against false positives due to conducting massive numbers of conditional independence tests; (8) showed the role of inclusion heuristics for computational efficiency; (9) demonstrated how perilous is to use non causal comparator methods to infer causality (something that GLL algorithms accomplish very well); and (10) showed the relatively large insensitivity of the algorithms to hyperparameter choice [1, 32].

Step 7. Empirically test algorithms in real life data with known answers/ solutions

This testing involves real data where known gold standard answers have been established by prior research. This is a very informative testing stage because a myriad of factors may exist in real data that have not been anticipated in theoretical analysis or in simulations. Conversely, it is also possible for real data to exhibit higher simplicity than what was anticipated by methods' developers which if true, typically leads to relaxing some of the related assumptions of the new method.

We re-iterate for emphasis that there are two reasons why we do not jump directly to step 7 (i.e., omitting empirical testing under controlled conditions):

First, real data does not afford *full control* of all relevant parameters that may influence the new method's performance. For example, we cannot arbitrarily control sample size, or signal strength, or dimensionality, or % of unmeasured variables, connectivity of the causal data generating process, etc. in real data since these factors have fixed and in many cases unknown characteristics in the available real datasets.

Second, real data with known high quality answers may be very limited and we do not wish to overfit the new method development to a small number of validation datasets (as will invariably happen, see chapter "Overfitting, Underfitting and General Model Overconfidence and Under-Performance Pitfalls and Best Practices in Machine Learning and AI" on overfitting).

Empirically testing new and existing methods with real data with known answers typically follows three designs:

1. **Centralized benchmark design.** A small group of expert data scientists organize and execute a series of tests of a new or existing method using several datasets and several state of the art alternative methods. Ideally all reasonable alternatives and baseline comparators including the best known methods for this type of problem are included and are executed according to the best known specifications (e.g., the specifications provided by their inventors). The datasets used are sufficient to cover a wide range of data typically encountered in the application domain. A multitude of factors are varied and their effects studied. Simulated and resimulated data may also be included a priori or ante hoc (e.g., to shed light on behaviors in real data). Example such studies are [1, 30–32, 37, 45–48, 51, 54–56, 59, 60].

2. **Distributed benchmark design.** This design is a variation of the centralized benchmark and typically occurs in the context of a scientific or industry consortium or coalition. A central team of experts organizes a benchmark similar to design 1 however analyses are conducted by several groups within the consortium. Each group may employ different methods, protocols, etc., and this natural variation is studied by the organizers who analyze results across participating teams. For an example of this design see [49].

3. **Public challenge design.** This design is a variation of the distributed benchmark and typically occurs in the context of a *participatory science* framework. A central team of experts or a challenge organization organizes the challenge typically with one or few datasets and a fixed data design. Analyses are conducted by volunteers across the globe. Each group may employ different methods, protocols, etc., and this natural variation is studied by the organizers who analyze results across participating teams. For an example of this design see [44].

Table 1 summarizes the characteristics of each design and points to strengths and weakness.

ML challenges serve two fundamental purposes. One is the *education* of scientists from different fields about the problems the challenge addresses and giving them data, and a platform to experiment. The second purpose is to explore which

Table 1 Empirical testing of AI/ML with real data and know answers: Three alternative designs (green: positive characteristics, red: weaknesses)

Characteristic	Challenges (ideally-conducted)	Centralized Benchmark Studies (ideally-conducted)	Distributed Benchmark Studies (ideally-conducted)
1. Led by	Academic groups or commercial companies	Academic groups (typically) or commercial companies (rarely)	Academic groups (typically) or commercial companies (rarely)
2. Conducted by	Many participants with varying (often not high) qualifications	Small teams of expert data scientists	Small teams of expert data scientists + Participant members of consortium
3. Participatory and open science	Strong	Limited	Limited
4. Educational intent	Yes	Secondary Focus	Secondary Focus
5. Empirical performance intent	Yes	Yes	Yes
6. Scope and representativeness of data	Very small/biased	High/unbiased	medium/ modestly biased
7. Updated over time by same or different groups	Almost never	Often	Almost never
8. Explore effects of data design	No	Yes	Yes
9. Explore effects of sample size	Almost never	Yes - controlled	Yes – as part of normal variation
10. Explore effects of model selection	Yes	Yes - controlled	Yes – as part of normal variation
11. Explore effects of error estimation	No	Yes - controlled	Possibly
12. Explore effects of algorithm choice	Yes	Yes - controlled	Yes – as part of normal variation
13. Suboptimal execution of algorithms and model selection	Common	Rare	Part of studied variation
14. Cost	Externalized to competitors	Internal to benchmark team	Distributed among consortium members

algorithmic methods are better at a particular point in time for a particular problem. Well-designed challenges can generate valuable information and enhance interdisciplinary engagement. Poorly-designed challenges (which in our estimation are the majority, currently) can be very misleading designs with respect to evaluating AI/ML methods. We elaborate in the following pitfall:

Pitfall 5.8

Issues and pitfalls of ML challenges. In many if not most cases, challenges suffer from **fixing the data design and the error estimation** thus *removing from consideration two out of the three determinants of ML success (i.e., data design, ML model selection and error estimation protocol, algorithm)*.

Challenges also routinely restrict the design of modeling by pre-selecting variables, and over-simplifying the statement of problems, sometimes to meaningless extremes.

Challenges also often suffer from *incomplete or highly biased representation in the competitor pool.* Typically participants in challenges are either students or interested scientists who have competencies in areas unrelated to AI/ML.

Another limitation is that *not all appropriate algorithms are entered in a challenge and when they enter, they are not necessarily executed according to optimal specifications.*

Finally, challenges typically involve a *very small number of datasets that do not represent a large domain.* Such representative coverage typically requires dozens of datasets or more *in the same comparison.*

Despite these limitations, a select number of challenges that are designed to a high degree of quality, when interpreted carefully and with the appropriate qualifications, can provide valuable empirical scientific information. For examples of well-designed, high quality, and carefully interpreted challenges the reader may refer to the challenges conducted by the ChaLearn organization [50].

Best Practice 5.6

The preferred design for validating AI/Ml methods with real life data with known answers is the centralized benchmark design. Distributed benchmark designs, whenever feasible, add value by exploring natural variation in how methods are applied by experts. Finally competitions have several intrinsic limitations and have to be interpreted carefully.

In-depth example for step 7 (Empirically test algorithms in real life data with known answers/solutions). Development or evaluation of scalable discovery methods of biomarkers and molecular pathways from high dimensional biomedical data, CONTINUED.

In our running example, of developing principled and scalable biomarker and pathway discovery algorithms all of the algorithms discussed in section "Over- and Under-Interpreting Results" were also tested extensively with real data where true answers were known or could be established via predictive verification. Statnikov et al. showed the superlative performance for biological local pathway discovery. Aphinyanaphongs et al. showed the performance in text categorization comparing with all major acedemic and commercial comparators of the time. Statnikov and Aliferis showed the massive gene expression signature equivalence classes in cancer microarray data. Alekseyenko, Statnikov and Aliferis evaluated in GWAS prediction signatures and causal loci discovery. Ma, Statnikov and Aliferis showed minimization of experiments in biological experimental data. Other benchmarks addressed additional microbiomic, cancer, and other types of data [1, 18, 22–24, 29–34, 37, 40, 41, 45–47, 52, 53].

Step 8. Empirically test algorithms in real life data without known answers/ solutions but where future validation can take place
In the final step of the new method development and validation process, the AI/ ML method and the models produced by it are tested in real data where the correct answers can be obtained but only prospectively: If the models are predictive we obtain true values and compare them to the predicted values. In causal modeling we conduct randomized controlled experiments and compare the effects of interventions against the algorithmic estimates for such effects. Other forms of validation designs are also possible depending on the nature of the AI/ML methods' goals and intended outputs.

We caution the reader that **only after successful completion of ALL prior steps** in the new or existing AI/ML method development or appraisal, is applying the method in real-life problems with any risk, warranted.

In-depth example for step 8 (Empirically test algorithms in real life data with unknown answers/solutions). Development or evaluation of scalable discovery methods of biomarkers and molecular pathways from high dimensional biomedical data, FINAL.

In our running example, the methods were deployed in several real-life projects related to basic and translational science discovery, experimental therapeutics, and healthcare improvements. Application areas included: (1) predicting risk for sepsis in the neonatal ICU; (2) diagnosing stroke from stroke-like syndromes using proteomic markers; (3) modeling the decision making and determining melanoma guideline non-compliance of dermatologists; (4) determining which patients with ovarian cancer will benefit from frontline Tx with bevacizumab; (5) understanding mechanisms and predicting outcomes in children with PTSD, (6) creating models that predict accurately citations of articles in deep horizons; (7) creating models that characterize the nature of citations; (8) creating models to classify articles for methodological rigor and content; (9) models that scan the WWW for dangerous medical advice; (10) models for diagnosis of psoriasis using microbiomic signatures from the skin; (11) multi-omic clinical phenotype predictions; (12) discovery of new targets for osteoarthritis; (13) detection of subclinical viral infection using gene signatures from serum; (14) analysis and modeling of longevity using clinical and molecular markers and (15) modeling of the mediating pathways between exercise and diet and cardiometabolic outcomes for drug target discovery [35, 36, 40, 51, 54–56, 59, 60–65].

In conclusion, the above interrelated case studies give an "insider's view" on, and showcase the feasibility and benefits of a complete rigorous development and validation approach for new methods using the example of local causal graph and MB algorithms and their extensions.

Similar in-depth rigorous development efforts have characterized the history of Bayesian Networks, SVMs, Boosting, Causal inference algorithms, and other methods (see chapters "Foundations and Properties of AI/ML Systems", "An Appraisal and Operating Characteristics of Major ML Methods Applicable in Healthcare and Health Science", and "Foundations of Causal ML"). However we do point out that unfortunately in many cases, widely-adopted methods and tools both in the academic and commercial realms lack many of the steps outlined here and therefore they have to be used with caution especially in high-stakes (high risk, high cost) application domains. The next section gives a highly condensed overview of properties of major AI/ML methods.

Best Practice 5.7
Develop and validate ML/AI methods using the following stages/steps:
- Step 1. Rigorous problem definition (in precise mathematical terms and establishing how the mathematical goals map to the healthcare or health science discovery goal).
- Step 2. Theoretical analysis of problem (complexity, problem space characteristics etc.).
- Step 3. First-pass algorithms solving the problem.

- Step 4. Theoretical properties of first pass algorithms: focus on representation power, soundness and completeness, transparency.
- Step 5. Algorithm refinements and optimizations.
- Step 6. Empirically test algorithms in controlled conditions .
- Step 7. Empirically test algorithms in real life data with known answers/ solutions.
- Step 8. Empirically test algorithms in real life data without known answers/ solutions but where future validation can take place.

Best Practice 5.8
Avoid evaluating methods by employing expert narratives showing "validity".

Best Practice 5.9
Do not reinvent the wheel. Verify that a new method does not solve a problem previously solved by a better performing method.

Best Practice 5.10
Create open box methods to the full extent possible. Do not pursue weak justifications that fail to translate the models to accurate human readable representations.

Best Practice 5.11
Do not confuse "open source" for "transparent" and "closed source" for black box".

A Concise Overview of Properties of Major AI/ML Methods

Table 2 gives a high-level, very concise view on properties of key families of AI/ML methods. A few observations are in order:

1. Heuristic systems by definition lack well-defined, well-understood or confirmed properties. We include them in the table only to remind the reader that they are seriously handicapped in that regard, and should not be used in high-stakes applications (until a better understanding of their risk and benefits is achieved).

Table 2 Map of properties of major AI/ML methods

Method	THEORETICAL PROPERTIES									EMPIRICAL PERFORMANCE		
	Representational Power	Semantic Clarity	Transparency	Soundness	Completeness	Computational Complexity	Space Complexity	Sample size	Probability Theory Compliance	Empirical Accuracy (in common use)	Empirical Accuracy (in recommended use)	Method misapplication in practice
Heuristic systems (i.e., pre-scientific AI/ML)	?	?	?	?	?	?	?	D	?	D	D	Common
Logics	+↑	+↑	+↑	+↑	+o	+↓	+↑	N/A	D	+↑	+↑	Uncommon
Rule Based Systems & Logic-derived	+o	+↑	+↑	+↑	+o	+↓	+↑	N/A	+↓	+o	+o	Uncommon
MEU Decision Theory	+o	+↑	+↑	+↑	+↑	+o	+↑	N/A	+↑	+↑	+↑	Uncommon
Search	+↑	+↑	+↑	D	D	D	D	N/A	D	+↑	+↑	Uncommon
OLS	+o	+↑	+↑	+↑	+↑	+↑	+↑	+↑	+o	+o	+↑	
GLM	+o	+↑	+↑	+↑	+↑	D	D	+↑	+↑	+↑	+↑	Uncommon
ANN/DL	+↑	+↑	+↓	+o	+↓	+↓	+o	+↓	+↑	+o	+↑	Common
SVM	+↑	+↑	D	+↑	+↑	+↑	+↑	+↑	+o	+↑	+↑	Uncommon
NB	+↓	+↑	D	+↑	+↑	+↑	+↑	+↑	+↑	+↓	+↓	Common
Bayes Nets	+↑	+↑	+↑	+↑	+↑	D	+↑	+o	+↑	+↑	+↑	Uncommon
KNN	+↑	+↓	+↑	+o	+↑	+↓	+↑	+↑	+o	+o	+o	Common
DT	+↑	+↑	+↑	+o	+o	+↑	+o	+o	+↑	+o	+↑	Uncommon
Clustering	+↑	D	+↑	+↓	+↓	+o	[o↓]	+↓	+↓	+↓	+o	Common
Stacking	D	D	+↓	D	+↑	[o↓]	[o↓]	+o	+[↑↓]	+↑	+↑	Uncommon
RF	+↑	+↑	+↓	+↑	+o	+o	+o	+o	+↑	+o	+↑	Common
Boosting	+↑	D	+↓	+↑	+o	+o	+o	+o	+↑	+↑	+↑	Uncommon
Penalized Regression	+o	+↑	+↑	+[↑o]	+↑	+o	+↑	+o	+[↑↓]	+↑	+↑	Uncommon
UAF	+↓	+↑	+↑	+↓	c	+↑	+↑	+↑	N/A	+↓	+o	Uncommon
SV-RFE	+↓	D	+↓	+↓	+↓	+↑	+↑	+↑	+↓	+↑	+↑	Uncommon
Markov Boundary Feature Selection	+↑	+↑	+↑	+↑	+↑	+↑	D	+↑	D	+↑	+↑	Uncommon
Embedded Feature Selection	+↓	+o	+↑	+↓	+↓	+↑	+↑	+↑	D	+↓	+↑	Common
Wrapper Feature Selection	D	D	D	+↓	+↓	D	D	D	D	+↓	+↓	Common
Kaplan Meier	+↑	+↑	+↑	+↑	+↑	↑	+↓	+o	+↑	+↑	+↑	Uncommon
Cox PH	+o	+↑	+↑	+↑	+↑	+↑	+↓	+o	+↑	+↑	+↑	Uncommon
AFT	+↓	+↑	+↑	+↑	+↑	+↑	+↑	↑	+↑	D	D	Uncommon
ANOVA	+↓	+↑	+↑	+↑	+↑	+↑	+↑	↑	+↑	+o	+↑	Common
(G)LMM	+o	+↑	+↑	+↑	+↑	+o	+↑	+o	+[↑o]	+↑	+↑	Uncommon
GEE	+o	+↑	+↑	+↑	+↑	+↑	+↑	+o	+[↑o]	+↑	+↑	Uncommon
SEM (linear)	+o	+↑	+↑	+↑	+↑	+↑	+↑	↑	+[↑o]	+o	+↑	Uncommon
PC	+↑	+↑	+↑	+↑	+↑	+↓	+↑	+↑	+↑	+↓	+↓	Common
FCI	+↑	+↑	+↑	+↑	+o	+↓	+↑	+↑		?	?	?
GFCI	+↑	+↑	+↑	?	+o	?	+↑	+↑	+↑	?	?	?
GES	+↑	+↑	+↑	+↑	+↑	+o	+↑	+↑	+↑	+o	+o	Uncommon
MMHC/LGL	+o	+↑	+↑	+o	+o	+↑	+↑	+↑	+↑	+↑	+↑	Uncommon

(continued)

Table 2 (continued)

Symbol Notation

+ = Properties are known. ? = Properties are unknown

↑ = strong; o = medium; ↓ = weak;

D depends on choice of algorithm, or problem;

[.] depicts range of values.

Color Notation

Green = strong; orange = medium; red = weak or property is unknown; gray = depends on choice
of algorithm, or problem; white = not applicable

2. Most methods that are widely used today have well understood properties, or at
   most a few gaps in the understanding of their properties.
3. There is no perfect method across all properties and problem types: every method
   has weak spots.
4. Some methods are compromised by being commonly used in problems that they
   should not (i.e., "user error"). In these cases there is always a better method for
   that problem category.
5. Statistical machine learning methods have stronger/better studied properties in
   general.
6. It is possible for some methods to have sub-optimal theoretical properties but
   exhibit excellent empirical performance in some problem categories and/or
   selected datasets.

Explanation of terms:

Representation	What kind of relationships can the method represent? In case of modeling methods, are the model assumptions restrictive? ↑ (strong): Any relationship (e.g. Universal Function Approximator) o (limited): Constrained functional form ↓ (weak): Restrictive assumptions apply D (Depends): Inherits property from an component method, has other kind of dependence (e.g. on an underlying distribution), or the properties varies across members of a broader category of methods
Semantic clarity	Is the method (or model) semantics clear? E.g. in case of a predictive model, is the meaning of the model components clear? ↑ (strong): Yes o (moderate): Some parts are not clearly defined ↓ (weak): Not having clear meaning
Transparency	Does the method semantics relate to real-world entities in a clear manner? Is it easily understood by humans? ↑ (strong): The relationship between real-world entities and method components can be explained. Humans easily understand method/models. ↓ (weak): Method is difficult to interpret, additional algorithms are needed to interpret o (moderate): Between ↑ and ↓

Soundness	*When the model assumptions are met*, are the results correct? (E.g. for a predictive model, is the model error optimal?) ↑ (strong): Yes, guaranteed (e.g. convex problem, Optimal Bayes Classifier, etc); o (medium): Trapped in local optima, only approximates target function to some acceptable degree; ↓ (weak): Output may considerably deviate from correct answer
Completeness	Will the method output correct answers for all problem instances? ↑ (strong): Yes, will produce correct answers for full problem space; o (medium): considerable but not full coverage of problem space; ↓ (weak): only small portions of problem space correctly answered, or very significant regions are omitted.
Compute	Computational complexity. For predictive models, it includes the complexity of both model construction and prediction. ↑ (strong): Very fast. E.g., for executing predictive models, linear in number of variables, and with a small hyperparameter space o (medium): May build multiple models. ↓ (weak): Requires extensive computing (e.g. immense hyper-parameter space, exponential in the number of variables, etc.) D (depends): Typical and worst-case are very different; can take advantage of properties of the problem (e.g. graph connectivity)
Space	Storage complexity required for the computation, or for storing the model (if there is a model) ↑ (strong): Approx. number of variables o (medium): linear in the number of variables ↓ (weak): super-linear in the number of variables or proportional to the data set size (if data set size exceeds order of number of variables)
Sample size	Sample size required to train the model (to an acceptable performance on problems that constitute the preferred use of this method) ↑ (strong): small sample size is sufficient (e.g. linear in the number of variables, in the number of effective parameters, support vectors, etc.) o (medium): moderate (e.g., low order polynomial) sample sizes required to number of effective parameters ↓ (weak): large sample sizes are required (e.g., super- or higher order-polynomial to number of effective parameters)
Probabilistic consistency	(1) Model can return probabilities (or output can be converted to probabilities) and (2) probabilistic output is calibrated or can be calibrated ↑ (strong): designed to be probabilistically consistent o (medium): output can be converted into probabilities ↓ (weak): not meant to produce probabilities and there is no easy way to convert predictions into consistent probabilities

Empirical accuracy in common use	In its common use, what is the method's empirical performance in terms of result accuracy (e.g. accuracy or AUC for classification models)? ↑ (strong): One of the strongest among methods that are best-of-class for this problem. (E.g. DL for imaging; Cox PH for time-to-event, etc.) o (medium): Performs noticeably worse than the best, but still outperforms several methods. ↓ (weak): Performs substantially worse than most applicable methods.
Empirical accuracy in recommended use	In its preferred use, what is the method's empirical performance in terms of result accuracy (e.g. accuracy or AUC for classification models)? ↑ (strong): one of best-in-class methods for this problem. (E.g. DL for images; Cox PH for time-to-event, etc.) o (medium): performs noticeable worse than the best-in-class, but still useful in some cases. ↓ (weak): Performs substantially worse than best and has no mitigating uses.
Method misapplication in practice	Common: The method is commonly used for tasks that is not best-in-class Uncommon: The method is seldomly used for tasks that is not best-in-class

We advise the reader to study this table and cross-reference with the description of methods and guidance for their use in chapters "Foundations and Properties of AI/ML Systems", "An Appraisal and Operating Characteristics of Major ML Methods Applicable in Healthcare and Health Science", and "Foundations of Causal ML".

A Worksheet for Use when Evaluating or Developing AI/ML Methods

It is highly recommended as new or existing methods are being evaluated to use a chart such as the one shown in Table 3. There are three purposes in this endeavor: (a) Remind the developer or evaluator about the necessary dimensions of validation/appraisal. (b) Maintain a record of progress as the various stages of evaluation are advancing. (c) Enforce due diligence both in an absolute sense but also in comparison to applicable alternatives. (d) Enforce honesty/reduce developer bias in assessing the added value of the evaluated method over established incumbents. (e) More objectively assess marketing claims about the strengths of commercial products.

Table 3 Worksheet for evaluating new and existing AI/ML methods

Method	Theoretical properties										Empirical performance		
	Representational Power	Semantic clarity	Transparency	Soundness	Completeness	Computational Complexity	Space Complexity	Sample size	Probability Theory Compliance		Empirical Accuracy(in common use)	Empirical Accuracy (in recommended use)	Method misapplication in practice
Method to be evaluated	OBTAIN BY THEORETICAL ANALYSIS PROPERTIES AND INSERT APPRAISAL IN EACH COLUMN										OBTAIN BY EMPIRICAL EXPERIMENTATION AND INSERT APPRAISAL IN EACH COLUMN		
Best-in-class known method #1 for that problem domain	SELECT FROM THE LITERATURE BEST KNOWN EXISTING METHOD FOR PROBLEM TYPE AND COPY ITS THEORETICAL PROPERTIES IN EACH COLUMN										COPY EMPIRICAL PROPERTIES IN EACH COLUMN		
Best-in-class known method #2 for that problem domain	SELECT FROM THE LITERATURE SECOND BEST KNOWN EXISTING METHOD FOR PROBLEM TYPE AND COPY ITS THEORETICAL PROPERTIES IN EACH COLUMN										COPY EMPIRICAL PROPERTIES IN EACH COLUMN		
Best-in-class known method #3 for that problem domain	SELECT FROM THE LITERATURE THIRD BEST KNOWN EXISTING METHOD FOR PROBLEM TYPE AND COPY ITS THEORETICAL PROPERTIES IN EACH COLUMN										COPY EMPIRICAL PROPERTIES IN EACH COLUMN		
Baseline comparator method for the problem domain	SELECT FROM THE LITERATURE BASELINE EXISTING METHOD FOR PROBLEM TYPE AND COPY ITS THEORETICAL PROPERTIES IN EACH COLUMN										COPY EMPIRICAL PROPERTIES IN EACH COLUMN		

Over-and Under-Interpreting Results

We conclude this chapter with a discussion of avoiding over-interpreting and under-interpreting AI/ML results.

A major principle for the scientifically valid use of AI/ML models is their proper interpretation for either driving healthcare decisions and improvements as well as for driving discovery in the health sciences. Two major and antithetical pitfalls are the over- and the under-interpretation of results given the data design (see chapter "Data Design") and the properties of the algorithms and protocols employed.

> **Pitfall 5.9**
> Interpreting results of a method's beyond what its known properties justify.

> **Pitfall 5.10**
> Interpreting results of a method's below what its known properties justify.

A few examples of the over-interpretation pitfall include:

(a) Interpreting weak predictive methods (and resulting models) as if they have much stronger accuracy (usually combined with omitting stating the weak aggregate signal of the method's models e.g., in the context of regression analyses of biomarkers).

(b) Assigning special biological or mechanistic significance to variables because they are stable in resampling or because they are ranked high according to univariate association with a response variable.

(c) Generally interpreting causally the findings of predictive methods (and resulting models).

(d) Failing to observe that some feature selection methods in omics data commonly do not, or marginally outperform random selection.

(e) Ignoring the possibility of hidden (aka unmeasured or latent) variables distorting the observed effects of measured variables.

(f) Ignoring effects of small sample size variation on results.

(g) Assuming (without proof) that case matching according to hypothesized confounders has controlled all confounding. Assuming in SEM modeling that the domain causal structure is known with certainty.

(h) Assuming that propensity scoring perfectly controls confounding.

(i) Treating coefficient values in regularized regression methods (Lasso family, SVMs, and other "penalty+loss" algorithms) as if they are equivalent to statistical conditioning (e.g., in classical regression).

(j) Assuming (without testing) that the assignment of subjects to treatment arms in trials from existing datasets is perfectly randomized and without bias. Etc.

A few examples of the under-interpretation pitfall include:

(a) Focusing on small individual variable effects without noticing that the aggregate signal over many variables is large (e.g., in GWAS studies).
(b) Focusing on small coefficient of variation of a model (i.e., total response variance explained) and failing to notice that some variables have strong individual effects (this is the reverse of the previous under-interpretation problem).
(c) Failing to pick up strong putative causal factors even when causal ML algorithms indicate their significance, because "correlation is not causation".
(d) Dismissing methods (and resulting models) because they are not statistically stable under resampling.

We will revisit these problems in subsequent chapters as they require a holistic understanding of data design and proper AI/ML algorithm design and execution. The best practice we will state at this point however is:

Best Practice 5.12
Interpret results of application of a method (and resulting models) at the level justified by its know properties.

Key Messages and Concepts Discussed in Chapter "Principles of Rigorous Development and of Appraisal of ML and AI Methods and Systems"

1. Establishing and knowing the properties of AI/ML methods enables informed assessments about the Performance requirements, the Safety requirements, and the Cost-effectiveness requirements of corresponding AI/ML solutions, and leads to building trust in the AI/ML solution.
2. A best practice workflow was presented, that can be used to establish the properties of any new or pre-existing method, tool or system, so that a rational, effective and efficient solution to the problem at hand can be identified.
3. The importance of rigorous problem definitions (in precise mathematical terms, and with precise correspondence to health care or health science objectives).
4. Re-inventing the wheel and why it is undesirable.
5. First-pass algorithms vs algorithm refinements and optimization.
6. Parallel algorithms, Distributed/Federated, Sequential, and Chunked algorithms.
7. Relaxing algorithmic assumptions/requirements.
8. Generalized algorithm frameworks and generalized conditions for performance guarantees.

9. What are AI/ML (or data science) Stacks.
10. "Pipelines", "Automodelers", and "Platforms".
11. Explanation, interpretability, and transparency: Black box AI/ML methods and/or models; Transparent (or open, or white, or clear) box.
12. Justification of a method or a model (and their outputs) vs high-fidelity explanation of a method or model (and their outputs) e.g., by functional equivalence.
13. Human-understandable models and formalisms.
14. Open source software vs Closed source (or proprietary) software.
15. The importance of testing algorithms in controlled conditions.
16. Simulated data; Label-reshuffled data; Re-simulated data, and their properties and use.
17. Real-life examples of using the new method development process to establish the properties of well known (new or pre-existing) methods, tools or systems.
18. Interpreting results of application of a method at the level justified by its known properties.

Pitfalls Discussed in Chapter "Principles of Rigorous Development and of Appraisal of ML and AI Methods and Systems"

Pitfall 5.1.: Developing methods with theoretical and empirical properties that are:
(a) Unknown, or
(b) Poorly characterized in disclosures and technical, scientific or commercial communications and publications, or
(c) Clearly stated (disclosed) but not proven, or
(d) Not matching the characteristics of the problem to be solved at the level of performance and trust needed.

Pitfall 5.2. Evaluating the success of methods with poorly defined objectives, by employing expert narratives showing "validity".

Pitfall 5.3. Defining the goals of methods in mathematical terms but without establishing how the mathematical goals map to the healthcare or health science discovery goal.

Pitfall 5.4. Reinventing the wheel: whereby a new method is introduced but it has been previously discovered yet ignored (willfully or not) by the "new" method developers.

Pitfall 5.5. Reinventing a method but make it worse to established methods (…"reinventing the wheel and making it square"!).

Pitfall 5.6. Providing peripheral/oblique and thus inadequate justifications of the model and its decisions which do not "open" the black box.

Pitfall 5.7. Confusing "open source" for "transparent" and "closed source" for black box".

Pitfall 5.8. Issues and pitfalls of ML challenges. In many, if not most cases, challenges suffer from fixing the data design and error estimation thus *removing from consideration, two out of the three determinants of ML success (i.e., data design, ML model selection and error estimation protocol, algorithm).*

Challenges also routinely restrict the design of modeling by pre-selecting variables, and over-simplifying the statement of problems, sometimes to meaningless extremes.

Challenges also often suffer from *incomplete or highly biased representation in the competitor pool.* Typically participants in challenges are either students or interested scientists who have competencies in areas unrelated to AI/ML.

Another limitation is that *not all appropriate algorithms are entered in a challenge and when they enter, they are not necessarily executed according to optimal specifications.*

Finally, challenges typically involve a *very small number of datasets that do not represent a large domain.* Such representative coverage typically requires dozens of datasets or more *in the same comparison.*

Pitfall 5.9.: Interpreting results of a method (and resulting models) beyond what its known properties justify.

Pitfall 5.10.: Interpreting results of a method (and resulting models) below what its known properties justify.

Best Practices Discussed in Chapter "Principles of Rigorous Development and of Appraisal of ML and AI Methods and Systems"

Best Practice 5.1. Methods developers should strive to characterize the new methods according to the dimensions of theoretical and empirical properties.

Best Practice 5.2. Methods developers should carefully disclose the known and unknown properties of new methods at each stage of their development and provide full evidence for how these properties were established.

Best Practice 5.3. Methods adopters and evaluators (users, funding agencies, editorial boards etc.) should seek to obtain valid information according to the dimensions of theoretical and empirical properties for every method, tool, and system under consideration.

Best Practice 5.4. Methods adopters and evaluators should map the dimensions of theoretical and empirical properties for every method, tool, and system under consideration to the problem at hand and select methods based on best matching of method properties to problem needs.

Best Practice 5.5. The properties of a ML algorithm can be negatively or positively affected by the ML protocol to extreme degrees (see chapter "Lessons Learned from Historical Failures, Limitations and Successes of AI/ML In Healthcare and the Health Sciences. Enduring problems, and the role of BPs." for several important case studies that show the immense and often under-appreciated practical consequences). Similarly the data design can negatively or positively affect the ML protocol and its embedded algorithms to extreme degrees. Therefore, it is imperative to design AI/ML methods taking into account any positive or negative interactions of data design with the protocols and embedded algorithms employed.

Best Practice 5.6. The preferred design for validating AI/Ml methods with real life data with known answers is the centralized benchmark design. Distributed benchmark designs, whenever feasible, add value by exploring natural variation in how methods are applied by experts. Finally competitions have several intrinsic limitations and have to be interpreted carefully.

Best Practice 5.7. Develop and validate ML/AI methods using the following stages/steps:
- Step 1. Rigorous problem definition (in precise mathematical terms and establishing how the mathematical goals map to the healthcare or health science discovery goal).
- Step 2. Theoretical analysis of problem (complexity, problem space characteristics etc.).
- Step 3. First-pass algorithms solving problem.
- Step 4. Theoretical properties of first pass algorithms: focus on representation power, soundness and completeness, transparency.
- Step 5. Algorithm refinements and optimizations.
- Step 6. Empirically test algorithms in controlled conditions.
- Step 7. Empirically test algorithms in real life data with known answers/solutions.
- Step 8. Empirically test algorithms in real life data without known answers/solutions but where future validation can take place.

Best Practice 5.8. Avoid evaluating methods by employing expert narratives showing "validity".

Best Practice 5.9. Do not reinvent the wheel. Verify that a new method does not solve a problem previously solved by a better performing method.

Best Practice 5.10. Create open box methods to the full extent possible. Do not pursue weak justifications that fail to translate the models to accurate human readable representations.

Best Practice 5.11. Do not confuse "open source" for "transparent" and "closed source" for "black box".

Best Practice 5.12. Interpret results of application of a method at the level justified by its known properties.

Classroom Assignments and Discussion Topics, Chapter "Principles of Rigorous Development and of Appraisal of ML and AI Methods and Systems"

1. Choose one ML/AI method of your choice and characterize it according to best practice 5.7. use any literature that is adequate for that purpose.

2. Choose a well-cited paper from health sciences or healthcare that uses AI/ML. Characterize the primary methods using best practice 5.7.

3. Can you describe a real-life example of over- or under-interpreting a type of AI/ML analysis or modelling?

4. Are there safeguards in human professional training and certification analogous to the best practices presented in this chapter?

5. Revisit the question of chapter "Artificial Intelligence (AI) and Machine Learning (ML) for Healthcare and Health Sciences: the Need for Best Practices Enabling Trust in AI and ML" stating: *"The so-called No Free Lunch Theorem (NFLT) states (in plain language) that all ML and more broadly all AI optimization methods are equally accurate over all problems on average. Discuss the implications for choice of AI/ML methods in practical use cases"* using the tools of the present chapter

6. Revisit the question of chapter "Artificial Intelligence (AI) and Machine Learning (ML) for Healthcare and Health Sciences: the Need for Best Practices Enabling Trust in AI and ML" stating: *"'It is not the tool but the craftsman'. Does this maxim apply to health AI/ML?"* using the tools of the present chapter.

7. Revisit the question of chapter "Artificial Intelligence (AI) and Machine Learning (ML) for Healthcare and Health Sciences: the Need for Best Practices Enabling Trust in AI and ML" stating: *"Construct a 'pyramid of evidence' for*

health ML/AI similar to the one used in evidence based medicine." using the tools of the present chapter.

8. Revisit the question of chapter "Artificial Intelligence (AI) and Machine Learning (ML) for Healthcare and Health Sciences: the Need for Best Practices Enabling Trust in AI and ML" stating:

    "You are part of an important university/hospital evaluation committee for a vendor offering a patient-clinical trial matching AI product. Your institution strongly needs to improve the patient-trial matching process to improve trial success and efficiency metrics. The sales team makes the statement that "this is a completely innovative AI/ML product; nothing like this exists in the market and there is no similar literature; we cannot at this time provide theoretical or empirical accuracy analysis however you are welcome to try out our product for free for a limited time and decide if it is helpful to you". The product is fairly expensive (multi $ million license fees over 5 years covering >1,000 trials steady-state).

    What would be your concerns based on these statements? Would you be in position of making an institutional buy/not buy recommendation?"

    Use the guidelines of the present chapter to compose a brief report and recommendations.

9. Revisit the question of chapter "Artificial Intelligence (AI) and Machine Learning (ML) for Healthcare and Health Sciences: the Need for Best Practices Enabling Trust in AI and ML" stating:

    "A company has launched a major national marketing campaign across health provider systems for a new AI/ML healthcare product based on its success on playing backgammon, reading and analyzing backgammon playing books and human games, and extracting novel winning strategies, also answering questions about backgammon, and teaching backgammon to human players.

    How relevant is this impressive AI track record to health care? How would you go about determining relevance to health care AI/ML? How your reasoning would change if the product was not based on success in backgammon but success in identifying oil and gas deposits? How about success in financial investments?

    Use the guidelines of the present chapter to compose a brief report and recommendations.

10. Revisit the question of chapter "Artificial Intelligence (AI) and Machine Learning (ML) for Healthcare and Health Sciences: the Need for Best Practices Enabling Trust in AI and ML" stating:

    "Your university-affiliated hospital wishes to increase early diagnosis of cognitive decline across the population it serves. You are tasked to choosing between the following five AI/ML technologies/tools:

    • *AI/ML tool A guarantees optimal predictivity in the sample limit in distributions that are multivariate normal.*

- *AI/ML tool B has no known properties but is has been shown to be very accurate in several datasets for microarray cancer-vs-normal classification.*
- *AI/ML tool C is a commercial offshoot of a tool that was fairly accurate in early (pre-trauma) diagnosis of PTSD.*
- *AI/ML tool D is an application running on a ground-breaking quantum computing platform. Quantum computing is an exciting and frontier technology that many believe has potential to make AI/ML with hugely improved capabilities.*
- *AI/ML tool E runs on a novel massively parallel cloud computing platform capable of Zettascale performance.What are your thoughts about these options?"*

Use the guidelines of the present chapter to compose a brief appraisal.

11. Revisit the question of chapter "Artificial Intelligence (AI) and Machine Learning (ML) for Healthcare and Health Sciences: the Need for Best Practices Enabling Trust in AI and ML" stating:

"The same question as #10 but with the following additional data:

- *AI/ML tool A sales reps are very professional, friendly and open to offering deep discounts.*
- *AI/ML tool B is offered by a company co-founded by a Nobel laureate.*
- *AI/Ml tool C is offered by a vendor with which your organization has a successful and long relationship.*
- *AI/Ml tool D is part of a university initiative to develop thought leadership in quantum computing.*
- *AI/Ml tool E will provide patient-specific results in 1 picosecond or less.How does this additional information influences your assessment?"*

Use the guidelines of the present chapter to compose a brief appraisal.

12. Comment on the representation power of the following methods and corresponding problems:

1. Decision Trees	$\longleftrightarrow$	predictive modeling
2. KNN	$\longleftrightarrow$	outlier detection
3. Deep Learning	$\longleftrightarrow$	pathway reverse engineering
4. Simple Bayes	$\longleftrightarrow$	simulating an arbitrary joint probability distribution
5. SVMs	$\longleftrightarrow$	predictive modeling with a random subset of the inputs missing
6. Regularized repressors	$\longleftrightarrow$	evaluate similarity of distributions

13. Rank the transparency and interpretability of the methods of question 12 for their preferred context of use.

14. Method X is correct whenever condition Y holds in the data. However, Y is not testable. Is X well characterized for soundness? Can it be?

Bonus add-on: comment along the same lines on the soundness of the Aracne algorithm' monotone faithfulness condition and of the Propensity Scoring's "ignorability condition".

15. How the notions of "heuristic power" and soundness relate?

16. A classifier model has acceptable error rate in 2/3 of the patient population. This subpopulation is identifiable by the model and its properties. What are its soundness and completeness? What would the soundness and completeness be if no one could identify the cases with unacceptable error margins?

17. Why worst-case complexity is less useful than "complexity in x% of problem instances"?

18. In some cases it is possible to use properties over the problem class to immediately determine properties of specific algorithms. Developer D introduces method M and claims it can solve a problem with known exponential worst case complexity in polynomial time. What can you immediately prove?

19. Can clustering methods be used to discover causality soundly and completely? Use your observations on its computational complexity and representational power to disprove this notion.

20. If discovering causal relations is worst-case exponential and regularized regression and SVMs are guaranteed quadratic time, what can you infer about the ability of regularized regression and SVMs for discovery of causality?

21. A faculty in a university brings forward a proposal to administration for installing a large compute cluster that has the compute power of 10,000 desktop computers. The faculty wishes to use brute force algorithms to discover non-linear discontinuous functions in the form of parity functions that have average case exponential cost to model to the number of variables. If a single desktop can solve such problems for up to 3-way variable interactions, what maximum degree interactions can be discovered with the proposed cluster?

22. How Bayesian Networks can reduce exponentially the model storage requirements compared to simple use of Bayes' theorem?

23. Suppose we store models that incorporate discrete conditional probability tables over binary variables. For a variable X that has parents P1, ..., Pk how does the storage complexity grows, as k grows? How is this complexity self-limiting if available sample size is relatively small?

24. In the 1980s a popular AI representation was the Certainty Factor Calculous (CFC, created by medical AI pioneers B.G. Buchanan and E. Shortliffe), a form of stochastic rules expert system representation. It was subsequently discovered by D. Heckerman et al. that unless limitations on the data distribution form were present, the CFC was not compatible with probability theory. Can you articulate when and why this might be a problem?

25. A commercial product promises that it can find "valuable insights" for health-care improvement. Can you translate this deliverable in mathematical comput-able terms? What does it mean in terms of guaranteed properties if this type of output cannot be formalized mathematically?

26. Discuss the (humorous) maxim: "2 months in the lab will save one 2 hours in the library".

27. Woods wrote a 1975 classic AI paper titled "What's in a link". In it he criticized the vague specification of the technical semantics of semantic networks (a prominent AI knowledge representation of his time derived from formal logic) and the impact that different semantics have on computability and complexity. Can you identify analogous problems in today's AI/ML? For example, consider the causal semantics (or lack thereof) in the field of network science and of the numerous biological pathway reverse engineering methods.

28. "Data Hubris" is described by the statement "Having lots of data is more impor-tant than choice of algorithm". What does this maxim means? Can you com-ment on the validity of this statement? What about if you add consideration of data design?

References

1. Aliferis CF, Statnikov A, Tsamardinos I, Mani S, Koutsoukos XD. Local causal and Markov blanket induction for causal discovery and feature selection for classification part II: analysis and extensions. J Mach Learn Res. 2010;11(Jan):235–384.
2. Shapere D. The concept of observation in science and philosophy. Philos Sci. 1982;49(4):485–525.
3. Van Fraassen BC. Scientific representation: paradoxes of perspective, vol. 70; 2010. p. 511–4.
4. Trujillo CM, Anderson TR, Pelaez NJ. A model of how different biology experts explain molecular and cellular mechanisms. CBE Life Sci Educ. 2015;14(2):ar20.
5. Goldfarb B, King AA. Scientific apophenia in strategic management research: significance tests & mistaken inference. Strateg Manag J. 2016;37(1):167–76.
6. Wagenaar WA. Appreciation of conditional probabilities in binary sequences. Acta Psychol. 1970;34:348–56.
7. Ramsey FP. On a problem of formal logic. Classic Papers in Combinatorics. 1987:1–24.
8. Frank R, Hargreaves R. Clinical biomarkers in drug discovery and development. Nat Rev Drug Discov. 2003;2(7):566–80.
9. Fleming TR, DeMets DL. Surrogate end points in clinical trials: are we being misled? Ann Intern Med. 1996;125(7):605–13.
10. Califf RM. Biomarker definitions and their applications. Exp Biol Med. 2018;243(3):213–21.
11. Kohavi R, John GH. Wrappers for feature subset selection. Artif Intell. 1997;97(1–2):273–324.
12. Pearl J. Probabilistic reasoning in intelligent systems, vol. 88, No. 3. San Mateo: Morgan Kaufmann; 2014.
13. Spirtes P, Glymour CN, Scheines R, Heckerman D. Causation, prediction, and search. MIT press; 2000.
14. Tsamardinos I, Aliferis CF. Towards principled feature selection: relevance, filters, and wrap-pers. In: Proceedings of the Ninth International Workshop on Artificial Intelligence and Statistics; 2003.
15. Winston WL. Operations research: applications and algorithms. Cengage Learning; 2022.

16. Cormen TH, Leiserson CE, Rivest RL, Stein C. Introduction to algorithms. MIT press; 2022.
17. Wolpert DH, Macready WG. No free lunch theorems for optimization. IEEE Trans Evol Comput. 1997;1(1):67–82.
18. Tsamardinos I, Aliferis CF, Statnikov A. Algorithms for large scale markov blanket discovery. In: Proceedings of the 16th International Florida Artificial Intelligence Research Society (FLAIRS) Conference; 2003. p. 376–80.
19. Koller D, Sahami M. Toward optimal feature selection. Stanford InfoLab; 1996.
20. Cooper GF, Abraham V, Aliferis CF, Aronis JM, Buchanan BG, Caruana R, Fine MJ, Janosky JE, Livingston G, Mitchell T, Monti S. Predicting dire outcomes of patients with community acquired pneumonia. J Biomed Inform. 2005;38(5):347–66.
21. Margaritis D, Thrun S. Bayesian network induction via local neighborhoods. Adv Neural Inf Proces Syst. 1999;12
22. Aliferis CF, Tsamardinos I, Statnikov A. HITON: a novel Markov blanket algorithm for optimal variable selection. In: AMIA annual symposium proceedings; 2003. p. 21–5.
23. Tsamardinos I, Aliferis CF, Statnikov A. Time and sample efficient discovery of markov blankets and direct causal relations. In: Proceedings of the 9th ACM SIGKDD International Conference on Knowledge Discovery and Data Mining; 2003. p. 673–8.
24. Tsamardinos I, Brown LE, Aliferis CF. The max-min hill-climbing Bayesian network structure learning algorithm. Mach Learn. 2006;65(1):31–78.
25. Upadhyaya SR. Parallel approaches to machine learning—a comprehensive survey. J Parallel Distrib Comput. 2013;73(3):284–92.
26. Verbraeken J, Wolting M, Katzy J, Kloppenburg J, Verbelen T, Rellermeyer JS. A survey on distributed machine learning. Acm computing surveys (csur). 2020;53(2):1–33.
27. Pérez-Cruz F, Figueiras-Vidal AR, Artés-Rodríguez A. Double chunking for solving SVMs for very large datasets. Proceedings of Learning; 2004.
28. Data Analysis Computer System and Method For Parallelized and Modularized Analysis of Big Data; Patent No.: US 9,720,940; August 1, 2017.
29. Statnikov A, Lytkin NI, Lemeire J, Aliferis CF. Algorithms for discovery of multiple Markov boundaries. J Mach Learn Res. 2013;14(Feb):499–566.
30. Statnikov A, Aliferis CF. Analysis and computational dissection of molecular signature multiplicity. (cover article). PLoS Comput Biol. 2010;6(5):e1000790.
31. Statnikov A, Ma S, Henaff M, Lytkin N, Efstathiadis E, Peskin ER, Aliferis CF. Ultra-scalable and efficient methods for hybrid observational and experimental local causal pathway discovery. J Mach Learn Res. 2015;16:3219–67.
32. Aliferis CF, Statnikov A, Tsamardinos I, Mani S, Koutsoukos XD. Local causal and Markov blanket induction for causal discovery and feature selection for classification part I: algorithms and empirical evaluation. J Mach Learn Res. 2010;11(Jan):171–234.
33. Statnikov A, Tsamardinos I, Dosbayev Y, Aliferis CF. Gene expression model selector (GEMS): a system for automated cancer diagnosis and biomarker discovery from microarray gene expression data. Int J Med Inform. 2005;74(7–8):491–503.
34. Fananapazir N, Statnikov A, Aliferis CF. The FAST-AIMS clinical mass spectrometry analysis system. Adv Bioinforma. 2009;2009:598241. http://www.hindawi.com/journals/abi/2009/598241/.
35. Saxe GN, Ma SS, Ren J, Aliferis CF. Machine learning methods to predict child posttraumatic stress: a proof of concept study. BMC Psychiatry. 2017;17:article # 223.
36. Saxe GN, Statnikov A, Fenyo D, Ren J, Li Z, Prasad M, Wall D, Bergman N, Briggs EC, Aliferis C. A complex systems approach to causal discovery in psychiatry. PLoS One. 2016;11(3):e0151174.
37. Statnikov A, Aliferis CF, Tsamardinos I, Hardin D, Levy S. A comprehensive evaluation of multicategory classification methods for microarray gene expression cancer diagnosis. Bioinformatics. 2005;21(5):631–43.
38. Gunning D, Aha D. DARPA's explainable artificial intelligence (XAI) program. AI Mag. 2019;40(2):44–58.

39. Murdoch WJ, Singh C, Kumbier K, Abbasi-Asl R, Yu B. Definitions, methods, and applications in interpretable machine learning. Proc Natl Acad Sci. 2019;116(44):22071–80.
40. Sboner A, Aliferis CF. Modeling clinical judgment and implicit guideline compliance in the diagnosis of melanomas using machine learning. In: AMIA Annual Symposium Proceedings. American Medical Informatics Association; 2005. p. 664–8.
41. Statnikov A, Aliferis CF, Hardin D, Guyon I. A gentle introduction to Support Vector Machines in biomedicine, vol. II. World Scientific Publishing Co. Pte. Ltd; 2013.
42. Aliferis CF, Statnikov A, Tsamardinos I. Challenges in the analysis of mass-throughput data: a technical commentary from the statistical machine learning perspective. Cancer Informat. 2006;2:133–62.
43. Aliferis CF, Statnikov A, Tsamardinos I, Schildcrout JS, Shepherd BE, Harrell FE Jr. Factors influencing the statistical power of complex data analysis protocols for molecular signature development from microarray data. PLoS One. 2009;4(3):e4922.
44. Guyon I, Aliferis C, Cooper G, Elisseeff A, Pellet JP, Spirtes P, Statnikov A. Design and analysis of the causation and prediction challenge. In: Causation and prediction challenge. PMLR; 2008. p. 1–33.
45. Aphinyanaphongs Y, Fu LD, Li ZG, Peskin ER, Efstathiadis E, Aliferis CF, Statnikov A. A comprehensive empirical comparison of modern supervised classification and feature selection methods for text categorization. J Assoc Inf Sci Technol. 2014;65(10):1964–87.
46. Statnikov A, Henaff M, Narendra V, Konganti K, Li ZG, Yang LY, Pei ZH, Blaser MJ, Aliferis CF, Alekseyenko AV. A comprehensive evaluation of multicategory classification methods for microbiomic data. Microbiome. 2013;1:23.
47. Narendra V, Lytkin NI, Aliferis CF, Statnikov A. A comprehensive assessment of methods for de-novo reverse-engineering of genome-scale regulatory networks. Genomics. 2011;97(1):7–18.
48. Statnikov A, Wang L, Aliferis CF. A comprehensive comparison of random forests and support vector machines for microarray-based cancer classification. BMC Bioinformatics. 2008;9(1):319.
49. Shi L, Campbell G, Jones WD. The MicroArray quality control (MAQC)-II study of common practices for the development and validation of microarray-based predictive models. Nat Biotechnol. 2010;28(8):827–38.
50. ChaLearn. http://www.chalearn.org.
51. Winterhoff B, Kommoss S, Heitz F, Konecny GE, Dowdy SC, Mullany SA, Park-Simon TW, Baumann K, Hilpert F, Brucker S, du Bois A, Aliferis C. Developing a clinico-molecular test for individualized treatment of ovarian cancer: the interplay of precision medicine informatics with clinical and health economics dimensions. In: AMIA annual symposium proceedings, vol. 2018. American Medical Informatics Association; 2018. p. 1093.
52. Ma SS, Kemmeren P, Aliferis CF, Statnikov A. An evaluation of active learning causal discovery methods for reverse-engineering local causal pathways of gene regulation. Sci Rep. 2016;6:22558.
53. Ray B, Henaff M, Ma S, Efstathiadis E, Peskin ER, Picone M, Poli T, Aliferis CF, Statnikov A. Information content and analysis methods for multi-modal high-throughput biomedical data. Sci Rep. 2014;4:4411. http://www.nature.com/articles/srep04411
54. Mani S, Ozdas A, Aliferis C, Varol HA, Chen QX, Carnevale R, Chen YK, Romano-Keeler J, Nian H, Weitkamp JH. Medical decision support using machine learning for early detection of late-onset neonatal sepsis. J Am Med Inform Assoc. 2014;21(2):236–336.
55. Fu LD, Aphinyanaphongs Y, Aliferis CF. Computer models for identifying instrumental citations in the biomedical literature. Scientometrics. 2013;97(3):871–82.
56. Aphinyanaphongs Y, Fu LD, Aliferis CF. Identifying unproven cancer treatments on the health web: addressing accuracy, generalizability and scalability. Stud Health Technol Inform. 2013;192:667–71.
57. Statnikov A, Alekseyenko AV, Li ZG, Henaff M, Perez-Perez GI, Blaser MJ, Aliferis CF. Microbiomic signatures of psoriasis: feasibility and methodology comparison. Sci Rep. 2013;3:2620.

58. Alekseyenko AV, Lytkin NI, Ai JZ, Ding B, Padyukov L, Aliferis CF, Statnikov A. Causal graph-based analysis of genome-wide association data in rheumatoid arthritis. Biol Direct. 2011;6(1):25.

59. Statnikov A, Lytkin NI, McVoy L, Weitkamp J, Aliferis CF. Using gene expression profiles from peripheral blood to identify asymptomatic responses to acute respiratory viral infections. BMC Res Notes. 2010;3(1):264.

60. Fu LD, Aliferis CF. Using content-based and bibliometric features for machine learning models to predict citation counts in the biomedical literature. Scientometrics. 2010;85(1):257–70.

61. Kraus VB, Ma S, Tourani R, Fillenbaum GG, Burchett BM, Parker DC, Kraus WE, Connelly MA, Otvos JD, Cohen HJ, Orenduff MC. Causal analysis identifies small HDL particles and physical activity as key determinants of longevity of older adults. EBioMedicine. 2022;85:104292.

62. Saxe GN, Ma S, Morales LJ, Galatzer-Levy IR, Aliferis C, Marmar CR. Computational causal discovery for post-traumatic stress in police officers. Transl Psychiatry. 2020;10(1):1–12.

63. Attur M, Krasnokutsky S, Statnikov A, Samuels J, Li Z, Friese O, Le MPH G-G, Rybak L, Kraus VB, Jordan JM, Aliferis CF, Abramson SB. Low-grade inflammation in symptomatic knee osteoarthritis: prognostic value of inflammatory plasma lipids and peripheral blood leukocyte biomarkers. Arthritis & Rheumatology. 2015;67(11):2905–15.

64. Attur M, Statnikov A, Samuels J, Li Z, Alekseyenko AV, Greenberg JD, Krasnokutsky S, Rybak L, Lu QA, Todd J, Zhou H, Jordan JM, Aliferis CF, Abramson SB. Plasma levels of interleukin-1 receptor antagonist (IL1Ra) predict radiographic progression of symptomatic knee osteoarthritis. Osteoarthr Cartil. 2015;23(11):1915–24.

65. Feig JE, Vengrenyuk Y, Reiser V, Wu C, Statnikov A, Aliferis CF, Garabedian MJ, Fisher EA, Puig O. Regression of atherosclerosis is characterized by broad changes in the plaque macrophage transcriptome. PLoS One. 2012;7(6):e39790.

The Development Process and Lifecycle of Clinical Grade and Other Safety and Performance-Sensitive AI/ML Models

Constantin Aliferis and Gyorgy Simon

Abstract

This chapter introduces the notion of "clinical-grade" and other sensitive, mission-critical models and contrasts such models with more fault-tolerant feasibility, exploratory, or pre-clinical ones. The steps outlined span from requirements engineering to deployment and monitoring and also emphasize a number of contextual factors determining success such as clinical and health economic considerations. AI's "knowledge cliff" is discussed and the need to operationalize AI/ML "self-awareness" and overcome its limitations to ensure generality and safe use. This chapter introduces many core pitfalls and best practices. The overarching concepts, pitfalls and BPs of the chapter will be elaborated further and implementation will be presented across the book and especially in chapters "Foundations and Properties of AI/ML Systems," "An Appraisal and Operating Characteristics of Major ML Methods Applicable in Healthcare and Health Science," "Foundations of Causal ML", "Model Selection and Evaluation", and in chapter "Overfitting, Underfitting and General Model Overconfidence and Under-Performance Pitfalls and Best Practices in Machine Learning and AI".

Keywords

Clinical-grade AI/ML model · High-stakes/risk AI/ML model · Lifecycle of and development/validation process for AI/ML models · Decision support · "Knowledge cliff" · Transparency and explanation · Model selection and error estimation protocols · Model equivalence classes

C. Aliferis (✉) · G. Simon
Institute for Health Informatics, University of Minnesota, Minneapolis, MN, USA
e-mail: constantinaibestpractices@gmail.com

© The Author(s) 2024

G. J. Simon, C. Aliferis (eds.), *Artificial Intelligence and Machine Learning in Health Care and Medical Sciences*, Health Informatics,
https://doi.org/10.1007/978-3-031-39355-6_6

Clinical-Grade and Other Mission-Critical AI/ML Models vs. Exploratory and Feasibility Models

As we have seen in chapter "Artificial Intelligence and Machine Learning for Healthcare and Health Sciences: the Need for Best Practices Enabling Trust in AI and ML", AI/ML is widely applicable across industries, endeavors, and objectives. One of the differentiating characteristics of biomedical AI/ML is the high cost of wrong decisions which is typically not shared with many other types of commercial AI/ML.

Examples of non-biomedical AI/ML tasks that have typically *low cost* of errors:

- Recommendation systems in online e-commerce platforms,
- Recommendation systems for digital media streaming,
- Ad dollar allocation to increase sales,
- Language filters in social media,
- Email spam detectors,
- Image recognition in search engines.

While some non-biomedical areas do have *high-risk applications* such as:

- Autonomous vehicles,
- Weapons and defense systems,
- Algorithmic trading,

these are relatively rare compared to healthcare and the health sciences, that are replete with tasks that have very high cost of failure, including in:

- Diagnosis of serious diseases,
- Choice of treatment in oncology and other life-threatening diseases,
- Differentiation of early signs of benign from malignant conditions or conditions that will progress to life-threatening stages or have other dire consequences if the right treatment is delayed,
- Generating hypotheses for re-organization of healthcare services and other interventions that may severely affect the cost-effectiveness and outcomes of a health system.

Even health science tasks that on the surface may seem tolerant of errors have important serious unintended consequences, for example in:

- Discovery of drug targets which if having many false positives, will lead to failed novel pharmaceuticals pipelines with up to multibillion-dollar losses,
- Conflating correlative with causal factors leading to pursuing expensive and risky interventions that cannot possibly improve outcomes,
- Low signal-to-noise ratio in the biomedical literature due to massive production of false results which disrupts progress in the health sciences,
- Failure to discover novel effective treatments and practice interventions.

Because the requirements of high-stakes models are very different than those of models with less severe costs and consequences, we differentiate between the following very different classes of models and place strong emphasis on the safe and effective development of high-risk models. We first crystalize the related key concept definitions:

Exploratory AI/ML models: models that test scientific hypotheses or generate new hypotheses but without linking critical patient, health system, or health sciences decisions to the quality of such models.

Feasibility AI/ML models: models that test the feasibility of constructing a certain type of model but without linking critical patient, health system, or health sciences decisions to the quality of such models.

Pre-clinical AI/ML models: models that test the feasibility of constructing (at a later stage) patient or health system critical models.

Clinical-grade and mission-critical AI/ML models: models with performance characteristics that allow for effective and safe use for patient, population, health system or health sciences-level decisions [1].

The delineation between exploratory, feasibility and clinical grade models is fundamentally a *risk* assessment process. Within the categories of feasibility and clinical-grade (or other mission-critical) models, further risk analyses will typically occur. These risks may involve model inaccuracy related risks, legal risks, ethical risks, financial risks, etc.

Risk assessment of health AI/ML models can greatly facilitated via application of the *risk management framework* provided by the **ISO 14971 standard** and/or by application of the **FDA criteria for regulated medical devices** (see chapter "Regulatory Aspects and Ethical Legal Societal Implications (ELSI)" for detailed discussion). Another useful high-level framework is the **translational science spectrum** [2] comprising steps T0 to T4. Exploratory and feasibility AI/ML would typically fall in stages T0-T1, whereas T2 and beyond corresponds to clinical-grade AI/ML.

T0 research: Basic biomedical research, including preclinical and animal studies, not including interventions with human subjects.

T1 research: Translation to humans, including proof of concept studies, phase 1 clinical trials, and focus on new methods of diagnosis, treatment, and prevention in highly-controlled settings.

T2 research: Translation to patients, including phase 2 and 3 clinical trials, and controlled studies leading to clinical application and evidence-based guidelines.

T3 research: Translation to practice, including comparative effectiveness research, post-marketing studies, clinical outcomes research, as well as health services, and dissemination & implementation research; and

T4 research: Translation to communities, including population level outcomes research, monitoring of morbidity, mortality, benefits, and risks, and impacts of policy and change.

Notice that *even if a model is not subject to regulatory oversight per se, it may still pose very significant risks.* Consider for example, a model for forecasting resource utilization/needs used by a hospital's administration business planning; or a model used by health insurers for contract pricing and reimbursability; or, finally a model that helps a pharmaceutical manufacturer prioritize its drug pipeline. It is entirely conceivable for errors in such models to lead to very substantial financial losses and/ or disruption of health services or of R&D and production, affecting the well-being not only of such organizations but of large populations of individuals as well.

Also notice that whereas a marketed/deployed AI/ML model may directly affect patients' outcomes and require regulatory approval, the pre-cursors of such models that investigate feasibility will not typically require such oversight (but be subject to other ethical and legal constraints).

The major (high-level) pitfalls that the present chapter addresses are:

Pitfall 6.1.1
Treating the development of clinical-grade or mission-critical AI/ML models as if they were exploratory, feasibility or pre-clinical ones.

Pitfall 6.1.2
Failing to establish and apply appropriate sufficient criteria and enforce BPs for model development, validation, and lifecycle support that will ensure safe and effective deployment in high risk settings.

Best Practice 6.1.1
Define the goals and process of AI/ML model building as either feasibility/ exploratory or as clinical-grade/mission-critical and apply appropriate quality and rigor criteria and best practices.

In the remainder of this chapter (as well in related chapters diving into technical details) we will expand and enrich these pitfalls and present corresponding BPs.

The Lifecycle of Clinical-Grade and Other Mission-Critical AI/ ML Models (with Indicative Real-Life Example References). A Development Process

Recall from chapter "Artificial Intelligence (AI) and Machine Learning (ML) for Healthcare and Health Sciences: the Need for Best Practices Enabling Trust in AI and ML" that learning and other AI methods produce decision support models focused on specific problem solving tasks. In chapter "Principles of Rigorous Development and of Appraisal of ML and AI Methods and Systems" we described a systematic process for designing or evaluating learning methods (algorithms, algorithm families, pipelines, and automodelers) in terms of desirable operating characteristics.

Here we focus our attention to the development process, *not of methods but of models* with desirable performance characteristics (aka assurances) [3] across the lifecycle of the AI/ML models or systems [4].

Conceptually, and similar to the method development and evaluation process of chapter "Principles of Rigorous Development and of Appraisal of ML and AI Methods and Systems," the described model lifecycle process combines elements of tested-and-true software and medical device development processes: the modified **waterfall development process** where iterative development is allowed (and here in addition, certain parts are occurring in parallel); and the **stage-gate development process** [5–7].

We will assume that the models will be based on existing or newly-developed and validated methods and will introduce pitfalls and a best practice process and steps, the purpose of which is to ensure that performance and safety goals are met. We discuss real life examples to ground the concepts in reality and make them clear. The overarching concepts and BPs of the present chapter are complemented by additional implementation details presented in chapters: "Foundations and Properties of AI/ML Systems," "An Appraisal and Operating Characteristics of Major ML Methods Applicable in Healthcare and Health Science," "Foundations of Causal ML", "Evaluation", and "Overfitting, Underfitting and General Model Overconfidence and Under-performance Pitfalls and Best practices in Machine Learning and AI" (Fig. 1).

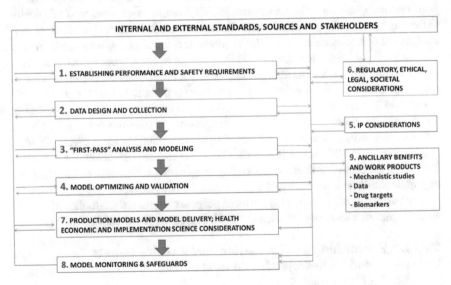

Fig. 1 Lifecycle of AI/ML models and a Best Practice workflow for their development. *Steps 6 and 5, 9 progress in parallel with steps 1–4, 7–8*

For each of the above steps/stages, we discuss where and how relaxing the stringency of requirements is warranted for feasibility, exploratory, or preclinical models.

Step 1. Establishing Performance and Safety Requirements

The first step of developing a new AI/ML model or system is deciding what its intended goal is and what other constraints should be considered. This step corresponds to the traditional *requirements engineering* process familiar in the development of practically any computer, IT or engineering system [8]. Requirements engineering for AI and ML is currently an emerging field and many challenges exist in identifying the categories of goals and the right processes for conducting successful requirements engineering in health AI/ML [9–11]. Various desired properties, such as accuracy, explainability, safety etc. are often discussed in this emerging literature. We will incorporate in the components of step 1 these concepts - using a healthcare and health sciences perspective - as well as concepts from the related literature on healthcare and life sciences analytics, clinical prediction modeling, and healthcare risk adjustment [12–14].

Step 1.1. Specifying Performance Targets
In order for AI/ML models to be effective there must be a *clear minimum set of performance goals that the successful models have to meet or exceed*. Typically these can be determined according to the need to meet some desired clinical outcomes goal *in either absolute or relative terms*. Indicative examples include: severe post-surgical infections less than 1/100 in surgeries of some type; reducing adverse events for some treatment used in patients with condition X by three-fold relative to current incidence; achieving diagnostic accuracy for condition X that is at least 50% better than current human error rates; improving current hypertensive medication compliance of patients by 30%; eliminating 1-month re-admissions in Medicare patients; controlling false positive biomarker identification for some disease X such that no more than 10% of newly identified biomarkers are statistical false positives; improving the cost-effectiveness of existing diagnostics, treatments, or other patient or population-level interventions by some specific margin, etc.

The various metrics often used for these purposes are part of the toolkit of AI/ML *model evaluation* and are discussed at length in chapter "Evaluation".

Step 1.2. Establishing and Evaluating Performance Targets in Real-Life and Multi-Objective Context of Use; Stakeholder Engagement
The target requirements represent meaningful goals in real-life discovery and health care settings as a function of the needs of a plurality of stakeholders and may be subject to objective or subjective judgments and values. Such judgment may originate by clinical experts, national guidelines, or may be tied to financial and payer expectations, and may also incorporate patient's and human subjects' perspectives

(e.g., about subjective quality of life in various health states, or expectations about privacy, health risks etc., respectively) and ELSI (Ethical, Legal, Social Implications) as well as JEDI (social Justice, health Equity, Diversity, Inclusion) criteria and desiderata (see chapter "Regulatory Aspects and Ethical Legal Societal Implications (ELSI))" for the importance and nature of ethical consideration and goals including extensive discussion of the important elements of health equity and elimination of unfair treatment of disadvantaged populations.

The context of these assessments has to be carefully constructed so that it is well-defined and facilitates the subsequent model development. By way of analogous examples, a well-defined context of model use may be similar to patient inclusion criteria specification for a clinical trial protocol, FDA contexts of use for biomarkers, FDA approved uses for drugs, etc.

Stakeholders and sources of guidance for developing a well-specified context of use of the sought models as well as performance requirements include:

(a) External (independent) or organizational (internal) clinical experts;
(b) Clinical service directors;
(c) The scientific literature, including science-driven hypotheses;
(d) National, state and organizational guidelines;
(e) Payers and contracts terms between providers and payers;
(f) Regulatory bodies and legal compliance experts;
(g) Ethics experts;
(h) Community representatives;
(i) Individual patients and patient advocacy groups;
(j) Professional and scientific societies;
(k) Scientific standards and standards groups;
(l) It is also possible for goals to be generated by data-driven opportunity identification by prior application of AI/ML technology.

The above serve as the most common important sources for setting quality and cost improvement initiatives in the context of QCI of health systems, Learning Health Systems initiatives, and academic and industry R&D initiatives where AI/ML can be an enabling technology. Especially with regards to general data and science standards, models and their underlying data both at development, validation and deployment stages ideally must follow:

(m) FAIR principles for scientific data and software (Findable Accessible Interoperable and Reusable data and software).
(n) TRUST data principles (Transparency, Responsibility, User focus, Sustainability, and Technology).
(o) *Open Science* practices including open access, open data, open source, and open standards for software, data and scientific findings.
(p) Data security and HIPAA and other compliance requirements for data privacy by virtue of state of the art IT security, de-identification, and secure management of all sensitive EHR, RCT and other data.

(q) Use of shareable and standardized terminologies and common data models (e.g., RxNorm, ICD9, ICD10, SNOMED CT, CPT, LOINC, HL7, OMOP, PCORnet CDM, i2b2, for research with clinical data; and OBI, GO, VariO, PRO, GO, CL, etc. for research with molecular data. See chapter "Data Preparation, Transforms, Quality, and Management" for detailed discussion and references for data requirements and practices).

An appraisal and synthesis of the above requirements may typically be undertaken by institutional AI/ML governance and oversight committees [15, 16].

Step 1.3. From Accuracy to Value Proposition and Health Economics

AI/ML loss functions and the general theory that governs AI/ML are typically constructed around predictivity measures (e.g., AUC, weighted accuracy, MSE etc., see chapter "Evaluation"). A *translation step* is typically needed to map predictivity measures and other model properties (e.g., cost of inputs to the model per application of the model) into downstream *value*.

In healthcare, generally there are four key business drivers of value: (a) revenue growth, (b) operating margins, (c) asset efficiency, and (d) organizational effectiveness. These drivers in turn impact three main business goals: (1) clinical performance, (2) operational performance, and (3) financial performance [4].

There are many metrics used to measure these goals and chapter "Evaluation" discusses both clinical outcome oriented metrics as well as health economic ones. We will briefly mention here that metrics exist that combine clinical with economic value, for example the metric of *Incremental Cost Effectiveness Ratio (ICER)* which is a typical and widely-used value assessment health economics tool based on economic cost (e.g., expenditure in dollars) per unit of effectiveness typically measured in Quality Adjusted Life Years (QUALYs) gained by use of some intervention, technology, medication, or in our case AI/ML model. The ICER and other cost-effectiveness metrics have several useful properties:

(a) They allow placing a variety of wildly heterogeneous possible improvements on current practices, in clinical care or science, in direct comparison to one another.
(b) They allow optimal allocation of limited resources to maximize the expected benefit across all possible mixtures of interventions.
(c) They enable specifying minimum performance requirements that are necessary for making the decision of incurring the costs required for developing and/or deploying the envisioned or existing AI/M model. See chapter "Evaluation" for details.

Step 1.4. System-Level Goals and interactions vs."Tunnel-Vision" Model Development

A common shortcoming of AI/ML model development practice is that they have performance requirements that are meaningful in a narrow context but are blind to *system-level consequences and interactions*.

As an example in clinical settings, consider the need to decide whether patients with COVID-19 infections should be admitted in the ICU versus the hospital clinic and the related problem of whether milder COVID cases should be hospitalized or sent home. AI/ML models focusing exclusively on eliminating the risk of bad outcomes for these patients would tend to overwhelm the hospital and ICU beds to the detriment of patients with other conditions. If a fixed number of hospital beds can be made available in some time horizon, and patients with different risks for dire outcomes are "competing" for the limited beds, sound development and evaluation of Covid admission models should take into account the patients with different conditions and the system of care holistically. *As of the time this book is written, the literature on AI/Ml decision support models strongly indicates that such system-level interactions are typically not considered, yet they are critical for the health system holistically.*

Step 1.5. Relaxing the Stringency of Requirements for Feasibility, Exploratory, or Pre-clinical Models. Proper Level of Interpretation

The above requirements can be relaxed when dealing with feasibility, exploratory or preclinical models. It is entirely appropriate for such models to have a combination of the following:

- Unspecified performance targets,
- Open-ended application contexts,
- To be driven by scientists' curiosity,
- To omit system-level interactions,
- To forego incorporation of health economics, and
- To not consider clinical-grade compliance and risk management.

However, even for such early efforts, the closer they are to the ideal specifications of clinical-grade and mission-critical models, the more informative and the closer they are to eventually leading to significant contribution to health care and the health sciences. Additionally, serious caution is warranted regarding the problem of producing too much "noise" in the literature resulting from models lacking or with loose requirements and purpose.

Finally, creators of feasibility, exploratory and pre-clinical models should not over-interpret them and exaggerate their significance. **The reader is referred to chapter "Principles of Rigorous Development and of Appraisal of ML and AI Methods and Systems," for guidance on over and under interpreting methods and models produced by them, which applies exactly here as well, and will not be repeated as it applies precisely as stated in section "Over-and Under-Interpreting Results," in the same chapter.**

We can therefore refine and expand pitfall 6.1. by including:

Pitfall 6.2.1.1
Failure to specify and evaluate meaningful performance targets and real-life context of use.

Pitfall 6.2.1.2
Failure to engage all appropriate stakeholders.

Pitfall 6.2.1.3
Failure to establish value targets and translate predictivity and other technical model characteristics into real-world value assessments.

Pitfall 6.2.1.4
Failure to consider broader interactions of envisioned models with the health system or with the system of science and of R&D. "Tunnel vision" evaluation with blind spots to the broader implications and consequences.

Pitfall 6.2.1.5
Failure to consider ELSI and JEDI desiderata and consequences.

Pitfall 6.2.1.6
Interpreting results of models beyond what their properties justify.

Pitfall 6.2.1.7
Interpreting results of models below what their known properties justify.

The corresponding best practices are:

Best Practice 6.2.1.1
When pursuing risk and performance-sensitive model development, specify concrete model performance targets for well-defined care or discovery settings.

Best Practice 6.2.1.2
When pursuing risk and performance-sensitive model development, engage all appropriate stakeholders.

Best Practice 6.2.1.3
When pursuing risk and performance-sensitive model development, translate model accuracy to value, establish value targets and translate predictivity and other technical model characteristics into real-world value assessments.

Best Practice 6.2.1.4
When pursuing risk and performance-sensitive model development, carefully consider and plan for system-level goals and interactions. Avoid too narrow ("tunnel vision") model development.

Best Practice 6.2.1.5
When pursuing clinical-grade and risk-sensitive model development, carefully consider ELSI and JEDI desiderata and consequences.

Best Practice 6.2.1.6
When pursuing feasibility, exploratory, or pre-clinical models, relax stringency of requirements applicable to clinical-grade models.

Best Practice 6.2.1.7
When pursuing clinical-grade and risk-sensitive model development, interpret models and models' decisions exactly as their known properties justify.

Step 2. Data Design and Collection

The second stage in the clinical-grade and mission-critical model development process is the careful data design that will facilitate data collection and modeling to enable meeting the model performance requirements. In chapter "Data Design" we cover extensively the most relevant data designs and their relative strengths and weaknesses, their connection to modeling methods, their biases, their effect on performance, and other important characteristics.

One of the fundamental premises of this book and of chapter "Data Design" in particular (also discussed in chapters "Foundations and Properties of AI/ML Systems," "Principles of rigorous development and of Appraisal of ML and AI Methods and Systems," and "Lessons Learned from Historical Failures, Limitations and Successes of AI/ML In Healthcare and the Health Sciences. Enduring Problems, and the Role of Best Practices"), is that the data design is, generally speaking, as important as the actual algorithms and AI/ML analytic protocols and stacks and many failures occur when the data design is deficient. In particular, powerful data designs may render the choice of algorithms inconsequential, and conversely a poor data design will increase the modeling work and difficulty exponentially, up to rendering the whole model development workflow infeasible.

Pitfall 6.2.2.1
Failure to create a rigorous and powerful data design which facilitates modeling that will meet performance and safety requirements.

For feasibility, exploratory, or pre-clinical modeling, on the other hand, developers can and often do utilize "convenience" datasets without extensive efforts for bespoke and optimized data sampling. In such cases the feasibility modeling has to be tailored to the limitations of the convenience datasets and the interpretation has to be careful to not overstate what can be developed with imperfect data designs.

Pitfall 6.2.2.2
Failure to consider and judiciously interpret the limitations of convenience data designs on the performance and meaning of feasibility and exploratory models.

Best Practice 6.2.2.1
When pursuing risk and performance-sensitive model development, create a rigorous and powerful data design which facilitates modeling that will meet performance and safety requirements.

Best Practice 6.2.2.2
When pursuing risk and performance-sensitive model development, judiciously interpret the limitations of convenience data designs for the performance and meaning of feasibility and exploratory models.

Step 3. First-Pass Analysis and Modeling

The next stage of clinical grade and mission-critical AI/ML model development is that of "first-pass" modeling before final optimized models are attempted. This stage essentially asks "how much signal seems to be in the data for the problem at hand, using the immediately-available data?". If the preliminary signal is high, then transition to high performance/low risk models will be easier, faster, and cheaper. If the preliminary signal is small, then major efforts may be needed in data collection, new method development, sophisticated modeling, etc. and still these efforts may not meet target requirements. In R&D designs where alternative projects compete for the same limited R&D funds, this stage may be the point where some of the projects will be "weeded out" in favor of more promising ones.

The first-pass modeling therefore must be rigorous and involves a number of activities that to large extent mirror aspects of rigorous methods development previously discussed in chapter "Principles of Rigorous Development and of Appraisal of ML and AI Methods and Systems":

(a) Literature review of what has been accomplished, and how, and what level of performance was reached by prior efforts;

(b) Theoretical analysis of the problem space and its characteristics;

(c) Available or easy /cheap to collect data for initial development and testing;

(d) Approaches and results previously explored both in terms of data design, algorithms and models;

(e) Verifying and reproducing prior literature findings/claims;

(f) Variation of data/populations used to derive prior models and how they match the population for the intended new models; and

(g) Preliminary estimates of predictivity of the first pass models and whether they meet requirements.

These considerations collectively establish that first pass modeling does not imply a haphazard and "anything goes" approach to modeling. Several criteria apply that **sharply differentiate feasibility modeling (which is not tied to a clinical-grade or mission-critical modeling) with first pass modeling (which is part of a R&D chain that intends to achieve, eventually, clinical-grade and mission-critical performance).**

Finally an important consideration is to avoid overfitting, which as we see in detail in chapter "Overfitting, Underfitting and General Model Overconfidence and Under-Performance Pitfalls and Best Practices in Machine Learning and AI", will occur when repeated rounds of modeling with additional methods in same data are conducted *without appropriate over-fitting avoidance protocols being in place.*

The steps in this stage can also serve, at the discretion of the data scientists and the project leaders, as a blueprint for strong exploratory modeling (always remembering that if exploration is the sole goal, then much lower data and performance and safety requirements can be pursued).

> **Pitfall 6.2.3.1**
> Failure to ensure the successful transition from first pass modeling to optimized clinical grade models by ignoring: the problem space characteristics; data available for development and testing; prior literature on approaches and results previously explored both in terms of data design, algorithms and models; forfeiting verification and reproducing prior literature findings/claims; and failure to obtain robust preliminary estimates of predictivity of the first pass models and whether they meet requirements.

Pitfall 6.2.3.2
Succumb to overfitting when repeatedly analyzing data from first pass to optimized modeling stages.

Best Practice 6.2.3.1
When moving from first pass modeling to optimized clinical grade models take into account: the problem space characteristics; data available for development and testing; prior literature on approaches and results previously explored both in terms of data design, algorithms and models; verification and reproducing prior literature findings/claims; obtaining robust preliminary estimates of predictivity of the first pass models and whether they meet requirements.

Best Practice 6.2.3.2
Avoid overfitting due to repeatedly analyzing data from first pass to optimized modeling stages.

An Important Protocol for Over-Fitting Resistant Model Selection, and Unbiased Model Error Estimation

Critical to a successful ML method is the choice of model selection and error estimation protocol. Such a protocol should support the following:

(a) Unbiased error estimation (i.e., estimate accurately the generalization error of the model in the large sample population).

(b) Avoiding overfitting the model to the training data, especially if dimensionality is high, sample size is small, and many methods are applied.

(c) Avoid missing strong models for the task at hand (i.e., avoid under-fitting).

Figure 2 depicts the core concept and simplified pseudo-code for a powerful such protocol that has great applicability across a wide range of biomedical ML modeling problems: the **Repeated Nested Balanced N-fold Cross Validation (RNBNFCV) protocol** [17]. The bottom part shows pseudocode for a bare-bones RNBNFCV. The top part demonstrates a simple example of operation of a three-fold cross validation optimizing two values (1,2) of one hyper-parameter (C) for one algorithm.

As can be seen the data is split randomly in 3 equal parts P1, P2, P3. Each part is stratified so that has equal number of positive and negative values of the binary response (i.e., the splits are balanced). For each of the P1, P2, P3 datasets, two parts are used for model selection and the remainder (third part) is used for error

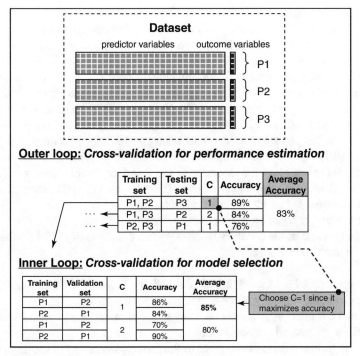

Fig. 2 Repeated Nested Balanced N-fold Cross Validation (RNBNFCV) protocol. *Top: simple example of operation of a three-fold cross validation optimizing two values of one hyper-parameter for one algorithm. Balancing labels, repeated application, and construction of final model not shown for simplicity. Bottom: pseudocode for bare-bones RNBNFCV. See text for details*

estimation. For example in split 1 {P1, P2} will be used for model selection and P3 for error estimation. We say that the error estimation occurs in the outer loop and the model selection in the inner loop. This is evident from both the graphic and the pseudocode.

Within each model selection part of a split, we use a random part for fitting a model and the rest for evaluating its performance. For example in inner split 1, P1 will be used to fit a model with hyper parameter $C = 1$ and tested on P2. Then in inner split 2, P2 will be used to fit a model with $C = 1$ and evaluated in P1. The average accuracy over the inner splits informs the merit of $C = 1$. We do the same for $C = 2$ and find out that $C = 1$ is the best value for the hyper-parameter. This terminates this most simplistic model selection. Now we join P1 and P2 and train a model with $C = 1$. We evaluate in P3 in the outer loop and record the accuracy (=89%).

We repeat this procedure for the other outer cross validation splits (i.e., P1,P3/P2 and P2,P3/P1). The trace of the model selection for these splits is not shown, but we can see that the best C for the second split was 2 and for the third split was 1. Based on these values for C, models are fit on {P1, P3} and {P2, P3} respectively, and accuracies estimated on P2, P1, respectively.

The average of these outer loop accuracies are then averaged to provide a final unbiased estimate of the accuracy that this protocol can identify (83%). What is not shown in this simplified figure is:

1. The final model is a model that we will fit from all data {P1,P2,P3} using $C = 1$. The estimated accuracy of 83% applies to this final model.
2. We can use many algorithms and many hyper-parameters with many values and let the protocol find the best model.
3. We can further reduce the variance of the final estimates and of the model selection by repeating the whole procedure and averaging the error estimates.

Step 4. Model Optimizing and Validation

Step 4.1. Modify or Enhance Data Design, Algorithms, and Protocols

Once a first-pass analysis has been completed and the data scientists have collected important information about the sufficiency of data (e.g., is there need to collect more variables, or larger sample size, to clean up and transform variables etc., or alter other data design aspects), as well as modeling (e.g., whether the algorithm and protocols applied seem sufficient or require inclusion of additional analytic methods and in some cases enhancing methods with new method development efforts), they can proceed with optimized model building and validation. This includes the following key steps:

Step 4.2. Obtain Performance Metrics and Meeting Targets

This is accomplished using *model selection* and *error estimation and evaluation designs and procedures* for appropriate performance metrics as explained in chapters "Foundations and Properties of AI/ML Systems" (fundamental methods), "Model Selection", "Evaluation", and the chapter on overfitting. The performance metrics can be estimated with purely statistical methods and/or with collection of new data and prospective validations. See chapter "Evaluation" for pros and cons of these approaches.

In case that further refinements are needed because performance targets are not fully met, this will trigger revisiting and iterating between steps 4.1.-4.2, and possibly new method development (chapter "Principles of Rigorous Development and of Appraisal of ML and AI Methods and Systems"). It is also possible that targets cannot be met despite efforts and therefore relaxing the original model specifications and re-architecting the whole problem solving effort toward more feasible goals, may be necessary.

Step 4.3. Uncertainty and Error

This step involves a thorough characterization of the optimized model's decision uncertainty and goes beyond establishing the main performance metrics. Examples of this step may include calculating: the robustness of model and its structure and parameters as a function of sampling variation (via resampling); sensitivity to modeling decisions (e.g., similarity distance metrics, kernel functions, algorithm families considered etc.); calibration; predictive intervals (measuring uncertainty of decisions). A related procedure at this stage is to "curve out" subpopulations in the model's inputs distribution space or the model's output using thresholding, clustering and other methods so that to define decision regions and populations that are characterized by high or low confidence. These steps are essential for managing misclassification risk and discussed further in chapter "Characterizing, Diagnosing and Managing the Risk of Error of ML and AI Models in Clinical and Organizational Application".

Step 4.4. Model Explanation/Interpretation

AI/ML Models are much more likely to be adopted and used if human stakeholders can understand their function and why they make the decisions they do. It is a critical element in making sure that AI/ML is safe and also commonly important for regulatory approvals. It is essential that **model explanations have high fidelity** (i.e., correspond precisely to how the AI/ML functions, and are not just persuasive but inaccurate justifications of the models [18]).

We have seen in previous chapters that some AI/ML methods are inherently understandable (e.g., logic, rule based systems, Bayes Nets, causal graphs, decision trees, linear regression etc.) while many other methods produce models that are black box and hard to understand.

The fields of explainable AI (XAI) and interpretable ML and their incarnations in health domains study methods to make black box models interpretable [19].

In this section we will delve into essential concepts and techniques for AI/ML interpretation.

Murdock et al. [20] define interpretation, in the context of ML, as producing insight from ML models. Specifically, they define interpretable machine learning as the extraction of relevant knowledge from a machine-learning model concerning relationships either contained in data or learned by the model. Other definitions include "*Interpretability is the degree to which a human can understand the cause of a decision*" [21].

Benefits of interpretable machine learning methods include: [21–23].

- Model interpretability allows the user of the model to investigate and understand why an unexpected prediction was made by the model.
- By extension, model interpretability allows us to debug models: the model developer can track down why the model made an erroneous prediction.
- Model interpretability can shed light on the data-generating mechanisms of the domain that is being modeled.
- Interpretable models offer a level of safety in that the user can anticipate model behavior.
- In the absence of strict standards that govern the interoperability of ML models (or ML models and humans), understanding exactly how the individual ML models operate, can increase trust in their effective co-operation.

As we discuss in Chapter "Regulatory Aspects and Ethical Legal Societal Implications (ELSI)", interpretable models also allow for the detection of biases present in the training data and are required for equitable and fair models.

A Taxonomy of AI/ML Interpretability

Methods for model interpretation can be categorized along the following dimensions [21, 24]:

- **Inherently interpretable vs. post hoc**. Models such as linear regression models, k-NN classifiers, decision trees are inherently interpretable; their language (see chapters "Foundations and Properties of AI/ML Systems", "An Appraisal and Operating Characteristics of Major ML Methods Applicable in Healthcare and Health Science", and "Foundations of Causal ML") is particularly suitable for human interpretation unless their size (e.g., number of leaves or number of variables) is excessive. In contrast, models such as kernel-SVM or Deep Learning are not easily interpretable, and the models are explained post hoc, after they have been constructed.
- **Global vs. local interpretability**. Global interpretation of a model attempts to explain the model in the entirety of the input space; local interpretation attempts to explain how the model operates in small part of the input space, possibly for individual instances. "Interpretation" generally refers to explaining how the model operates, while "explanation" generally refers to explaining how a model made a decision (or prediction) for a particular instance.
- **Model-agnostic vs. model-specific interpretation**. Model-specific interpretation techniques require that the model to be interpreted is a specific type of model, while model-agnostic interpretation methods aims to explain any type of models.

Properties of Interpretation Methods

Numerous properties for interpretation methods have been defined [24, 25]. Below we list some; the reader is referred to [24, 25] for a more complete list.

Accuracy is the extent to which the explanation model accurately predicts unseen instances.

Fidelity refers to the extent to which the model is able to accurately imitate the black-box predictor to be explained.

Consistency (among explanation methods) shows how similar explanations are from different methods for the same task.

Stability is the degree to which similar explanations are generated for similar instances.

Figure 3 depicts the taxonomy of interpretation method. We have already discussed the inherently interpretable methods in chapters "Foundations and Properties of AI/ML Systems," "An Appraisal and Operating Characteristics of Major ML Methods Applicable in Healthcare and Health Science," and "Foundations of Causal ML". We will provide some additional detail on the local and global model-agnostic methods and their properties.

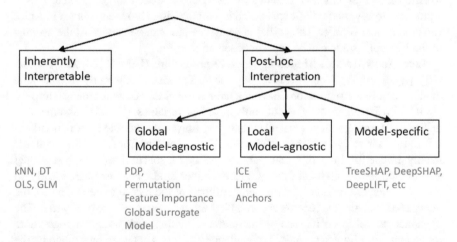

Fig. 3 Taxonomy of interpretation methods (with example methods in blue text underneath)

Partial Dependence Plots (PDPs) [26] is a methodology for visualizing the effect of predictor variables on an outcome in a reduced feature space. For a feature S of interest, and for each unique value s it takes, the partial dependence is the average effect of the remaining variables (keeping S = s fixed). The partial dependence plot depicts the predicted outcome as a function of S and can be converted into feature importance by computing the feature's deviation from the average effect or by taking the difference between the maximal and minimal effects.

Properties. PDP is a global method. The marginalization is over the remaining variables, which prevents the user from detecting "local" effects, that is relationships between S and the outcome that hold true only in a subspace. PDP is a plot, offering an intuitive interpretation. The method makes the assumption of independence between S and the remaining variables. Under this assumption, the interpretation is that the partial dependence is the marginal effect of S on the outcome.

Individual Conditional Expectation (ICE) [27] plot visualizes the dependence of the predicted outcome on a feature S for each instance i separately, resulting in one line per instance. The curve for instance i is created by fixing all features except S at their actual values and varying the value for S according to a grid of feature values. The predicted outcomes for different i's at the minimal value of S can differ, making it difficult to visually inspect a large set of curves at the same time. The centered ICE brings all the curves together to a common starting point.

Properties. ICE is a local method, providing a curve for each individual instance. Relationships that only hold true in parts of the input space can be detected. This is a plot, so the key method of explanation is visualization. Too many curves in a plot can create visual clutter. The partial dependence plot can be viewed as the average of the ICE curves and can be superimposed on the plot.

Local Interpretable Model-Agnostic Explanations (LIME) [28] and Anchors [29]. <u>Rationale:</u> (a) Even if a modeling method produces inherently interpretable models (e.g. linear regression), having a large number of variables erodes interpretability. The explainer model should only have few variables. (b) LIME assumes that in the local context of a particular instance, only few variables are particularly impactful. These locally impactful variables can differ from variables that are locally impactful in a different part of the input space. The explainer model should then have high local fidelity. The explainer model is constructed locally on records generated randomly in the neighborhood of the record to be explained, the query record q, and the records are weighted according to their proximity to q. The explainer model is an inherently interpretable model, such as linear regression, trained on the weighted records. The explanation for q is obtained by explaining the explainer model.

<u>Anchors</u> is an extension to LIME, which instead of building a local surrogate model, constructs an IF-THEN rule. They are called "anchors", because they sufficiently "anchor" the prediction locally – such that changes to the rest of the feature values of the instance do not matter; i.e., similar instances covered by the same anchor have the same prediction outcome. Two advantages of anchors over LIME include (1) the improved interpretability the rules and (2) scoping: while the scope of a LIME explanation is not always clear, anchors have a clearly delineated scope.

Properties of LIME. It is a local, model-agnostic method. The explainer model can be any interpretable model; the choice of model can be tailored to the audience. The explainer model can utilize features that the original model does not. These features must use the same instances (sampling units) as the original data set.

Permutation Feature Importance. Rationale: if information in features that are useful for prediction is destroyed by randomly shuffling the feature values, the predictive performance of the model should decrease. If the decrease is small, then the information in the original predictor wasn't very impactful; if the decrease is large, then the information in the original predictor had a large impact on the predictions. A model is constructed on the training set and the importance of feature S is estimated by comparing the predictive performance (or error) of the model on a test set with and without permuting S.

Note. Many variants of the method exist depending on (1) whether they use the training or test set, and (2) whether they re-train the model after permuting the feature values. Originally, Breiman [30] used the out-of-bag samples for variable importance estimation.

Properties. This is a global, model-agnostic method. It is computationally efficient: the model does not need to be retrained. This definition of importance relates to predictive performance instead of the effect of the variable on the outcome. The feature importance depends on how the underlying learning method attributes the effect of sets of collinear features to the individual features. Whether the model is retrained after feature value permutation or not, will particularly affect the importance of collinear features.

Conversion of black model to decision trees of other interpretable global surrogate model via meta-learning. This is a global model-agnostic method whereby the black box model is sampled for a large number of inputs (that must follow a modeled joint distribution of inputs or from a random sample from the population) and a new dataset, Dsam, is created. The response in this new dataset is the black box model's predictions (not the original response variables). This dataset is then processed with a Markov Boundary feature selector so that the input variables are reduced to the smallest set of features that carry maximum explanatory signal for the black box model's behavior. Then decision trees or other interpretable models are built on the projection of Dsam on the Markov Boundary features. The method can be used to explain human decision as well, (if we first construct an accurate model of the human decision which we can sample as much as we need). Figure 4 demonstrates the process and resulting decision trees in a project where the goal was to explain physician diagnostic decisions for differentiating melanomas from benign skin lesions [31]. The method can be combined with equivalence class modeling of all equivalent Markov Boundaries so that an unbiased and complete view of the black model can be generated. Notice that separate interpretable models have been constructed for each physician. Moreover we can use the interpretable models to identify guideline compliance for each physician. Caveats and caution when using this approach are: we may not be able to create an accurate approximation of the original black box model (or the human subjects we are studying). Application of Markov Boundary feature selection may not retain all original

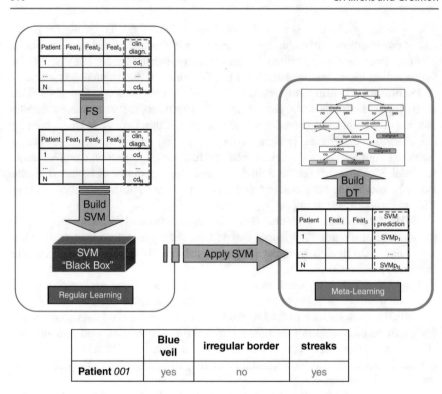

	Blue veil	irregular border	streaks
Patient *001*	yes	no	yes

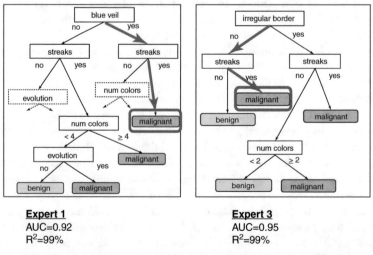

Fig. 4 Explanation by meta learning, Markov Boundary feature extraction and conversion to interpretable models. *Example in explaining physician diagnostic decisions for differentiating melanomas from benign skin lesions. Top: Original data from human decisions are feature-selected, then an accurate (but black box) model is created, then we sample the black model and create a dataset on which meta learning produces interpretable models (decision trees in this instance). Bottom: For a particular patient, we see key characteristics and how the interpretable model for expert physician 1 (left) compares with the model of physician 3 (right). In this case we can see that they agree, but with substantially different reasoning*

signal. Decision trees are sensitive to the order of variables so we need ensure that when some variables do not appear in a subtree that they are indeed ignored locally. Finally when equivalence classes exist, we need examine all equivalence classes. These caveats apply in general to all model-agnostic surrogate methods, however.

> **Explaining human decision making.** Once we create accurate models of human decision making, in principle all XAI methods discussed in this chapter can be used to explain human decision making (not just AI/ML models). This is a valuable technique that should be kept in mind when "Human-in-the-loop" systems are at play [32, 33]. See also chapter "From 'Human versus Machine' to 'Human with Machine'".

Pitfalls of Using Shapley Values (and Derivative Methods) for AI/ML Explanation

Shapley Values (SVs) is a framework for allocating rewards among agents who participate in collaborative coalitions to produce economic value that needs to be distributed fairly. This framework was devised by Lloyd Shapley who received the Nobel prize in economics for his discovery [34]. In economic game theory it has been shown that this framework has a number of desirable and unique properties and its value is undisputed. However it has been adopted rather uncritically first for explaining regression models [35] and then, more recently for explaining ML models [36]. As shown in an important recent work by Ma and Tourani [37] Shapley Values exhibit a number of severe shortcomings when it comes to explaining ML models:

1. SVs do not explain properly even linear models.
2. To calculate SVs one needs to build models that are unrelated to the model that needs be explained.
3. If SVs are calculated by data imputation and not de novo model rebuilds, the choice of imputation greatly affects the calculated values.
4. SVs for variables conditionally independent of T given blocking variable sets are (falsely) non zero.
5. SVs for variables not in the Markov Boundary of the response are non zero.
6. Causal effects of variables given their confounders are not monotonic to SVs.
7. SVs do not respect the causal Markov Condition and thus cannot be used to explain causal models.
8. SVs for a variable set L with less information content than that of set S can be larger than those of S. SVs are thus not monotonic to information content.
9. SVs are an improper measure of feature relevance (i.e., weakly relevant features can have higher SV than strongly relevant features).

Pitfalls of using feature-importance methods. In general these, just like Shapley Values methods, attempt to summarize the importance of features using a single summary value. This is a very problematic endeavor when dealing with complex multifaceted models. For example, they do not separate the unique, overlapping, and non-linear interaction information content of the variables in conjunction with other features in the model with which they may have overlapping content, or interact non-linearly to produce strong signal when jointly observed. See chapter "Foundations and Properties of AI/ML Systems" (section on feature selection, for more insight). They also cannot explain the causal effects of features under different conditioning, manipulation and observational setups (see chapter "Foundations of Causal ML" for insight). Finally these methods are not modeling effects of equivalence classes in the models.

Pitfalls of Explaining Transparent But Very Large Models

While a method may be entirely transparent for small scale models, the produced models may be very hard to interpret when they grow very large, because of the limits of human memory and cognition. Examples include large causal graphs, large decision trees, linear models with numerous variables with each one having a very small coefficient, large bagged model ensembles, boosted models, etc. Explaining such large models can be tailored to the specifics of each model family, or addressed with the usual array of surrogate models (i.e., as if the original model was a black box model). Table 1. shows example approaches, as indicative examples of the former approach.

Pitfalls of humans explaining models. Humans experts are often engaged (especially in the health sciences) for interpreting models. It is important to verify generalizable fidelity of human expert surrogate models.

Pitfalls 6.2.4.1 in Explanation of AI/ML
1. Using black box models is an obstacle to adoption and trust.
2. Shapley values (and derivative methods) have several severe shortcomings for AI/ML explanation.
3. Feature importance methods, that attempt to compress complex model behaviors into single values per variable, lack the necessary information capacity and may be inconsistent with feature selection theory and causality.
4. Inherently transparent but very large models often resist interpretability.
5. Human experts explaining models must be evaluated for validity just like ML surrogate models.

Table 1 Interpretation strategies for interpretable but very large models

Very large model family	Interpretation strategies
Linear regression and other GLM	• Group variables and examine their aggregate effects. • Create composite scores from large number of variables using dimensionality reduction or supervised regressors.
Decision trees	• Pre-process with maximally compact feature selection. • Prune trees to trade off accuracy with simplicity.
Causal graphs	• Eliminate all variables not leading to outcomes of interest. • Extract local causal neighborhoods and Markov Boundaries. • Extract causal paths from exposures of interest to outcomes of interest.
Bagged models	• Median, average, and ranges of distribution (across the model bag) of variable contributions to predictions within each model.

Best Practices for Explanation of AI/ML:

Best Practice 6.2.4.1. Everything else being equal, prefer interpretable model families when interpretability is desired.

Best Practice 6.2.4.2. Use standardized coefficients (if applicable) when comparing feature contributions in linear models.

Best Practice 6.2.4.3. Very large models, even when produced with intrinsically interpretable methods, may still be hard to interpret because of sheer scale. Isolating critical information from large models or simplification are recommended.

Best Practice 6.2.4.4. Apply feature selectors that maximally reduce dimensionality without loss of predictivity. Compact models are always easier to explain. Combine with interpretable model families or surrogate models as appropriate.

Best Practice 6.2.4.5. If accuracy is of paramount importance and if the black box models have significant accuracy advantages over the best interpretable models you can build, then use the black box model but apply explanation methods:
- Global surrogate models aiming to have high fidelity everywhere in the input space over all patterns that will be classified by the model. Verify generalizable fidelity of surrogate model before using.
- Local surrogate models aiming to have high fidelity in the local input space for every pattern pi that will be classified by the model. Verify generalizable fidelity of surrogate model before using.
- Human expert surrogate models which must be high fidelity everywhere in the input space and over-fitting resistant. Verify generalizability and fidelity of human expert explanations of models.

Best Practice 6.2.4.6. Shapley values, Shapley value approximations and feature importance methods that try to summarize complex model behaviors in one or few values are not advised as general or routinely used methods for explaining ML models.

A Note on Over- and Under-Interpreting Models

The structure and operating characteristics of AI/ML models offer important information about the data generating processes they model. This is especially important for discovery in the health sciences but also instrumental when we try and understand and improve systems and processes of healthcare. The appropriate interpretation of models refers to not deriving more or less (or more or less general or specific) conclusions than what the actual models entail. Because the appropriate model interpretation stems directly from the properties of the model family, knowledge of the model families (chapters "Foundations and Properties of AI/ML Systems," "An Appraisal and Operating Characteristics of Major ML Methods Applicable in Healthcare and Health Science," and "Foundations of Causal ML") is essential for proper model interpretation. See chapter "Principles of Rigorous Development and of Appraisal of ML and AI Methods and Systems" also for examples of appropriate and inappropriate model interpretation.

Step 4.5. Modeling Equivalence Classes

An extremely common pitfall in AI/ML modeling practices is that of ignoring equivalence classes of models. In order to understand the nature of this pervasive problem, and how to address it, we will present a simplified example.

Consider Fig. 5 where a system under study has the causal structure depicted. The outcome of interest is depicted in green. This is a terminal variable which means that no variables relevant to the system are measured (or have importance) after it (e.g. of such a biological terminal variable is death). Red variables are measured direct causes. Purple variables are measured indirect causes. Grey variables are unmeasured ("hidden" aka "latent") variables. Uncolored variables are confounded variables to the outcome (via measured or unmeasured confounders). Finally " ' " (prime) variables (A', C1', C2') have the same information about the outcome as (i.e., they are *information equivalent* with) the corresponding non-prime variables, e.g. A and A' are information equivalent about the outcome.

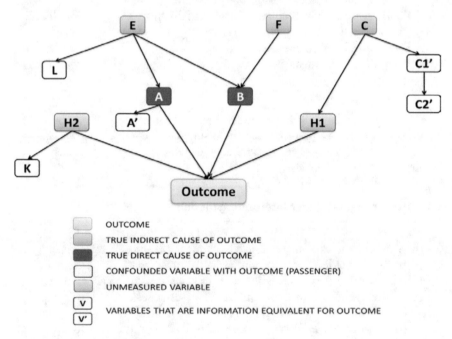

Fig. 5 Demonstration of problems in a domain with equivalence classes. Data generating structure. See text for details

Formally, information equivalency of two variables with respect to a third variable is defined as follows:

Definition
Target Information Equivalency (TIE) of variables A, A' with respect to variable T, (simplified definition that can be used to understand the example presented, adapted from [38]):

$A \text{ TIE}_T A' \leftrightarrow [(A \not\perp T), (A' \not\perp T), (A \perp\!\!\!\perp T \mid A'), (A' \perp\!\!\!\perp T \mid A')$

$\leftrightarrow$ denoting equivalence
$\not\perp$ denoting dependence
$\perp\!\!\!\perp$ denoting independence

In words:
Information_equivalent (A, A') with respect to T iff:
- Not Independent (A, T),
- Not Independent (A', T),
- Independent (A, T), given A' and
- Independent (A', T) given A.

In other words, A and A' have exactly the same (and non-zero) information about T.

Note 1:A, A' do not need to be strongly correlated (i.e., co-linear) or strongly associated. They can be TIE with respect to T even with small mutual association or correlation.

Note 2:A, A' may have different information content for other variables (different than T).

As can be seen in the example of Fig. 5, the minimum set of maximally predictive features in the data generating function is {A, B, H1, H2} and its equivalent {A', B, H1, H2}. This is because we can substitute A with A' and vice versa since they are equivalent with respect to the outcome. In the measured data (because of hidden variables) there are 6 Markov Boundaries and this set can be precisely discovered also (Fig. 6).

Note 3: In [38] more general definitions of information equivalency are presented that admit sets of equivalent variables, equivalences involving more than two

INFERRED MARKOV BOUNDARIES EQUIVALENCE CLASS

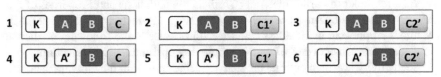

TRUE MARKOV BOUNDARIES EQUIVALENCE CLASS IN MEASURED DATA

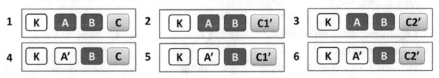

Fig. 6 Demonstration of equivalence class - related problems. Equivalence class consequences on predictive modeling. See text for details

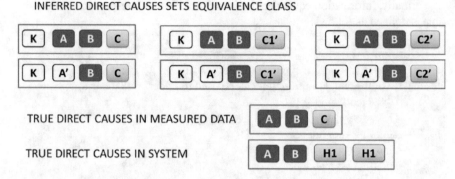

Fig. 7 Demonstration of equivalence class -related problems. Equivalence class consequences on local causal structure discovery. See text for details

equivalent sets, conditional independence with respect to arbitrary sets, and context-Independent equivalence (holding given any subset of other, non-equivalent variable sets). The simplified form of information equivalency covered here for conveying the basic idea of predictive equivalence, is considerably simpler than these more general cases.

The situation is similarly complicated for causal discovery. As seen in Fig. 7 direct causes of the outcome are {A, B, H1, H2}. In the measured data the apparent direct causes (barring successful application of latent variable detection algorithms) has an equivalence class with 3 members.

When the outcome is a terminal variable (e.g., death), and if no unmeasured confounders exist, and no information equivalencies, then the (single) Markov Boundary contains precisely the set of direct causes of the outcome.

If information equivalencies exist, without unmeasured variables, then one Markov Boundary member of the equivalence class will contain the direct causes precisely. When unmeasured variables exist in addition to equivalences, Markov Boundaries will contain a mixture of direct causes, indirect causes and non-causal confounded variables. Notice that when a variable appears in *all* Markov Boundaries then in the absence of latents it is guaranteed to be a direct cause (e.g. B).

As a reminder of earlier material (Chapters "Foundations and Properties of AI/ML Systems" and "An Appraisal and Operating Characteristics of Major ML Methods Applicable in Healthcare and Health Science"), the following predictive modeling errors may **occur when not employing optimal feature selection**:

1. Predictivity less than optimal predictivity achievable with the measure data.
2. Predictor model size larger than most parsimonious model among maximally predictive ones.

The following **additional causal modeling errors may occur when not employing causal methods**:

3. Including variables that are not causal although their confounders are fully measured (e.g., E, L, A and B in a SVM or PCA model although causal algorithms

detect that only A, B (and their equivalents) can be direct causes and E, L (and their equivalents) may be indirectly causal or confounded.

4. Discarding maximum causal effect variables in favor of ones with smaller causal effects (e.g. preferring E over A and B because it may have larger effect than either A or B alone, known as "information synthesis", for example in decision trees and other machine learning methods).

5. Failure to discover confounding by latents although it is discoverable.

We can now see the importance of not modeling equivalence classes which adds to the above errors:

Pitfall 6.2.4.2
Additional predictive modeling errors in analyses where the equivalence class of the optimal feature sets (Markov Boundaries) are not inferred.

1. The predictor model will be a random member of the Markov Boundary equivalence class. This may not be the cheapest, easiest or most convenient model to deploy clinically.

2. In domains with large equivalence classes, intellectual property cannot be defended since a third party can use an equivalent Markov Boundary and easily bypass a patent or other IP protections.

Pitfall 6.2.4.3
Additional causal modeling errors in analyses where equivalence classes of Direct Causes are not inferred.

1. Discarding causal variables in favor of non-causal ones (e.g., discarding A because its correlation with outcome vanishes when we include non-causal but information equivalent A' in a regression model).

2. Over-interpreting models: e.g., believing that because A' is a model returned by an algorithm, without equivalence class modeling, and A is not, then A' is biologically more important than A.

Because the size of the equivalence classes can be immense (i.e., exponential to number of variables see chapters "Foundations and Properties of AI/ML Systems" and "An Appraisal and Operating Characteristics of Major ML Methods Applicable in Healthcare and Health Science") finding the true causes when selecting a random member (as all algorithms not equipped for equivalence class modeling do) amounts to "playing a lottery ticket" with astronomical odds against the analyst. Similarly, finding the feature set that is most suitable for clinical application is astronomically unlikely if the Markov Boundary equivalence class is large and is not modeled.

Best Practice 6.2.4.7

(a) Use equivalence class modeling algorithms for discovering the equivalence class of optimally accurate and non reducible predictive models. E.g. TIE* instantiated with GLL-MB or other sound Markov boundary subroutines [38] (see chapter "An Appraisal and Operating Characteristics of Major ML Methods Applicable in Healthcare and Health Science").

(b) Use equivalence class modeling algorithms for discovering the equivalence class of direct causes. E.g. TIE* instantiated with GLL-PC or other sound local causal neighborhood subroutines (chapter "An Appraisal and Operating Characteristics of Major ML Methods Applicable in Healthcare and Health Science").

(c) When experiments can be conducted, consider using ML-driven experimentation algorithms that model equivalence classes. Experimentation may be needed to resolve the equivalence classes and unmeasured confounding. Such algorithms minimize the number of experiments needed. E.g., ODLP* algorithm [39].

Pitfall 6.2.4.4

Omit important steps in optimizing model performance and characterizing error and other properties that are essential for safe and effective deployment.

Best Practice 6.2.4.8

When pursuing risk and performance-sensitive model development: optimize model performance verifying that targets are met; otherwise modify or enhance data design, algorithms, and protocols, or relax requirements; once modeling is complete characterize error and other properties that are essential for safe and effective deployment and explain models and check their face validity.

Step 5. IP Considerations

Throughout the model development process, and depending on organizational policies regarding intellectual property (IP), close collaboration with commercialization experts and IP legal counsel may be needed. These experts may decide to file for patents and other forms of IP protection at various steps of the model development effort (and the same applies as well to method development efforts). The data scientists are essential part of this process as they have to provide technical details, text, data, and to teach the working of methods and models to the IP experts. This process involves several challenging aspects:

1. First the potential tension (and occasional controversy) between open science and open access principles with inventor or institutional desires for IP protection. On one extreme, lies the position that all IP protection must be avoided. On the other

extreme, lies a very strict sense of proprietary ownership of methods and models and complete lack of transparency about how methods and models work.

In between these extremes lie more balanced approaches where, for example, it may be acknowledged that certain inventions can work best (e.g. reach patients most effectively) via productization which requires commercial investment, which in turn often relies on some form of robust IP.

Simultaneously, this does not preclude, for example, allowing non-profit use of methods and models openly and without restrictions.

Patents (and patent applications even when not issued) of algorithms and models typically require "opening up" the new technology to scrutiny and understanding. This is true even if the patent applications are rejected by the USPTO or other (international) patent-issuing bodies. On the contrary, if a patent application is not pursued, the "trade secret" nature of the technology (unless of course disclosed openly) hides critical details from scientific inspection and opens up the possibility for errors and risk that would be entirely avoidable.

To complicate matters further, sound science and technology requires the ability to stabilize methods and model implementations such that they are not perpetually subject to unavoidable re-implementation or modification errors. Open source is, unfortunately, particularly vulnerable to such errors. "Locking" models and methods and their implementation is necessary if absolute certainty that their properties hold exactly as established by their validation studies.

2. If patent protection of AI/ML algorithms is desired, the inventors must understand that in recent years it has become increasingly hard to obtain such protection (i.e., ~5% issuance rate) since the SCOTUS has issued rulings that impose significant hurdles on grounds that the patentable inventions are not seen by patent examination as abstract ideas, or laws of nature. The USPTO has become increasingly resistant to granting patents on highly mathematical inventions such as AI/ML ones and often these have to be filed, e.g., in the form of tangible systems.

3. While AI/ML models and systems are much easier to patent than algortihms, a major hurdle lies with the (occasionally vast) equivalence classes of models with optimal or near–optimal performance. As explained previously, ML model M1 for optimal treatment of condition X may have an equivalence class with infinite size (just the number of fully information equivalent optimal and minimal predictor variables sets grows exponentially to the number of variables in the data). In such cases IP protection of the general methodology of producing the models may be pursued. Alternatively, a much newer approach relies on filing for IP protection of the equivalence class of optimal and near-optimal models. This latter approach requires specialized algorithms that derive the full equivalence class such as the ones described in (see comparisons of multiple methods in [38] and also discussion in chapters "Foundations and Properties of AI/ML Systems" and "An Appraisal and Operating Characteristics of Major ML Methods Applicable in Healthcare and Health Science").

Pitfall 6.2.5.1
Establish and exercise IP rights that defy fundamental principles of scientific reproducibility, openness to model and method scrutiny, and validation.

Pitfall 6.2.5.2
Failing to establish IP rights that are critical for successful dissemination and benefit from AI/ML innovation.

Pitfall 6.2.5.3
Failing to protect IP rights from bypassing IP by exploiting model equivalence classes.

Best Practice 6.2.5.1
Do not establish and exercise IP rights in ways that undermine fundamental principles of scientific reproducibility, openness to model and method scrutiny, and validation.

Best Practice 6.2.5.2
Establish IP rights that are critical for successful dissemination and patient and society benefit from AI/ML innovation.

Best Practice 6.2.5.3
Protect IP rights from "bypassing" that exploits model equivalence classes.

Step 6. Regulatory, Bias, ELSI, JEDI Considerations

Throughout all stages in the design, development, validation and deployment of clinical-grade and error-sensitive AI/ML models there are important considerations that cover legal compliance, and social and ethic dimensions. These are covered in chapter "Regulatory Aspects and Ethical Legal Societal Implications (ELSI)". At a high level in addition to regulatory approval, major legal issues are liability, and conformance to data privacy laws. With regards to ethics and health equity, access by all patients who might need the technology, eliminating various racial and other medically unjustified biases from the data and the models, are major concerns and specific techniques and practices (detailed in chapter "Regulatory Aspects and Ethical Legal Societal Implications (ELSI)") should be used to address these important dimensions.

As usual, these requirements can be relaxed (but not ignored) for pure feasibility and exploratory models.

Pitfall 6.2.6.1

Failing to address regulatory, legal, bias, ethical, social justice, and health equity requirements from design to clinical-grade and mission-critical model development validation and deployment.

Best Practice 6.2.6.1

When developing clinical-grade and mission-critical models address regulatory, legal, bias, ethical, social justice, and health equity issues.

Step 7. Production Models and Model Delivery. Health Economic and Implementation Science Considerations

Step 7.1. Converting Optimized Models to Production-Level Models

Very often, development of models is conducted with vast numbers of data inputs and resulting models may be impractical to deploy either because of the sheer complexity of the resulting decision support, or because of cost of measuring necessary inputs or cost of extracting those with bespoke interfaces to the EHR or other data sources. An essential aspect is the application of strong feature selection that maintains the full information content of the data, but discards all unnecessary information. This leads to more cost-effective and easy to deploy CDS (clinical decision support) or RDS (research decision support).

Another aspect of model inputs is whether they are objective or subjective. Examples of objective data inputs are: body measurements (e.g., weight, height) taken with standardized instruments and protocols or obtained from formal sources (e.g., age, death status, marital status); clinical labs; medications prescribed; psychological, cognitive and other questionnaires/instruments; gene and protein measurements; genetic polymorphisms (germline) or tumor mutations; and so on.

Subjective data inputs examples include: surgeon's assessment of degree by which all tumor tissue was removed; radiology interpretative reports (although many radiological findings can be very objectively measured); psychiatric mood evaluation; determination by dermatologist of color or smoothness of a skin lesion, etc.

In many situations it is possible for AI/ML model developers to **choose between objective and subjective data inputs that convey the same information.** Such choice then can be driven by how practical is the use of each data element, what is the cost, whether there are concerns that a model user may attempt to (intentionally or due to implicit biases) "game" the model by skewing subjective data inputs, whether the use of models needs to be fully automated and reproducible, or whether it is used in conjunction with human judgment, and so on.

Especially in the research realm, the effort to use as much objective data inputs as possible, is crucial to the reproducibility of the model's encapsulated knowledge and scalable application for discovery.

Step 7.2. Workflow Integration

Integrating AI/ML models to clinical or research workflows is another important element of successful deployment. The classical example often mentioned in "informatics 101" courses or discussions, is that of a care provider who has to stop and spend hours to input numerous data elements about a patient in a decision support AI/ML tool. Such a setup is entirely disruptive and unworkable and will lead to failure of adoption of that tool with very high degree of probability. Newer developments in digital health data harmonization and interoperability address this issue by use of standardized terminologies, and protocols that use those to provide seamless access to EHR so that AI/ML and other clincial decision support (CDS) can be integrated in practice easily. Still, there are many aspects of workflow integration that need be addressed and these require close collaboration of the AI/ML team with the clinical teams and the IT departments of care provider organizations.

Along these lines the sought integration may be "loose integration", or "tight integration". Loosely-integrated CDS often exists in the form of web-services that are being contacted by a hospital or other provider IT system using an asynchronous query-response protocol. More tightly-integrated CDS is typically part of the EHR, the computerized provider order entry (CPOE), the various alerting and guideline systems in active use, and may support both "push" and "pull" operating modes.

Step 7.3. Sandboxing

Sandboxing refers to the safe pre-deployment testing of an AI/ML model decision support in real-life settings but without affecting directly or indirectly critical patient care decisions. The sandboxing ensures both integration aspects, especially for proper data access, and many other elements of prospective validation and risk management (see chapter "Characterizing, Diagnosing and Managing the Risk of Error of ML and AI Models in Clinical and Organizational Application"). Recent regulatory efforts in the EU have elevated sandboxing into a legal requirement serving as a precursor to safe delivery of health AI/ML (see chapter "Regulatory Aspects and Ethical Legal Societal Implications (ELSI)").

Step 7.4. Scaling of CDS

The ability to scale the deployment of a CDS is critical when large numbers of patients are to be managed with input by the AI/ML model or when many providers across geographical regions are supported, and when the response time and availability of the decision support are critical. Fundamental aspects of scalability include horizontally and vertically scalable architectures. An overview of these and many other aspects of scalability are described in [40] and will not be elaborated here further.

Step 7.5. Implementation Science Aspects and Checklist

Another lens to successful deployment of AI/ML model is that of *Implementation Science* (IS), [41] a new field aiming to improve the *speed of innovation adoption*. Some notable IS key elements that we have covered in this chapter and throughout the book include:

1. Ensuring that the various models have been built to the specifications of stakeholders,
2. User and stakeholder education,
3. Cost-effectiveness and value of AI/ML decision support,
4. Sustainability, and
5. Rapid but rigorous validation in increasing degrees of proximity to the ultimate deployment setting.

The above requirements of step 7 are typically not strictly needed for feasibility, exploratory, or pre-clinical models.

Pitfall 6.2.7.1
Failing to pay attention to critical issues of implementation including: (1) conversion to practical, inexpensive, objective production models; (2) ensuring sustainability via reimbursement, cost reductions etc.; (3) demonstrating to stakeholders of meeting clinical or research needs and adding value; (4) providing user education and support; (5) ensuring community and patient buy-in; (6) sandboxing CDS while it is evaluated in care environment; (7) ensuring scaling of CDS; (8) integration to clinical, research and R&D workflows as appropriate.

Best Practice 6.2.7.1
When developing clinical-grade and mission-critical models, address critical issues of implementation including: (1) conversion to practical, inexpensive, objective production models; (2) ensuring sustainability via reimbursement, cost reductions etc.; (3) demonstrating to stakeholders of meeting clinical or research needs and adding value; (4) providing user education and support; (5) ensuring community and patient buy-in; (6) sandboxing CDS while it is evaluated in care environment; (7) ensuring scaling of CDS; (8) integration to clinical, research and R&D workflows as appropriate.

Step 8. Model Monitoring and Safeguards

From the very early AI research years, and especially expert system research, the problem of the AI's "knowledge cliff" was defined as a major problem with AI systems and a major departure from how humans think and solve problems.

"Knowledge cliff" of an AI system: the boundary of expertise, knowledge or problem solving ability of that system. Within this boundary the system will perform well, while outside this boundary performance may drop significantly and abruptly.

Pitfall 6.2.8.1
Creating and deploying AI/ML models and related decision support that lacks protections against falling out of the model's knowledge cliff.

In the chapters discussing data quality and management and characterizing, and managing the risk of error of ML and AI Models, we will describe in detail practical strategies for creating and deploying AI/ML that stays within their knowledge boundaries. We will also cover important concepts such as: outliers, safe and unsafe decision regions, calibration and recalibration, incorporating patient preferences, data shifts and model performance shifts & monitoring, distribution checking, causes of data shifts and how to address them, population mixture changes, seasonality and trends, epidemic dynamics, various interventional externalities (e.g., changes in standards of care, new vaccines, new populations, new treatments). We will also address data, and model variants and invariants, pristine vs. noisy inputs, model input mapping and harmonization, missing input values and rebuilding models.

Best Practice 6.2.8.1
When developing clinical-grade and mission-critical models ensure that the AI/ML models will stay within their knowledge boundaries by addressing: outliers, safe and unsafe decision regions, calibration and recalibration, incorporating patient preferences, managing data shifts and model performance shifts, population mixture changes, seasonality and trends, epidemic dynamics, various interventional externalities (e.g., changes in standards of care, new vaccines, new populations, new treatments). Carefully consider how models can successfully generalize from the original data/populations used for model development and validation to other populations and settings and address pristine vs. noisy inputs, model input mapping and harmonization, missing input values and rebuilding models.

Step 9 Ancillary Benefits and Work Products

During the course of architecting modeling efforts to address clinical and research problems, creating data designs and collecting data, developing, validating and deploying models several ancillary, several secondary objectives and work products can be produced including: mechanistic studies, reusable data gathering, drug target and biomarker discovery. Ideally there should be a plan on how to benefit from those, staring from capturing and eventually sharing the underlying data and findings for future or parallel use by the same groups and others.

Pitfall 6.2.9.1
Creating and deploying AI/ML models without consideration of ancillary and secondary objectives, benefits and work products preservation and management.

Best Practice 6.2.9.1
When developing clinical-grade and mission-critical models ensure that ancillary and secondary objectives, benefits and work products are managed and preserved.

Best Practices 6.2.9.2
Documentation. Throughout the model development process complete and thorough documentation must be maintained. Key elements of this documentation include:
1. Model goals.
2. Risk assessments.
3. Key interactions and input from stakeholders.
4. AI/ML governance and oversight committee deliberations.
5. Software documentation.
6. Data design documentation.
7. Data documentation.
8. IP documentation.
9. Legal and compliance documentation.
10. User guides and training documentation.
11. Ancillary work products documentation.
12. Checklists and worksheets (e.g., ones provided in this book to keep track of following relevant best practices).

Ideally the above documentation should include both raw information and distilled summaries, time-indexed and observing data privacy, and other appropriate laws and regulations.

This concludes the description of AI/Ml lifecycle stages and related pitfalls and best practices. Chapters "Foundations and Properties of AI/ML Systems" (foundational methods), "Evaluation" (evaluation metrics and designs), "Overfitting, Underfitting and General Model Overconfidence and Under-Performance Pitfalls and Best Practices in Machine Learning and AI" (overfitting) and "Characterizing,

Diagnosing and Managing the Risk of Error of ML and AI Models in Clinical and Organizational Application" (model debugging and managing risk) elaborate practically and theoretically on how one can implement them.

Key Concepts Discussed in Chapter "The Development Process and Lifecycle of Clinical Grade and Other Safety and Performance-Sensitive AI/ML Models"

Exploratory AI/ML models.
Feasibility AI/ML models,
Pre-clinical AI/ML models,
Clinical-grade and mission-critical AI/ML models,
Lifecycle of clinical-grade and other mission-critical AI/ML models,
Targeting model accuracy vs. targeting value proposition,
First-pass analysis and modeling,
IP considerations and tradeoff of different IP strategies,
Ancillary work products,
Health economic and implementation science considerations,
Production-level models,
Clinical and other decision support encapsulating AI/MLM models,
Sandboxing models,
Workflow integration,
Scaling model-based decision support,
Implementation science aspects and checklist,
Monitoring models,
"Knowledge cliff" of an AI system,
Model interpretability and explanation strategies,
Modeling equivalence classes,
Documentation practices.

Pitfalls Discussed in Chapter "The Development Process and Lifecycle of Clinical Grade and Other Safety and Performance-Sensitive AI/ML Models"

Pitfall 6.1.1: Treating the development of clinical-grade or mission-critical AI/ML models as if they were exploratory, feasibility or pre-clinical ones.

Pitfall 6.1.2.: Failing to establish and apply appropriate sufficient criteria and enforce BPs for model development, validation, and lifecycle support that will ensure safe and effective deployment in high risk settings.

Pitfall 6.2.1.1: Failure to specify and evaluate meaningful performance targets and real-life context of use.

Pitfall 6.2.1.2.: Failure to engage all appropriate stakeholders.

Pitfall 6.2.1.3.: Failure to establish value targets and translate predictivity and other technical model characteristics into real-world value assessments.

Pitfall 6.2.1.4.: Failure to consider broader interactions of envisioned models with the health system or with the system of science and of R&D. "Tunnel vision" evaluation with blind spots to the broader implications and consequences.

Pitfall 6.2.1.5.: Failure to consider ELSI and JEDI desiderata and consequences.

Pitfall 6.2.1.6.: Interpreting results of models beyond what their properties justify.

Pitfall 6.2.1.7: Interpreting results of models below what its known properties justify.

Pitfall 6.2.2.1: Failure to create a rigorous and powerful data design which facilitates modeling that will meet performance and safety requirements.

Pitfall 6.2.2.2: Failure to consider and judiciously interpret the limitations of convenience data designs on the performance and meaning of feasibility and exploratory models.

Pitfall 6.2.3.1.: Failure to ensure the transition from first pass modeling to optimized clinical grade models by ignoring: the problem space characteristics; data available for development and testing; prior literature on approaches and results previously explored both in terms of data design, algorithms and models; forfeiting verification and reproducing prior literature findings/claims; and failure to obtain robust preliminary estimates of predictivity of the first pass models and whether they meet requirements.

Pitfall 6.2.3.2.: Succumb to overfitting when repeatedly analyzing data from first pass to optimized modeling stages.

Pitfalls 6.2.4.1 in Explanation of AI/ML
1. Using black box models is an obstacle to adoption and trust.
2. Shapley values (and derivative methods) have several severe shortcomings for AI/ML explanation.
3. Feature importance methods, that attempt to compress complex model behaviors into single values per variable, lack the necessary information capacity and may be inconsistent with feature selection theory and causality.
4. Inherently transparent but very large models often resist interpretability.
5. Human experts explaining models must be evaluated for validity just like ML surrogate models.

Pitfall 6.2.4.2: Additional predictive modeling errors in analyses where the equivalence class of the optimal feature sets (Markov Boundaries) are not inferred.

1. The predictor model will be a random member of the Markov Boundary equivalence class. This may not be the cheapest, easiest or most convenient model to deploy clinically.
2. In domains with large equivalence classes, intellectual property cannot be defended since a 3rd party can use an equivalent Markov Boundary and easily bypass a patent or other IP protections.

Pitfall 6.2.4.3.: Additional causal modeling errors in analyses where equivalence classes of Direct Causes are not inferred:

1. Discarding causal variables in favor of non-causal ones (e.g., discarding A because its correlation with outcome vanishes when we include non-causal but information equivalent A' in a regression model).
2. Over-interpreting models: e.g., believing that because A' is a model returned by an algorithm, without equivalence class modeling, and A is not, then A' is biologically more important than A.

Pitfall 6.2.4.4.: Omit important steps in optimizing model performance and characterizing error and other properties that are essential for safe and effective deployment.

Pitfall 6.2.5.1.: Establish and exercise IP rights that defy fundamental principles of scientific reproducibility, openness to model and method scrutiny, and validation.

Pitfall 6.2.5.2.: Failing to establish IP rights that are critical for successful dissemination and benefit from AI/ML innovation.

Pitfall 6.2.5.3.: Failing to protect IP rights from bypassing IP by exploiting model equivalence classes.

Pitfall 6.2.6.1.: Failing to address regulatory, legal, bias, ethical, social justice, and health equity requirements from design to clinical-grade and mission-critical model development validation and deployment.

Pitfall 6.2.7.1.: Failing to pay attention to critical issues of implementation including: (1) conversion to practical, inexpensive, objective production models; (2) ensuring sustainability via reimbursement, cost reductions etc.; (3) demonstrating to stakeholders of meeting clinical or research needs and adding value; (4) providing user education and support; (5) ensuring community and patient buy-in; (6) sandboxing CDS while it is evaluated in care environment; (7) ensuring scaling of CDS; (8) integration to clinical, research and R&D workflows as appropriate.

Pitfall 6.2.8.1: Creating and deploying AI/ML models and related decision support that lacks protections against falling out of the model's knowledge cliff.

Pitfall 6.2.9.1: Creating and deploying AI/ML models without consideration of ancillary and secondary objectives, benefits and work products preservation and management.

Best Practices Discussed in Chapter "The Development Process and Lifecycle of Clinical Grade and Other Safety and Performance-Sensitive AI/ML Models"

Best Practice 6.1.1.: Define the goals and process of AI/ML model building as either feasibility/exploratory or as clinical-grade/mission-critical and apply appropriate quality and rigor criteria and best practices.

Best Practice 6.2.1.1: When pursuing risk and performance-sensitive model development specify concrete model performance targets for well defined care or discovery settings.

Best Practice 6.2.1.2: When pursuing risk and performance-sensitive model development engage all appropriate stakeholders.

Best Practice 6.2.1.3: When pursuing risk and performance-sensitive model development translate model accuracy to value, establish value targets and translate predictivity and other technical model characteristics into real-world value assessments.

Best Practice 6.2.1.4: When pursuing risk and performance-sensitive model development carefully consider and plan for system-level goals and interactions. Avoid too narrow ("tunnel vision") model development.

Best Practice 6.2.1.5: When pursuing clinical-grade and risk-sensitive model development, carefully consider ELSI and JEDI desiderata and consequences.

Best Practice 6.2.1.6: When pursuing feasibility, exploratory, or pre-clinical models relax stringency of requirements applicable to clinical-grade models.

Best Practice 6.2.1.7: When pursuing clinical-grade and risk-sensitive model development interpret models and models' decisions exactly as their known properties justify.

Best Practice 6.2.2.1: When pursuing risk and performance-sensitive model development create a rigorous and powerful data design which facilitates modeling that will meet performance and safety requirements.

Best Practice 6.2.2.2: When pursuing risk and performance-sensitive model development judiciously interpret the limitations of convenience data designs on the performance and meaning of feasibility and exploratory models.

Best Practice 6.2.3.1.: When moving from first pass modeling to optimized clinical grade models take into account: the problem space characteristics; data available for development and testing; prior literature on approaches and results previously explored both in terms of data design, algorithms and models; verification and reproducing prior literature findings/claims; and obtaining robust preliminary estimates of predictivity of the first pass models and whether they meet requirements.

Best Practice 6.2.3.2.: Avoid overfitting due to repeatedly analyzing data from first pass to optimized modeling stages.

Best Practice 6.2.4.1. Everything else being equal, prefer interpretable model families when interpretability is desired.

Best Practice 6.2.4.2. Use standardized coefficient (if applicable) when comparing feature contributions in linear models.

Best Practice 6.2.4.3. Very large models even when produced with intrinsically interpretable methods may still be hard to interpret because of sheer scale. Isolating critical information from large models or simplification are recommended.

Best Practice 6.2.4.4. Apply feature selectors that maximally reduce dimensionality without loss of predicivity. Compact models are always easier to explain. Combine with interpretable model families or surrogate models as appropriate.

Best Practice 6.2.4.5. If accuracy is of paramount importance and if the black box models have significant accuracy advantage over the best interpretable models you can build, then use the black box model but apply explanation methods:

(a) Global surrogate models aiming to have high fidelity everywhere in the input space over all patterns that will be classified by the model. Verify generalizable fidelity of surrogate model before using.

(b) Local surrogate models aiming to have high fidelity in the local input space for every pattern pi that will be classified by the model. Verify generalizable fidelity of surrogate model before using.

(c) Human expert surrogate models which must be high fidelity everywhere in the input space and over-fitting resistant. Verify generalizability and fidelity of human expert explanations of models.

Best Practice 6.2.4.6. Shapley values, Shapley value approximations and feature importance methods that try to summarize complex model behaviors in one or few values, are not advised as general or routinely used methods for explaining ML models.

Best Practice 6.2.4.7.

(a) Use equivalence class modeling algorithms for discovering the equivalence class of optimally accurate and non reducible predictive models. E.g. TIE* instantiated with GLL-MB or other sound Markov boundary subroutines [38] (see chapter "An Appraisal and Operating Characteristics of Major ML Methods Applicable in Healthcare and Health Science").

(b) Use equivalence class modeling algorithms for discovering the equivalence class of direct causes. E.g. TIE* instantiated with GLL-PC or other sound local causal neighborhood subroutines (chapter "An Appraisal and Operating Characteristics of Major ML Methods Applicable in Healthcare and Health Science").

(c) When experiments can be conducted, consider using ML-driven experimentation algorithms that model equivalence classes. Experimentation may be needed to resolve the equivalence classes and unmeasured confounding. Such algorithms minimize the number of experiments needed. E.g., ODLP* algorithm [39].

Best Practice 6.2.4.8. When pursuing risk and performance-sensitive model development: optimize model performance verifying that targets are met; otherwise modify or enhance data design, algorithms, and protocols or relax requirements; once modeling is complete characterize error and other properties that are essential for safe and effective deployment and explain models and check their face validity.

Best Practice 6.2.5.1.: Do not establish and exercise IP rights in ways that undermine fundamental principles of scientific reproducibility, openness to model and method scrutiny, and validation.

Best Practice 6.2.5.2.: Do establish IP rights that are critical for successful dissemination and patient and society benefit from AI/ML innovation.

Best Practice 6.2.5.3.: Protect IP rights from "bypassing" that exploit model equivalence classes.

Best Practice 6.2.6.1.: When developing clinical-grade and mission-critical models address regulatory, legal, bias, ethical, social justice, and health equity issues.

Best Practice 6.2.7.1.: When developing clinical-grade and mission-critical models address critical issues of implementation including: (1) conversion to practical, inexpensive, objective production models; (2) ensuring sustainability via reimbursement, cost reductions etc.; (3) demonstrating to stakeholders of meeting clinical or research needs and adding value; (4) providing user education and support; (5) ensuring community and patient buy-in; (6) sandboxing CDS while it is evaluated in care environment; (7) ensuring scaling of CDS; (8) integration to clinical, research and R&D workflows as appropriate.

Best Practice 6.2.8.1.: When developing clinical-grade and mission-critical models ensure that the AI/ML models will stay within their knowledge boundaries by addressing: outliers, safe and unsafe decision regions, calibration and recalibration, incorporating patient preferences, managing data shifts and model performance shifts, population mixture changes, seasonality and trends, epidemic dynamics, various interventional externalities (e.g., changes in standards of care, new vaccines, new populations, new treatments).

Carefully consider how models can successfully generalize from the original data/populations used for model development and validation to other populations and settings and address pristine vs. noisy inputs, model input mapping and harmonization, missing input values and rebuilding models.

Best Practice 6.2.9.1.: When developing clinical-grade and mission-critical models ensure that ancillary and secondary objectives, benefits and work products are managed and preserved.

Best Practices 6.2.9.2. Documentation. Throughout the model development process complete and thorough documentation must be maintained. Key elements of this documentation include:

1. Model goals.
2. Risk assessments.
3. Key interactions and input from stakeholders.
4. AI/ML governance and oversight committee deliberations.
5. Software documentation.
6. Data design documentation.
7. Data documentation.
8. IP documentation.
9. Legal and compliance documentation.
10. User guides and training documentation.
11. Ancillary work products documentation.
12. Checklists and worksheets (e.g., ones provided in this book to keep track of following relevant best practices).

Classroom Assignments and Discussion Topics, Chapter "The Development Process and Lifecycle of Clinical Grade and Other Safety and Performance-Sensitive AI/ML Models"

1. How does training of human clinical experts teach them to understand the limits of their expertise and how to refer problems outside their expertise to other experts? Which of these approaches could be incorporated in clinical grade AI/ML systems?

2. How does training of human scientist experts teach them to understand the limits of their expertise and how to refer problems outside their expertise to other experts? Which of these approaches could be incorporated in mission-critical AI/ML systems supporting health science discovery?

3. Conversely, some human experts (including physicians) are notoriously mis-calibrated. How does AI/ML models can address human cognitive decision making errors?

4. You are a study section member reviewing a study proposal that reads like the following vignette:

   "The PI of the present proposal has devoted her career in exploring Boosting-based predictive models in healthcare. Our overarching goal is to create powerful models to predict readmissions. We will use our novel methodology of BoostedBoostBoosting (B³) on readmission data from the ED of Hospital X. Deploying such models in practice has the potential to reduce the readmissions for a range of disorders reducing thus the costs and increasing the quality of care."

   Would you say this proposal is:

   (a) Biased in its choice of methods?
   (b) Well thought-out?
   (c) Compelling in its logic?
   (d) Likely to succeed in its stated goals?
   (e) Likely to yield useful results for clinical science?
   (f) Likely to yield useful results for patients?
   (g) Likely to yield useful results for AI/ML science (methods)?
   (h) Has hedged its bets on the new methods in case they are not as successful as hoped for?

   Use what you learnt in chapters "Foundations of Causal ML" and "Principles of Rigorous Development and of Appraisal of ML and AI Methods and Systems" to answer the above.

5. Can you improve the proposal vignette description to address any problems you identified in #4?

6. Consider a publication that describes a AI/ML regression model for risk of developing high blood pressure using a number of risk factors as inputs to the model. The overall explained variance (aka coefficient of variation) of the model is low, however one of the risk factors X has an odds ratio of 10 for high blood pressure. Is this model and risk factor X useful?

7. Consider an AI/ML risk model for developing Rheumatoid Arthritis incorporating GWAS data inputs (polymorphisms). None of the polymorphisms has an odds ratio with absolute value larger than 1.5 (i.e., the univariate effects are very small). Can this model be useful? How?

8. Consider the case of a very rare outcome Ox for patients with condition X. The probability of Ox in patients with X is 0.001. A new AI/ML model M has been developed recently that identifies patients with X who will develop Ox with probability 0.01 (i.e. a ten-fold increase in risk). At the same time the model has a false positive probability of 0.01. What are the challenges of incorporating this model in clinical practice?

9. Your university-affiliated hospital wishes to increase early diagnosis of cognitive decline across the population it serves. You are tasked to help choose between the following AI/ML technologies/tools for early detection of cognitive decline:

   (a) AI/ML tool A is 99% accurate.
   (b) AI/ML tool B has sensitivity 99% and specificity 99%.
   (c) AI/ML tool C has AUC 99%.
   (d) AI/Ml tool D has physician satisfaction 99%.
   (e) AI/ML tool E has 99% uptime.

   Do you have a preference for these tools? Which one will be most useful clinically? If you need additional information, what this might be?

10. An AI/ML classifier model has acceptable error rate in 2/3 of the patient population. This subpopulation is identifiable by the model and its properties. How would you address decisions in the 1/3 of the population for which the model is insufficiently accurate?

11. As explained in chapter "Foundations and Properties of AI/ML Systems" Bayesian Networks (BNs) have great flexibility in expressing flexible-input queries:

    (a) How can this be used to deal with incomplete evidence at decision making time?
    (b) For the same type of outcome, depending on the inputs used, the same model can have a wide range of errors. How would you characterize them as safe or not when there are so many of them?
    (c) How would you create safeguards for clinical-grade use of a BN model?

12. Some critics of Bayesian classifiers have criticized them on grounds that they may impose unrealistic data assumptions (for example the simple Bayes classifier), and that the error of output is multiplicative to errors of parameter specification (e.g., in BNs). How, in general, does the accuracy of model parameters relate to overall model error? Demonstrate cases where these criticisms are valid and cases where they are not.

13. Claim: it is always desirable to "bag" a variety of AI/ML models (i.e., build several models using repeated sampling or resampling and average them out). Similarly, any new model X should be a bagged classifier over all model families we can fit with our data.
    Are these statements true or false?

14. Claim: it is theoretically optimal to use Bayesian Model Averaging (BMA) over all possible models. Thus our new model X should be the BMA over the top 100 models (by predictivity or posterior probability given the data). True or false?

15. Friedman has proposed the following adage which he coined "the fundamental theorem of informatics": "*A computer decision model + human expert is better than either one of them*" (paraphrased here for clarity).
    Strictly speaking, this statement is neither a mathematical theorem nor it is always true in the absence of well-defined premises (see chapter "From 'Human versus. Machine' to 'Human and Machine'" for details).
    However, this statement implies useful guidance about:

    (a) The need to consider the success of models in a human system/context.
    (b) The need to integrate models in a workflow.

    Can you elaborate?

16. Identify 3 serious negative consequences that new knowledge discovery AI/ML model errors may have on each one of the following areas:

    (a) Scientific literature.
    (b) Drug discovery and Pharma.
    (c) Environmental policy.
    (d) Health crisis management.
    (e) Vaccination hesitancy and adoption.

17. Among the various stakeholders (patients, providers, health systems, payers, regulators) in development of AI/ML models, the same model errors may have *asymmetrical costs* (i.e., a large cost for stakeholder A may be small for B and medium for C and so on). The same is true for benefits.

    (a) Can you think of examples?
    (b) What principles and what methods do you think could/should be used to reconcile asymmetrical costs and asymmetrical benefits across multiple stakeholders?

18. AI/ML models with errors often translate to important *opportunity costs* (i.e., costs incurred by not taking a particular action such as administering useful medical interventions). Can you think of examples of opportunity costs stemming from model errors in the healthcare domain as well as in the research domain?

19. In engineering, machines, buildings, electronics, and other artifacts are expected to have well-defined parameters of safety and function. For example:

    (a) Bridges, have well specified weight loads, structural integrity in case of winds, earthquakes etc.
    (b) Cars have well-defined fuel efficiency, braking ability, acceleration, collision safety etc.
    (c) Electronics have well-defined power supply inputs, are guaranteed to not cause fires, and so on.
    (d) Maintenance schedules describe how long engineering artifacts can go without service, when they need replacement, what the service should be at specific intervals, etc.
    (e) Warrantees ensuring that in case of failure, the seller of the technology will incur replacement or repair costs.
    (f) In case of negligent construction of the products, the manufacturers are liable.
    (g) Similarly drugs come with labels that specific the intended usage, dosage, side effects, etc.

    In 2023 commercial and academic AI/ML models as well as AI/ML model-producing methods do not typically come with such well-defined and regulated guarantees. Consider the following questions:

    (a) Would the users of AI/ML models benefit if they would come with precise performance and safety guarantees?
    (b) Are there downsides to that?
    (c) What would it take to transition the current way AI/ML is marketed and used, into a better-regulated, and guarantees-driven technology?
    (d) If, hypothetically, at this time some of the AI/ML technologies and products cannot be provided with performance and safety guarantees, does this imply that they are *pre-scientific*? What might be the consequences of such a state of affairs?

20. As mentioned in chapter "Artificial Intelligence (AI) and Machine Learning (ML) for Healthcare and Health Sciences: the Need for Best Practices Enabling Trust in AI and ML", one of the most important and impressive AI effort was the INTERNIST-I expert system (by Miller, Myers and Pople Jr) which performed diagnosis across the full spectrum of internal medicine with accuracy meeting or exceeding those of attendant-level diagnosticians in very challenging diagnostic cases (NEJM's clinico-pathologic challenge cases). Neither this

system or its successor QMR (Miller et al) or offshoots such as DxPlain, (Barnet et al) managed to gain wide and long-lasting traction among working internists and health systems, however.

(a) If one considers these systems as clinical-grade, then explain this failure in terms of relevant pitfalls discussed in the present chapter.

(b) Provide an alternative evaluation of these weaknesses If one considers these efforts as exploratory, feasibility, or pre-clinical AI/ML.

21. A non-profit health system has operating margin of $10million in the last financial year and its Board of Directors decides to use it to improve health outcomes in the next financial year. The available options are as follows:

(a) *Intervention 1*, is a AI/ML-based precision medicine test for breast cancer treatment with ICER=$50,000 per QUALY gained. The applicable population is forecasted to be 500 individuals in the next FY. Each test (ordered once per patient) costs $5000.

(b) *Intervention 2*, is a new Covid-19 infection antiviral with ICER=$100,000 per QUALY gained. The applicable population is forecasted to be 300 individuals in the next FY (which will be the frame of decision making for this exercise). Each treatment regime (administered once per patient) costs $50,000.

(c) *Intervention 3*, is an AI/ML intervention to increase compliance to high blood pressure medication with ICER=$10,000 per QUALY gained. The applicable population is forecasted to be 1000 individuals in the next FY. Each intervention (applied once per patient) costs $1000.

Answer the following:

1. How many QUALYs would be gained by applying these interventions if unlimited funds were available?

2. Describe an optimal allocation of the available (limited) funds so that QUALYs gained are maximized.

3. If a new AI/ML technology would be employed that would lead to a new ICER of $25,000 for intervention 1, how would that affect the optimal allocation policy of funds and improvement in total QUALYs gained?

4. Comment on the interaction of technology improvement in the AI/ML of intervention 1 with the benefits from intervention 3 in the context of the global optimal funds allocation of (3).

5. Not all patients that could benefit from each intervention will receive them because of limited funds. What may be ethical and social justice principles to decide which patients receive a particular intervention and which do not?

6. The health system's AI/ML unit proposes an R&D project that will improve the accuracy of the models yielding new ICER for improved intervention 1 of $20,000. The cost of the project is a one-time

$1million to be covered by the $10million funds pool. The project can be executed immediately if funded.

- Should this R&D proposal be approved?
- What if the estimated risk for failure to obtain the targeted improvement is 50%?
- What is the break-even point of the risk of failure for the proposed R&D?

7. Can you outline a possible process and give a concrete numerical example of how the AI/ML unit may have calculated the expected ICER for intervention 1 based on anticipated model predictivity improvements?

References

1. da Silva LM, Pereira EM, Salles PG, Godrich R, Ceballos R, Kunz JD, Casson A, Viret J, Chandarlapaty S, Ferreira CG, Ferrari B. Independent real-world application of a clinical-grade automated prostate cancer detection system. J Pathol. 2021;254(2):147–58.
2. National Center for Advancing Translational Science (NCATS), NIH. Translational Science Spectrum. https://ncats.nih.gov/translation/spectrum.
3. Ashmore R, Calinescu R, Paterson C. Assuring the machine learning lifecycle: desiderata, methods, and challenges. ACM Computing Surveys (CSUR). 2021;54(5):1–39.
4. De Silva D, Alahakoon D. An artificial intelligence life cycle: from conception to production. Patterns. 2022;3(6):100489.
5. Munassar NMA, Govardhan A. A comparison between five models of software engineering. IJCSI. 2010;7(5):94.
6. Ruparelia NB. Software development lifecycle models. ACM SIGSOFT Software Engineering Note. 2010;35(3):8–13.
7. Pietzsch JB, Shluzas LA, Paté-Cornell ME, Yock PG, Linehan JH. Stage-gate process for the development of medical devices. J Med Device. 2009;3(2):021004.
8. Van Lamsweerde A. Requirements engineering in the year 00: a research perspective. In: Proceedings of the 22nd international conference on software engineering; 2000. p. 5–19.
9. Belani H, Vukovic M, Car Ž. Requirements engineering challenges in building AI-based complex systems. In: 2019 IEEE 27th international requirements engineering conference workshops (REW). IEEE; 2019, September. p. 252–5.
10. Villamizar H, Escovedo T, Kalinowski M. Requirements engineering for machine learning: a systematic mapping study. In: 2021 47th Euromicro conference on software engineering and advanced applications (SEAA). IEEE; 2021, September. p. 29–36.
11. Vogelsang A, Borg M. Requirements engineering for machine learning: perspectives from data scientists. In: 2019 IEEE 27th international requirements engineering conference workshops (REW). IEEE; 2019, September. p. 245–51.
12. Steyerberg EW, Steyerberg EW. Applications of prediction models. New York: Springer; 2009. p. 11–31.
13. Duncan IG. Healthcare risk adjustment and predictive modeling. Actex Publications; 2011.
14. McNeill D. Analytics in healthcare and the life sciences: strategies, implementation methods, and best practices. Pearson Education; 2013.

15. Cihon P, Schuett J, Baum SD. Corporate governance of artificial intelligence in the public interest. Information. 2021;12(7):275.
16. Cihon P, Maas MM, Kemp L. Should artificial intelligence governance be centralised? Design lessons from history. In: Proceedings of the AAAI/ACM conference on AI, ethics, and society; 2020. p. 228–34.
17. Statnikov A. A gentle introduction to support vector machines in biomedicine: theory and methods, vol. 1. World Scientific; 2011.
18. Papenmeier, A., Englebienne, G. and Seifert, C., 2019. How model accuracy and explanation fidelity influence user trust. arXiv preprint arXiv:1907.12652.
19. Payrovnaziri, S.N., Chen, Z., Rengifo-Moreno, P., Miller, T., Bian, J., Chen, J.H., Liu, X. and He, Z., 2020. Explainable artificial intelligence models using real-world electronic health.
20. Murdoch WJ, Singh C, Kumbier K, Abbasi-Asl R, Yu B. Definitions, methods, and applications in interpretable machine learning. Proc Natl Acad Sci. 2019;116(44):22071–80.
21. Molnar C. Interpretable machine learning. 2nd ed. Leanpub; 2022.
22. Afchar D, Guigue V, Hennequin R. Towards rigorous interpretations: a formalisation of feature attribution. In: International conference on machine learning. PMLR; 2021, July. p. 76–86.
23. Kim, B., Khanna, R. and Koyejo, O.O., 2016. Examples are not enough, learn to criticize! Criticism for interpretability. Adv Neural Inf Proces Syst, 29.
24. Guidotti R, Monreale A, Ruggieri S, Turini F, Giannotti F, Pedreschi D. A survey of methods for explaining black box models. ACM computing surveys (CSUR). 2018;51(5):1–42.
25. Robnik-Šikonja M, Bohanec M. Perturbation-based explanations of prediction models. In: Zhou J, Chen F, editors. Human and Machine Learning, Human–Computer Interaction Series, Chapter 9. Springer; 2018.
26. Friedman JH. Greedy function approximation: a gradient boosting machine. Ann Stat. 2001;29:1189–232.
27. Goldstein A, Kapelner A, Bleich J, Pitkin E. Peeking inside the black box: visualizing statistical learning with plots of individual conditional expectation. J Comput Graph Stat. 2015;24(1):44–65.
28. Ribeiro MT, Singh S, Guestrin C. "Why should i trust you?" Explaining the predictions of any classifier. In: Proceedings of the 22nd ACM SIGKDD international conference on knowledge discovery and data mining; 2016, August. p. 1135–44.
29. Ribeiro, M.T., Singh, S. and Guestrin, C., 2018. Anchors: high-precision model-agnostic explanations. In Proceedings of the AAAI conference on artificial intelligence 32(1).
30. Breiman L. Random forests. Mach Learn. 2001;45:5–32.
31. Statnikov A, Aliferis CF, Hardin DP, Guyon I. Gentle introduction to support vector machines in biomedicine, A-volume 2: case studies and benchmarks. World Scientific Publishing Company; 2013.
32. Zanzotto FM. Human-in-the-loop artificial intelligence. J Artif Intell Res. 2019;64:243–52.
33. Stead WW. Clinical implications and challenges of artificial intelligence and deep learning. JAMA. 2018;320(11):1107–8.
34. Shapley LS. A value for n-person games. Princeton University Press. 1953;2(28):307–17.
35. Lipovetsky S, Conklin M. Analysis of regression in game theory approach. Appl Stoch Model Bus Ind. 2001;17(4):319–30.
36. Erik Štrumbelj and Igor Kononenko. "Explaining prediction models and individual predictions with feature contributions". In: Knowledge and information systems 41.3 (2014), pp. 647–65.
37. Ma S, Tourani R. Predictive and causal implications of using Shapley value for model interpretation. In: Proceedings of the 2020 KDD workshop on causal discovery. PMLR; 2020, August. p. 23–38.
38. Statnikov A, Lemeir J, Aliferis CF. Algorithms for discovery of multiple Markov boundaries. The Journal of Machine Learning Research. 2013;14(1):499–566.

39. Statnikov A, Ma S, Henaff M, Lytkin N, Efstathiadis E, Peskin ER, Aliferis CF. Ultra-scalable and efficient methods for hybrid observational and experimental local causal pathway discovery. The Journal of Machine Learning Research. 2015;16(1):3219–67.
40. Adam T, Aliferis C. Personalized and Precision Medicine Informatics. Health Informatics Series. Basel, Springer Nature Switzerland; 2020.
41. Bauer MS, Damschroder L, Hagedorn H, Smith J, Kilbourne AM. An introduction to implementation science for the non-specialist. BMC Psychol. 2015;3(1):1–12.

Data Design in Biomedical AI/ML

Gyorgy Simon and Constantin Aliferis

Abstract

Data Design refers to the systematic choice of what data are modeled for analysis and how these data and the model output(s) are mapped between the Problem Space (real-world) and the Model Space (features for the ML modeling). ML data design is an essential element of ML modeling. ML data design differs from classical statistical, epidemiological etc. study designs in that (a) ML data design relies heavily on the existence of digital data repositories that are created independently of the problem solving intent at hand, (b) ML modeling is highly scalable and mostly automated, (c) when using experimental data, ML data design may be used to guide the experiments conducted, (d) uses a richer set of data representations that transcend the classical design matrices such as text, relational databases, graphs etc.; and (e) ML modeling has its own distinct capabilities, limitations and other properties and these are reflected in the data design choices. The present chapter covers tried and tested strategies and protocols that contribute to successful data designs and addresses a number of important biases that threaten validity and generalizability of results. Lower level data transformations, data storage, and security aspects are covered in the "Data Preparation, Transforms, Quality, and Management" chapter.

Data Design Overview

Figure 1. provides the context for Data Design by depicting the process of problem solving via ML modeling. Elements in black outlines are naturally occurring phenomena (i.e. occurring outside the control of problem solving team); elements in

G. Simon (✉) · C. Aliferis
Institute for Health Informatics, University of Minnesota, Minneapolis, MN, USA
e-mail: constantinaibestpractices@gmail.com

© The Author(s) 2024
G. J. Simon, C. Aliferis (eds.), *Artificial Intelligence and Machine Learning in Health Care and Medical Sciences*, Health Informatics,
https://doi.org/10.1007/978-3-031-39355-6_7

341

green outlines are controllable by the analyst/scientist involved in the ML-based problem solving. ML-based problem solving involves two steps. The first one is high-level **data design**, where one or more **problem solving data sets** are constructed. These data contain the subjects and data elements relevant to the problem, and are either extracted from a repository of naturally-collected data (i.e. without the control of the ML-based problem solving team—top branch in the figure) or collected specifically for the purpose of the modeling (lower branch). In the second step, **modeling data sets** are constructed, upon which machine learning algorithms can operate.

The goal of data design. A ML model can be viewed as a function that maps inputs to outputs. The inputs to the ML model are ML features, which exist in the *ML model space*. ML features don't always have one-to-one correspondence to real-world entities or to the naturally-collected data elements. These entities and data elements exist in the real-world *problem space*. Similarly, the model output, which exists in the model space, needs to be mapped to the real-world entities in the problem space. The goal of data design is to create this mapping between the real-world problem space and the model space in a manner that after mapping the real-world entities onto the ML model space, then solving the problem in ML model space, and finally mapping the ML solution from the model space back to the real-world (problem space), we obtain a correct solution to the real-world problem.

Figure 2 depicts the context around data design from the perspective of the ML modeling process. It presents an overview of the ML modeling process and its iterative interaction with modeling. The blue rectangle highlights the elements of the modeling steps that fall under data design, and these are the elements that are discussed in this chapter. Elements outside the blue box, namely, data transformations, model fitting, evaluation and iterative improvement of the model are covered in other chapters ("The Development Process and Lifecycle of Clinical Grade and

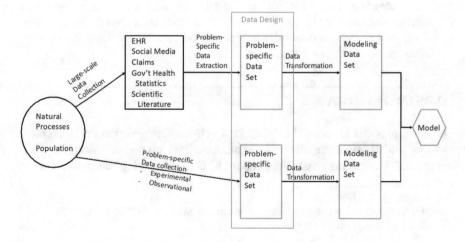

Fig. 1 Overview of problem solving using ML modeling

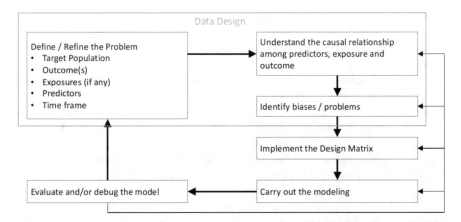

Fig. 2 Overview of the modeling process. Steps of the Data Design are highlighted inside the blue rectangle

Other Safety and Performance-Sensitive AI/ML Models," "Data Preparation, Transforms, Quality, and Management, " and "Evaluation") of this book.

> **Data design** is the process of creating a formal specification of project goals and variables and establishing a bidirectional mapping between the real-world entities (and data elements) in the problem space and the ML features in the ML model space. ML then provides the function approximation models of the real-world data generating process that can be used along with the aforementioned mapping to solve problems in the real world by first solving them in the ML model.

The first step in ML-based problem solving is to define the problem to be solved according to the following five elements:

1. **Outcome.** What clinical outcomes are we considering? If we consider multiple outcomes, which is the primary outcome and which are secondary?
2. **Exposure/Intervention**. Is there a particular exposure or intervention that we wish to estimate the effect of?
3. **Predictor variables** (aka independent non-interventional variables). Which variables are relevant to this analysis and we want to include? Which variables are confounders and we absolutely must include? Which variables must we omit?
4. **Target population**. Which patients should the answer hold true for?
5. **Time frame.** When should the answer hold true? When do we plan to intervene, apply the model, or use the knowledge that we gained from this analysis? How long does it take for the outcome to manifest itself?

The above 5 elements describe the real-world solutions we wish to obtain and the data elements needed to obtain them.

As part of the data design, we also need to consider potential *data design biases*. Data design biases are systematic errors in the choice of data sources, including variables and samples, as well as mismatch of data to the modeling methods to be used.

Classical statistical study design vs. data design. In classical statistical study design the data representation for modeling is a matrix (the "design matrix" in statistical terminology), often a two-dimensional table of numbers. In ML however, we often deal with other data representations such as higher-dimensional matrices (tensors), graphs, sequences, text documents, images, combinations of the above, etc. The data design methods we describe here are generally applicable, although for simplicity we give examples based on flat matrix representations.

Defining the Problem

At the initiation of a ML project, usually, only a rough clinical or health science question and the context of use of the results are known. The objective of this step is to refine the rough problem statements into a more precise, formalized and operationalizable format. By *precise*, we mean that problem statement contains all and only the information we need to solve it; by *formalized*, we mean that the answer to the problem can be expressed as an *estimand* (a computable quantity); and by *operationalizable*, we mean that we can compute the answer in terms of the available data elements. In the following sections, we describe the setting, the five elements that make problem statements precise, and the most commonly used estimands. Afterwards, we describe common data design types to which we can map our problem, and in the last section of this chapter, we describe the inference process and explain what a "valid answer" means.

Setting

The first critical junction in defining the problem statement is to decide the operative **setting**. We consider three broad settings. First *clinical settings*, where the problem concerns clinical decision making, including risk models, estimates of effects of exposures, targeting interventions, and timing of interventions. Such clinical models ideally will directly inform patient care or otherwise become part of health care delivery.

The second type of setting is *operational settings*, where the results from the analysis are not directly used for treating patients, but rather for managing the system of health care.

The third type of setting is *health science research*. ML models can be used for a broad array of research problems, which include biomarker discovery, optimized treatment protocols based on biomarkers, discovering biological causal pathways, clinical trials, etc. *Translational research* contexts bridge the health sciences with the health care problem solving domains.

The setting in which the modeling results are used entails many attributes of the data design and modeling. For example, evaluation of health care-oriented ML models needs to take patient safety into account. Clearly, the direct risk of harm to patients is highest in the clinical setting and lowest in the research setting. The scope of populations involved in health care versus health science modeling can vary from very narrow to full-population studies. However, health care modeling is often restricted to specific health systems with or without examination of translation across systems.

Setting refers to context in which the modeling results will be used. We broadly distinguish between three settings: clinical, operational and research. Different settings impose different requirements towards the steps of the modeling process.

Best Practice 7.1.1
The ML data design needs to take the operative setting of the ML models into account.

Elements of the Problem Statement

As we discussed earlier, the modeling project is typically motivated by a clinical question, an operational opportunity, or a research need. This initial motivation offers only a rough outline for the problem statement.

The five elements of a problem statement (Outcome, Exposure/Intervention, Predictor variables, Target population, Time frame) help make a rough problem statement more precise. [1].

Example 7.2.1
As a hypothetical example, experts in a health system may believe that "*starting diabetes treatment earlier could improve major cardiac events*".

The rough problem statement is "*Does starting diabetes treatment earlier reduce major cardiac events?*". This question is not precise: how much earlier should we start? It is not formalized: what metric (estimand) for outcomes should we compute? It is also not operationalizable: how do we define "diabetic" using the available data elements?

To make the question more precise, we need to define 5 elements. Not all elements are needed for all questions, but most questions need most of these elements.

Target Population

The **target population** is the set of patients to which the problem statement applies.

If we construct a clinical risk model, the target population consists of patients to whom we are going to apply the resulting model. All patients in the target population must be at risk of developing the outcome in the problem statement. If the problem concerns an interventional treatment, the target population is patients who are eligible for the treatment. If the problem concerns the study of a biological function, then the target population is the set of research subjects in which this biological function exists.

Example 7.2.1
The example problem statement is related to the patient population of the health system in question, so the target population is the patient population (1) served by the hypothetical health system (2) who would be considered for diabetes treatment, or who could conceivably benefit from earlier diabetes treatment. So the example question is further refined to: *"Can earlier initiation of diabetes treatment in diabetic patients eligible for it reduce major cardiac events in this health system?"*

Exposure/Intervention

Some studies are concerned with the effect of an intervention or of an exposure (defined below). Not all studies have an intervention of interest, but if there is one, we need to specify it. The intervention in our running example is the earlier initiation of diabetes treatment.

The intervention or exposure divides the population into two groups.

The patients receiving the therapeutic interventions are referred to as **treatment group**, while the remaining (untreated) patients are referred to **untreated** patients (also as **control**s if untreated *and* similar to the treated ones before treatment).

In case of an exposure to a naturally-occurring factor, patients with the exposure are referred to as the **exposed group** and the remaining patients form the **unexposed group** (or **controls** if similar to the exposed group before exposure).

In non-designed data (e.g., collected from routine care records) therapeutic interventions may be considered as exposures. It is also common to collect data about interventions and multiple exposures and model them simultaneously. Note that classical study design does not distinguish between exposure and treatment, and refers to both as 'exposure'.

Outcome

Not all analyses have a designated response variable (e.g., clinical outcome of interest). For example, finding comorbidities in older diabetic patients does not have a designated outcome of interest. However, the product of the analysis still needs to be specified. In this example, this product is the set of common comorbidities. Commonly, studies may also have multiple outcomes which are then categorized as primary and secondary.

> The **primary** outcome(s) is (are) the main focus of interest; other outcomes are called **secondary** outcomes.

> **Example 7.2.1**
> In our running example, the main and only outcome is major cardiac events (MACE). Additional (secondary outcomes) could also be of interest, e.g., health care utilization or quality of life.

> Patients with the outcome in question are referred to as **cases**, while patients without the outcome are referred to as **controls**.

Notice that the meaning of 'control' depends on the comparison being made: it can refer to two different groups, either those without the outcome or those without the intervention/exposure [2].

Time Period

Time period is the time frame encompassing the data to be modeled. Such time frames may concern, e.g., the time point at which the intervention is carried out (or a decision support model is used); or the time period during which the outcomes develop. There could also be a time period for collecting information before the intervention is applied.

> **Example 7.2.1**
> In our running example, for a retrospective analysis aiming to establish the effects of early diabetes treatment on MACE, we can use a design in which we collect historical patient data covering a 10 year time window starting 10 years before analysis and ending at time of analysis. MACE occurs 5–10 years after diabetes, hence the choice of time window length. Note that there are alternative designs to accomplish this modeling that will be discussed later.

Predictor (Non-Outcome) Variables

Predictor variables are all the data (in addition to outcomes) that could possibly be relevant to our modeling task. Predictor variables include demographics (age, sex or gender as appropriate), risk factors, exposures, interventions, social behavioral data, images, genetic information, etc. At a minimum, we need to include exposure variables that are known to influence the outcome(s) (if there are any), the interventions of interest (if there are any), those variables that are suspected to influence the exposure and outcome(s) of interest (i.e., potential confounders), and any other variable that we wish to adjust for.

There are also variables we should generally *not* include. (1) In a regression or SEM model that estimates causal effects, variables that must be excluded are (a) the causal descendants of the outcome and (b) variables on the causal chain between the exposure and the outcome. More details about causal modeling are provided in chapter "Foundations of Causal ML". (2) In a predictive model, variables that are associated with the outcome and occur after it, must be excluded if model application is desired before the outcome occurrence. More generally, variables that would be measured after the model application should not be included.

Common Metrics

There are a number of measures we use to estimate "risk" or "effect size" and they fall into three broad categories that are frequently confused. These are proportions, ratios and rates.

Proportion is the number of elements with a particular property divided by the total number of elements.

For example, the prevalence of the diabetes in a community, is a *proportion*, where the "particular property" is having diabetes and "elements" are patients. Thus, the prevalence of diabetes is the number of patients with diabetes in this community divided by the total number of members in the community.

Ratio: The number of elements with a particular property divided by the number of elements without the particular property.
OR (equivalently)
$p / (1-p)$,
where p is the proportion of elements with a particular property.

Rate: the number of measured events over a unit time period.

All these three types are fractions. Proportion and ratio have the same numerator, but differ in their denominators: for proportions, the elements in the numerator are included in the denominator, while for ratios, the elements in the numerator are excluded from the denominator. The proportion of diabetics in a population is the number of patients who are diabetic among all members of the population. Patients in the numerator (diabetic patients) are included in the denominator (all members). In contrast, the ratio of diabetic patients is the number of diabetic patients divided by the number of non-diabetic individuals. The numerator (diabetic patients) are excluded from the denominator (non-diabetic idividuals). The range of a proportion is between 0 and 1, while the range of the ratio is between 0 and infinity.

Rate differs from the other two types in that it has a time component: it measures the number of events over a unit period of time. For example, the rate of developing diabetes in the US is 1.4 million people *per year.*

Commonly used metrics include:

- **Prevalence**: the proportion of patients with a disease in the population at a point in time. This is often expressed as a percentage (number of diseased patients per 100 individuals); or in epidemiology, prevalence is more commonly expressed as number of diseased patients per 10,000 individuals.
- **Incidence**: the proportion of patients newly diagnosed with a disease in the population over a unit period of time. This is a rate often measured as number of new cases within 10,000 individuals over a year.
- **Probability** of an event.
- **Odds** of an event. Odds is a ratio: probability of an event divided by one minus the probability of that event.
- **Risk**: measures how likely it is for an undesirable event to happen. It can be measured as an actual probability, as hazard, log hazard, etc., within a time period.
- **Relative risk** is a fraction of an observed quantity divided by an expected (baseline) quantity. These quantities can be number of events, proportions, probabilities, rates (with the same time period for the observed and expected quantities).
- **Hazard and hazard ratio** are formally defined in the "Time-to-Event Outcomes," section of the "An Appraisal and Operating Characteristics of Major ML Methods Applicable in Healthcare and Health Science" chapter.
- **Average Treatment Effect** (ATE): average difference in therapeutic effect between comparable treated and untreated patients.
- **Average Treatment Effect in the Treated (ATT):** average effect of the treatment in a treated sample of patients (average difference of effect of treatment between treated patients vs without the treatment).
- **Individual treatment effect (ITE)**: the effect of treatment in a patient (difference in likelihood of an outcome with and without treatment).

Types of Modeling Problems

As we discussed in chapter "Artificial Intelligence (AI) and Machine Learning (ML) for Healthcare and Health Sciences: the Need for Best Practices Enabling Trust in AI and ML", AI/ML have an extraordinary range of applications. Thankfully the vast majority of problems fall into only a handful of common categories.

> Because the majority of problems fall into a few types, and each type can be addressed by a small number of data designs, **a few data design templates suffice for solving most problems encountered in health sciences and health care**.

Below we list the most commonly-encountered and broadly applicable problem classes.

Diagnostic problem class. This is the problem of assigning patients to diagnostic categories. It is solved by developing diagnostic models, hand-crafted or machine-learnt. An important aspect of the diagnostic problem is that it is concerned with diseases (or clinical conditions) that *currently* exist in the patient [3].

Screening problem class. A special case of the diagnosis problem where disease has not manifested clinically and needs to be detected as early as possible. Different from the diagnostic tests, screening tests are applied to a much greater number of patients. Mammography is an example of a screening test, aimed at identifying patients with breast cancer. When the screening test reports a positive result, a more reliable diagnostic test is then used to determine whether the subject indeed has the disease. Compared to diagnostic tests, screening tests are often less expensive, less harmful (have fewer side effects or lower risk to health) and thus can be deployed at a larger scale than a diagnostic test. Screening tests often suffer from producing a large number of false positives which is a consequence of the low prevalence of the tested condition in the broad population where the test is applied. ML modeling can help with implementing high quality scalable screening tests (e.g., radiology ancillary finding interpretation).

Risk prediction. This problems deals with forecasting patients' future risk of developing a disease or a disease related outcome. Risk models differ from screening or diagnostic models in two important ways. First, screening and diagnostic models are concerned with diseases that the patient already developed or is in the process of developing, while risk models are concerned with events that may occur in the future. Second, diagnostic tests are often confined to diseases, while the risk models can be used more broadly, such as to assess the risk of future re-hospitalization, ICU admission, prolonged illness, etc.

Prognostic problems. Prognosis usually refers to forecasting outcomes of interest in patients with a disease (or simply the likelihood of recovery from the disease) [3]. In molecular precision oncology commonly *predictive* (instead of prognostic) refers to the likelihood of outcomes given a treatment. ML models can perform these forecasts (and in some cases, e.g., high-throughput-based molecular oncology, they provide the primary means for this task).

Estimating treatment efficacy. The goal of this class of problems is to estimate the effect of an intervention on an outcome. This outcome can be an event (e.g. a disease or re-hospitalization) or a quantity (e.g. systolic blood pressure reduction in hypertensive patients). While it is sufficient for the relationship between the predictor features and the outcome of interest to be associative (correlational) for diagnostic, screening, and risk models; treatment efficacy estimation needs to be based on causal relationships (especially when changes in treatment practices are contemplated).

Biomarker or risk factor discovery. Biomarkers are a very diverse group of entities that include: (1) any correlate of a phenotype or outcome of interest; (2) complex computable models (aka "signatures") that can be used to diagnose, prognosticate or treat phenotypes/patients; (3) substitutes (proxy outcomes) for longer term outcomes in clinical trials; and (4) drug targets for new therapeutics. Accordingly, a variety of ML models can serve such discovery: for (1), predictive modeling; for (2), predictive, prognostic or causal ML modeling; for (3) and (4), causal ML modeling [4].

Operational problem solving. These models relate to the management and administration of health organizations, often involving resource planning and allocation. Examples include hospital bed allocation, ordering supplies, managing personnel, billing and reimbursement, etc.

Economic evaluations. These pertain to understanding the economic impact of clinical and administrative decisions. ML-enabled economic evaluations can be used to compare two treatments of the same disease and study their outcomes in light of their costs. They can also be used to inform resource allocation across multiple diseases by comparing health benefits of a new treatment of one disease versus the health benefits of a new treatment of a different disease. At an even higher level, they guide policy decisions about allocating funds to health care initiatives and prioritize investments [5].

Subpopulation discovery. This class of problems is closely related to (1) precision health, (2) poor average effects of treatments, and (3) population mixtures. With respect to (1), precision treatments target subgroups that will benefit from the treatment and protect subgroups that are more susceptible to toxic side effects. Regarding (2), often, RCTs reveal that the average effect of a new treatment in the general population of patients may be small, however, it is possible for the treatment to be optimally effective in a subgroup. In case (3), where an apparently homogeneous population in reality comprise subpopulations with different underlying disease mechanisms or physiology, it is often useful to de-mix these subpopulations and apply subpopulation-appropriate health interventions.

Inference: What Is a Valid Solution?

Effective ML-based problem-solving must ensure the validity of the produced solutions. In this section, we elaborate on solution validity. Every problem at hand concerns a particular patient population, the **target population**. The solution of the problem is **valid** if it holds true in the target population. It is very rare that we have

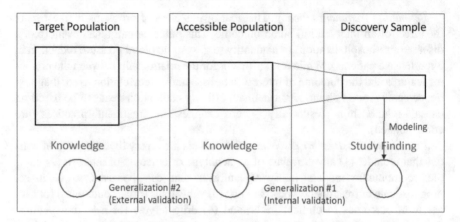

Fig. 3 Inference. We estimate a quantity in the target population using a discovery sample

data for the entire target population. Instead we often have access to a different population called the **accessible population**. Because it is impractical to collect data about all members in the accessible population, we draw a **discovery sample** from the accessible population (Fig. 3). Thus, ML models are derived from the discovery sample and not the target population and not even from the entirety of the accessible population. We must thus ensure that the solutions produced by the models generalize to the accessible population and then further to the target population [1].

> A **valid solution** is one that is true in the discovery sample and remains true in (i.e., generalizes to) the accessible and target populations.

Therefore central to validity is **generalizability**. The typical generalizability discussed in machine learning textbooks is *internal validity* referring to the requirement that a solution that is valid (holds true) in the discovery sample must generalize to the accessible population. Generalizability further to the target population is a type of *external validity*. The goal of using design protocols and best practices is to help achieve both types of validity.

Let us illustrate this concept through an example: consider the hypothetical question of whether aggressive management of high cholesterol helps reduce heart disease incidents. If this is a research question, then we may wish the answer to generalize to a very broad patient population such as all patients who have high cholesterol in the entire nation. The target population is all patients with high cholesterol in the nation (who have not had heart disease yet). Suppose, we conduct this study in a consortium of academic health centers located in a handful of states. Our accessible population then consists of patients with high cholesterol who are typically seen at these specific academic centers and have health data recorded in the corresponding EHRs. Further assume that we have analytic access to a small portion of health records (our discovery sample).

Assuming that the discovery sample is a random sample from the accessible population and that the resulting model is applied close to the time frame when the discovery sample was drawn, the results from the discovery sample will generalize to the accessible population as long as we do not have modeling issues such as overfitting (chapter "Overfitting, Underfitting and General Model Overconfidence and Under-Performance Pitfalls and Best Practices in Machine Learning and AI"). However, the accessible population (individuals seen at academic health centers) and the target population (general USA population with high cholesterol) likely systematically differs and full generalizability of the results from the accessible population to the target population is unlikely. To address this problem, the original accessible population should be constructed in a way that better represents the general population. If that is not feasible then use of the models should be restricted to the accessible population only. Other more sophisticated techniques may also correct the generalizability issues. The general rule of thumb is that an imperfect design will require immense modeling efforts to rectify its biases (and may still not achieve the desired generalizability).

Best Practice 7.2.1
Seek to ensure validity and generalizability with good data design first. Resort to analytic corrections of biases only to the extent that optimal design is not attainable.

Now let us consider the same question in a narrower context with some important biases present: does aggressive management of high cholesterol help reduce heart disease incidents in the patient population of a specific health system? The target population is patients in this singular health system with high cholesterol. As before we may draw a random discovery sample of patients from the electronic health record (EHR) system to answer this question. Our accessible population appears to be the same as the target population. Assume further that not all patients are included in the EHR and that the patients in the EHR differ from the patients not in the EHR. For example patients in the EHR can have lower or higher cholesterol levels than those not in the EHR. Also assume that patients not in the EHR, predominantly receive their high cholesterol treatments in a different health system. Under these and many similar conditions, even when we build models for a single health system using data strictly from said health system, the target and accessible populations can differ. Such differences can impact generalizability and thus validity. A model that is valid in a data rich environment could perform poorly in a data poor environment when selection bias is present. Whether a model generalizes can be determined, of course, and can be made to generalize better through careful data design.

Pitfall 7.2.1
A random sample from a registry or an EHR is not necessarily a random sample from the patient population.

Best Practice 7.2.2
Ensure that the accessible population is representative of the target population.

Best Practice 7.2.3
Ensure that the discovery sample is representative of the accessible (and target) populations.

Data Design

In the previous section, we started with a rough question and transformed it into a problem statement. We specified the operative setting (clinical, operational, research) and made the problem statement more *precise* (than the rough question) by describing five major elements: (1) target population, (2) intervention, (3) outcome, (4) time period and (5) predictor variables. We also defined an estimand, a computable metric that solves the problem. In this section, we focus on the "How?", how the problem can be solved.

Data designs provide a framework within which different problem types can be carried out while ensuring validity.

In this book, we focus mostly on observational studies, where data is already generated and we have no influence over how patients are treated or how their data is captured in sources like the EHR, but we do have influence over how data is sampled from such sources and in some cases how data will be collected specifically for modeling. These foci reflect the majority of practical situations and are harder than having full control over data generation and collection.

In the following sections, we describe the data design hierarchy, which allows us to answer a few simple questions about exposure, outcome and temporal relationships and arrive at a data design. We describe the most common data designs in detail, providing concrete examples. After we describe the data designs, in Table 1, we relate them to the problem types from section "Types of Modeling Problems" and to the metrics from section "Common Metrics" thus connecting the data design process with problem solving requirements.

Table 1 Mapping of problem types to appropriate data designs, analytic methods and measures. "Any" data design means, that the simplest data design depends on whether the problem at hand is temporal and not, and whether an outcome exists and whether it is rare

Problem Type	Simplest design serving this goal	Analytic methods [and metrics]
Association between risk factor and outcome	Cross-sectional	Classification [odds ratio, relative risk, etc]
Summarizing patient info	Cross-sectional or cohort	Clustering
Summarizing patient info with respect to a particular outcome	Cross-sectional	Classification, regression
Subpopulation discovery	Cross-sectional or cohort	Clustering or specialized method [Meaningful metrics depend on the definition of subpopulation]
Subpopulation discovery with respect to a specific outcome	Cross-sectional or cohort	Classification, regression, time-to-event, causal modeling, followed by post-hoc analysis of ML models
Diagnosis/screening/risk model/ risk score	Cohort	Classification, regression, time-to-event [Incidence, relative risk, hazard, etc]
Diagnosis/risk model/risk score when outcome is rare	Case-control	Classification, regression, [odds ratio]
Biomarker discovery/risk factors	Cohort	Classification, time-to-event, causal modeling
Disease trajectory	Cohort	Sequence mining, repeated measures modeling (e.g. GEE), recurrent neural networks (RNN)
Forecasting (utilization, cost, lab results)	Cohort	Regression modeling, VAR, RNN, time series modeling
Longitudinal risk models	Cohort	Repeated measures, recurrent networks,
Treatment effect estimation	Cohort	Causal ML, SEM, regression (after confounder identified)
Causal structure discovery	Cross-sectional or cohort	Causal ML
Effect of complex treatment protocols	Cohort	Structural marginal, RNNs, [ITE, ATE, ATT]
Density estimation	Any	
Outlier detection	Any	Model-based outlier detection, Parzen windows, KNN, 1-class SVM

Data Design Hierarchy

Experimental Data Designs: these involve generation of data by manipulating some of the variables. From the perspective of the ML problem-solving team using the methods of this book, the team may have control over these interventions (we call this a **primary experimental data**) or, alternatively they may be given access to data in which someone else conducted interventions and the team had no control over these interventions (we call this **secondary experimental data**).

Observational Data Designs: these involve data that was measured/generated by the ML problem-solving team (we call this a **primary observational data),** or alternatively the team may be given access to data that someone else measured and the team had no control over such observations (we call this **secondary observational data).**

For example, if the problem-solving ML team is given access to previously conducted randomized clinical trials, the interventions had been assigned by the RCT experimenters; patients were randomized into groups receiving intervention (treated) or being controls (untreated). Similarly, if the problem-solving ML team is given access to EHR data, interventions occurred before the ML modeling starts and thus the team can only observe these interventions. However, in contrast to RCT data, the nature of interventions in EHR data does not involve randomization or controlled interventions.

Figure 4, adopted from [6], describes how several prototypical data designs ensue under the above conditions.

If an analysis starts with an exposure and follows subjects to determine the outcome, it is called a **cohort design**. Conversely, when the analysis starts with an outcome, identifying subjects with (and without) an outcome, and proceeds backwards in time to establish their plausible causes, then it is termed a **case-control design**. Finally, if the exposures and outcomes are determined at a single time point (cross section), then it is called a **cross-sectional design.**

Cross-sectional design. The exposure and outcome are observed in the same cross section. With the existence of exposed and unexposed groups, the association between the exposure and the outcome can be measured, but since they are

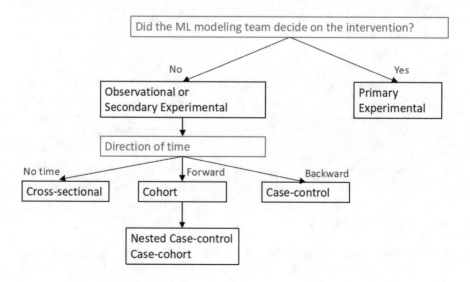

Fig. 4 Data design hierarchy

measured in the same cross section, the temporal relationship between them cannot be readily observed (but may be inferable with causal ML see chapter "Foundations of Causal ML"). The date of the cross section is the **index date**.

> **Best Practice 7.3.1**
> A cross-sectional data design suffices if one can solve the problem using the *prevalence* of the outcome in the exposed and unexposed groups.

> **Pitfall 7.3.1**
> A cross-sectional design is inappropriate if there is a time gap between the exposure and the outcome and is important, or if incidence of the outcome is of interest.

Cohort design. The logic of the analysis follows the passage of time: it progresses from the exposure towards the outcome. A cohort of patients with a particular exposure is identified, and a second comparison cohort without the exposure can also be observed (if needed by the problem at hand). These two cohorts are followed forwards in time determining their outcomes. The date of the exposure and the date when unexposed patients are included is the **index date**. The time period during which the cohort is followed is the **follow-up period**. Since patients did not have the outcome at the time of exposure, this design allows for measuring incidence rates and relative risks [7].

> **Pitfall 7.3.2**
> A cohort design falls short when the outcome is rare or if it takes a long time for the outcomes to develop.

Case-control design. Here we start with identifying a group of subjects with the outcome (cases) and another group of subjects without the outcome (controls). Then the analysis progresses backwards in time, looking for exposures in the records of the subjects. When a comparison group (unexposed patients) exists, associations can be measured. However, without knowledge of the prevalence of the outcome, incidence rates and hence relative risks cannot be computed in absolute terms. The critical part of this design is the choice of controls (or, equivalently, the availability of reliable ML algorithms that control analytically possible confounding) [8].

Relationship Between Problem Type and Data Design

> **Best Practice 7.3.2**
> Use the easiest/most economical data design that can solve problem. The mapping of the problem to a problem type can help find the best design.

Refining the Discovery sample—Use of Inclusion/Exclusion Criteria

The discovery sample is defined using a set of inclusion and exclusion criteria. As their names imply, inclusion criteria select patients to be included in the cohort and exclusion criteria exclude patients from the cohort.

> The objective of the inclusion/exclusion criteria is to create a discovery sample that resembles the target population as closely as possible.

As we described in section "Inference: What Is a Valid Solution?," modeling allows inferences, in which knowledge/models generated in a discovery sample are used in the target population (after sufficient validation). The discovery sample comes from the accessible population, which can be different from the target population and even the discovery sample can be different (not a random sample) from the accessible population. Our goal with the inclusion/exclusion criteria is to make the discovery sample representative of the target population.

A common starting point is the description of the target population as an inclusion criterion. Next, we refine it by specifying additional inclusion or exclusion criteria.

Exclusion criteria describe patients in the accessible population who are either unlikely to contribute to the validity of the findings, or are excluded so that the accessible population resembles the target population better. Common reasons for exclusion include:

1. Patients are not at risk of the outcome. For example, when studying the risk of falling in the elderly, patients who are bed-bound should be excluded because they have an artificially low risk of falling.
2. A special case of not being at risk is having a pre-existing outcome when we try to measure the incidence rate of a phenomenon. Patients who already have the outcome at baseline or are very likely to have the outcome (albeit being undiagnosed) at baseline are excluded.
3. Patients who are very unlikely to receive the intervention. Patients who are not at risk of or are at very low risk of the outcome should be excluded from modeling that determines the effect of an intervention. The intervention in such patients

(if ethical) would show little (if any) efficacy and these patients would very rarely (if ever) receive this intervention.

4. Patients who have a different disease mechanism than the one under study.
5. Patients having a pre-existing condition that precludes the results from holding true. For example, models in which heart rate is a risk factor may not hold true in patients with pacemakers (heart rate is artificially controlled).
6. Insufficient data. Patients with insufficient data can be excluded, however, doing so can introduce biases.
7. A special case of insufficient data is insufficient follow-up. Patients with insufficient follow-up can be excluded, but doing so may introduce biases.

We will discuss discovery sample construction further in the context of the data design types.

Example of a Cohort Design

Cohort studies are arguably the most common data designs in clinical analytic models.

> The defining characteristics of a **cohort study** are that (1) a **cohort** of patients are selected and (2) the cohort is followed *forward* in time to determine the outcomes.

In this exposition, we will focus on two kinds of cohort studies. The first one does not have a specific intervention, we merely measure the association between baseline exposures with the incidence of an outcome and construct a risk model. The second has a specific intervention.

Cohort Studies without a Specific Intervention of Interest

Example 7.3.1
Let's consider development of a clinical risk model for assessing a patient's 7-year risk of diabetes. Our hypothetical health system plans to apply this model every time a patient undergoes blood sugar testing. Patients that are found to have high risk of diabetes are referred to a diabetes prevention clinic.

Study type. This is a risk model (Table 1) and cohort study is appropriate. We are interested in measuring the 7-year risk of developing diabetes (incidence of diabetes), so hazard, hazard rate, probability, and possibly other measures are appropriate (Table 1).

Index date. To determine an index date, we take its intended clinical application into account. When a new blood sugar test result becomes available, the model will be applied to determine whether the patient needs to be referred to a diabetes prevention clinic. Patients can have multiple blood glucose tests, so we can simply take a cross-section of the eligible population at a random time and use their most recent test result, provided it is sufficiently recent. The criterion for "sufficient recent" is determined based on clinical knowledge; the objective is to ensure that if the blood glucose measurement had been taken exactly on the index date, we would *not* expect it to be meaningfully different from this "sufficiently recent" measurement.

Defining the target population. The target population consists of patients who are at risk of developing incident diabetes and have received blood glucose test(s) before the index date. Patients with pre-existing diabetes are no longer at risk of developing *incident* diabetes.

Inclusion/exclusion. The objective is to ensure that the discovery sample is not significantly different from the target population, which consists of patient who undergo blood sugar test(s). The discovery sample comes from the accessible population, which may be different from the target population. We can use inclusion/exclusion criteria to modify the discovery sample to better resemble the target population. Concerning the selection of the accessible population, we can use any convenient population, as long as it is not significantly different from the target population. For example, if we wish to apply the model to patients in 2020 and forward, then we could select patients (say) with blood sugar test(s) between 2005 and 2015, assuming that the criterion for ordering a blood glucose test has remained reasonably unchanged during this period (2005–2020). Conversely, we would not use patients only from (say) the obesity clinic as the accessible population, because obesity is a risk factor of diabetes and thus patients in the obesity clinic can have already progressed further towards diabetes than the general patient population with blood sugar measurements. We also have to be mindful to exclude patients who may have had their blood glucose taken for reasons other than suspecting diabetes (e.g. application for life insurance)—the resulting model will not be applied to these patients.

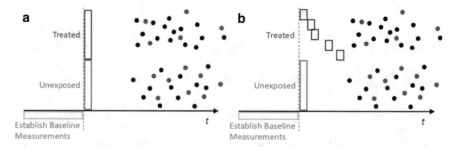

Fig. 5 Illustration of cohort data designs. Panel A represents a cohort design with a single cross-section, where treatment status does not change after the index date. Panel B shows a cohort design with staggered exposure. The horizontal axis is time, black dots represent censored patients (dropped out without an event) and red dots represent patients who suffered events

Cohort Studies with an Intervention of Interest

Figure 5 shows an illustration of different types of cohort studies with an intervention of interest. The horizontal axis represents time and the dashed vertical line is the index date where we start following patients. Each dot represents a patient. Black dots are censored patients (dropped out without an event) and red dots are patients with an event. The location of the dot shows the time of the event or censoring.

The vertical axis denotes treatment status. Panel A shows a simple design, with a single cross section, where patients' treatment status does not change after the index date. Panel B shows a staggered treatment design, where the treatment status of some patients changes over time. These two designs solve different problems.

> **Example 7.3.2**
> We suspect that the prolonged (at least 6 months) use of a hypothetical drug has an adverse effect that increases the risk of mortality in diabetic patients. We wish to measure the effect size.

Problem type. This is a treatment effect estimation problem (Table 1) and we are going to use a cohort design with an intervention of interest (the particular drug). Since no particular time frame is specified for the outcome, hazard (time-to-event outcome) is appropriate for measuring the "risk of mortality". (Had the problem specified 7-year mortality, we could have also used probability or death in 7 years.)

Exposure. Exposed patients are those who have used this drug for at least 6 months. We have multiple options for unexposed patients. If the clinical question places an emphasis on prolonged use as opposed to short-term use, then an appropriate control (unexposed) group is patients who took the drug for less than 6 months. If the comparison really is about being exposed to the drug at all, then an appropriate comparison group is patients who never took this drug.

Index date. The question does not specify any timing information, so we can take a cross section of patients at a random date and use this date as the index date. Some of the patients in this cross section will have already taken the drug for 6 months, other patients have not, and some patient will never take it.

Target population. Patients with diabetes who may be considered for intervention through this drug.

Inclusions/exclusions. Considerations for the construction of the analytic cohort are similar to those in the previous example. However, patients unexposed at the index date may later become exposed to the drug. In that case, this patient can be excluded; or the patient can be included but censored at the time of exposure to the drug. Caution is required with the latter approach, because censoring can be informative.

Predictor variables and confounding. The outcome, mortality, depends on factors other than exposure to the drug. Some of these factors can also influence exposure to the drug, thus they can be confounders. These confounders, if known with certainty, must be accounted for, for example, by including them as covariates or by balancing them between exposed and unexposed patients using propensity matching. If confounders are not known but are measured, we can discover them using causal ML methods.

Predictor variables of mortality are evaluated at the index date. If a patient has taken the drug for 6 months before the index date, the drug may have adversely affected some of the predictor variables by the index date. If these predictor variables are on the causal chain between the drug and the outcome they *must* be excluded.

If some variables are affecting the outcome but are not on the causal chain between treatment and outcome, they *should* be included.

Determining the precise location/role of such variables requires extensive domain knowledge or application of causal ML techniques that can place variables in the correct causal role category.

This is merely an illustrative design. Many other (possibly more appropriate) designs are also possible.

> **Example 7.3.3**
> Let us estimate the effect of a hypothetical diabetes drug on reducing the risk of mortality. Let us assume that this drug can be prescribed to all diabetic patients.

Clinical use. We assume that this model will be applied to patients, who are diabetic and are not yet on this drug (and possibly not on other drugs that target the same disease). Assume that every time such a patient interacts with the health system, the model will be applied. If the predicted risk exceeds a certain level, the patient is given the drug; otherwise, the patient will not receive the drug. This process repeats until the patient falls outside the inclusion criteria (e.g. gets this drug, gets a different drug for the same disease, is lost to follow-up, or dies).

Problem type. This is also a treatment effect estimation problem (Table 1) and we are going to use a cohort design with an intervention of interest (the particular drug). Similar to Example 7.3.2., since no particular time frame is specified for the outcome, hazard (time-to-event outcome) is appropriate for measuring the "risk of mortality".

Exposure. Exposed patients are those taking the drug and unexposed patients are those who do not take any drugs for this disease.

Index date. For exposed patients, the index date is the date of their first prescription. There are multiple options for the choice of controls. First, we can take a sample of eligible patients at a date who did not receive the drug yet at that date. This date can be chosen randomly or as the median date of the exposed patients' index dates. When a control patient receives any drug for the same disease (either the drug in question or a different drug for the same disease), the patient is censored.

Inclusion/exclusion. Considerations for the construction of the analytic cohort are similar to those in the previous example. If the drug is contraindicated for some patients for reasons unrelated to the outcome, these patients can be included (as untreated patients); if the drug is contraindicated for the presence of a complication that increases mortality (the outcome), these patients should be excluded as they increase the risk of mortality in the untreated group.

Predictor variables. We must include all confounders and we can include variables that cause the treatment or the outcome. We should not include variables that are descendants of the outcome, nor variables that are on the causal chain between the treatment and the outcome.

Merits and Demerits of Cohort Studies

Best Practice 7.3.3
Cohort studies are straightforward and necessary if the time gap between the index date and the outcome cannot be ignored.

Best Practice 7.3.4
Cohort studies allow us to estimate the prevalence and/or incidence of outcomes, separately for exposed and unexposed patients (if an intervention is considered).

Being able to estimate the prevalence or incidence of outcomes, separately for exposed and/or unexposed patients, allows us to compute a multitude of measures, including relative risks, hazard ratios, as well as odds ratios.

Pitfall 7.3.2
Cohort studies are less practical if the outcome is rare or if the outcome takes a long time to develop.

The key challenge to a cohort design is rare outcomes and outcomes that develop over very long periods of time. EHR systems track a great number of patients, but patients can be lost to follow-up over time. When the time gap between the index date and the outcome is long, we may not find sufficiently many cases due to the follow-up constraint.

In the case when outcomes are rare, a very large cohort may be necessary to contain a sufficiently high number of cases (patients with confirmed positive outcome). When some of the important variables need to be collected, ascertained or processed in a way that increases cost, doing this for a very large cohort is not cost effective. Additionally, if the outcome is very rare, a single cross section may not yield sufficient number of possible cases.

Case-Control Design

Case/control studies start from the outcome. Cases (patients with positive outcome) and controls (patients without an outcome) are identified and possibly sampled. Patient records for this sample are then examined moving backwards in time, recording the exposures (or treatments) they experienced.

Pitfall 7.3.3
When we sample cases or controls in a case/control design, we have to do so without any regard to the exposure. Whether a patient is selected into the cohort or not must be independent of the exposure(s)/treatment(s).

Best Practice 7.3.5
Whenever possible, the use of clinical trial data is recommended for case/control studies.

In observational data with complex causal structure and potentially unobserved confounders, we may inadvertently select patients based on criteria that are linked to the exposure/treatment. In clinical trial data, the exposure/treatment is not caused by any of the variables. Observe, however, that putative causes of the outcome (other than the randomized treatment) can be confounded in a RCT design (Fig. 6).

Merits and Demerits

Best Practice 7.3.6
Case/control design is best suited when the outcome is rare, but the exposures/treatements are relatively frequent.

Case-control designs have smaller sample requirements and depending on the costs of collecting or measuring variables they can substantially reduce total data cost.

The key demerit lies in creating a discovery sample with artificial distribution of cases and controls. When the data is sampled de novo for analysis (as opposed to pre-existing e.g. in an EHR) this leads to difficulties in optimizing model use according to loss functions that are prior-dependent (because the natural prior is not known).

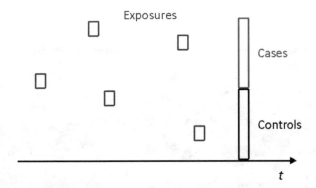

Fig. 6 Illustration of a case-control data design. The horizontal axis represents the passage of time and patients are listed vertically. Purple boxes are the exposures (or treatments) that some of the patients had. The design starts with the selection of a set of cases (red rectangle representing a number of patients) and a set of controls (black rectangle). Then patient history is examined retrospectively (backwards in time) looking for and recording exposures (or treatments)

> **Pitfall 7.3.4**
> Case/control studies do not measure the prevalence of the outcome, which makes computing measures other than odds ratios non-trivial.

Case/control studies do not measure the prevalence of the outcome, thus we can only estimate odds ratios. Luckily, for rare outcomes, the odds ratios and relative risks are similar.

Nested Case-Control Design and Case-Cohort Design

These two designs attempt to merge the benefits of the cohort design with the case-control design. We would conduct a regular cohort design, but embed a case/control design. In the cohort, we select all cases (patients with the outcome) and match them to controls (patients without the outcome) based on their baseline characteristics. One benefit of this approach is that the exposure/treatment needs to be ascertained only for the cases and the selected controls, not all patients, yet because it is a cohort design, we can estimate prevalence of the outcome [1, 9].

A nested case-control and a case-cohort designs are both case/control designs nested into a cohort design. They differ in the way controls are selected. Nested case/control studies match cases with controls individually, while case-cohort studies simply take a random sample of the non-cases in the cohort as the control group.

The key limitation of these designs is the same as the case/control design: finding appropriate controls is error-prone and difficult to automate.

Biases

In statistics, bias refers to a systematic tendency which causes differences between results and facts [10, 11].

> In the context of data design, bias are systematic deficiencies in the design that lead to errors in the produced models and corresponding problem domain solutions.

> A bias is *systematic* if it is not arising purely through randomness. Many different types of bias exist. For example, in case of *measurement bias*, the systematic error exists between the measured and the actual values of a variable; similarly, in case of an *estimation bias*, the systematic error is between the estimate and the true value. In the context of drawing a sample from a population, *sampling bias* [11] occurs when some characteristic in the sample is over- or underrepresented relative to the population.

Broader uses of the term bias are also common. For example, an *evaluation bias* arises when the estimated performance of a model systematically differs from the actual performance often due to a flawed evaluation metric or method. *Social biases*, such as *racial bias*, arise when a systematic difference that cannot be attributed to a morally and scientifically justifiable reason between social groups (e.g. races or ethnicities) exist in terms of some desirable or undesirable metric (e.g. employment, compensation, incarceration rate). Analogously, *health equity bias* arises when health related measures, such as unjustifiable mortality rate, access to health care or health care utilization systematically differ across groups of patients. *Analytic bias* happens when the inference of the relationship between outcome and exposure/treatment is incorrect: the estimate of the relationship from the sample systematically differs from the true relationships in the population [12].

A particularly bad case of an analytic bias is when the direction of the relationship reverses, as it can happen in case of the **Simpson's paradox**.

Even broader use of the term also exists where bias refers to a systematic preference of one option versus another. For example,

Inductive bias of a machine learning algorithm is the preference that the algorithm has for certain models over others. This is the only common use of the term bias that has a positive connotation.

Cognitive biases are systematic propensities of human decision making that lead to errors in decision making. Such cognitive biases may be the result of evolutionary adaptations that require rapid action based on heuristic or limited analytical reasoning.

In this section, we focus on biases that we encounter in data design. These are mainly estimation biases, including sampling and analytic biases as well as Simpson's paradox. Other kinds of biases are discussed in the appropriate sections. Inductive bias is discussed in the "Foundations and Properties of AI/ML Systems" chapter, measurement bias in the "Evaluation" chapter,, and human biases in judgement and decision making in the "From 'Human versus Machine' to 'Human with Machine'" chapter.

Commonly Encountered Biases in Data Design

Confounding bias. When the purpose of the analysis is to quantify the relationship between an exposure and an outcome, confounding, latent or observed, can distort this relationship. The confounding factor can take many forms and some of the common confounding forms have their own name. When the confounding factor is the missingness of data, we have *information bias;* when the factor is a latent factor causing certain patients in the target population to be excluded from the sample, we have *selection bias*; or when a factor is an indication for the exposure (treatment in this case) of interest and independently causes the outcome, we have *confounding by indication* [13].

Selection bias occurs when a (typically latent) factor causes certain patients to be excluded from the discovery sample who are part of the accessible population or from the accessible population who are part of the target population. Analysis is valid (unbiased) if the accessible population is a random sample from the target population and the discovery sample is a random sample from the accessible population. Violation of this assumption can affect the external validity (discovery sample or accessible population is not a random sample from the target population) or the internal validity (discovery sample is not a random sample from the accepted population) [11].

Selection bias can affect the analysis by creating an artifactual difference between cases and controls or between exposed and unexposed patients. In the former case, estimates of the prevalence of the outcome will be biased, which will transcend to any metric, such as relative risk, that relies on prevalence; in the latter case, the relationship between the exposure and outcome will be biased.

Information bias. Information bias occurs when the information is available differentially between cases and controls or between exposed and unexposed patients. The former biases prevalence estimates and the latter biases estimates of the association between exposure and treatment. *Recall bias* is a special case of information bias, where cases and control recall (remember) exposures differently [11].

Confounding by indication. This is another special case of confounding bias, where a confounder is an indication for the treatment and can independently cause an outcome. For example, infection may cause fever and thus use of paracetamol as well as it may be a cause for asthma later in life, thus it can distort the association between paracetamol use and asthma [13, 14].

Ascertainment bias. Certain exposures cause the outcome to be ascertained at a higher probability. For example, having eye problems may trigger a diabetes test (diabetic retinopathy) leading to the discovery of diabetes which may remain undiscovered in patients without eye problems. In some cases, when the proportion of patients with and without the exposure is "unlucky", Simpson's paradox combines with ascertainment bias and reverses the direction of the association between the exposure and outcome. This latter form of ascertainment bias is *Berkson's bias* [15]. We discuss Simpson's paradox later in Section "Simpson's Paradox".

Informed presence bias. Related to ascertainment bias, patients who have frequent encounters may have more problems documented that would remain undiscovered otherwise.

Non-contemporaneous control bias. If the comparison group is selected from a different time frame from the cases or the exposed group, they no longer represent a random sample from the accessible population (or the target population) leading to biases [16].

Reverse causation. Cause and effect may appear reversed in association. For example, when sedentary lifestyle is associated with increased death rate, sedentary lifestyle may not be the cause of death; quite on the contrary, a deadly disease may have caused the sedentary lifestyle and ultimately the death [17].

Simpson's Paradox

Consider two factors, A and B, both binary for simplicity. Further, consider that we are studying the probability of the outcome in the four groups defined by the two factors. Figure 7 provides an illustration of the results. There are four circles in the figure representing the four groups. The radius of the circles is proportional to the number of subjects in the group. The horizontal layout of the circles relates to factor B: the two circles on the left lack factor B (i.e. B = 0) and those on the right have

Fig. 7 Illustration of Simpson's paradox

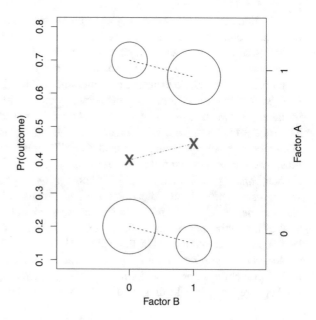

factor B (i.e. B = 1). The vertical position of the circles relates to factor A: the two circles on the top have factor A = 1, while the bottom two circles have A = 0. The vertical axis represents the probability of outcome. Clearly, factor A is associated with higher probability of outcome, as the two circles with A = 1 are higher than the two with A = 0. The two X's in between the top and bottom circles represent the average probability in the sample when B = 0 (on the left) and when B = 1 (on the right).

Let us consider patients with A = 1. They are located in the top two circles. We can see that the probability of outcome is lower when B = 1. The 80 patients with A = 1 and B = 0 (top left circle) have an average probability of outcome of 0.7, which is higher than the average probability of 0.65 in the group of 120 patients with A = 1 and B = 1 (top right circle). Similarly, let us consider the remaining patients, those with A = 0 (the bottom two circles). The probability of outcome is again lower for patients with B = 1. The 120 patients with A = 0 and B = 0 (bottom left circle) have an average probability (for the outcome) of 0.2, which is higher than the average probability of 0.15 in the group of 80 patients with A = 0 and B = 1 (bottom right circle). Paradoxically, when we look at all patients with B = 0, they have an average probability of 0.4 (left X), which is lower(!) than the average probability of 0.45 (right X) for patients with B = 1.

The interested reader is referred to [18] for more details and to [19] for a causal interpretation of the Simpson's Paradox.

Best Practice 7.4.1
If you see an unexpected effect direction, always consider the possibility of Simpson's paradox and Bergson bias.

Key Messages and Concepts Discussed in Chapter "Data Design"

Data design is an iterative process that transforms available data elements into an analytic matrix. The analytic matrix is a data set, on top of which ML algorithms can be directly executed. A successful data design allows for the ML algorithms to produce a valid solution to an ML problem.

A solution is valid if it holds true in the discovery sample that it was computed from and generalizes to the target population. The target population is the population, in which we want to use the modeling results (model, knowledge, etc).

Setting refers to the context in which the modeling result will be used. We broadly distinguish between three settings: clinical, operational and research. The setting will determine the requirement towards the data design, and more broadly, the entire analytic process.

The components of the data design include (1) defining an analytic question, (2) designing the analytic matrix (data design), (3) executing the modeling, (4) debugging and evaluating the model. The process is iterative.

The analytic question starts with a rough question that prompted the analytic project and is refined to be precise, formalized and operationalizable.

To make an analytic question precise, we commonly define five elements: (1) target population, (2) intervention, (3) outcome, (4) time period and (5) predictor variables.

The analytic question is formalized if its answer can be expressed as a computable estimand. The section "Common Metrics" list several such estimands (metrics).

Most analytic questions map to a small number of study types which are listed in the "Types of Modeling Problems" section. This allows us to develop templated solutions to these questions. These templates are the data designs.

Data designs form a hierarchy and by answering some questions about exposure, outcome and their temporal relationship, we arrive at a data design.

In this book, we focus on observational studies and we considered three main data designs: (1) cross-sectional, (2) cohort, and (3) case/control. In addition, nested designs, such as case/control nested into a cohort study or case/cohort are also discussed.

Concrete data design examples are shown and the merits and demerits of the various data designs are elaborated on.

Biases are systematic differences between two quantities. Often, one of these quantities are estimates (or measurements) and the other is observed. Biases that are common in data designs are presented. We discuss Simpson's paradox.

Best Practice Recommendations and Pitfalls, Chapter "Data Design"

Best Practice 7.1.1. The ML data design needs to take the operative setting of the ML models into account.

Best Practice 7.2.1 Seek to ensure validity and generalizability with good data design first. Resort to analytic corrections of biases only to the extent that optimal design is not attainable.

Best Practice 7.2.2 Ensure that the accessible population is representative of the target population.

Best Practice 7.2.3 Ensure that the discovery sample is representative of the accessible (and target) populations.

Best Practice 7.3.1. A cross-sectional study suffices if you can answer the analytic question with the *prevalence* of the outcome in the exposed and unexposed groups.

Best Practice 7.3.2. Use the simplest data design that can answer your analytic question. The mapping of an analytic question to a study type can help find the simplest design.

Best Practice 7.3.3. Cohort studies are very straightforward and necessary if the time gap between the index date and the outcome cannot be ignored.

Best Practice 7.3.4. Cohort studies allow us to estimate the prevalence and/or incidence of outcomes, separately for exposed and unexposed patients (if an intervention is considered).

Best Practice 7.3.5. Whenever possible, the use of clinical trial data is recommended for case/control studies.

Best Practice 7.3.6. Case/control design is best suited when the outcome is rare, but the exposures are relatively frequent.

Best Practice 7.4.1. If you see an unexpected effect direction, always consider the possibility of Simpson's paradox.

Pitfall 7.2.1. A random sample from a registry or an EHR is not necessarily a random sample from the patient population.

Pitfall 7.3.1. A cross-sectional study is inappropriate if a time gap between the exposure and the outcome is expected and important or if incidence of the outcome is of interest.

Pitfall 7.3.2. Cohort studies may not be appropriate if the outcome is rare or if the outcome takes a long time to develop.

Pitfall 7.3.3. When we sample cases or controls in a case/control study, we have to do so without any regard to the exposure. Whether a patient is selected into the cohort or not must be independent of the exposure(s).

Pitfall 7.3.4. Case/control studies do not measure the prevalence of the outcome, which makes computing measures other than odds ratios non-trivial.

Classroom Assignments and Discussion Topics, Chapter "Data Design"

1. Consider the problem of predicting the risk of a disease in a clinical setting and in a research setting. Can you think of some differences in the data design for these two settings in terms of (1) the purpose of the model, (2) data sources, (3) target population, (4) choice of modeling algorithm, and (5) evaluation?

2. Consider the problem of predicting the probability of discharge from the hospital in 4 days for a patient, in two settings: clinical setting and operational setting. Can you think of clinical and operational questions that could require these probabilities? How would the resulting models be different?

3. Suppose you have a discharge model that is being used in a clinical setting. For each patient, it predicts the probability of discharge in 10 days. You are asked to estimate the number of beds that will be available in 10 days. Would you use the clinical model or would you build a model specifically to estimate the number of available beds?

4. You are tasked with predicting the 7-year risk of diabetes.
   (a) Is the outcome prevalence or incidence of diabetes?
   (b) Is there an exposure of interest? Comparison groups?
   (c) Is a cohort study an appropriate data design? Could you make a cross-sectional design work?
   (d) What is the eligibility criterion and what is the target population? (You need to make some assumptions.)
   (e) Suppose the model will be used in obese patients. How did the eligibility criterion (and the target population) change?
   (f) Is obesity an "exposure of interest" and would the study require a comparison between obese and non-obese patients?
   (g) If you use a cohort study, how would you construct your cohort? What would be the index date? Accessible population? Exclusion criteria? Please elaborate.
   (h) Suppose the model is used only once, precisely at the moment a patient first becomes obese. How would you change your design? (Hint: a cross-section at a random date will probably not yield a sufficient number of patients.)
   (i) Suppose now that your outcome is a very rare form of diabetes. Is a cohort study still appropriate?

5. A hypothetical diabetes drug came to market 10 years ago. It is intended for diabetic patients to reduce the risk of major cardiac events. You are tasked to evaluate this drug in terms of its real-world effect (as seen in EHR data) to reduce major cardiac events and mortality.
   (a) What type of problem is this?
   (b) What is the outcome?
   (c) Is there an exposure/intervention of interest?
   (d) What are the comparison groups? (You have to make assumptions. Discuss how these assumptions affect your answer.)
   (e) What are potential confounders? How would you adjust for confounding? The question is intentionally underspecified. Feel free to make several assumptions and discuss how different assumptions affect your design.

6. You are building a model that advises clinicians on the expected effect of a hypothetical diabetes drug on major cardiac events (MACE). This model computes the risk of MACE and if the predicted probability exceeds a certain (clinically determined) threshold, the patient is given the drug. The model is applied to diabetic patients at every encounter until the patient either receives a diabetes drug or has achieves a normal blood sugar level.
   (a) Is there an exposure/intervention of interest?
   (b) What are the comparison groups (if any)?
   (c) What is the eligibility criterion and the target population?
   (d) Is a cohort study appropriate?
   (e) How would you determine the index date?

7. What is the simplest data design to
   (a) Determine whi0ch is more common: high blood pressure or high cholesterol
   (b) Determine whether the prevalence of major cardiac event is more common among patients with or without diabetes?
   (c) Determine whether the incidence of major cardiac event is more common among patients with or without diabetes?
   (d) Assess the effect of obesity on diabetes?
   (e) Compare the effect of two diabetes drugs on major cardiac events?
   In *your(!)* opinion, when is a data design "simple"?

8. Can you use Cox model with cross-sectional design?

9. How do you handle confounders in a deep learning model?

10. Consider a machine learned diabetes risk calculator. This model would predict patients' 7-year risk of diabetes based on some commonly available data elements in non-diabetic patients. It would be applied to patients with high blood pressure, high blood cholesterol or obesity.
    (a) Can you think of a choice of accessible population that would cause selection bias?
    (b) Can you give an example of information bias in this context?
    (c) You find that heart disease is negatively associated with diabetes in this model. Can you explain this finding using Ascertainment bias? Berkson's bias?

11. Consider the diabetes risk calculator from the previous question. Assume that this calculator now tries to predict the risk of a very rare form of diabetes.
    (a) Design a case/control study for developing this model. Who are the cases? Who are the controls? When do you evaluate the baseline predictor variables?
    (b) Can you give an example of non-contemporaneous control bias in this context?

12. "I prefer chocolate over vanilla ice cream." Can you rephrase this statement using the term "bias". Can you explain how this is a bias?

13. Can you explain why systematic racism is a bias using the definition of bias?

References[1]

1. Hullet SB, Cummings SR, Browner WS, Grady DG, Newmann TB. Designing Clinical Research. 3rd ed. Wolters Kluwer Health; 2001.
2. Mann CJ. Observational research methods. Research design II: cohort, cross sectional, and case-control studies. Emerg Med J. 2003;20:54–60.
3. Cook NR. Statistical evaluation of prognostic versus diagnostic models: beyond the ROC curve. Clin Chem. 2008;54(1):17–23. https://doi.org/10.1373/clinchem.2007.096529.
4. Lukač N. Adam T, Aliferis C, editors. Personalized and precision medicine informatics: a workflow-based view. Croat Med J. 2020;61(6):577–8. https://doi.org/10.3325/cmj.2020.61.577. Springer Nature Switzerland AG; 2020; print ISBN 978–3–030-18,625-8; online ISBN 978-3-030-18626-5. PMCID: PMC7821372.
5. Drummond MF, Sculpher MJ, Torrance GW, O'Brien BJ, Stoddart GL. Methods for the economic evaluation of health care programmes. 3rd ed. Oxford University Press; 2005.
6. Grimes DA, Schulz KF. An overview of clinical research: the lay of the land. Lancet. 2002;359(9300):57–61. https://www.thelancet.com/series/epidemiology-2002
7. Grimes DA, Shulz KF. Cohort studies: marching toward outcomes. Lancet. 2002;359(9303):341–5.
8. Grimes DA, Shulz KF. Case-control studies: research in reverse. Lancet. 2002;359(9304):431–4.
9. Kulathinal S, Karvanen J, Saarela O, Kuulasmaa K. Case-cohort design in practice - experiences from the MORGAM Project. Epidemiol Perspect Innov. 2007;4(4):15. https://doi.org/10.1186/1742-5573-4-15.
10. Bias. Wikipedia. https://en.wikipedia.org/wiki/Bias_(statistics)14.
11. Jager KJ, Tripepi G, Chesnaye NC, Dekker FW, Zoccali C, Stel VS. Where to look for the most frequent biases? Nephrology (Carlton). 2020 Jun;25(6):435–41. https://doi.org/10.1111/nep.13706.
12. Kramer MS. Analytic bias. In: Clinical epidemiology and biostatistics. Berlin, Heidelberg: Springer. https://doi.org/10.1007/978-3-642-61372-2_5.
13. Kyriacou DN, Lewis RJ. Confounding by indication in clinical research. JAMA. 2016;316(17):1818–9.
14. Aronson JK, Bankhead C, Mahtani KR, Nunan D. Confounding by indication. In: Catalogue of Biases; 2018. https://catalogofbias.org/biases/confounding-by-indication/.
15. Berkson J. Limitations of the application of fourfold table analysis to hospital data. Biometrics. 1946;2(3):47–53.
16. Catalogue of Bias Collaboration, Spencer EA, O'Sullivan J. Informed presence bias. In: Catalogue of bias; 2017. https://catalogofbias.org/biases/informed-presence-bias/.
17. Sattar N, Preiss D. Reverse causality in cardiovascular epidemiological research. More common than imagined? Circulation. 2017;135:2369–72.
18. Agresti A. Categorical data analysis. 2nd ed. Wiley; 2002. p. 51.
19. Pearl J. Understanding Simpson's Paradox. Technical Report R-414,. UCLA; 2013.
20. Grimes DA, Shulz KF. Descriptive studies: what they can do and cannot do. Lancet. 2002;359(9301):145–9.
21. The catalog of bias collaboration. https://catalogofbias.org/about/.

---

[1] For details on data design, classical statistical study design, and, more broadly, on research design, the interested reader is referred to a series of articles in the Lancet [6–8, 20] and to [1], which is a textbook. A comprehensive catalog of biases is available at [21].

Data Preparation, Transforms, Quality, and Management

Steven G. Johnson, Gyorgy Simon, and Constantin Aliferis

Abstract

Data preparation and feature engineering transform source data elements into a form that can be used by analytic and machine learning methods. Raw source data elements are transformed into data design features that are specified in the data design through an iterative process of mapping data elements to concepts, value sets, and phenotype expressions. Data that meet the data design criteria are extracted into a data mart where the quality of the data can be assessed. Once data are of sufficient quality and meet expectations, ML features are developed for use in machine learning models.

Keywords

Data warehouse/data mart/dataset · Feature engineering · Data quality · Missing data · AI/ML ecosystems

Overview

ML modeling requires sophisticated data transformations of the data extractions or samples collected to serve the needs of an application according to the specifications of the data design (Chapter "Data Design", Fig. 1.) The current chapter is concerned with this lower-level mapping (aka data transformation), of raw data elements into features suitable for ML modeling.

S. G. Johnson (✉) · G. Simon · C. Aliferis
Institute for Health Informatics, University of Minnesota, Minneapolis, MN, USA
e-mail: joh06288@umn.edu

G. J. Simon, C. Aliferis (eds.), *Artificial Intelligence and Machine Learning in Health Care and Medical Sciences*, Health Informatics,
https://doi.org/10.1007/978-3-031-39355-6_8

377

The raw data is transformed into the modeling data set in two steps. In the first step, the raw data is transformed into features, **data design features**, that the data design utilizes; and in the second step, the data design features are further transformed into **ML features** that the learning algorithm can operate on.

The key difference between the two steps is that the first step is independent of the learning algorithm and simply implements the study design, while the second step transforms the features specifically for the learning algorithm.

Figure 1 presents an outline of this process. Progressing from left to right, we start with the raw data elements in one or more source data repositories. The block labelled "Prepare Data" represents the first step, where we transform the raw data elements into data design features as specified by the data design. The target population, outcomes and covariates of interest are expressed in terms of the data design features. Data for these features are stored in a data mart. The next large block represents the second step and is labelled "Feature Engineering", in which data design features are refined to ensure they represent what the modeling team intended and ML features are created. Converting raw data into ML features is an iterative process. Both steps (Data Preparation and Feature Engineering) iterate internally until sufficient data quality is achieved. When data quality issues cannot be resolved, there may be a need to move backwards, stepping back from Feature Engineering to Data Preparation or from Data Preparation to find new raw data elements. The block at the bottom of Fig. 1 is the "Data Ecosystem", which is a collection of tools that

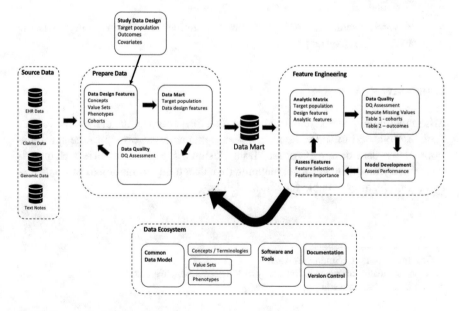

Fig. 1 Feature engineering architecture

support the entirety of the data transformation process. Data Ecosystem contains information about data mapping (from raw data to real-world entities), the tools necessary for the transformation, and other ancillary functions such as documentation and version control.

The chapter starts by defining data and related concepts (section "Working with Data"). Section "Constructing the Design Features" describes the first step (Data Preparation) and section "Modelling Dataset and Feature Engineering" describes the second step (Feature Engineering). Due to its importance, data quality assurance receives a section on its own (section "Data Quality") and section "Missing Data" discusses the missing data problem. Finally, in section "Data Processing Stacks" we review popular data processing ecosystems.

Working with Data

During the process of transforming raw data into an ML modeling dataset, we face a number of challenges. These challenges include:

1. The data in the EHR (and possibly other system) were designed with documentation of care in mind and their design may not be optimal for our purpose.
2. Data may be coming from different sources and each source may use a different terminology to denote the same real-world entity (e.g. "Systolic blood pressure", "Blood pressure, systolic").
3. Related to different terminologies, measurement units could also differ (e.g. temperature can be measured in F versus C).
4. Data quality issues abound: formatting issues, out of bound measurements, invalid characters, etc.

Common to many of these challenges is differences in mapping data in the data sources to real-world entities. In what follows, we describe terminologies related to the real-world (Problem Space in Chapter "Data Design") entities.

> A (biomedical) **concept** is a real-world clinical entity, such as a diagnosis, a medication, or a lab result.

"Blood pressure", "Systolic Blood Pressure", "Blood pressure medication", "Diagnosis of high blood pressure" are all concepts and so are "Patient", "Diagnosis", "Medication", etc. However, the blood pressure reading of "140 mmHg", is *not* a concept; it is an *observation* for the concept "Blood Pressure".

> A **vocabulary** is the collection of all terms that a domain addresses.

This definition has two parts. First, there is a domain. A vocabulary for heart disease medications will contain all terms related to heart disease medications, but will (mostly) *not*(!) contain terms for unrelated domains, such as cancer diagnostic procedures, or will contain them at very high levels without any details. Second, a vocabulary contains *all* terms related to a domain, including synonyms (e.g. "Systolic blood pressure", "Blood pressure, systolic").

A **terminology** is a standardized vocabulary that represents a system of concepts.

For example, the International Classification of Diseases, revision 10 (ICD-10) is a terminology that represents the system of all diseases. Within this terminology there is an entry, "I21 Acute Myocardial Infarction", for heart attack.

Property: entries in a terminology are unique. Terminologies do not contain synonyms, so in ICD-10, for instance, there is no entry such as "Heart attack". The lack of synonyms makes terms corresponding to a concept unique, and thus terminologies are used to assign unique IDs to concepts.

An **ontology** is a representation of a domain of concepts, comprising (1) concepts and their formal names (i.e. terminology), (2) attributes of the concepts, and (3) relationships among the concepts.

The types of **relationships** ontologies encode depend on the domain and the ontology. For example, the National Drug File Reference Terminology (NDF-RT) is an ontology for pharmaceuticals and it defines relationships such as "has_ingredient", "has_MOA" (mechanism of action), "may_treat", "may_prevent", etc. Most ontologies, however, define the ISA (taxonomy or containment) relationship: e.g. A beta blocker ISA ("is an") anti-hypertensive medication, which ISA ("is a") cardiovascular medication.

Attributes of concepts in the NDF-RT are, for example, whether a drug is meant for human use, available dosages, available routes (e.g. oral, topical, injectable), etc.

In mapping the raw data to real-world entities, the smallest unit is a data element.

A **data element** represents a singular concept.

For example, a birthdate, lab test result or a patient's name are data elements. Data elements are also called fields, columns or attributes.

Data elements can be brought together into a dataset to answer a specific analytic question.

A **dataset** is a collection of data elements that groups related concepts together.

For example, yesterday's claims or a copy of an EHR are datasets. Datasets can have other containment structures such as tables, rows, databases, etc.

A modeling problem can utilize several datasets, each dataset representing some aspect of the modeling.

It is common practice for an organization to bring all the data it needs into a common location, called a **data warehouse** (or data repository) (Fig. 2).

When an analytic project is carried out, data elements required by the analytic project are extracted and stored into a **data mart**.

A **data mart** is an extract of a subset of data from a data warehouse that is built for a specific project or for a group of related projects and contains only the data elements and patients/subjects of interest.

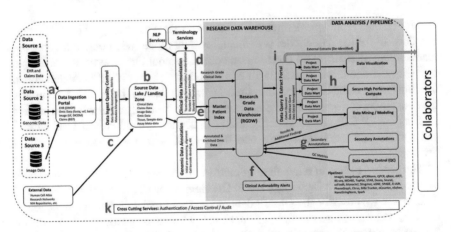

Fig. 2 Architecture of a Research Data Warehouse (RDW). (**a**) incoming data flows from assay labs, plus data sources external to the institution; (**b**) data landing zone; (**c**) data input quality control processes; (**d**) terminology harmonization and standardization; (**e**) linkage to health record data and master subject index; (**f**) return of actionable results and generation of related alerts; (**g**) primary and secondary meta data and annotations; (**h**) secure transfer channels to supercomputing; (**i**) data portal with search, visualization, data extraction and analysis functions; (**j**) data flows to external and internal collaborating researchers; and (**k**) authentication, access control and audit services/layers

Datasets and data marts differ in two ways. First, a data warehouse (and to a certain degree a data mart, as well) are created for a broad purpose; while a dataset is created for a specific purpose. For example, a data mart for all hospitalizations may exist. From this data mart, a dataset for studying care pattern variations after heart attack can be extracted. Naturally, only a fraction of hospitalizations and a fraction of data elements (procedures, treatments, lab results, diagnoses, etc.) are related to heart attack. Thus, the resulting data set is both narrower in focus and smaller in size than the original data mart. Second, a data mart is typically standardized in terms of the terminologies it uses for various concepts. In contrast, a dataset might span multiple data warehouses and may therefore rely on different terminologies, or it may contain unstandardized data that do not conform to any particular terminology.

The linkage between the raw data and the real-world entities is provided by the data model.

> The **data model** is an abstract model that defines data elements and standardizes how these data elements relate to each other and to real-world entities (clinical concepts, in our case).

Thus, a data model plays three roles. The first role is to catalog all data elements. If a domain for the data model is defined, the data model will contain all data elements in that domain. If no domain is specified, as could be case for the main data repository, the implicit domain is all clinical affairs, the set of all data elements in the data model is the entirety of the clinical concepts that can be modeled. Naturally, the data model can be expanded if necessary; in fact, publicly available data models, such as the OMOP model (described later in section "Standardized Data Models and Ontologies for Health Care and the Health Sciences") undergoes regular reviews.

The second role is to relate data elements to each other. Later in this chapter (in section "Standardized Data Models and Ontologies for Health Care and the Health Sciences"), we describe the OMOP data model in more detail, but in the meantime consider the caricature example of "patients" who have "encounters" and during these encounters, they may receive diagnoses of "diseases". Words in quotes are both data elements and clinical concepts. The data model will indicate relationships between "patients" and "encounters" and between "encounters" and "diseases".

The third role of a data model is to establish a mapping between the data elements and the real-world clinical entities. Terminologies serve this role. For each data element, for which terminologies exist, a terminology is selected. That data element is now standardized to a particular terminology. Continuing with the above caricature, we can assume that no terminology is needed for the data elements "patient" and "encounter", but several terminologies exist for diseases. We can elect to use ICD-10 to describe diseases. Although "encounter" does not have a terminology on its own, it may have an attribute, say "encounter type", which can still have a well-defined vocabulary (containing terms such as "emergent", "urgent", or "elective"). The data model can still specify that the "encounter type" attribute of the data element "encounter" must use this vocabulary.

Related to a data model is a data dictionary.

> A **data dictionary** is an inventory of all data elements and their "meta-data", which comprises (a) the type of a data element (e.g. date, string, integer, real-value numeric), (b) expectations of the data (e.g. feasible values, range), (c) the terminology it is mapped to (if any), and (d) usually a brief narrative of what the data is supposed to represent.

A data dictionary is essentially a documentation of parts of the data model. Additionally, it is also complementary to it. When a data element cannot be mapped to a terminology, the data dictionary will contain metadata about that data element. For example, to the best of our knowledge, no terminology exists for "birthdate" (because it would be merely list of all dates and a term conveying that it is unknown). We still need to document the format of the date (e.g. yyyy-mm-dd), whether a date may be missing, a NULL value for missing dates if missingness is allowed (or the fact that missingness is not allowed), and possibly ranges of acceptable birthdates.

> **Best Practice 8.2.1**
> It is a best practice to use a data dictionary to define each data element in the dataset that we are working with.

Every organization or even every project can define its own data model. However, having several, potentially incompatible data models hinders sharing data, expertise, and models across organizations or even across projects within the same organization. It also leads to waste, as the same terms need to be redefined for every project or organization.

> A **common data model** describes a standard data model that a data warehouse and derivative data marts conform with. This is used in projects and research networks and to foster interoperability of healthcare data across organizations.

Finally, we can define data. The fundamental raw material for developing AI and machine learning models is data. There are several definitions for **data** [1] with a practical definition being that "data" is the lowest level, initial ingredient on the path to information, knowledge and wisdom [2].

> **Data** are what we are given at the start of our analytic modeling and represent observations about the real-world.

In healthcare, data can come from electronic health records (EHR), claims, research data registries, wearables, and patient reported data. Not all information is available in electronic format; some information that might be useful must be first transformed into something a computer can work with. For example, paper forms, clinical expertise, or patient's genome must be processed into useful features.

> For our purposes, we will use a practical definition of **data** as anything in electronic form that a computer can process.

Data model vs data design. Both data model and data design create a mapping from raw data to features used in modeling. Data design uses higher-level semantics. While a data model is primarily concerned with mapping real-world entities into data elements, a data design is concerned with the role the data elements plays in the analysis (outcome, exposure/intervention, predictor variable), the time-frame within which we consider the data element, the subjects/patients we need data from, etc.

Standardized Data Models and Ontologies for Health Care and the Health Sciences

As we discussed earlier, data models represent the linkage between the data in the data warehouse and the clinical context and are essential for the data to have meaning. *Common data models* differ from (regular) data models in that their definitions and specifications are shared across projects and possibly organizations. Several common data models exist within healthcare, including OMOP [3], i2b2 [4], HL7 FHIR [5], PCORNet [6], and others. Each of the EHR vendors has their own data model and research collaboratives have also developed their own data models. This proliferation of data models means that many projects have to spend a substantial amount of time converting from different source data formats into whichever model was used by the study team. This is inefficient and may also cause semantic data translation errors when moving from one format to another.

Table 1 Standardized ontologies for harmonizing data

Data type class	Standard ontologies for data mapping
Molecular and cellular data	
Assay results meta data	Ontology for biomedical investigations (OBI)
Transcriptomics Genetics variants Epigenetics	GO, VariO
Proteomics	PRO
Metabolomics	Chemical entities of biological interest ontology (ChEBI), gene ontology (GO)
Cellular types	CL
Clinical Data	
Pharmacological treatments	RxNorm
Comorbidities	ICD9, ICD10, SNOMED CT
Procedures	CPT
Laboratory tests	LOINC, HL7

While it isn't right for every situation, the Observational Medical Outcomes Partnership (OMOP) Common Data Model (CDM) is gaining momentum and a number of research collaborations have decided to standardize on it including the National Institutes of Health All Of Us initiative [7], National COVID Cohort Collaboration (N3C) [8] and the eMerge network [9]. As more and more healthcare organizations develop and maintain an OMOP version of their healthcare data, they can more easily contribute to these research initiatives and researchers can better trust that the data from different organizations mean the same.

Table 1 shows key standardized ontologies for harmonizing data across domains, research sites, groups etc. Harmonization works by mapping data elements to standardized ontologies, thus ensuring (a) bringing same variables and values to common computer readable codes, (b) accurate search for data elements, and (c) interoperability across groups and sites.

There are hundreds of ontologies and terminologies that are used to represent healthcare data, and more are being added every year. Table 1. contains some of the most commonly used ontologies and terminologies both in health sciences data, specifically in molecular and cellular, and in clinical data.

Even within a type of data (i.e. clinical vs. molecular), different domains use different terminologies.

For **molecular and cellular data**, these include the Ontology for Biomedical Investigations [10] for terminology related to assay results, Gene Ontology (GO) [11, 12], genetics variants VariO [13], metabolomics [14], and the Cell Oontology (CL) [15]. Commonly used **clinical data** terminologies for medications include RxNorm [16] and NDF-RT [17]; for laboratory tests LOINC [18]; for diagnoses ICD-10-CT [19], DRG (specifically for reimbursement) [20]; for procedures CPT [21] and ICD-10-PCS [19].

For any research study, a significant amount of work is required in standardizing the data and ensuring terminologies are consistently and correctly applied within the dataset.

Several tools exist that help with this translation. The Unified Medical Language System (UMLS) offers its Metathesaurus as a way to cross-walk between equivalent concepts [22]. In terms of tools, the Observational Health Data Science and Informatics (OHDSI) program [3] offers a single vocabulary service, named Athena, that provides a translation between common healthcare vocabularies.

As healthcare knowledge in medicine continues to advance, new terms need to be created to represent concepts in the data. The common data model may also need to evolve to accommodate new information and new types of data such as genomic, image, and unstructured note data. The OMOP data model itself has gone through a number of versions and the most recent version (5.4) does supports these new data types. Similarly, vocabularies also continue to evolve. As new concepts are created, they must be added to terminologies and be connected together across related terminologies. Both the Athena vocabularies and the UMLS Metathesaurus are continuously maintained to ensure new terms and linkages are up-to-date.

Constructing the Design Features

As we discussed earlier, the transformation from raw data to a modeling dataset consists of two main steps. First, the raw data elements in the data warehouse relevant to the analytic question are transformed into *data design features*; and in the second step these design features are further transformed into *ML features* that the learning algorithm can operate on. In this section, we focus on the first step. Specifically, we discuss the following tasks (1) extract the data elements from the warehouse that are necessary for the study, (2) transform them in a manner that is agnostic of the learning algorithm into the set of design features, and (3) using the inclusion/exclusion criteria from the study design, create a cohort of patients who are subjects in the study.

We defined **concept** in Section "Working with Data" as a real-world clinical entity, such as a diagnosis, a medication, or a lab result.

A **feature** represents a concept. A **data design feature** represents a concept in the data design; and an **ML feature** (variable) in the ML modeling dataset.

The difference between concept and feature is that features are those concepts that are referenced in the study design. There are numerous other features in the data model that are not referenced in the study design. These concepts do not need to be used in the analysis and will not be turned into features.

In this book, we refer to the concepts that appear in the data design as **(data) design features**.

Sometimes, for a concept in the study design, there exists a data element in the data mart that has a one-to-one correspondence. However, often, multiple data elements need to be combined to accurately represent a concept.

Example 8.3.1
Suppose we are interested in the side effects of a particular drug and we are constructing a cohort consisting of patients currently taking this particular drug. This drug is a concept, it is referenced by the data design (as an inclusion criterion), and thus, needs to become a data design feature. Due to the terminology we use, this drug has a one-to-one correspondence with the data in the medications table. In this case, the design feature is the corresponding drug in the medications table.

Example 8.3.2
Consider the concept of a "diabetic patient". This concept could be defined as a patient with a diagnosis code that indicates diabetes. Under this definition, the design feature would be the presence of any diabetes-related diagnosis code. Diabetes is known to be underdiagnosed, thus using this definition could lead to false negatives. If the requirements of the modeling problem are sensitive to false negatives (and less sensitive to false positives), we may need to cast a wider net and define "diabetic patient" as patients with any indication of diabetes. In this case, the design feature could be created using a simple algorithm which checks whether the patient has a diabetes-related diagnosis code, a (possibly preventive) prescription of anti-diabetic drugs, or a periodic measurement of blood glucose (indicating suspicion of diabetes). In both cases, the design feature requires transformations of the data elements in the dataset. In the first case, the design feature maps to a set of diagnosis codes (called a value set); in the second case, a simple algorithm (called a phenotyping algorithm) transforms the original data elements into the design feature. Also note, that the amount of transformation the raw data needs to undergo depends on the requirements of the study.

The raw data may come from a variety of sources, but it was often collected for some purpose other than research. In some cases, such as randomized control trials, data may be collected specifically for a study and therefore already be perfectly tailored to what that modeling problem needs. However, in most cases, the raw data will need to be transformed into a form that is required to implement the data design. These transformed forms are given names such as features, variables, phenotypes, predictors, etc. and are often used interchangeably. In the subsequent sections we are going to discuss phenotypes, and value sets as two prominent ways of transforming the raw data elements into design features.

As transformations occur, information about inputs, the transformations themselves, and their outputs should be documented as meta-data. Not only is this required to reproduce results, but it is also necessary to ensure that researchers that use the resulting output understand how and why the data was produced and that it can therefore be trusted.

> **Data provenance (or data lineage)** is the meta-data that describes data transformations. A complete set of data lineage information helps researchers know that the data that they are using in their study or for their model are correct.

In the remainder of this chapter, we will describe specific ways to construct the design features and also discuss cohort construction.

Phenotypes

Simple algorithms, like the one in the diabetes example (Example 8.3.2), are referred to as **phenotyping algorithms**. In genetics, a phenotype is an individual's observable traits [23]. We will use the term phenotype to refer to the traits of the individuals represented in our data.

> A **phenotype** is an algorithm or expression that defines a feature and is specified at a sufficient level of detail to be computable.

When we're working with data transformations, we need to define the phenotypes computed from the source data in such a way that they can be consistently applied by anyone trying to reproduce the study. We will create these computable and reproducible phenotype definitions using concepts, value sets, cohorts, covariates and combinations of these that can be combined into complex expressions to define exactly the concept that we wish to represent. Some phenotypes are simple.

For example, a patient that has had a heart attack will have a single diagnosis code that indicates they had that event as part of their record (for example, an ICD10 code of I21). Other phenotypes may be more complex. For example, a patient will be considered as a Type II diabetic patient if they have at least two diagnosis codes in their record within the prior 2 years (e.g. descendants of ICD10 code E11), at least one diabetes medication prescribed (e.g., metformin) and at least one HgA1c measure above 6.5 in the past 2 years.

Value Sets

Value sets, sometimes called concept sets, are lists of concept codes that further define a phenotype of interest by enumerating all of the codes that comprise that phenotype.

Only in simple cases will a single concept code identify the concept that a researcher is interested in. For example, in the case of atrial fibrillation, a researcher may just be interested in chronic atrial fibrillation and therefore will use SNOMED concept code 4141360. But more often, a list of the different concept ID's that describe the intended phenotype is required. The UMLS value set authority (VSAC) [24] was created to allow organizations to develop and maintain lists of concept codes that define very specific phenotypes of interest. But finding all of the codes for the intended definition is still difficult. For example, within the VSAC, there are 62 different definitions of an atrial fibrillation concept set (Fig. 3).

It is still a difficult task for a researcher to find a version of atrial fibrillation that defines their intended definition of atrial fibrillation. Even though the VSAC was created to provide a mechanism to share concept sets, it is still hard to know what phenotype a particular set of concepts really refers to and reusing these concepts sets can be problematic. In many cases researchers still end up defining their own set of codes.

☐ Atrial Ablation	ICD10PCS SNOMEDCT	Grouping	The Joint Commission	2.16.840.1.113883.3.117.1.7.1.203	19
☐ Atrial Ablation	SNOMEDCT	Extensional	The Joint Commission	2.16.840.1.113883.3.117.1.7.1.243	13
☐ Atrial fibrillation	SNOMEDCT	Intensional	Optum	2.16.840.1.113762.1.4.1078.17	15
☐ Atrial Fibrillation	ICD10CM	Extensional	Change Healthcare	2.16.840.1.113762.1.4.1182.275	4
☐ Atrial Fibrillation	ICD9CM	Extensional	ACEP/AMA-PCPI	2.16.840.1.113883.17.4077.2.1003	1
☐ Atrial Fibrillation	ICD10CM	Extensional	ACEP/AMA-PCPI	2.16.840.1.113883.17.4077.2.1004	6
☐ Atrial Fibrillation	SNOMEDCT	Extensional	ACEP/AMA-PCPI	2.16.840.1.113883.17.4077.2.1005	13
☐ Atrial Fibrillation	ICD10CM SNOMEDCT	Grouping	ACEP/AMA-PCPI	2.16.840.1.113883.17.4077.3.1001	19
☐ Atrial Fibrillation/Flutter	ICD10CM ICD9CM SNOMEDCT	Grouping	The Joint Commission	2.16.840.1.113883.3.117.1.7.1.202	30
☐ Atrial Fibrillation/Flutter	ICD9CM	Extensional	The Joint Commission	2.16.840.1.113883.3.117.1.7.1.244	2
☐ Atrial Fibrillation/Flutter	ICD10CM	Extensional	The Joint Commission	2.16.840.1.113883.3.117.1.7.1.245	9
☐ Atrial Fibrillation/Flutter	SNOMEDCT	Extensional	The Joint Commission	2.16.840.1.113883.3.117.1.7.1.246	19
☐ Atrial Fibrillation/Flutter	SNOMEDCT	Extensional	The Joint Commission	2.16.840.1.113883.3.117.1.7.1.249	2
☐ Body Site Value Set	SNOMEDCT	Intensional	HL7 Terminology	2.16.840.1.113883.3.88.12.3221.8.9	40253

Fig. 3 Examples of atrial fibrillation value sets. (Screenshot taken from https://vsac.nlm.nih.gov/valueset/expansions?pr=all)

There are common pre-defined value sets for us to use. Although ICD codes form a taxonomy, it is imperfect. There are codes that describe multiple diseases (e.g. diabetic retinopathy, hypertensive kidney), yet they appear only once in the ICD hierarchy; and conversely, codes indicative of a certain disease can appear in different parts of the taxonomy (e.g. pre-existing diabetes in pregnancy does not appear under the diabetes codes). This motivated the creation of the Clinical Classification Software Refined (CCSR) [25], which creates value sets of ICD-10-CT codes for different diseases, regardless of where the code resides in the ICD-10 hierarchy. Another example of value sets is the Elixhauser comorbidities. Suppose we wish to estimate the effect of an exposure (e.g. lead poisoning) on mortality. To elicit the effect of lead poisoning, we need to adjust for the patient's general state of health, because other severe comorbidities the patient may have could also influence mortality risk. Elixhauser comorbidities are such severe comorbidities, and for each comorbidity, a value sets of ICD-10 codes is predefined [26].

Modeling Dataset and Feature Engineering

In the current section, we focus on the second step of transforming raw data into ML features, namely the transformation of the data design features into ML features. Recall that ML features are specific to the learning algorithm and allow them to operate on these features optimally. In this section we describe (1) the modeling dataset, (2) transformation of the data design features into ML features, (3) feature selection, and (4) feature importance.

ML Modeling Dataset

Now that we have defined the features, variables, phenotypes and the discovery sample, we can put this information into a format that is more easily consumed by our analysis and modeling software.

> An **ML Modeling Dataset** is a data structure that contains information about the cohort and is in a convenient input format for the ML algorithm we selected for use.

The classical modeling dataset, also known as design matrix or analytic matrix, is typically a two-dimensional structure with one row for each subject (or observation) and a column for each variable/feature. Modern ML methods, in addition to analytic matrices, can also utilize higher dimensional tables (tensors), as well as non-tabular data sets (graphs, sequences, images, text, etc.).

> A ML modeling dataset can contain classical analytic tables, data sets in more modern data formats, or a combination of these.

In this section we will examine best practices for producing these data extracts that will be consumed by our ML software. We will first examine the different types of fact tables defined as the "long" vs the "wide" data formats.

Classical Analytic Table Formats

Ultimately, data science projects need a way to represent all the information about each person that is part of each cohort in the study. Most data science projects use a simple spreadsheet-like fact table.

The **format** of the table is how the rows and columns of the table are laid out.

Typically, the table is arranged such that each row represents a person and the columns represent features (or facts) about that person.

In **wide** format, there is one row per patient/subject/sampling unit and facts about the subject are laid out in columns; in the **long** format, there is one fact/ observation per row and each patient/subject/sampling unit can have multiple rows.

Example 8.4.1
Consider a cohort of patients. We collect facts about these patients and each lab result is a fact. In the wide format, we have one row per patient and the different lab tests are the columns. Not all patients have results for all tests; thus, some fields in a row will be empty. In the long format, the different lab results the patient has are the rows. The columns could be patient id, date, lab type, lab result.

Table normalization and pivoting. Suppose that in the domain of the data model, several different lab tests can be administered, including cholesterol tests (LDL, HDL, TG), glucose test (FPG), kidney function tests (creatinine), inflammation, etc. We could store these results in a "wide" table, with columns patient id, result date, LDL, HDL, TG, FPG, etc. Given that the LOINC terminology for laboratory results identifies 56,000 different lab tests, this would result in a table with 56,000 columns, which is a problem by itself. Compounding this problem is the fact that for each patient at each encounter (which is a row in this wide table), only a few tests are administered, thus the vast majority of the columns in each row would have missing value (NULL). Storing all these NULL values, wastes space. To prevent this waste, the table is *normalized* into a "long" format, where the columns are patient id, result date, lab type, lab result and a row is generated only for those tests that were actually administered. This way no NULL values need to be recorded.

Most analytic software however expect *unnormalized* ("wide") tables, where lab results that could have been administered (but maybe not for this patient) are columns. The operation to covert a normalized (long) table into unnormalized (wide) table is called **pivoting**. The pivot operator takes a column ("lab type" in this example), creates new columns for (potentially user-selected) unique values of this column, and populates these new columns with values taken from another original column ("lab result"). When there is no data for a particular lab test on a particular date, the corresponding field is set to NULL.

Laboratory results are not the only normalized columns. The same normalization takes place for other data elements, such as diagnoses, medications, etc.

Longitudinal data. Longitudinal observations arise in several settings, including routinely collected data in the healthcare setting and clinical trials. These two settings can have different characteristic affecting the format in which the data is stored.

In a clinical trial setting, repeated measures may be taken following a particular schedule. All trial subjects are administered the same battery of tests at the same time point (where time may be measured related to entry into the trial, rather than calendar time). Suppose, two lab tests, LDL and creatinine, are measured for each subject on days 1, 5, and 30, then the data may be stored a "wide" format, having columns patient id, ldl_day1, ldl_day5, ldl_day30, creatinine_day1, creatinine_day5, creatinine_day30. In the longitudinal data analysis literature, this format is called **person-level** format.

Alternatively, in a routine healthcare setting, the schedule at which lab results are collected varies from person-to-person. Attempting to store such data in person-level format would yield an excessive number of columns: there would be a column for every date when a lab test was administered (for any patient) and every lab test. Instead, a "longer" format, called the **person-event** format (also known as **counting process** or lifetable format in the survival literature; see Chapter "Methods Summary") is used. In the person-event format, there is a row for each patient at each time point when *that patient* has a lab test administered. Suppose, we measure cholesterol (LDL, HDL, TG) and kidney function (creatinine), a table in the person-event format would have columns patient id, result date, LDL, HDL, TG, creatinine.

Note that the person-event format is not a normalized format. Although it has a row for every time point when a test was administered (to *that person*), not all lab tests may be administered at that time. Tests that were not administered would have NULL values.

Relationship between analytic software and analytic table format. Almost all analytic software expect unnormalized tables (i.e. wide format, person-event or person-level format). From the perspective of normalization, the analytic software determines the format of the analytic table. In contrast, in the case of longitudinal data, analytic method (and software) is selected based on the data format. Data in person-level format versus person-event format yield different models with different interpretation.

Best Practice 8.4.1
Whether the data need to be pivoted or not depends on the software that will be used for modeling. Almost always, the software will expect pivoted (wide) data.

Best Practice 8.4.2
The choice between person-level and person-event format is driven by the analytic need and the analytic software (model) is chosen accordingly.

Feature Engineering

As we discussed earlier, data design features are transformed into ML features to better suit the ML algorithm. What we have not discussed earlier are the benefits of these transformations. These benefits include:

1. Models can become more interpretable (e.g. transform non-linear features, de-skew distributions),
2. Predictive performance can improve as the transformation can reduce bias, variance and noise (e.g. scaling continuous variables, remove outliers, autoencoders),
3. The transformation can combine existing features into features that are easier to use (e.g. single variable for complex diabetes phenotypes),
4. Summarize other features in a more meaningful way (e.g. summarize comorbidities into a risk index or severity index)
5. Make the modeling possible (e.g. using natural language processing to extract features from narrative text, dimensionality reduction).
6. The transformation can also be specifically aimed at reducing the dimensionality of the problem (i.e. the number of variables)

Featuring engineering is the process of transforming existing variables, or developing additional variables, or features, from the source data that can enable the use of a particular learning algorithms, improve its performance, or interpretability.

Feature engineering also involves understanding how all of the features are related so that irrelevant and redundant features can be removed and the most important features are identified for subsequent analysis and model development.

In the following, we review several techniques for transforming the design features into ML features.

Scaling. Several techniques, including neural networks, perform best when variables are brought to the same scale. Scaling helps prevent variables that are vastly different numerically, such as creatinine levels (between 0 and 2) and weight in pounds (between 0 and 500) from overwhelming an analysis, although some analytical techniques can deal with large scale differences. Variables can be brought to the same (or similar) scale by (1) simply normalizing them to be between (say) 0 and 1 (and possibly trimming some outliers), or (2) standardizing the features (subtracting the mean and dividing by the standard deviation).

Addressing Non-linearity. Some algorithms assume a linear relationship between the predictor variable and its effect on the outcome. Features that do not satisfy this assumption can be transformed. Common transformations include expanding the features into a polynomial (adding the squared, cubed, and higher order versions of the same feature), taking the square root or log of the feature, or more broadly, transforming it through a non-linear function. Alternatively, continuous features can be *binned.* This involves splitting the variable range into a number of categories or *bins.* For example, "age" can be split into bins of "0–16", "17–65" and ">65" in an analysis.

Indicator variables. Many algorithms (e.g. regression, SVM, neural networks, etc.) operate exclusively on numeric variables. Some implementations of these algorithms may accept categorical variables, but will internally encode them into numeric variables. The key to converting categorical variables into numeric is that binary variables are often implemented as integer 0 or 1 values, thus they *appear* numeric. Although they may not have distributional characteristics that typical numeric variables have, from a technical perspective they appear numeric in the sense that they support numerical operators, such as addition and multiplication that the fitting algorithms rely on.

One-hot encoding. This is the simplest way to convert categorical variables into indicator variables. Each *level* (unique value) of a categorical variable becomes its own new variable. For example, the source data may have a variable named "eye_color" that contains the items "blue", "brown", "green", or "black". Each of these items becomes an ML feature, which could be named, for instance, "eyes_blue", "eyes_brown", "eyes_green", and "eyes_black" and each would have a value of 0 or 1.

Binning. Continuous variables can also be converted into a set of indicator variables through binning. We discussed binning as a way of handling non-linear effects, but it can also help interpretability. There are several strategies to binning, including equi-depth and equi-width binning. In case of equi-depth binning, the number of observations in all bins will be as close to equal as possible. In case of equi-width binning, the range of values covered by each bin will be roughly equal. For example, categorizing age as 20–40, 40–60, 60–80 is equi-width, because all three bins cover a range of 20 years of age.

Contrast coding. When (ordinal or nominal) categorical variables are transformed into a set of indicator variables chiefly for the purpose of improving interpretation, *contrast coding* is used. The name comes from the property that levels of the categorical variable are encoded into indicator variables in such a way that the effect of each level is *contrasted* against another level or a reference level. When used in a regression model, the use of contrast coding schemes also has implications on the meaning of the intercept of the model.

Treatment coding is the simplest contrast coding scheme. It considers one level as the reference level and encodes all other levels using one-hot-encoding. In a regression model, the effect of each level on the outcome is measured relative to the reference level and the effect of the reference level on the outcome becomes part of the intercept. Other encodings, that offer different guarantees for the intercept and different interpretations for the effect sizes, include the Sum, Deviation, Helmert, Orthogonal Polynomial, Forward Difference, and Backward Difference (see [27–30] for details) codings. Creating contrasts manually can capture complex semantic relationships among levels of a categorical variable. Some coding schemes are most meaningful for ordinal variables.

Example 8.4.2
Consider a blood pressure variable with levels "normal", "pre-hypertensive", "hypertensive, grade 1", "hypertensive, grade 2". This is an ordinal variable, where "normal" < "pre-hypertensive" < "hypertensive, grade 1" < "hypertensive, grade 2" in terms of blood pressure: patients whose blood pressure is "normal" have lower blood pressure than patients whose blood pressure is "pre-hypertensive". If we encode this variable into four indicator variables, such as 'Is blood pressure normal?' or 'Is blood pressure pre-hypertensive?', the ordering among these four indicator variables will not be explicit to the learning algorithm. If, instead, we encoded these variables as 'Is blood pressure at least "hypertensive, grade 2"?', then it is explicit to the learning algorithm that "grade 2" should carry higher risk than "grade 1", because every patient with "grade 2" also has "grade 1", and, in fact, they have already exceeded "grade 1". If the learning algorithm is a linear regression algorithm, the interpretation of the coefficient of "grade 2" becomes the excess risk associated with having grade 2 hypertension relative to grade 1 hypertension.

Pitfall 8.4.1
If ordinal variables (or more generally, variables with semantic relationships among their levels) are encoded using one-hot-encoding, the semantic relationships will be hidden from the modeling algorithm.

Best Practice 8.4.3
If categorical variables with sematic relationships among their levels need to be converted into a set of indicator variables, design an encoding scheme (if possible) that makes this semantic relationship explicit to the learning algorithm.

Missingness indicators. We will discuss handling missing values later in Section "Missing Data". When the missingness of data for a design feature carries information, *missing feature indicators* can be defined for each such features. The missingness indicator takes the value 1 if a variable is missing and 0 if it is present. The indicator allows the learning algorithm to assign an effect size to the missing feature.

Combining features to reduce dimensionality. It is often desirable to combine existing features into new features to make a particular analysis or model easier to build or understand. This is called dimensionality reduction. Dimensionality reduction is discussed in Chapter "Methods Summary".

Scores. A supervised way of combining features is to create scores. A **score** is often a weighted sum of several features, where the weight can be assigned fully manually [30], semi-manually by converting regression weights into—supposedly more easily applicable—integer weights [31], and fully computationally, where regression weights are used as is [32].

Automated feature engineering. There are also methods to automatically engineer features by using software to create hundreds or thousands of features based on data elements. This saves the researcher from having to devise features that they think will be helpful for the model and instead generates a large set of potentially useful features. Feature selection techniques can then be used to find a subset of features for a more efficient but high performing model. Automated feature engineering algorithms apply mathematical functions to information about the relationship between data elements in a database or correlations between features to generate new features [33–35]. Automatic feature generation can save time and may even propose novel features, but a big issue is that the methods will generate a very large number of features, most of which will not be useful. Efficient feature selection algorithms must then whittle the set of features down to an optimal set. Domain experts hand crafting a set of features can usually do better than the automated algorithms [34].

Deep Feature Synthesis [34] is an automated feature generation method that operates on relational databases using the entity-relationship models and generates features that span multiple tables. The "depth" of the features is the number of entities that were used to create the features and is a user parameter.

Autoencoders aim to create new features, collectively called a data representation, such that the original data features can optimally be reconstructed from these new features. Autoencoders use deep learning to learn this representation and the objective is to minimize the so-called reconstruction error, which is the difference between the input data reconstructed from the new representation and the actual input data [36], given the architecture, including the size of the new representation (number of new features). If the resulting representation is of lower dimensionality than the original data, then this is also a dimensionality reduction technique (see chapter "Methods Summary"). We also discussed in Chapter 3 transfer learning, where a pre-trained model is used (after removing its output layer) as a new data representation. This new data representation can be viewed as a set of automatically engineered new features.

There are many commercial tools that can automatically generate features as well as a few open source tools for Python (e.g. autofeat [37] and Featuretools [38]) and for R (e.g. tsfeaturex [39]).

Knowledge-based automated features. Another common way to generate features is to use external knowledge, for example, a physical equation, to generate these features or to train a model to learn these features and apply these models to training data set thereafter to generate the new features for the training data. Some of the clinical scores, where the scores were computed on an external data set, unrelated to the training data, are special cases of this approach. For a more complete review of example of knowledge-based features, the reader is referred to [40].

Data Quality

Data quality is the degree to which a dataset meets a user's requirements [41] and is fit for the purpose it is intended [42]. Whether the data was collected for the purpose of the modeling task (primary use of the data) or for a different purpose and the modeling task just uses the data as a convenience sample (secondary use of the data), data quality issues can exist and can impact the modeling and its results.

Consequences of data quality issues range from benign to catastrophic.

For example, from a modelling perspective, when a lab result is missing for a patient because of an accidental loss of data, this is typically benign: the issue is known and many modeling methods can correct for it. If a dataset has unknown biases, these biases can invalidate a model—*unbeknownst to the modeling team*—leading to potentially incorrect clinical predictions or findings.

When researchers try to make use of this data, such as research studies and quality initiatives, the first thing they need to do is to understand the quality of the information, what the data represents and mitigate any issues or gaps in what they require from the data.

While all modeling, even outside healthcare, can be impacted by data quality issues, data quality issues are exacerbated in healthcare due to (1) lack of standards for describing or dealing with data quality issues within healthcare data, (2) the lack of a common EHR data model, (3) a preponderance of vocabularies and terminologies to represent data types and the complexity of healthcare data, (4) the continuing evolution of additional medical concepts procedures and conditions as new medical knowledge is discovered.

Pitfall 8.5.1
There a fallacy that "Because of data quality issues in EHR data, they cannot be used for discovery".

Best Practice 8.5.1
EHR data can be used for discovery, but be aware of the quality issues and select modeling methods that can correct for the relevant and potentially consequential issues.

Data Quality Standards

One major issue is that there are no standard ways of describing data quality. Until recently, there have not been standard ways of even consistently referring to different issues and aspects of data quality. A number of frameworks have tried to standardize the terms that are used to describe data quality issues, and a distillation of that work resulted in harmonized terminology for data quality [43]. The primary dimensions of data quality are Plausibility (*are data believable?*), Conformance (*do data values conform to standards?*) and Completeness (*are there missing data?*).

We can categorize the many different types of data quality issues that arise into the following groups. If we can identify data quality issues, then we can potentially apply mitigation strategies to deal with the issues, which are described in Table 2, which lists data quality dimensions with examples of the types of data quality issues that can arise.

There is a growing body of work to develop frameworks of data quality rules that can be used to assess the quality of a specific dataset or cohort.

Table 2 Examples of data quality issues

Data quality dimension	Description	Example issues
Value conformance	Values conform to formatting constraints	Dates have invalid formats such as "Jan 1 1998"
Relational conformance	Values follow relational constraints	There exist visit records that don't have an associated patient record
Computational conformance	Computed values follow specifications	BMI is computed using any height measurement in the record instead the one paired with the weight
Completeness	Absence of values agrees with expectations	Diagnosis codes for COVID don't exist before 1/1/2020
Uniqueness plausibility	Values identify a single object	Patients from a single institution that have multiple MRNs
Atemporal plausibility	Data values and distributions agree with independent measurement or clinical knowledge	Measurement error when nurse takes BP readings, data entry errors BMI > 100
Temporal plausibility	Values conform to temporal expectations	Admission date after discharge date Antibiotic prescribed before admission date

Assessing Data Quality

There is software that implements some of the data quality assessments. For example, the Data Quality Dashboard (DQD) [44], which is one of the data quality tools within the OHDSI toolset, assesses data quality along the dimensions of Completeness, Plausibility and Conformance. The DQD uses the harmonized data quality terminology and implements data quality rules to provide a system that can evaluate an OMOP formatted dataset and provide a set of metrics that be used to compare across datasets or for a single dataset across time (Fig. 4).

The DQD encapsulates expectations as data quality rules that can be executed against the data to produce reports to show the overall data quality of the dataset. Importantly, it provides a quantitative score for the dataset that can be tracked over time (to see if changes are improving data quality) and across datasets (to ensure that datasets across organizations are of similar quality). Figure 5 lists examples of the type of rules and metrics that are computed by the data quality dashboard.

While these quantitative data quality metrics are useful, they only assess overall data quality. One important exercise is for the researcher to explicitly define the

	Verification				Validation				Total			
	Pass	Fail	Total	% Pass	Pass	Fail	Total	% Pass	Pass	Fail	Total	% Pass
Plausibility	159	21	180	88%	283	0	283	100%	442	21	463	95%
Conformance	637	34	671	95%	104	0	104	100%	741	34	775	96%
Completeness	369	17	386	96%	5	10	15	33%	374	27	401	93%
Total	1165	72	1237	94%	392	10	402	98%	1557	82	1639	**95%**

Fig. 4 Example of a data quality dashboard [44]

STATUS	CONTEXT	CATEGORY	SUBCATEGORY	LEVEL	DESCRIPTION	% RECORDS
⊞ FAIL	Validation	Completeness	None	TABLE	The number and percent of persons in the CDM that do not have at least one record in the DEVICE_EXPOSURE table (Threshold=0%).	100.00%
⊞ FAIL	Validation	Completeness	None	TABLE	The number and percent of persons in the CDM that do not have at least one record in the VISIT_DETAIL table (Threshold=0%).	100.00%
⊞ FAIL	Validation	Completeness	None	TABLE	The number and percent of persons in the CDM that do not have at least one record in the NOTE table (Threshold=0%).	100.00%
⊞ FAIL	Validation	Completeness	None	TABLE	The number and percent of persons in the CDM that do not have at least one record in the SPECIMEN table (Threshold=0%).	100.00%
⊞ FAIL	Validation	Completeness	None	TABLE	The number and percent of persons in the CDM that do not have at least one record in the PAYER_PLAN_PERIOD table (Threshold=0%).	100.00%

Showing 1 to 5 of 1,639 entries   Previous 1 2 3 4 5 ... 328 Next

Fig. 5 Examples of data quality rules implemented in a data quality dashboard [44]

expectations that they have of the data that is relevant to their particular research question. Even if a dataset is of high quality in general, it may not be for certain research questions.

> **Best Practice 8.5.2**
> Provide a minimal set of data quality metrics for Completeness, Plausibility and Conformance.

Missing Data

> A data element is **missing**, if no data value is stored for a variable (features).

There are three general reasons why data may be missing. First, and arguably most common in healthcare, is *structural missingness*, where the data was not supposed to be collected in the first place. For example, we would not expect cholesterol data to be collected at an encounter for vaccination. The second general reason is inadvertent missingness. There was a reason to collect the data, but for example, the test failed to yield result. A third reason is data quality issues. Relevant data quality issues include not Plausible data elements (for example, BMI > 100), or values with formatting errors that impact data quality (Conformance).

Informative missingness. One important attribute to missingness is whether it is informative. Missingness is informative, if missingness of a data element is predictive of the outcome in question. One important consequence of informative missingness is that it can confound the relationship between (observed) predictors of the outcome.

Types of missingness. Data can be missing **completely at random** (MCAR), **missing at random** (MAR) or **missing not at random** (MNAR). If the probability that a particular piece of data is missing is independent of any other variables as well as the true (unobserved) value of the missing variable, then it is missing completely at random (MCAR). In this case, the reasons that the data are missing are not related to the missing data itself and every observation has an equal chance of being missing. This allows us some freedom to deal with that missing data. Unfortunately, most data is not missing completely at random.

If the probability that a particular piece of data is missing depends only on other observed variables and does not depend on the true (unobserved) missing value (given the other observed variables), then the data is **missing at random (MAR)**.

In this case there is a relationship between one or more observed pieces of data that is associated with the missing data. We can use the observed data to help us adjust for the missing data. Unfortunately, there is not usually an easy way to confirm that the missing data is only a function of the observed data.

Table 3 Types of missing data with examples

Missing data type	Description	Example issues
Missing completely at random (MCAR)	The reason that the data are missing are not related to the missing data itself and every observation has an equal chance of being missing	A lab test did not produce a result or an automated blood pressure cuff does not record results periodically
Missing at random (MAR)	There is a relationship between one or more observed pieces of data that is associated with the missing data	A patient has no HgA1c results (because they are not diabetic)
Missing not at random (MNAR)	The probability that data is missing depends on the data itself	A patient does not report a quality of life score (because they are depressed)

Finally, if the probability that a particular piece of data is missing depends on the unobserved data itself, then the data is **missing not at random (MNAR).** Missing not at random is the most complicated situation and there is no way to confirm if missing data is MNAR without knowing the values of the missing data (which, of course, are missing). One of the only ways to mitigate MNAR data is to try to identify and resolve reasons for the cause of the missing data (Table 3).

Handling missingness. Missing and implausible data can be handled in a number of different ways [45]. Traditional methods of dealing with missing data have assumed the data are MAR or MCAR. But if data are MNAR, those methods will produce biased estimators [46].

Complete data analysis, listwise deletion. Complete data analysis (aka listwise deletion) removes all of the data for any patient that has missing values. This is easy to implement, but can result in biased data if it is not truly MCAR or when the complete data is not a random sample from the analytic sample (or population). This approach also wastes data and reduces the population for modeling.

Single imputation methods calculate a replacement value for the missing data. Single imputation produces a set of complete data, but it has a few disadvantages. Most of the methods introduce bias, and only stochastic regression produces an unbiased dataset. Single imputation methods include using the mean (or median) of the complete data as a replacement for the missing values, hot-deck imputation (replacing missing values using values from "similar" patients), and last observation forward imputation (for longitudinal data, taking the last measured value and using for remaining missing values). Stochastic regression is the recommended single imputation method since it produces unbiased data for MAR and MCAR data. Stochastic regression involves developing a regression model to predict values for incomplete variables (using complete variables) and then adding a normally distributed residual term to the values in order to add the proper variance into the missing variables [45].

Multiple imputation methods create multiple copies of the dataset and compute estimates for the missing values. This technique replaces missing values in multiple copies of the original dataset and then analyzes each copy to produce model parameter estimates and standard errors. All of the model estimates are then pooled to produce a final set of model parameters and error estimates. There are a number of ways that the missing values can be estimated and the model parameters pooled. There are R (Mice) and Python (Scikit-learn, IterativeImputer) packages that implement these techniques.

Pattern-based modeling. When missingness follows only a few patterns, namely when only a few combinations of variables with simultaneously missing data exist, an alternative to imputation is to build models for each pattern separately. This method results in a collection of models (rather than a single model), one for each missingness pattern, but may produce unbiased estimates even for MNAR data.

Data Processing Stacks

In order to process and transform data, we need to use a set of tools. There are many data environments and software for working with data, including several excellent commercial environments, but there are also freely available open source tools.

As organizations continue to create an exponentially expanding amount of new data, there has been more focus on inventorying, describing and governing that data. Processes that transform data should use FAIR principles for scientific data and software (Findable Accessible Interoperable and Reusable data and software) [47, 48] and TRUST data principles (Transparency, Responsibility, User focus, Sustainability, and Technology) [49].

> A **data processing stack** is a group of related tools that are designed to work together well and which form an ecosystem for efficiently working with data.

The qualities that are required in an effective data processing stack are:

1. Support for a common data model (CDM), which is a data model that is common across projects and researchers, promoting the sharing of artifacts and expertise in a community of researchers
2. Efficient and flexible access to databases and data storage structures (SQL, csv, flat file, etc.)
3. Tools to document data transformation steps and track data lineage
4. Support for using a complete programming language (e.g. R, Python, Julia, etc.) not just a data access language (e.g. SQL)
5. Rich packages and libraries to help with data transformations, data quality assessment, visualizations, feature engineering and model performance assessment
6. Support for the FAIR and TRUST principles

Documenting Data Transformations

> **Best Practice 8.7.1**
> It is a best practice to document all data transformations so that the entire process can be reproduced from scratch if necessary.

The documentation tool should ideally allow for mixing narrative text to describe each step of the data pipeline with the actual code that implements the transformations so that everything is in once place. In addition to data artifacts, the pipeline will also produce data quality assessments, summary tables and visualizations of the data and meta-data. The documentation environment should make it easy to keep all of these artifacts connected together and easily viewable. Feature engineering is an iterative process and the data pipeline will change quite often. The documentation and data pipelines should have a version control ability to track changes and allow for rollback of the undesired changes. The documentation is also something that should be easily shared within the project and across projects, ideally in a way that the documentation can collaboratively be edited and shared.

If the project does not require a specific documentation tool, an excellent place to start are Jupyter notebooks. They serve as documentation and as a development environment to write and execute code. Jupyter is an open-source web application that allows for creating and sharing documents that contain live code, equations, visualizations and narrative text [50]. Alternatives with similar capabilities include Zeppelin, R Studio, etc.

Common Data Processing Stacks

Structured Query Language (SQL) is a language for low-level data manipulation and transformation. Many SQL engines are designed to achieve very high performance on retrieving data elements from large data warehouses or data marts, but lack features for sophisticated feature engineering, such as missing value imputation, etc.

Spark is an open-source data science ecosystem, with implementations of SQL standards, offering powerful data transformation and feature engineering capabilities. Emphasis is placed on computational scalability, optimization, and load-balancing across potentially very large number of compute nodes. Spark also has ML modeling capabilities and some Spark environments, such as Zeppelin, support visualization. Programming languages supported by Spark include Scala (its native language), Java, Python, R, etc.

R is an open-source, primarily statistical programming language. As such, it natively supports tasks related to feature engineering, statistical modeling, and visualization. It is highly extensible, and packages implement all major population ML algorithms. With its origins in statistical processing, its data extraction and transformation capabilities were designed for smaller, in-memory data sets, however, packages have been developed to interface with database engines. It is not the first choice tool for data extraction.

Python is an open-source, interpreted, high-level, dynamically typed, general-purpose programming language created by Guido van Rossum in 1991. It has developed into one of the first-choice environments for data science activities, with extension packages covering an extremely broad range of areas including numerical computation, manipulation of tabular and graphical data, ML modeling, visualization, etc.

Matlab is a commercial language, originally for high-performance matrix manipulations and visualization. Major machine learning methods have been implemented for Matlab.

Table 4 summarizes how well each data stack addresses different tasks.

Best Practices 8.7.2
The minimum set of tools to learn is a common data model, at least one of the data science programming languages, and data access using SQL.

Data Pipelines

A **data pipeline** is a set of software programs that convert the raw data in the data sources into a modeling dataset that ML algorithms can directly operate on.

A data pipeline differs from a data processing stack, in that a data pipeline is a project-specific while a data processing stack is still general-purpose. Data processing stacks were implemented to be, after project-specific customizations, broadly applicable to a wide range of projects. The data pipeline, on the other hand, is fully implemented by the modeling team and its main purpose is specifically to produce the modeling data set. Often, data pipelines are implemented using data processing stacks.

Table 4 Some common data processing stacks. Notation: '-': not designed to perform this task; 'O': possible to perform the task but not recommended; '+' good at performing the task; '++' designed specifically for efficiently performing this tasks

Task	SQL	Spark	R	Python	Matlab
Data extraction from a warehouse or data mart	++	++	O	+	O
Data transformation (creating data design features)	+	++	+	+	+
Feature engineering	−	++	++	++	++
Modeling	−	+	++	++	++
Visualization	−	O	++	++	++

Data science projects usually have quite a few data transformation steps. In fact, data manipulation, transformation, quality assessment and standardization consume most of the effort in a typical data science project. It is critical that data transformation steps be well defined, well documented, and reproducible. As we have discussed earlier, it is critical to document all of the steps of the data transformations in a project. Most projects will have many steps that need to be executed in a certain order in order to reproduce all of the features used in a project.

> **Best Practice 8.7.3**
> Every project should create and maintain a data pipeline, which is a repeatable process that performs all of the steps required to transform data from the source data to the final analytic fact table that is used as input for the analytic and modeling part of the project.

The team should be able to recreate the modeling dataset from scratch using only the source data and the data pipeline. It is also critical that metadata about when these transformations occurred on which source datasets and the characteristics of the data at that time are documented.

We discussed data lineage or data provenance (e.g. when did the transformation happen and what were the source input data) in section "Constructing the Design Features". The data lineages help researchers know how the data that they are analyzing was created. It helps other researchers and collaborators reproduce the steps with their own data set, and it helps all of the stakeholders trust that the data was transformed in a manner that was expected and supports the analytic process. In commercial data science systems data lineage capabilities may be built into their products. For researchers using open source software, they usually have to cobble together their own solutions. Recently, there are a number of open source projects emerging that help to document data lineages (e.g. Amundsen, Datahub and Marquez).

> **Best Practice 8.7.4**
> Ensure that meta-data associated with phenotypes and variables contains enough information to allow for the re-creation of the phenotypes/variables from source data.

It is also important that as the definitions of the phenotype and variables change, the version of those definitions that was used to compute the variable is also recorded. Using a version control system for the definitions is also a best practice. You can check-in the code from your Jupyter Notebooks, Python or R programs in order to maintain a reproducible data pipeline.

A data pipeline is also a convenient place to insert data quality assessments. Information about the source data and its impact on the transformed data is important metadata that can help researchers to debug any analytic issues. These projects record data quality metadata of the source data longitudinally. They currently do not have very good mechanisms for assessing the data quality of transformed data elements, so researchers may have to develop their own assessments.

It is also useful to automate data pipelines and allow them to be executed when the source data changes. It may often be expensive in time and money to run entire pipelines on very large datasets in full, so it is useful to understand how source data updates impact downstream variable transformations. This allows software to only execute the parts of the pipeline that are necessary to regenerate the downstream elements and if certain source data does not change it may not affect other downstream elements, which is more efficient.

The result of the data pipeline should be the creation of your modeling data set. Some data ecosystems have tools to support this process. For example, OHDSI has the Atlas tool that takes as input a cohort definition (using the web UI or via a JSON definition file) and creates an analytic cohort from the criteria. Atlas supports defining variables as single concepts or via value sets. At this time, Atlas does not support defining more complex phenotype expressions, which need to be handled outside of the tools using a programming language or SQL.

Key Concepts in Chapter "Data Preparation, Transforms, Quality, and Management"

Biomedical concept, vocabulary, terminology, ontology.
Data element, dataset, data warehouse, data mart.
Data model, data dictionary, common data model.
Data provenance (lineage).
Phenotyping algorithm, value set.
Feature, variable.
ML Modeling Dataset.
Classical analytic table format: wide and long tables.
Variable types: numeric, binary, categorical (nominal and ordinal).
Feature engineering.
Data quality, data quality standards.
Missing Data, informative missingness, Types of missingness (MCAR, MAR, MNAR).
Data processing stack, ecosystems, data pipelines.

Pitfalls and Best Practices in Chapter "Data Preparation, Transforms, Quality, and Management"

Pitfall 8.4.1. If ordinal variables (or more generally, variables with semantic relationships among their levels) are encoded using one-hot-encoding, the semantic relationships will be hidden from the modeling algorithm.

Pitfall 8.5.1. There a fallacy that "Because of data quality issues in EHR data, they cannot be used for discovery".

Best Practice 8.2.1. It is a best practice to use a data dictionary to define each data element in the dataset that we are working with.

Best Practice 8.4.1. Whether the data need to be pivoted or not depends on the software that will be used for modeling. Almost always, the software will expect pivoted (wide) data.

Best Practice 8.4.2. The choice between person-level and person-event format is driven by the analytic need and the analytic software (model) is chosen accordingly.

Best Practice 8.4.3. If categorical variables with sematic relationships among their levels need to be converted into a set of indicator variables, design an encoding scheme (if possible) that makes this semantic relationship explicit to the learning algorithm.

Best Practice 8.5.1. EHR data can be used for discovery, but be aware of the quality issues and select modeling methods that can correct for the relevant and potentially consequential issues.

Best Practice 8.5.2. Provide a minimal set of data quality metrics for Completeness, Plausibility and Conformance.

Best Practice 8.7.1. It is a best practice to document all data transformations so that the entire process can be reproduced from scratch if necessary.

Best Practices 8.7.2. The minimum set of tools to learn is a common data model, at least one of the data science programming languages, and data access using SQL.

Best Practice 8.7.3. Every project should create and maintain a data pipeline, which is a repeatable process that performs all of the steps required to transform data from the source data to the final analytic fact table that is used as input for the analytic and modeling part of the project.

Best Practice 8.7.4. Ensure that meta-data associated with phenotypes and variables support at some basic aspects such as the date of the transformation and the version of the source data that was used to compute that variable.

Questions for Class Discussion and Assignments Chapter "Data Preparation, Transforms, Quality, and Management"

1. The International Classification of Diseases, Revision 10 (ICD-10) is often used for documenting the diagnosis of diseases in the electronic health records. How many codes can you find that indicates type-2 diabetes mellitus among the ICD-10 codes?

   https://www.icd10data.com/ICD10CM/Codes/E00-E89/E08-E13

   (The above link takes you to the diabetes subtree of the ICD-10 hierarchy.)

   The Clinical Classification Software (CCS) reorganizes ICD-10 codes into diseases (with overlaps) so that they better represent diseases. Look at the ICD-10 codes under the type-2 diabetes CCS category (END005). Did you find any ICD-10 codes that are not in the E11 branch?

   (CCS is available from https://www.hcup-us.ahrq.gov/toolssoftware/ccsr/dxccsr.jsp)

2. Look at the RxNorm or NDF-RT terminologies. Where would you find insulin?

3. Creatinine in the bloodstream is one of the indicators of kidney disease. Which creatinine codes from LOINC can you use? How do they differ? [Hint: Beware of creatinine in urine.]

4. We aim to build a diabetes risk prediction model for adult (age >18) patients with elevated fasting plasma glucose (FPG) levels (at least 100 mg/dL). Exclude patients with pre-existing diabetes (as indicated by the presence of a diabetes diagnosis code, FPG >125 mg/dL, or prescription of an anit-diabetic drug). As predictors, we use specific vital signs and lab results: systolic and diastolic blood pressure, pulse, body mass index (BMI), cholesterol levels (LDL, HDL, TG), and FPG.

   (a) What are you design features? (Hint: Do not forget features in the inclusion and exclusion criteria and outcome.)

   (b) Assuming your institution uses ICD-10 for documenting diagnoses, how would you define 'pre-existing diabetes'? Hints: Use the term "value set".

   (c) You can cross-check your value set with CCS or CCSR for ICD-10-CT. https://www.hcup-us.ahrq.gov

      Hint: Use CCS or CCSR for ICD-10-CT (clinical terminology CT; not procedure codes PC)

   (d) Based on the description in the question, how would you define the phenotyping algorithm for 'pre-existing diabetes'? For this question, you may assume that a value set for "diabetes medication" already exists. You can also use the vital signs and lab test names, you do not need to look up their LOINC codes.

   (e) Phenotype for the outcome. How is it different from your answer for question (d)?

5. Suppose you implement your risk model using GLM.

(a) What would be your ML features? [Hint: Is pre-existing diabetes going to be turned into ML features?]

(b) Do you need to transform your lab results in any way?

(c) Due to inclusion and exclusion criteria, FPG will be truncated to a range between 100 and 125 mg/dL. Will this cause any problems?

(d) Assume that age below 45 has no effect, between 45 and 65 have moderate effect and above 65, age has a very pronounced effect. How would you turn age into ML features?

(e) Suppose we wish to add anti-hypertensive (blood pressure) medications as predictors. Further assume for simplicity that we only have three anti-hypertensive subclasses (ACE, ARB and BB). How would you encode these drugs into ML features? [Hints: Some patients do not take anti-hypertensive drugs.]

(f) If I told you that ACE and ARB have roughly the same effect, but BB is more potent, would you change your encoding?

(g) How would you change your encoding if I told you that BB can be added to an ACE/ARB regimen for even greater (i.e. interaction) effect? [Hint: there are two solutions; one of them does not require new ML features.]

6. Suppose you implement your risk model from Question 4 using neural networks? How would your answers to Question 5 change?

7. While implementing your model from Question 5 (using GLM), you find that some of the blood pressure measurements are missing. How do you handle the situation under the following conditions? Would you delete patients with missing blood pressure? Would you impute? Would you create a missingness indicator variable? Is the missingness informative?

(a) All blood pressure measurements were collected, but a technician accidentally forgot to transfer some of them. Whether a blood pressure measurement was transferred or not is random.

(b) Some blood pressure measurements are not collected because the patient is young, and BMI as well as all lab results indicate that the patient is healthy.

(c) The missing blood pressure measurements are not collected because the patient is obviously healthy. For the same reason, other labs are missing, too.

8. Suppose observations for blood pressure are missing completely at random (a technician forgot to transfer them to you). Since they are missing completely at random, you decide to impute the population mean value.

(a) Will this impact the predictions from your model?

(b) Does this change the variance of the blood pressure in the sample? (Hint: use the formula for sample variance.)

(c) Would this affect the estimated error of the prediction from your model? Would this effect the significance of the coefficient for blood pressure?

(d) How can you compensate for this possible change in variance? (Hint: stochastic regression.)

9. Consider an ordinal categorical variable with four levels, A < B < C < D. How do I encode this variable into ML features to achieve the desired interpretation?

   (a) I wish to know the effect of B, C, D relative to A.
   (b) I wish to know the effect of B relative to A, the effect of C relative to B and the effect of D relative to C.
   (c) Some values are missing. I wish to know the effect of all levels and the effect of missingness relative to A. How do I define the ML features and the missingness indicator?
   (d) Some values are missing. I wish to know the effect of B relative to A, the effect of C relative to B, the effect of D relative to C, and the effect of missingness relative to D.

10. Consider an ordinal variable with three levels: A < B < C. Let $\alpha_0, \alpha_B, \alpha_C$ denote the intercept and the coefficients quantifying the effects of B relative to A and C relative to A in a regression model. In an alternative encoding, let $\beta_0, \beta_{AB}, \beta_{BC}$ denote the intercept, the effect of B relative to A and the effect of C relative to B. Can you express α_c in terms of β's? (Hint: You can consider a simple model with a single predictor, the variable in question. You can now express the prediction from both models in terms of their respective coefficients when the observation (for your only predictor) is A, B and C. Can the predictions differ between the two models?)

11. Consider a caricature problem of predicting mortality based on predictors related to blood pressure (systolic and diastolic blood pressure, presence of blood pressure medications) and cholesterol (LDL, HDL, TG, presence of cholesterol medications). Two models are considered. The first one, model A, uses all 7 predictors to predict mortality. The second, alternative model, is a stacked model, where the first layer consists of a blood-pressure score, which is implemented as the predictions from a logistic regression model that predicts mortality using the 3 blood pressure related variables; and a cholesterol score that is implemented as a logistic regression model predicting mortality using the 4 cholesterol-related variables. The second layer is also a logistic regression model that predicts mortality based on the blood pressure score and cholesterol score. Are these models (model A and the stacked model) different? Is one of the models more constrained? Can you think of situations when one model performs better than the other?

12. The Charlson comorbidity score [51] is a weighted sum of the presence of comorbidities that predicts 1-year mortality. It is frequently used to adjust for a patient's state of health. What is the benefit from using such a score versus using the individual comorbidities? Is there a disadvantage?

References

1. Witten, Frank, Hall, Pal, Data (2005) Practical machine learning tools and techniques. Data Min Knowl Disc.
2. Matney S, Brewster PJ, Sward KA, Cloyes KG, Staggers N. Philosophical approaches to the nursing informatics data-information-knowledge-wisdom framework. ANS Adv Nurs Sci. 2011;34:6–18.
3. Stang PE, Ryan PB, Racoosin JA, Overhage JM, Hartzema AG, Reich C, Welebob E, Scarnecchia T, Woodcock J. Advancing the science for active surveillance: rationale and design for the observational medical outcomes partnership. Ann Intern Med. 2010;153(9):600–6.
4. Murphy SN, Weber G, Mendis M, Gainer V, Chueh HC, Churchill S, Kohane I. Serving the enterprise and beyond with informatics for integrating biology and the bedside (i2b2). J Am Med Inform Assoc. 2010;17:124–30.
5. HL7. Fast Healthcare Interoperability Resources (FHIR). https://hl7.org/fhir/. Accessed 1 Jul 2022.
6. Fleurence RL, Curtis LH, Califf RM, Platt R, Selby JV, Brown JS. Launching PCORnet, a national patient-centered clinical research network. J Am Med Inform Assoc. 2014;21:578–82.
7. All of Us Research Program. The "all of us" research program. N Engl J Med. 2019;381:668–76.
8. Haendel MA, Chute CG, Bennett TD, et al. The national COVID cohort collaborative (N3C): rationale, design, infrastructure, and deployment. J Am Med Inform Assoc. 2021;28:427–43.
9. Hripcsak G, Shang N, Peissig PL, et al. Facilitating phenotype transfer using a common data model. J Biomed Inform. 2019;96:103253.
10. Bandrowski A, Brinkman R, Brochhausen M, Brush MH, Bug B, Chibucos MC, Clancy K, Courtot M, Derom D, Dumontier M, Fan L, Fostel J, Fragoso G, Gibson F, Gonzalez-Beltran A, Haendel MA, He Y, Heiskanen M, Hernandez-Boussard T, Jensen M, Lin Y, Lister AL, Lord P, Malone J, Manduchi E, McGee M, Morrison N, Overton JA, Parkinson H, Peters B, Rocca-Serra P, Ruttenberg A, Sansone SA, Scheuermann RH, Schober D, Smith B, Soldatova LN, Stoeckert CJ Jr, Taylor CF, Torniai C, Turner JA, Vita R, Whetzel PL, Zheng J. The ontology for biomedical investigations. PLoS One. 2016;11(4):e0154556. https://doi.org/10.1371/journal.pone.0154556;eCollection2016.
11. Ashburner M, et al. Gene ontology: tool for the unification of biology. Nat Genet. 2000;25(1):25–9.
12. Gene Ontology Consortium. The Gene Ontology resource: Enriching a gold mine. Nucleic Acids Res. 2021;49(D1):D325–34.
13. Vihinen M. Variation ontology for annotation of variation effects and mechanisms. Genome Res. 2014;24(2):356–64.
14. Hastings J, Owen G, Dekker A, Ennis M, Kale N, Muthukrishnan V, Turner S, Swainston N, Mendes P, Steinbeck C. ChEBI in 2016: improved services and an expanding collection of metabolites, vol. 44. Nucleic Acids Res; 2016. p. D1214–9.
15. Diehl AD, Meehan TF, Bradford YM, Brush MH, Dahdul WM, Dougall DS, He Y, Osumi-Sutherland D, Ruttenberg A, Sarntivijai S, Van Slyke CE. The cell ontology 2016: enhanced content, modularization, and ontology interoperability. J Biomedical Semantics. 2016;7:1–10.
16. RxNorm. https://www.nlm.nih.gov/research/umls/rxnorm/overview.html.
17. National Drug File Reference Terminology (NDF-RT™) Documentation U.S. Department of Veterans Affairs, Veterans Health Administration. 2015. https://evs.nci.nih.gov/ftp1/NDF-RT/NDF-RT%20Documentation.pdf.
18. Logical Observation Identifiers Names and Codes (LOINC). https://loinc.org/about/.
19. World Health Organization. International Statistical Classification of Diseases (ICD) and related health problems. https://www.who.int/standards/classifications/classification-of-diseases.
20. Centers for Medicade & Medicare Services. Medicare Severity Diagnosis Related Groups (MS-DRG). https://www.cms.gov/medicare/medicare-fee-for-service-payment/acuteinpatientpps/ms-drg-classifications-and-software.

21. American Medical Association. Current Procedural Terminology (CPT®). https://www.ama-assn.org/amaone/cpt-current-procedural-terminology.
22. Bodenreider O. The unified medical language system (UMLS): integrating biomedical terminology. Nucleic Acids Res. 2004;32:D267–70.
23. Phenotype. In: Genome.gov. https://www.genome.gov/genetics-glossary/Phenotype?id=152. Accessed 8 Aug 2022.
24. Bodenreider O, Nguyen D, Chiang P, Chuang P, Madden M, Winnenburg R, McClure R, Emrick S, D'Souza I. The NLM value set authority center. Stud Health Technol Inform. 2013;192:1224.
25. Healthcare Cost and Utilization Project (HCUP). Clinical classification software refined. https://www.hcup-us.ahrq.gov/toolssoftware/ccsr/ccs_refined.jsp.
26. Healthcare Cost and Utilization Project (HCUP). Elixhauser comorbidities. https://www.hcup-us.ahrq.gov/toolssoftware/comorbidityicd10/comorbidity_icd10.jsp.
27. UCLA Statistical Consulting Group. R Library Contrast Coding Systems for Categorical Variables. https://stats.oarc.ucla.edu/r/library/r-library-contrast-coding-systems-for-categorical-variables/.
28. Lisa DeBruine, Anna Krystalli, Andrew Heiss. Contrasts. https://cran.r-project.org/web/packages/faux/vignettes/contrasts.html.
29. Patsy: contrast coding system for categorical variables. https://www.statsmodels.org/dev/contrasts.html.
30. Ngufor C, Caraballo PJ, O'Byrne TJ, Chen D, Shah ND, Pruinelli L, Steinbach M, Simon G. Development and validation of a risk stratification model using disease severity hierarchy for mortality or major cardiovascular event. JAMA Netw Open. 2020;3(7):e208270. https://doi.org/10.1001/jamanetworkopen.2020.8270. PMID: 32678448; PMCID: PMC7368174.
31. Wilson PWF, Meigs JB, Sullivan L, Fox CS, Nathan DM, D'Agostino RB. Prediction of incident diabetes mellitus in middle-aged adults: the Framingham offspring study. Arch Intern Med. 2007;167(10):1068–74. https://doi.org/10.1001/archinte.167.10.1068.
32. Huang IC, Frangakis C, Dominici F, Diette GB, Wu AW. Application of a propensity score approach for risk adjustment in profiling multiple physician groups on asthma care. Health Serv Res. 2005;40(1):253–78. https://doi.org/10.1111/j.1475-6773.2005.00352.x. PMID: 15663712; PMCID: PMC1361136.
33. Kaul A, Maheshwary S, Pudi V. Autolearn—Automated feature generation and selection. IEEE International Conf Data Mining; 2017.
34. Kanter JM, Veeramachaneni K. Deep feature synthesis: towards automating data science endeavors. In: 2015 IEEE international conference on Data science and advanced analytics (DSAA). ieeexplore.ieee.org; 2015. p. 1–10.
35. Katz G, Shin ECR, Song D (2016) ExploreKit: automatic feature generation and selection. In: 2016 IEEE 16th international conference on Data mining (ICDM). ieeexplore.ieee.org. pp 979–984.
36. Goodfellow I, Bengio Y, Courville A. Chapter 14 Autoencoders. In: Deep Learning. MIT Press; 2016. http://www.deeplearningbook.org.
37. Horn F, Pack R, Rieger M. The autofeat python library for automated feature engineering and selection. In: Machine Learning and knowledge discovery in databases. Cham: Springer International Publishing; 2020. p. 111–20.
38. Alteryx Featuretools. https://github.com/alteryx/featuretools. Accessed 1 Jul 2022.
39. Roque NA, Ram N. Tsfeaturex: an R package for automating time series feature extraction. J Open Source Softw. 2019;4:1279. https://doi.org/10.21105/joss.01279.
40. Willard J, Jia X, Xu S, Steinbach M, Kumar V. Integrating scientific knowledge with machine Learning for engineering and environmental systems. ACM Comput Surv. 2022;55(4):37. https://doi.org/10.1145/3514228.
41. Ehsani-Moghaddam B, Martin K, Queenan JA. Data quality in healthcare: a report of practical experience with the Canadian primary care sentinel surveillance network data. Health Inf Manag. 2021;50:88–92.

42. Johnson SG, Byrne MD, Christie B, Delaney CW, LaFlamme A, Park JI, Pruinelli L, Sherman SG, Speedie S, Westra BL. Modeling flowsheet Data for clinical research. AMIA Jt Summits Transl Sci Proc. 2015;2015:77–81.
43. Kahn MG, Callahan TJ, Barnard J, et al. A harmonized Data quality assessment terminology and framework for the secondary use of electronic health record Data. EGEMS (Wash DC). 2016;4:1244.
44. OHDSI (2019). The book of OHDSI: observational health Data sciences and informatics.
45. Enders CK. Applied missing Data analysis. 2nd ed. New York: Guilford Publications; 2022.
46. Rubin DB. Inference and missing data. Biometrika. 1976;63:581–92.
47. Wilkinson MD, Dumontier M, Aalbersberg IJJ, et al. The FAIR guiding principles for scientific data management and stewardship. Sci Data. 2016;3:160018.
48. Lamprecht A-L, Garcia L, Kuzak M, et al. Towards FAIR principles for research software. Data sci. 2020;3:37–59.
49. Lin D, Crabtree J, Dillo I, et al. The TRUST principles for digital repositories. Sci Data. 2020;7:144.
50. Kluyver T, Ragan-Kelley B, Pérez F, et al. Jupyter notebooks-a publishing format for reproducible computational workflows. International Conference on Electronic Publishing; 2016.
51. Charlson ME, Pompei P, Ales KL, MacKenzie CR. A new method of classifying prognostic comorbidity in longitudinal studies: development and validation. J Chronic Dis. 1987; 40(5):373–83.

Evaluation

Gyorgy Simon and Constantin Aliferis

Abstract

The purpose of model evaluation is to assess the model's suitability for the intended purpose. In the evaluation of clinical models, we consider three levels of evaluation. At the core, we are concerned with predictive performance, namely whether the model we constructed has sufficiently high predictive ability. On the next level, we are concerned with generalizability. We wish to ensure the model is robust to changes over time and we may wish to know whether the model can generalize to different demographics at different geographic locations or to a different service with different disease severity. Finally, on the third level, we evaluate the model from the perspective of achieving the clinical objective and doing so at a cost that is acceptable to the health system.

The purpose of evaluating a clinical model is to ensure that a model has sufficient performance, is valid in the target population (and any other population of interest), and is capable of achieving the clinical objectives at a cost that is acceptable to the health system.

We consider three levels of model evaluation. Let us illustrate these levels through the hypothetical example of developing a screening test. Suppose a diagnostic test for a disease exists, it is reliable, but invasive and can cause serious adverse events. We wish to develop a machine learning based screening model that determines whether a patient needs to undergo this invasive diagnostic test. We evaluate this screening model.

G. Simon (✉) · C. Aliferis
Institute for Health Informatics, University of Minnesota, Minneapolis, MN, USA

© The Author(s) 2024

G. J. Simon, C. Aliferis (eds.), *Artificial Intelligence and Machine Learning in Health Care and Medical Sciences*, Health Informatics,
https://doi.org/10.1007/978-3-031-39355-6_9

415

On the first layer, we have to ensure that the model can predict the outcome and has sufficiently high predictive performance to capture patients at high risk of the outcome who really need to undergo the invasive diagnostic test.

On the second layer, we are concerned with the validity of the model. As we discussed in chapter "Data Design", the model is developed on a discovery sample with the intent of applying it in the target population. We discussed two kinds of validations. First, *internal validation* is concerned with generalization from the discovery sample to the accessible population; and *external validation* is concerned with generalizability to the target population and other populations of interest. More formally, external validation refers to validating a model in a setting that is different from the setting of the accessible population. The setting can differ, for example, in the time frame, geographic location, data collection method, or clinical setting (clinical application).

Finally, on the third layer, we wish to ensure that the model achieves the health objective of reducing adverse events from the invasive test without missing too many patients with the disease. We wish to do this at a reasonable cost; ideally, the added cost of the ML-based screening test is offset by the savings on the invasive diagnostic test and its adverse events.

Section "Evaluating Model Performance" focuses on the core evaluation, where we discuss the predictive performance of a model. In sections "Clinical Usefullness" and "Health Economic Evaluation", we evaluate the clinical utility and health economic impact of the model. Finally, in section "Estimators of Model Performance", we discuss internal and external validation, as well as "estimators", methods for estimating model performance in the context of generalizability.

Evaluating Model Performance

In this section, we focus on common measures (or metrics) of model performance. In the course of writing this book, we found over 30 different measures of model performance just for time-to-event outcomes alone, many of which were proposed recently. Therefore, complete coverage of the measures in existence is impractical. Instead, we aim to provide an extensive overview of measures, and we specifically strive to include measures that measure different aspects of model performance, that have different properties, or measures that are derived from different principles (e.g. how close is the estimate to the actual value; how does the estimate co-vary with the actual value, or how well does the model fit the data). Not all of these measures are commonly used. For example, among the 30 performance measures for time-to-event outcomes, one measure, Harrell's C statistic, covers 63% of the published literature [1]. To guide the reader, we will indicate which measures are commonly used, which combinations of measures provide complementary information and under what conditions is a combination preferable over another.

> **Best Practice 9.1.1**
> Use evaluation metrics appropriate for the outcome type.

> **Best Practice 9.1.2**
> Multiple metrics are needed to cover different aspects of model performance. Use sets of measures that provide complementary information.

We present the measures organized by model outcome types. In this section, we discuss measures for categorical (including binary and multinomial); in the subsequent two sections, we discuss continuous (Gaussian and non-Gaussian) and time-to-event outcomes. Finally, we discuss calibration in section "Calibration", which applies to all of the above outcome types.

Model Performance Metrics for Classification

We grouped measures of classification performance into two groups. The first group is directly based on the contingency matrix (and thus misclassifications). These methods typically require the prediction, which is often a score or a probability, to be converted into an actual predicted class label. The second group, which we call discrimination-based measures, do not require the conversion of a score into predicted class labels.

Performance Metrics Based on the Contingency Matrix
At the core of the first group of evaluation metrics lies the contingency table (sometimes called the misclassification table or confusion matrix) depicted in Table 1 [2–4]. In binary (two-class) classification problems, a subject can be *predicted* to be positive or negative. If the subject is predicted positive, they fall into the first column; if predicted negative, into the second column. In reality, the subject can be positive or negative. If the subject is a positive, they fall into the first row of the table (actual positive, AP), and if they are actual negative, they fall into the second row (actual negative, AN). Subjects who are predicted to be positive (first column) and are actually positive (first row) are true positives (TP); subjects who are predicted

Table 1 Sample contingency table

Actual	Predicted		Total
	Positive	Negative	
Positive	TP	FN	AP = TP + FN
Negative	FP	TN	AN=FP + TN
Total	PP = TP + FP	PN=FN + TN	Grand total = N

positive (first column) but are actually negative (second row) are false positives (FP). Analogously, subjects who are predicted negative (second column) and are actually positive (first row) are false negatives (FN); and subjects who are predicted to be negative (second column) and are actually negatives (second row) are true negatives (TN).

Based on the contingency table, the following measures can be defined (Table 2).

A number of additional measures can also be defined (Table 3) and these are used in some fields of study.

Mathematically related measures. Table 3 contains measures in pairs, where the top measure is mathematically related to the measure below. They describe the same aspect of a classifier. For example, true positive rate TPR is the proportion of true positives among the actual positives. Since the actual positives are TP + FN, the false negative rate (FNR), which describes the false negatives among the actual positives, is simply 1-TPR. FNR offers no information about the classifier beyond what TPR already offered.

Complementary measures. Each pair of complementary measures describes different aspects of the classifier. For example, one measure can describe how well the classifier performs on actual positive subjects, while the second measure can describe how well the classifier performs on actual negative subjects. Common pairs include precision and recall. Precision describes how selective the classifier is for positive subjects, but does not tell us what percentage of the actual positives we selected. A classifier that only classifies a single subject as positive, and that subject

Table 2 Commonly used measures of classifier performance based on contingency tables

Accuracy, % correctly classified, weighted 0/1 loss	
(TP + TN)/N	Proportion of subject correctly classified
Precision, predicted positive value (PPV)	
TP/PP=TP/(FP + TP)	Proportion of true positives (actual positives) among predicted positives
Recall, sensitivity, true positive rate (TPR)	
TP/AP=TP/(TP + FN)	Proportion of true positives (predicted positives) among actual positives
Specificity, true negative rate (TNR)	
TN/AN=TN/(TN + FP)	Proportion of true negatives (predicted negatives) among actual negatives

Table 3 Additional measures of classifier performance, their definitions and mathematical relationships

True positive rate (TPR)	TP/AP = TP/(TP + FN)
False Negative Rate (FNR)	FN/AP=FN/(TP + FN) = 1-TPR
True Negative Rate (TNR)	TN/AN = TN/(TN + FP)
False Positive Rate (FPR)	FP/AN=FP/(TN + FP) = 1-TNR
Predicted Positive Value (PPV)	TP/PP = TP/(TP + FP)
False Discovery Rate (FDR)	FP/PP=FP/(TP + FP) = 1-PPV
Predicted Negative Value (PNV)	TN/PN = TN/(FN + TN)
False Omission Rate (FOR)	FN/PN=FN/(FN + TN) = 1-PNV

is actually positive, has a precision of 1 (100%) but is very likely useless, since it fails to identify the vast majority of the positive cases. In a complementary manner, recall provides exactly this missing piece of information. Similarly, sensitivity and specificity are a commonly used pair. Sensitivity tells us what percentage of the actual positives the classifier classified as positive, while specificity tells us the percentage of actual negatives classified as negative. A trivial classifier, which classifies every subject as positive, has sensitivity of 1 (100%), but is useless. In a complementary manner, specificity would show that this classifier captured none of the actual negatives, thus it has specificity of 0. A third complementary pair that is commonly used is bias and discrimination, which we will describe later.

Pitfall 9.1.1
Don't use mathematically related measures together. They do not provide additional information.

Best Practice 9.1.3
Common complementary pairs of classifier performance evaluation metrics include: (1) precision/recall; (2) specificity/sensitivity; (3) bias/discrimination.

Measures that Describe the Performance with Respect to Both Positives and Negatives

Given these complementary pairs of measures, it is reasonable to ask whether there are measures that can do both: describe positives *and* negatives. There are two commonly used measures that achieve this goal. First is **accuracy** (percent correctly classified).

$$Acc = \frac{TP + TN}{N}$$

While accuracy involves both the true positives and negatives, as a percentage of the entire population, it is very sensitive to the distribution of actual positives and negatives in the population. Suppose only 1% of the population is positive, then a trivial classifier, which classifies nobody as positive, achieves a seemingly very high 99% accuracy, yet this classifier is completely uninformative.

Pitfall 9.1.2
Accuracy is very sensitive to the prevalence of actual positives and negatives.

Another measure that combines performance with respect to positive and negative subjects is F-measure

$$F1 = \frac{2 * \text{prec} * \text{recall}}{\text{prec} + \text{recall}} = \frac{2 * TP}{2TP + FP + FN}$$

where 'prec' denotes precision (predictive positive value). One drawback of the F-measure (specifically the $F1$ measure) is that it assigns equal importance to precision and recall.

Weighted Confusion Matrices

In some applications, the cost of misclassification can be different between false positives and false negatives. For example, in case of a screening test, the harm caused by false positives (the screening test incorrectly reports the patient as having the disease) is often lower than the harm caused by false negatives (the screening test missed a case completely). In the former case, the patient may undergo a more invasive diagnostic test that determines that the patient does not actually have the disease, while in the latter case, the patient may remain undiagnosed for possibly a long period of time, suffering the consequences of the undiagnosed disease.

The confusion matrix can be element-wise multiplied with the weight matrix (Table 4) and weighted versions of the measures from Tables 2 and 3 can be computed. For example, a weighted version of accuracy would become

$$\text{weighted acc} = \frac{w_{TP}TP + w_{TN}TN}{w_{TP}TP + w_{FP}FP + w_{FN}FN + w_{TN}TN}$$

When different types of misclassifications have different consequences, the TP, TN, FP and FNs can be assigned weights in the computation of the evaluation measures based on contingency tables.

Measures of Discrimination

Many classifier models produce a score or a probability of a subject belonging to one class versus another. Confusion matrices require that we dichotomize the score into a predicted class: subjects with a score above a threshold are considered positive, those with a score below the threshold are classified as negative. The values in the confusion matrix, namely the number of TP, TN, FP, NF are influenced by this threshold, and thus the metrics we compute from the confusion matrix are

Table 4 Correct and misclassification weights for measures based on confusion matrices

Actual	Predicted	
	Positive	Negative
Positive	w_{TP}	w_{FN}
Negative	w_{FP}	w_{TN}

influenced by this threshold. Consequently, when we compare two classifiers, our preference for one over the other may also be influenced by this threshold.

For classifiers that output a score or probability of an instance belonging to the positive class, measures of classifier performance in Tables 2 and 3 require the specification of a threshold for classifying an instance positive (above the threshold) or negative (at or below the threshold). This threshold influences the performance measurements.

In this section, we look at measures of discrimination, the classifier's ability to distinguish between the two classes, without requiring such a threshold.

Concordance

Concordance operates directly on the score without having to threshold it into a decision. **Concordance** (**C-statistic** or **discrimination** by other names) is the probability that in a randomly selected pair of patients, one actual positive and one actual negative, the actual positive patient has a higher score than the actual negative patient. For binary classification, the C-statistic can be computed as the area under the ROC (to be described next) and thus it is also known as Area Under the ROC (**AUC**).

Concordance is related to the measures based on the confusion matrix. Consider every distinct score S a classifier produces. We use each score as the threshold for determining a predicted label: patients with scores above this threshold are predicted positive (PP) and at the score or below are predicted negative (PN). We can now compute the true positive rate (TPR) and the false positive rate (FPR). The S different thresholds result in S different TPR-FPR pairs, which we can plot. The resulting curve is called the **Receiver Operating Curve** (ROC).

Example 9.1.1
Consider a hypothetical classifier that produced the following predictions on a hypothetical data set (0.01, 0.02, 0.05, 0.19, 0.21, 0.3) with the corresponding true outcomes being (0, 1, 0, 1, 0, 1). These six distinct predicted probabilities yield seven different thresholds as summarized in Table 5.

Table 5 Shows a hypothetical data set with six observations and six distinct predicted probabilities of outcome (shown in the text) yielding seven different possible cutoffs. For each cutoff, the number of true positive (TP), false positive (FP), true negative (TN), and false negative (FN) classifications are shown. The corresponding sensitivity and specificity values are also shown

Threshold	TP	FP	FN	TN	Sens.	Spec.	1-Spec.	Remark
0.00	3	3	0	0	1.00	0.000	1.00	Everyone is predicted positive
0.01	3	2	0	1	1.00	0.333	0.667	
0.02	2	2	1	1	0.667	0.333	0.667	
0.05	2	1	1	2	0.667	0.667	0.333	
0.19	1	1	2	2	0.333	0.667	0.333	
0.21	1	0	2	3	0.333	1.00	0.000	
0.30	0	0	3	3	0.000	1.00	0.000	Nobody is predicted positive

With a cutoff of 0, observations with predicted probability >0 are classified as positive. In this case all observations have predicted probability >0, thus all observations are predicted positives. Among these 3 are actual positive and 3 are actual negative observations. Therefore, we have 3 true positives (TP = 3) and 3 false positives (FP = 3). The sensitivity is 3/3 = 1 and the specificity is 0/3 = 0.

When we increase the cutoff to 0.01, the one observation with predicted probability of 0.01 becomes predicted negative and all other observations (with predicted probability >0.01) remain predicted positives. Given that this observation is an actual negative, the number of true negatives increases (to 1) and the number of false positives decreases (to 2). This yields a sensitivity of 3/3 = 1 and a specificity of 1/3 = 0.333.

As the cutoff increases to 0.02, one actual positive patient gets reclassified from predicted positive to predicted negative, thus sensitivity becomes 2/3 = 0.667 and specificity remains 1/3 = 0.333. Proceeding in the same manner, the last cutoff is 0.3. At this cutoff, nobody is classified as predicted positive (since no predicted probability > 0.3), thus sensitivity is 0 and specificity is 1.

The ROCs are plots of the classifier's performance at various thresholds (for classifying an instance positive). Sensitivity is plotted against 1-specificity.

The ROC for this example is shown in Fig. 1. The seven rows of the table correspond to the seven points in the plot, with the first row being the lightest blue and the last row being the darkest blue.

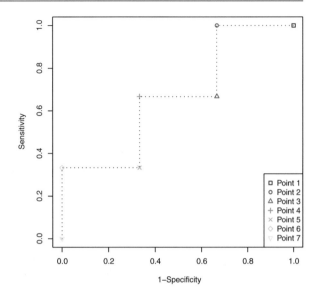

Fig. 1 The ROC based on Table 5. The point corresponding to the first row of the table is the darkest blue and the last row is the lightest blue

The ideal classifier has a FPR of zero, meaning that none of the actual negative subjects were classifiers as (false) positives. It has a TPR of 1, meaning that every actual postive patient is classified as positive. The ideal classifier would reside in the top left corner of the ROC. A completely uninformative classifier resides on a diagonal line from (0, 0) to (1, 1) with an AUC of 0.5.

Interpretation of the ROC. Figure 2 depicts two classifiers, Model 1 and 2, built on the same data set, having the same AUC of 0.7, but different characteristics. The horizontal axis is (1-specificity), also known as the false positive rate, which is the proportion of false positives among the actual negatives. The vertical axis is sensitivity (also known as recall), which is the proportion of true positives among the actual positives. When the false positive rate is low (1-Specificity < 0.5), Model 1, depicted in blue, achieves higher sensitivity, than Model 2 (depicted in orange). Conversely, when the false positive rate is high, Model 2 has higher sensitivity. If the application of the modeling requires low false positive rate, then Model 1 is preferable; but if for a different application, false positives are less of a concern than false negatives, then we may prefer Model 2. For example, Model 1 is preferable as a risk model, which targets an intervention to a small portion of the population at high risk, while Model 2 would be preferable as a screening model, where the main objective is to identify as many true positives as possible.

Fig. 2 Comparing the ROCs for two models built on the same data set that achieve the same AUC (of 0.7) but have different characteristics

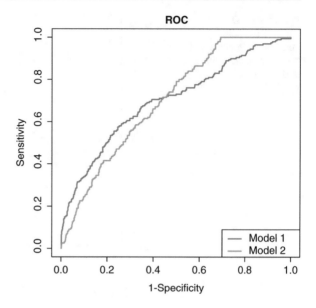

In addition, the following **probabilistic relationships are valid interpretations of the AUC ROC**:

- The probability that a random positive case is ranked before a random negative case. (= probability that a random pair with one positive and one negative case are ranked correctly).
- The proportion of positives ranked before a random negative case.
- The proportion of negatives ranked after a random positive case.
- The expected true positive rate if the ranking is split just before a random negative case.
- The expected false positive rate if the ranking is split just after a uniformly drawn random positive.

Lorenz Curve

Lorenz curves [5] were originally introduced in econometrics in 1905 to depict the distribution of wealth. The horizontal axis shows the cumulative distribution of the population in increasing order of wealth and the vertical axis corresponds to the cumulative distribution of wealth. The Lorenz curve has been adapted to health sciences.

Fig. 3 Comparing the
Lorenz curves of the two
models from Fig. 2. The
two models were built on
the same data set, achieve
the same AUC (of 0.7) but
have different
characteristics

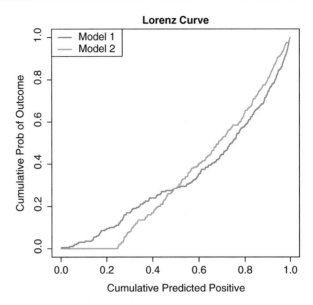

The Lorenz curve depicts classifier performance. The horizontal axis represents the cumulative distribution of observations that are predicted positives ordered in increasing order of risk and the vertical axis is the cumulative distribution of positive outcomes.

Other parameterizations of the axes are possible: patients could be ordered in decreasing order of risk and the vertical axis could represent the cumulative distribution of the missed negatives (false negatives).

Interpreting the Lorenz curve (Fig. 3). The interpretation of the Lorenz curves is more straightforward than that of an ROC. The horizontal axis corresponds to the cumulative proportion of the population classified as positive when ordered in increasing order of risk. In plain English, the value p on the horizontal axis corresponds to the $100p$ percent of patients with the lowest predicted risk. The vertical axis is sensitivity (recall). The orange line, corresponding to Model 2, shows that the 30% of the population with the lowest predicted risk (0.25 on the horizontal axis) contains no actual positives (sensitivity = 0), while the blue line (corresponding to Model 1) indicates that Model 1 included 10% of the positives. If we used 0.25 as the classification threshold, namely, subjects with predicted probability of outcome in excess of 0.25 are predicted positives, classification by Model 1 would have resulted in 10% false negatives and no false negatives by Model 2. Again, Model 2 (orange) is better at identifying low risk patients, while Model 1 (blue) is better at identifying high risk patients.

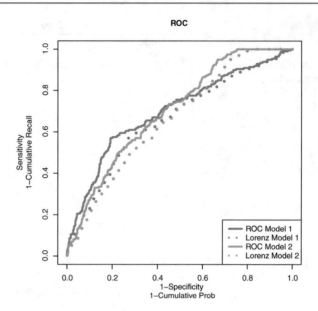

Fig. 4 Comparison of the ROCs for the two models from Fig. 2 along with the "inverted" Lorenz curves. The "inverted" Lorenz curve is "flipped" along both axes

Comparing the ROC and the Lorenz Curves

Figure 4 depicts the ROC for the two models and also the "inverted" Lorenz curve, where the Lorenz curve is "flipped" along both axes. We can see that the "inverted" Lorenz curve and the ROC are very similar. Also, the differences between the two models are also very similar regardless of which curves we use.

Lorenz curves offer two key benefits. (1) Their interpretation is more straightforward than that of ROCs. (2) The Lorenz curves are advantageous when we are interested in predictive performance on low-risk patients. Predictive performance for the high-risk patients looks very similar to the ROC, and we can thus approximately interpret the ROC as a Lorenz curve with respect to the high-risk patients.

> The Lorenz curves and the ROC contain similar information and are generally similar.

> **Best Practice 9.1.4**
> The ROC is much more commonly used than the Lorenz curve and is more familiar to many readers.

For both ROC and Lorenz curves, the uninformative model, i.e. model with AUC of 0.5, is a diagonal line from (0, 0) to (1,1). The ideal point on an ROC curve is where the false positive rate is 0 and the sensitivity is 1. This is the top left corner. The ideal point on the Lorenz curve is where the model classifies all negatives as negative without any false negatives. This point is (1-prevalence) on the horizontal axis and 0 on the vertical axis.

Another consequence of the dependence on the outcome prevalence is that Lorenz curves are only comparable within the same population (or populations with the same outcome prevalence). Generally, models are compared within the same population, so this is more of a theoretical limitation.

Precision-Recall (PR) Curve and AUC-PR
The precision-recall (PR) [6] curve plots the performance of a classifier in a way that is similar to the ROC. The horizontal axis is recall and the vertical axis is precision. Each point corresponds to a classification threshold. Recall that for classifiers that produce a score, observations with a score above the threshold are classified as positive and (at or) below the threshold as negative.

Analogously to AUC for the ROC, the PR curve also has a summary statistic, which is the area under the PR curve (AUC-PR, also known as AUPRC).

Multi-Class Classification
Confusion matrices for the multi-class classification setting with k classes (typically, k>2) will have k columns corresponding to the k predicted labels and k rows corresponding to the k actual labels [7].

A measure like accuracy can be computed in a straightforward manner, representing the proportion of subjects correctly classified.

A key disadvantage of accuracy, as we discussed earlier, is that it is affected by the prior probabilities of the classes. Cohen's kappa is a measurement of agreement between two sets of classifications (the predicted and the true in this application). Unlike accuracy, Cohen's kappa takes the agreement that arises by chance between the two classifications into agreement [7]. However, under some unbalanced conditions, it has been shown to be *incoherent*, assigning better score to the worse classifier [8].

While additional metrics that are specific to multi-class classification exist (e.g. Matthews Correlation Coefficient; MCC [8]), in the followings, we focus on general strategies to convert the evaluation of multi-class classification into a sequence of binary classifications. This strategy has the advantage that it can be used with virtually all of the above measures.

> In a multi-class classification problem with k classes, the computation of most performance measures requires that the multi-class problem is broken down into a series of binary classifications following one of two main strategies, One-Vs-One or One-vs-All.

These strategies perform a sequence of evaluations. In the One-Vs-One strategy, each evaluation corresponds to a pair of class labels, measuring the model's ability to classify one of these two classes versus the other. One evaluation is carried out for all pairs of classes. In the One-Vs-All strategy, each evaluation measures the model's ability to classify one class versus all other classes [9].

The binary classification metrics are computed for each comparison and are averaged. For example, computing the precision of a k-class classification model using the One-vs-All strategy will initially result in k precision values which are later averaged. Averaging can be done by computing the arithmetic mean of the k performance metrics or by computing the weighted average of these metrics, where the weight is proportional to the number of instances belonging to the class.

To incorporate the cost of misclassification, the multi-class confusion matrix can be element-wise multiplied by a k-by-k weight matrix, where each cell contains the weight associated with the misclassification cost.

Model Performance Measures for Continuous Outcomes

> Measures of predictive model performance for continuous outcomes fall into two groups: those that examine the residuals (difference between the prediction and the actual value) and aggregate them into an overall value; and (2) metrics that measure how well the prediction covaries with the actual value.

The first group is (somewhat) analogous to the misclassification-based measures, while the second group is analogous to concordance in classification [10]. We explore these two groups in the following two sections.

Residual Based Metrics

Let $\hat{y}_i$ denote the prediction from a model and let y_i denote the actual value. The **squared residual** (squared error; SE) is defined as

$$r_i^2 = \left(\hat{y}_i - y_i\right)^2 .$$

Because of the square, large residuals contribute disproportionately (quadratically) large errors. The **absolute error** (absolute deviation) is defined as the absolute value of the residual $|r_i| = \left|\hat{y}_i - y_i\right|$ and all residuals have a proportionate contribution. In some cases, it is useful to make the error proportional to the amplitude of the prediction, so that the same deviation contributes less error if the predicted value is higher. The **Pearson residual** is defined as

$$r_{pearson} = \frac{\left(\hat{y}_i - y_i\right)^2}{\hat{y}_i}$$

Based on these residuals, we can define the following commonly used metrics (Table 6).

Variations of these measures are also in use. For example, sum squared error (SSE) is $N \times MSE$, and root mean squared error (RMSE) is $\sqrt{MSE}$.

Concordance-Analogue Metrics

The next set of metrics measure how well the predictions co-vary with the actual values.

The most fundamental such metric is R^2 and it measures linear correlation between the predicted and actual values

$$R^2 = 1 - \frac{MSE}{\frac{1}{N}\Sigma_i \left(\hat{y}_i - \bar{y}\right)^2}$$

An R^2 of 0 indicates random prediction while an R^2 of 1 indicates that the prediction is perfectly (positively) correlated with the actual value.

Ideally, R^2 is computed on a validation set. When no validation set is available, R^2 can be adjusted for model complexity, penalizing large numbers of predictors relative to the number of observations. The adjusted R^2 is defined as

Table 6 Common residual-based measures for predictive model performance for continuous outcomes

Mean Squared Error (MSE)	$\frac{1}{N}\sum_i r_i^2$
Mean Absolute Error (MAE)	$\frac{1}{N}\sum_i |r_i|$
Median Absolute Deviation (MAD)	$\text{median}_i \, |r_i|$
Mean Pearson Residual	$\frac{1}{N}\sum_i |r_{pearson,i}|$

$$R_{adj}^2 = 1 - \frac{(1-R^2)(N-1)}{N-K-1}$$

where N denotes the number of observations and K the number of predictors.

The main drawback of R^2 is that it measures a linear relationship. When linearity is undesirable, Spearman correlation can be used instead.

Example 9.1.2
[Influence of outliers in Gaussian data.]

In the absence of outliers and extreme values (that are highly unlikely under the model), the relationship between the predicted values and the actual values can be assumed linear when the data generating process is approximately Gaussian. However, outliers introduce outsized residuals and possibly quadratically disproportionate errors (if we are using squared errors), breaking the linear relationship between predicted and actual values. In this example, we study how the outliers influence various metrics.

Using an arbitrary known linear function $f(x)$ we generated predictor x and outcome y pairs with standard normal noise added: $y \sim f(x) + \varepsilon$, $\varepsilon \sim Normal(0, \sigma)$. We used the true generating function as the "model". We then mixed in 0, 1, 5 and 10% outliers. For the outliers, their "predicted" value is the prediction from the "model" $f(x)$ and their actual value is the 99.9th quantile of the possible predicted values under the "model" given the predictors, that is the 99.9th percentile of $Normal(f(x), \sigma)$. We evaluated the predictions using the above metrics and summarized the results in the Table 7 below.

The interpretation of the table is as follows. If we use the true "model" on a test set without outliers, it achieves an MSE (second row) of 0.933 (second column), but if we add 1% outliers to the test data sets, the apparent MSE of the model increases to 1.019 (column 3). This 9% difference is solely due to outliers and does not actually reflect a difference in the goodness of the model: the model is the same true data generating model but evaluated on a data set that contains outliers.

Table 7 Example 9.1.2—Influence of outliers in Gaussian data

Metric	Outlier percent			
	0%	1%	5%	10%
MSE	0.933	1.019	1.344	1.716
MAE	0.773	0.796	0.884	0.984
MAD	0.676	0.679	0.708	0.744
Pearson	0.018	0.181	0.236	8.563
R^2	0.575	0.598	0.647	0.685
Spearman	0.662	0.649	0.618	0.589

As expected, with increasing outliers, the apparent model performance decreases the most when we use MSE as the evaluation metric. Adding 1% outliers increases the MSE by 9%, adding 5% outliers by 44% and adding 10% outliers increases the MSE by 84%. In comparison, when we used MAE as the evaluation metric, the corresponding changes were 3%, 14.3% and 27.2%; and when we used MAD, the difference further decreased to 0%, 4.6% and 9.9%. MAE and MAD are indeed more robust in face of outliers.

The use of the Pearson residual is not ideal for Gaussian data. It utilizes squared error (it is sensitive to outliers) and is normalized by the prediction. If an outlier has an expected value close to 0, the Pearson residual can become very large, because a large squared residual is divided by a value close to 0.

The R^2 statistic indicates *better* model performance in the presence of outliers than in their absence. This is merely a coincidence. The outliers are chosen to be incongruent with the data generation process, so we should not see an improvement in the model performance.

The Spearman correlation became worse in the presence of outliers, showing a decrease of 2, 6.7 and 11.1%.

Best Practice 9.1.6
All of these measures are appropriate for Gaussian data.

Best Practice 9.1.7
MSE is more sensitive to outliers than MAD.

Pitfall 9.1.4
Pearson residual is sensitive to small predictive values.

Example 9.1.3
[Non-gaussian Data]

Another assumption that many of the residuals and the R^2 statistic makes is homoscedasticity: the variance of an observation is constant across the observations. This assumption does not hold for many exponential family distributions, including the Poisson distribution which we often use to model counts.

Given predictors x, and a generating function f, in this example, we generated Poisson outcomes y as $y \sim \text{Poisson}(\lambda = f(x))$. To this data, we fitted an ordinary

Fig. 5 Comparison of three common types of residuals plotted against the log of the true value

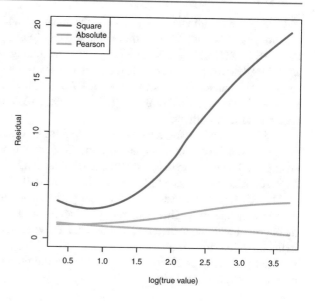

least-square (OLS) regression model and a Poisson model. We also generated an independent test set and evaluated the two models on this test set using the above metrics.

Figure 5 shows a smoothed plot of the residuals of the test set against the log of the true value for three commonly used residuals: square, absolute and Pearson. We can see that both the squared and the absolute residuals increase as the true value y increases. This suggests that in the evaluation, observations with large true values have an outsized impact. Note, that this not large *errors* having an outside impact; this is large *true values* having an outsized impact. In contrast, the Pearson residual remains mostly flat, because the residual is normalized with respect to the predicted value. This suggests that no particular range of the true outcome has an outsized impact. As a side note, notice that the log (true value) starts at 0.5 and thus the predicted values are ~1.5. If the predicted values were close to 0, dividing by the predicted value could create unduly large Pearson residuals (as we saw in the previous example).

In Gaussian regression, observations are assumed homoscedastic: all observations are assumed to have the same variance. In contrast, when we model counts, the variance of the observations is related to their predicted values: the variance of the Poisson distribution is the same as its mean. Therefore, higher predicted values have higher variance. The Pearson residual is the squared residual divided by the variance, thus it is the square of the residual measured in standard deviations.

Pitfall 9.1.5

When the outcome is not homoscedastic, some ranges of the outcome value (larger values) can dominate the evaluation.

Best Practice 9.1.8
When evaluating predictive model with continuous outcomes that are heteroscedastic, consider using a residual that normalizes the expected variance (such as the Pearson residual for counts) or at least for the predicted value.

Pitfall 9.1.6
R^2 is designed to measure the linear correlation between the predicted and actual values. When this is not linear, R^2 is inappropriate.

Best Practice 9.1.9
When the relationship between the predicted and actual values is not linear, consider using a rank-based measure such as Spearman or Kendall correlation.

Time-to-Event Outcomes

The evaluation of time-to-event models differs from the evaluation of models for categorical or continuous outcomes in two ways. First, the outcome is time-dependent: the state of the outcome changes over time. A subject without an event at the beginning of the follow-up period may develop an event over time. Second, the outcome is not observable for censored patients.

The prediction from the time-to-even model can also differ. Some predictions are time dependent (e.g. survival probability or cumulative hazard), while other predictions are not (e.g. (log) risk score from a Cox proportional hazards model). Time-dependent and independent predictions require different evaluation methods.

Several factors complicate the evaluation of time-to-event models: (1) the true outcome is time dependent, (2) the prediction itself can be time-dependent, and (3) subject may be lost to follow-up.

Time-independent predictions can be transformed into time-dependent predictions and vice versa.

For example, a time independent measure, specifically the risk score, can be converted into a time-dependent measure by multiplying it with a (time-dependent) baseline hazard. When a software package (e.g. a deep learning package) only provides risk scores, a Cox model can be fit with the risk score as the sole independent variable to obtain the baseline hazard function. With the baseline hazard function in hand, survival probabilities can be computed. Conversely, a time dependent measure can be converted into "time-independent" by taking its value at a single clinically relevant time point. Alternatively, the time-dependent measure can be integrated over time [1].

Survival Concordance. This is an extension of the concordance measure (C-statistic) to time-to-event outcomes.

> The C-statistic is the probability that in a randomly selected pair of patients, where one had an event earlier than the other had the event or got censored, the one with the event has a shorter predicted time to event.

Several versions of the C-statistic for time-to-event models exist, chiefly differing in the way they address censoring.

The most commonly used C-statistic is Harrell's C. The scikit documentation [11] and the vignette for the random survival forest R package [12] provide an exact algorithm for the respective implementations. Harrell's C has been shown to depend on the censoring distribution of the training data and to be biased when the proportion of censored subjects is high (~50% or above). Uno's C statistic [13] addresses this issue by using inverse probability of censoring weighting.

Measures based on prediction error: IAE, ISE, Brier Score, and IBS. When the prediction from the time-to-event model is a (time-dependent) survival probability, the **prediction error** at the time can be computed as

$$PE(t)_i = \widehat{S(t)}_i - S(t)_i,$$

where $\widehat{S(t)}_i$ is the predicted survival probability of subject i at time t and $S(t)_i$ is the actual survival curve for subject i; or as

$$PE(t)_i = \widehat{S(t)}_i - \delta(t)_i,$$

where $\delta(t)_i$ is the disease status of subject i at time t. Using the prediction error as a residual in conjunction with a loss function (such as absolute error or squared error) and integrating it over time yields **the Integrated Absolute Error** (IAE), $\int |PE(t)_i| \, dt$, which uses the absolute prediction error, and similarly, **the Integrated Squared Error** (ISE), $\int PE(t)_i^2 \, dt$, which uses the squared prediction error.

To address censoring, the individual time points can be weighted by the inverse propensity of censoring. The **Brier Score**, at a time point t, is essentially an inverse propensity of censoring weighted squared prediction error

$$BS(t) = \frac{1}{N} \sum_i \left(S(t)_i^2 \, \delta(t)_i \, G(t)^{-1} + \left(1 - \hat{S}(t)_i\right)^2 \, I_{T_i > t} G(t)^{-1} \right),$$

where T_i is the time of event for subject i, $G(t)$ is the propensity of censoring as estimated through a Kaplan-Meier estimator [12]. The BS can be integrated over time to obtain the Integrated Brier Score (IBS), which is no longer time-dependent.

Time-dependent ROC and iAUROC. ROCs are useful tools for evaluating classifiers. The time-dependent ROC analysis views time-to-event modeling as a sequence of binary classification tasks evaluated either at a single clinically meaningful time point or at multiple time points. For this analysis, at a time point t, the prediction from the time-to-event model needs to be converted into a classification outcome. Heagerty and Zheng [14] have proposed three main strategies: cumulative/dynamic (C/D), incident/dynamic (I/D), and incident/static (I/S) that chiefly differ in the definition of a case, a control and the risk set. In case of C/D, at a time t, a case is a subject with an event time < = t (but after time 0), a control is a subject with follow-up up to t and no event, and the risk set consists of all cases and controls. This is "cumulative" because patients with events accumulate and is "dynamic" because the risk set depends on t. The I/D strategy defines a case as a patient who suffered an event exactly at time t; and defines controls as subjects remaining event-free at time t. This strategy excludes patients who developed an event before t. Finally, the I/S strategy defines cases identically to I/D but the risk set is static; it consists of all patients present at a separate time point t*, the time point when the cohort is defined.

Based on the definitions of cases/controls, the specificity and sensitivity can be computed, the ROC curve can be drawn, and the AUC can be computed.

Similarly to C-statistic, the sensitivity in the AUC computation can be weighed by the inverse propensity of censoring to make the estimates more robust in face of censoring. The AUC values at different time points can be integrated over a preselected set of time points to obtain the integrated AUROC or (iAUROC).

Best Practice 9.1.10
The most common evaluation metric of a time-to-event model is Harell's C statistic (survival concordance) [13].

Pitfall 9.1.7
When a model produces time-dependent predictions, these need to be summarized into a single value before the C statistic can be computed.

Best Practice 9.1.11
Time-dependent predictions can be summarized into a single value as (1) survival probability at the end of the study, (2) survival probability at the median survival time, (3) or survival probability at some clinically relevant time.

> **Best Practice 9.1.12**
> If an ROC is desired, time-to-event prediction can be converted into classification outcomes at a specific (clinically relevant) time point using the C/D strategy to plot the ROC.

Calibration

Discrimination tells us how well the model can rank patients on their risk of outcome. Calibration tells us complementary information [2, 3, 15, 16].

> Calibration tells us how reliable the estimates are in different ranges of the predicted risk of outcome.

> There are four types of calibrations: mean, weak, moderate and strong, satisfying increasingly stringent criteria.

Mean calibration, also known as **calibration-in-the-large**, simply ascertains that the mean of the predicted risk of outcome coincides with the mean observed outcome in the sample. Many algorithms, including regression models, guarantee mean calibration in the development sample, thus discrimination is more important. On the other hand, in an external sample, the model may not be mean-calibrated.

Weak calibration assures that the model does not provide overly small or large predictions (relative to the actual incidence or prevalence) or that the model is not too close to the mean event rate (or prevalence). The principal tool for weak calibration is the calibration model, which is a regression model, regressing the observed outcome on the predicted risk. For continuous outcomes, the **calibration model** takes the form

$$y \sim \beta_0 + \beta_y \hat{y}$$

where $\hat{y}$ is the prediction from the model, β_0 is the **calibration intercept** and β_y is the **calibration slope**. In a well-calibrated model, the slope is 1 and the intercept is 0.

When the outcome is binary, Cox's method is used, where the calibration model takes the form of

$$\text{logit}(y)\beta_0 + \beta_y \text{logit}\left(\hat{y}\right) + \text{offset}(\text{logit}\left(\hat{y}\right))$$

Weak calibration suffers from several shortcomings.

Pitfall 9.1.8
Weak calibration can only detect miscalibrations that are affine, involving a shift or a scale.

Pitfall 9.1.9
A model, that is well calibrated by the weak calibration criterion, does not guarantee to be well calibrated in all regions of the predicted outcome.

Hosmer-Lemeshow test. Both of these limitations stem from the fact that the calibration model is a (generalized) linear model. The ***Hosmer-Lemeshow* test** has been proposed to overcome these limitations. It performs a chi-square test comparing the sum predicted probability of outcome with the sum of the events in the 10 deciles of the predicted probability range. The test has 8 degrees of freedom internally and 9 externally. The chi-square test does not rely on the linearity assumption, however, it is not powerful and requires a certain minimum sample size.

Moderate calibration checks whether the model is unbiased over the entire range of the predicted probabilities. Typically, a flexible calibration curve, such as local polynomial regression (loess), is used to model the observed outcome as a function of the predicted risk. Figure 6 shows the calibration curve of a model on a hypothetical data set.

Fig. 6 Calibration curve of a model

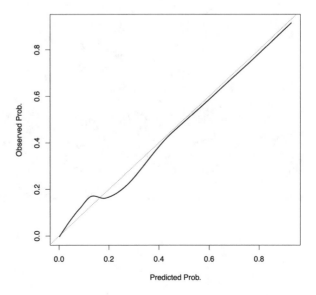

In the figure, the horizontal axis corresponds to the predicted probabilities of the outcome and the vertical axis to the observed probabilities. The diagonal dashed line represents a perfectly calibrated model, one where the predicted and observed probabilities always coincide. The model slightly underestimates the risk when the predicted probability is between 10 and 20% and slightly overestimates the risk when the predicted probability is between 20 and 40%.

It may be desirable to summarize the calibration curve into a single number. Let $\hat{y}$ denote the probability of outcome predicted by the model, y_c denote the smoothed observed probability of outcome (when the predicted probability is y) and $f()$ the density of $\hat{y}$. The **Integrated Calibration Index (ICI)** is defined as

$$\int |\hat{y} - y_c| f(\hat{y}) d\hat{y},$$

the absolute difference between the predicted and (smoothed) observed probability is integrated over the range of predicted probabilities weighed by the density of the predicted probability.

Another summary statistic of the calibration curve is **Harrell's E**. Harrell's E(q) is the qth quantile of the $|\hat{y} - y_c|$ distribution. For example, E50 is the median difference between the predicted and (smoothed) observed probabilities of outcome.

Pitfall 9.1.10
Flexible calibration curves depend on the smoothing applied to the curve.

Strong calibration ensures that the model predictions are unbiased for every possible input combination. This is often impossible to achieve in practice.

Example 9.1.4 [Weak calibration]
We created a synthetic data set with 10 predictors, 1000 observations and outcome prevalence of 20%. We first checked calibration-in-the-large. The mean predicted probability in the entire training sample was 0.199, while the mean outcome was 0.2 (p-value 0.99).

Next we checked weak calibration. The model

$$\text{logit}(y) \sim \beta_0 + \beta_y \text{logit}(\hat{y}) + \text{offset}(\text{logit}(\hat{y}))$$

yielded $\beta_o = 0.063$ (p-value 0.61) and $\beta_y = 0.063$ (p-value 0.440). With both the calibration intercept and slope being non-significant, the model is considered well-calibrated in the weak calibration sense.

Example 9.1.5 [Poorly calibrated models]
To illustrate the effect of the calibration intercept and slope, we took the above well-calibrated model and intentionally mis-calibrated it by adding +1 and − 1 to the intercept and using 1.5 and 0.5 as the slope. Figure 7 shows the resultant calibration curves. These are flexible (loess) curves.

Blue lines in Fig. 7 show curves with non-zero calibration intercept. This makes the model consistently over- or underestimate the risk over the entire range of predicted probabilities. Orange curves represent miscalibrations where the calibration slope is not 1. When it is larger than 1, the model produces more extreme estimates: it underestimates the risk in the low probability range and overestimates the risk for higher predicted risks. Conversely, when the calibration slope is less than 1, the model produces estimates that are closer to the prior probability of the outcome.

Fig. 7 Shows flexible calibration curves. The gray dashed line represents perfect calibration and the black curve is a well-calibrated model from Example 9.1.5. The blue curves are miscalibrated, the calibration intercepts are + 1 (dashed line) and − 1 (solid line). The orange curves are also miscalibrated, their calibration slopes are 0.5 (solid line) and 1.5 (dashed line)

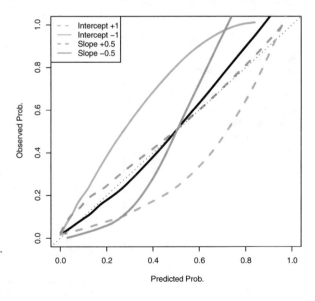

Example 9.1.6 [Sensitivity of moderate calibration to smoothing]
We created a synthetic data set with 10 predictors and 1000 observations and
fit a model to this data. We checked moderate calibration on the training data.
For the calibration curve, we used local weighted least squares smoothing
(loess) with four different smoothing parameters. Figure 8 shows the resulting
calibration curves.

In Table 8, we show the ICI, E50 and E90 for the model. These are the calibration indices of the same model; they only differ because of using a different smoothing parameter for the flexible calibration curve.

Table 8 shows the effect of varying the smoothing parameter on the Integrated
Calibration Index (ICI), Harrell's E50 and E90. These calibration indices
were calculated for the same model; they only reflect changes in the smoothing parameter. The empirical confidence interval of ICI (at smoothing of 0.7)
was computed using the data generating distribution of the outcome risk and
was 0.011 to 0.041. Thus all ICI values, regardless of the smoothing parameter, fall into the confidence interval.

Fig. 8 The calibration
curve for a single model
using different smoothing
parameters. Darker blue
indicates more smoothing;
the default value is 0.7.
The black dashed line
represents perfect
calibration

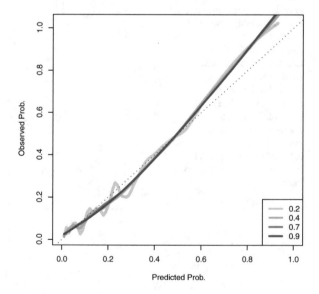

Table 8 Illustration of sensitivity to smoothing in moderate calibration. The ICI, E50 and E90 values were computed for the same model using four different smoothing parameters

Smoothing parameter	ICI	E50	E90
0.2	0.027	0.030	0.104
0.4	0.022	0.029	0.107
0.7	0.018	0.025	0.110
0.9	0.020	0.027	0.111

Clinical Usefulness

The measures discussed in section "Evaluating Model Performance" describe how well a model can predict but give us very little information about how useful a model would be in practice.

There are two critical concerns regarding the clinical utility of a model. First, the different types of misclassification errors a model makes can have different consequences and a balance has to be struck between the benefits and the adverse consequences of using the model. Second, when the model relates to treatment (or intervention), the effectiveness of this intervention needs to be evaluated.

Weighted Specificity/Sensitivity, Weighted Precision/Recall

One consideration is that the two kinds of errors a model may make can have different consequences. In an example of a cancer screening test, false positives, patients where the test erroneously predicted a healthy patient to have cancer can have less grave consequences than false negatives, where patients with cancer are erroneously reported as being cancer-free. We have discussed weighted confusion matrices earlier in this chapter as a means for taking the different consequences of false positives and false negatives into account.

Measures Related to Effectiveness

The expectation from an intervention is that it reduces some adverse outcome or increases some beneficial outcome. Measures of effectiveness compare rates of events among treated and untreated (control) patients.

The top portion of the Table 9 shows the number of patients with an event ('Event') and without an event ('No-Event') among the treated (column 'Treated') and untreated (column 'Control').

Absolute risk is the proportion of patients in the treated (ART) or control (ARC) groups with an event. This is a dimensionless measure ranging from 0 to 1. The

Table 9 Commonly used measures of clinical effectiveness

	Treatment	Control
Event	TE	CE
No-event	TN	CN
Total (sum)	TS	CS
Absolute risk (AR)	TE/TS	CE/CS
	Absolute Risk in the treatment group (ART) = TE/TS	Absolute Risk in the control group (ARC) = CE/CS
Absolute risk reduction (ARR)	ARC-ART	
Relative Risk (RR)	ART/ARC	
Relative risk reduction (RRR)	(ARC-ART)/ARC = 1-RR	
Number need to treat (NNT)	1/ARR	
Odds ratio (OR)	$\dfrac{TE/TN}{CE/CN}$	

difference between ART and ARC is the **Absolute Risk Reduction** (ARR), which directly relates to the effectiveness of treatment in absolute terms: an ARR of 0.09 reduces the risk of event by 0.09 in the treatment group relative to the control group. However, ARR offers no information about which part of the risk scale either the treatment or the control group lies. For example, the same reduction of 0.09 can be more meaningful when ART = 0.01 and ARC = 0.10, corresponding to ten fold reduction in risk, as compared to the case when ART = 0.40 and ARC = 0.49.

Number needed to treat (NNT) is the reciprocal of ARR. The desired interpretation of NNT is the number of patients needed to receive the treatment to prevent one event that would have happened otherwise. This interpretation is attractive in clinical practice because it is absolute and in a unit that is easy to interpret (number of patients). The interpretation of NNT, however, depends on clinical context, namely, the disease prevalence and consequences of leaving the disease untreated. Therefore direct comparison of NNT is only appropriate across treatments of the same disease with respect to the same outcome.

NNT and ARR are equivalent, but NNT suffers from a number of drawbacks that ARR does not. NNT is dimensioned (number of patients) while ARR is not; the range of NNT is unbounded, while ARR is in the range of −1 to 1. When the treatment is ineffective, ARR = 0. Testing the significance of ARR is straightforward by checking whether its confidence interval contains 0. Conversely, when the treatment is ineffective, NNT has a singularity. Therefore, statistically testing whether a treatment is effective is problematic with NNT. Moreover, the range of NNT has a "hole": NNT cannot take values between −1 and 1. Computing the confidence interval of NNT is possible by inverting the upper and lower bounds of the confidence interval of ARR, but this does not yield a correct confidence interval.

Relative risk (RR) operates on the proportional scale as opposed to ARR's absolute scale. RR thus eliminates the problem of having a particular absolute difference reflect very different effectiveness when clinical risk ranges are very different, but

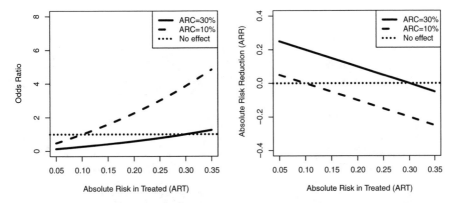

Fig. 9 Odds Ratio compared to Absolute Risk Reduction. Number of treated and control patients is fixed at 1000. ART is varied from 5% to 35% and ARC is fixed at 30% (solid line) and at 10% (dashed line). The dotted line represents ineffective treatment

introduces a similar problem: the same RR in patients with low risk could correspond to a clinically meaningless risk reduction, while the same RR in higher risk patients can be very meaningful. It is therefore recommended to report both RR and ARR.

Since the measures form two large groups, OR and measures around ARR (including RR, RRR, and NNT), in Fig. 9, we compare the behavior of OR and ARR. We simulated two datasets. Both have 1000 patients in the treatment as well as the control groups. In one data set, we fixed the number of control patients with an event at 100 (corresponding to 10% ARC) and in the other we fixed it at 300 (30% ARC). We varied the number of patients with event in the treatment group from 50 to 350 (corresponding to ART of 5–35%). More effective treatments have lower ART. The left panel depicts the odds ratio (OR) and the right panel depicts absolute risk reduction (ARR). Note, that RRR is ARR/ARC, thus with fixed ARC, RRR is just a scaled version of ARR. Similarly, NNT is the reciprocal of ARR.

OR and ARR are consistent: when OR indicates better performance for the treatment (lower OR), ARR also indicates better performance (higher ARR). The event rate in the control group creates only a shift in ARR, while it shifts as well as scales OR. The same difference between two treatment effectiveness results can appear as a numerically larger difference in OR. This has shown to have influenced treatment decision,

Measures of effectiveness fall into two groups: odds ratio (OR) and measures related to absolute risk reduction (ARR) (including RRR, RR, NNT). Both are invariant to scaling the number of treated or control patients, but OR is also invariant to scaling the number of controls (relative to the patients with events).

Pitfall 9.2.1
In case/control studies, measures of effectiveness that depend on the prior of classes, are misleading when the balance of cases to controls in the samples differs from the balance in the target population.

Best Practice 9.2.1
For case/control designs, use OR.

Relative risk (RR) and relative risk reduction (RRR) are relative measures while absolute risk reduction (ARR) and number needed to treat (NNT) are absolute.

Best Practice 9.2.2
Absolute and relative risk measures provide complementary information, so whenever possible, both should be reported.

Best Practice 9.2.3
ARR and NNT convey the same information and differ in interpretation. ARR is dimensionless, while NNT is measuresd in number of patients and is preferred in clinical practice.

Pitfall 9.2.2
The range of NTT has a "hole". This makes significance testing and constructing confidence intervals difficult.

Net Benefit

Net benefit is a measure of the clinical utility of a model, which takes into account not only the predictive ability of the model but also the potential harm the application of a model can cause in practice.

Let us consider the scenario of a screening test, where patients with positive screening result undergo a more invasive but more reliable diagnostic test, while patients with negative screening result are not considered further. The use of the screening test can cause (at least) two kinds of harm. First, false negatives, patients who have the disease but received a negative screening result, are left undiagnosed and consequently untreated, thus they have higher risk of harm from the disease. Second, false positives are patients who received a positive screening result, underwent the invasive diagnostic procedure, incurring the risk of adverse events associated with the diagnostic test, and were found disease free. Harm from diagnostic procedure can include avoidable stress, infection, or sepsis. Relative to applying the diagnostic test to every patient, using a screening test can reduce the number of patients who undergo the diagnostic test and thus reduces the harm associated with the diagnostic test, but increases the risk of leaving the disease undiagnosed (in false negative patients) and thus increases the risk of harm associated with the undiagnosed disease. The **net benefit** is defined as

$$\mathrm{Net\,Benefit} = \frac{TP}{N} - w\frac{FP}{N},$$

where N is the total number of patients, TP and FP denote the (number of) true and false positives, respectively, and w is a weighing factor representing the tradeoff between the harm caused by false positives and false negatives. The weighing factor is determined by expert opinion, by physician-patient joint decision making, or by cost analysis.

Interpretation. The interpretation of net benefit is the increase in TP as a proportion of the population (or sample) after accounting for the risk of harm both from false positives and false negatives.

Example 9.2.1 [Net benefit]
Consider a population of 1000 patients and a disease with 20% prevalence. There are 200 patients with the disease and 800 without. Further, consider a screening test that reported a positive result for 500 patients and 160 of them were true positives (and 340 were false positives). There are 40 false negatives. A second test would report a positive result for 400 patients, 150 of them true positives and 250 false positives, yielding 50 false negatives.

The second test has 10 more false negatives than the first test but it has 90 fewer false positives. Suppose false negatives are very dangerous and false positives are trivial, say false negatives are 20 times more costly than false positives, then the net benefit of the first test is TP/N−w FP/N = 160/1000−1/20 * 340/1000 = 0.143. This is higher than the net benefit of the second test, which is 150/1000−1/20 * 250/1000 = 0.1375. Conversely, suppose that the screening test is repeated annually and the disease takes years to progress. In that case, the risk of false negatives can still be higher than the risk of false positives, but to lesser extent than in the previous example, say false negatives are "only" five times as costly as false positives. In that case, the net benefit of the first test is 160/1000−1/5*340/100 = 0.092, which is lower than the net benefit of the second test, which is 150/1000−1/5*250/100 = 0.10.

Decision Curve

Consider a screening test which yields a probability of outcome. To obtain a positive/negative classification, the probability is dichotomized using a threshold p: patients with predicted probability of disease above p are positive and undergo the diagnostic procedure, while patients with predicted probability of disease with less than (or equal to) p are declared free of disease and are not considered further. As we have already seen in this chapter, the choice of threshold p influences the predicted positives, TP and FP, thus it influences net benefit. In other words, a net benefit value can be computed for each possible (and reasonable) threshold p and FP-FN tradeoff w.

The threshold p and w are related. Consider a threshold, slightly higher than p. Without loss of generality, assume that reducing this threshold to p increases the number of predicted positives by one patient. If the model is well calibrated, then this patient has probability p of being a case (actual positive) and 1-p of being a control (actual negative). If the patient is an actual positive, then the number of true positives increased by one (with probability p). If the patient is an actual negative, then the number of false positives increased by one (with probability $(1-p)$). At equilibrium,

$$\frac{TP}{N} - w\frac{FP}{N} = p - w(1-p) = 0$$

yielding the relationships between p and w

$$w = \frac{p}{1-p} \quad \text{and} \quad p = \frac{w}{1+w}$$

When the output from a predictive model needs to be thresholded into a clinical decision, (a) net benefit depends on this threshold and (b) the threshold can be computed based on the assumed ratio of harm caused by the two kinds of misclassifications, false negatives and false positives.

Example 9.2.2

Returning to the net benefit example, if the first test results in probabilities, and we believe that the consequence of false negatives is 20 times worse than that of false positives, then $w = 1/20$, and we should set the classification threshold to $p = w/(1 + w) = 1/21$.

Decision curves plot the net benefit as a function of p along with two default policies, Treat All and Treat None.

Figure 10 shows a decision curve for a hypothetical screening model.

The horizontal axis corresponds to the classification threshold p, and the vertical axis is the net benefit. The three lines represents three policies. The blue solid line represents the policy of interest, which is based on a machine learnt model. The model estimates the probability of outcome in each patient. Patients with probability above the threshold receive the invasive diagnostic test ("treatment"), those below do not. The other two models are two default policies. The horizontal black line is the "Treat none" policy, where no patient is given the diagnostic test, while orange dashed line represents the "Treat all" policy where every patient is given the invasive diagnostic test ("treatment").

Since net benefit measures the true positives treated under a policy as a proportion of the entire sample minus the risk of harm, the "Treat None" policy yields no true positives treated nor does it cause harm from treatment, since nobody is treated. The orange line represents the "Treat All" policy. Since we treat everyone, one would not expect the net benefit to depend on the threshold, however, the threshold is determined by the ratio of harm caused by false positives versus false negatives, denoted by w in earlier sections. Net benefit does depend on w. When the threshold is 0, $p = 0$, we assume that the treatment causes no harm $w = p/(1-p) = 0$, and thus the net benefit is the prevalence of disease in the sample. When the threshold is the prevalence of disease, 0.2 in this example, $w = 0.2/0.8 = \frac{1}{4}$, meaning that false negatives cause four times as much harm as false positives. In this case, the net benefit for the Treat All policy is TP/N - w FP/N = $p - p/(1-p) (1-p) = 0$. As the threshold

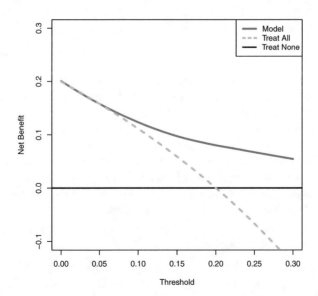

Fig. 10 Decision Curve for a hypothetical screening model. Horizontal axis denotes the classification threshold p, the vertical axis shows Net Benefit. The blue (solid) line represents the decision curve for the model, the orange (dashed) line represents the decision curve for the "Treat All" policy and the horizontal line (at 0) represents the decision curve for the "Treat None" policy

exceeds the prevalence, in other words the ratio of harm from false negatives versus false positives exceeds $p/(1-p)$, the Treat All policy has a negative net benefit.

The blue line has a similar interpretation. If we believe that the harm caused by false negatives is w times higher than the harm caused by false positives, we select $p = w/(1 + w)$ as the threshold and the net benefit can be seen in the graph. For example, when the harm caused by false negatives versus false positives is 1:4, $w = \frac{1}{4}$, $p = w/(1 + w) = 0.2$ and the net benefit is 0.80. This is substantially higher than the other two policies, both of which have net benefit of 0.

The figure shows that the model-based policy (blue line) has superior net benefit over the two default policies over the entire range of FN:FP harm ratio, and consequently, the entire range of classification thresholds.

Relationship Between Net Benefit and AUC

Figure 11 depicts the relationship between AUC and decision curves. The three panels correspond to three different disease prevalence: 10%, 20% and 40% from left to right. Each panel is a decision curve plot, analogous to Example 9.2.2, comparing three model-based policies, based on models with AUC of 0.6, 0.7, and 0.8, and two default policies: "Treat All" and "Treat None". The horizontal axis is the classification threshold p and the vertical axis is Net Benefit. Since the maximal net benefit (achievable when treating the false positives cannot cause harm) varies by the prevalence of disease, the vertical axis in the three panels use different scales, namely 0 to disease prevalence.

Generally, higher AUC results in higher Net Benefit regardless of disease prevalence.

However, even models with reasonable AUC can underperform a default policy of "Treat All". For all three prevalence, the model-based policy based on AUC of 0.6 performed worse than the "Treat All" policy. When the prevalence is low (left panel), the extent to which it underperformed (relative to the maximal achievable Net Benefit) is greater than when the prevalence is high (right panel). Similar to the "Treat All" policy, the model-based policy, even when based on a reasonable model (AUC > 0.5), can have negative net benefit. This happens when the cost of false positives is high and the predicted positives do not have sufficient true positives to compensate for the risk of harm from false positives.

Pitfall 9.2.3
Even models with reasonable AUC can underperform a default policy of "Treat All".

To further explore the relationship between Net Benefit and AUC, Net Benefit can be expressed in terms of sensitivity and specificity.

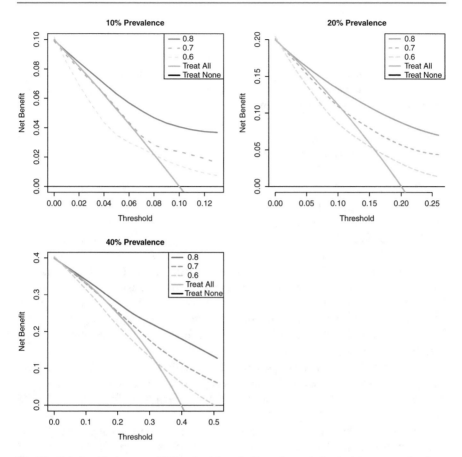

Fig. 11 Relationship between AUC and net benefit. In each panel, the decision curves for three model-based policies, based on models with AUCs of 0.6, 0.7, and 0.8, and the two default policies are plotted. The three panels represent three diseases with prevalence of 10%, 20% and 40%. Note that the scale of the vertical axis is different across the three panels

$$NB = sensitivity * prevalence - w(1 - specificity) * 1 - prevalence$$

This shows that similarly to AUC, NB is also balancing between sensitivity and 1-specificity, however it adjusts for the prevalence of the outcome and also for the ratio of harm caused by the two kinds of misclassifications (false positives and false negatives).

Key references for clinical effectives are (chapter "Regulatory Aspects and Ethical Legal Societal Implications (ELSI)" in [2], [17–20].

Health Economic Evaluation

In this section, we provide an overview of evaluating the health economic effect of a new model or intervention [21–23]. Health economic evaluations focus on evaluating health-related actions, such as new models, interventions, therapies, practices, or policies, in terms of their cost and consequences. Without loss of generality, we call these actions "interventions". Consequences include health benefits or disbenefits from the new interventions, their side effects, and effects this new intervention may have on other parts of the health system.

> Health economic evaluations aim to evaluate the health benefits and disbenefits of an intervention taking their cost into account.

Several kinds of health economic evaluations exist. **Cost effectiveness analysis** (CEA) compares interventions that relate to a single common effect that may differ in magnitude between alternative interventions. For example, two treatments of the same disease may both extend life (common effect) but to varying degrees at varying costs. Analyzing the degree of extending life as a function of costs incurred constitutes a CEA.

Although technically not a CEA, **Cost Minimization Analysis** (CMA) is related. CMAs are applicable when two treatments achieve the same outcome (to the same degree) but at different costs. In this case, the treatment with the lower cost would be chosen.

The second type of health economic analysis is **Cost Utility Analysis** (CUA). Similarly to CEAs, CUAs also compare two interventions in terms of costs and health consequences, but unlike CEAs, the health consequences of the interventions do not need to be common. Instead of a specific clinical endpoint, CUAs utilize generic measures of health gain, making the consequences comparable. This allows for the comparison of programs across different areas of health care, where a common clinical endpoint would not make sense. When a new program is implemented, often another area needs to be disinvested. CUAs also allows for accounting for health lost in the disinvested area in comparison to health gained in the new program on the same scale. Such generic measures of health include Quality-Adjusted Life Years (QALY), Disability-Adjusted Life Years (DALY), and Healthy years equivalent (HYE), which we introduce in the next section.

The final type of health economic analysis we look at is **Cost Benefit Analysis** (CBA). CBAs compare interventions, more generally, policies, in terms of their costs and consequences, where the consequence is also expressed in monetary terms. This can be useful for policy decisions, where one of the interventions is not health-related and thus a health-related consequence is inappropriate. Such analyses require quantifying the monetary value of health, which is a complex topic in its own right. In this section, we do not consider CBAs any further and focus on CUAs,

Table 10 Comparison of health economic evaluations

Type of analysis	Clinical end-points	Measure of consequence
Cost effectiveness analysis	Common across the compared interventions	A natural measure for that common clinical end-point
Cost minimization analysis	Common across the compared interventions	Interventions achieve the same consequence; they only differ in terms of cost
Cost utility analysis	Clinical end-points for the compared intervention can be the same, but does not have to be	Generic measure of health (QALY, DALY, HYE)
Cost benefit analysis	Clinical end-points for the compared intervention can be the same, but does not have to be. The end-point of some of the interventions do not even have to be clinical	Monetary value

which are the most common types of health economic evaluations, and CEAs, which are common when two treatments of the same disease are compared (Table 10).

Components of a CEA and CUA

Health economic analyses have three main components: (1) alternative interventions compared, (2) estimation of costs, and (3) estimation of benefit (consequence).

Alternative Interventions

To determine whether a new intervention is to be adopted, it needs to be compared with alternative interventions. One of the alternatives can be the current standard of care. Different alternatives can be mutually exclusive, in which case they can be compared directly. The new intervention can be used together with alternatives (adjuvant therapy), in which case comparisons can be made among combinations of treatments or sequences of treatments.

Care must be taken to include all relevant alternatives. The proposed new intervention may outperform some but not all alternatives. Many cost effectiveness measures posit that the new intervention can only be adopted if it outperforms all alternatives.

Best Practice 9.3.1
Include *all* alternative interventions in a health economic evaluation.

Estimating Costs

Estimating costs naturally includes the direct cost of the intervention. In an environment, where resources are limited, there is also an opportunity cost associated with the intervention. When resources are allocated for a particular intervention/program, other interventions/programs may have to be disinvested. These disinvested programs give up benefits, which is an opportunity cost, and it also needs to be included in the cost calculation.

> **Best Practice 9.3.2**
> Include the opportunity cost as cost of intervention/program in a health economic evaluation.

Measures of Benefit

CEAs and CUAs both measure the benefit of a new intervention in terms of health gained. CEAs use more direct clinical outcomes, while CUAs use generic measures of health. In this section, we review metrics of health.

> **Direct clinical outcomes** are very similar to clinical trial endpoints and are usually natural measures of the outcome of interest.

For example, for lipid lowering drug, the clinical endpoint could be reduction of major cardio-vascular events and a natural measure of that could be 8-year incidence of major cardio-vascular events.

A common direct clinical outcome is mortality. Several natural measurements exist for mortality including the extension of life in years (a time to event outcome) or an incidence (e.g. 8-year mortality risk).

When the clinical outcome of interest takes place in a long time frame that makes analysis impractical, an intermediate end-point and its natural measure can be used. Continuing with the lipid-lowering example, an intermediate endpoint can be cholesterol reduction achieved and its natural measure is the corresponding lab result. Another kind of intermediate measures include cases detected in a screening test, or process measures of diabetic control (such as percentage of patients with a1c measured, feet examined, etc). Intermediate measures have to be linkable to the clinical outcome of interest and the quality of these measures depends on how strongly the intermediate outcome is linked to the actual clinical outcome of interest.

> **Best Practice 9.3.3**
> Do not use intermediate end-points unless they are very strongly linked to the outcome of interest.

Health is multidimensional and the above clinical outcome measures typically capture one aspect of it: either the length of life or an aspect that relates to the disease of interest. Generic health scores have been proposed to measure multiple aspects of health simultaneously.

Health related quality of life (HRQoL) scores are generic health scores that measure a patient's health from multiple perspectives and do not concentrate on specific diseases.

A commonly used measure HRQoL is the Short Form 13 (SF-13) consisting of 13 multiple choice questions and the SF-36 consisting of 36 questions [24]. Both cover major health domains including whether health problems limit patients' daily activity, mental health problems limiting daily activity, level of pain, vitality, and how patients perceive their health. One problem with such multidimensional measures is that the different dimensions, or the answers to the 36 questions, often need to be summarized into a single value for analysis.

Another problem with the current measures is that quality of life and length of life can represent a tradeoff. For example, a cancer patient may select a treatment that offers better quality but shorter life over another treatment with longer but lower-quality life. Ideally, a health measure can capture both of these aspects of health into a single value. The solution is to adjust the life years for quality of life giving rise to the following measures.

Quality Adjusted Life Years (QALY) is a measure that weighs each remaining life year proportionally to the quality of life. The weight is determined by patient preference. QALY is a continuous valued measure, where, by convention, 0 often represents death and 1 perfect health. This is an interval measure, where 0 is arbitrary and health states worse than death can take negative values.

Disability Adjusted Life Years (DALY) weighs each remaining life year proportional to (the lack of) disabilities. Weights are determined by a committee and are fixed. DALY is a discrete measure that can only take seven different values.

Healthy Years Equivalent (HYE) creates a mapping, based on patient preferences, from years remaining to equivalent years of completely healthy life. The mapping can be determined, for example, by using a series of questions asking the patients whether they prefer y years ($y > 1$) in their current health or 1 year completely healthy life. When the patients are indifferent, that is the equivalence point.

Generic measure of health that summarize a patient's health into a unidimensional measure include QALY, DALY, and HYE.

Decision Making Using CEA and CUA

Once alternative treatments are identified, associated costs are estimated and a measure of benefit is selected, we now continue to describe how these can be used for decision making.

Consider two treatment alternatives, A and B; B is the new treatment and A is an alternative treatment such as the current standard of care.

Incremental cost Δ_C is the difference in cost between A and B. It includes the additional acquisition cost of B (vs A) and any and all additional opportunity costs. The incremental cost is not necessarily positive: the new treatment can save cost or even an expensive new pharmaceutical may lower opportunity costs. **Incremental health benefit** Δ_h is the difference in health outcomes between A and B. If health benefit is measured in QALYs, this represents the extra QALYs achieved by using B over A.

Incremental cost effectiveness ratio (ICER) is the ratio Δ_c/Δ_h, which quantifies the cost increase (Δ_c) incurred to achieve a unit health gain (e.g. 1 QALY).

A treatment is deemed **cost effective** if ICER $< k$, where k is the cost-effectiveness threshold. The cost effectiveness threshold means that diverting k units of health care resources from other parts of the healthcare system to the new intervention is expected to displace 1 QALY of health elsewhere in the health system.

Example 9.3.1 [Cost effectiveness]
Suppose treatment B has an incremental cost of \$20,000 and an incremental benefit of 2 QALYs. When the cost effectiveness threshold k is \$20,000/ QALY, we expect to lose 1 QALY in the health system per every \$20,000. Therefore, using treatment B at the incremental cost of \$20,000, we expected to lose 1 QALY elsewhere in the health system. Now, B also provides us health benefits. The incremental health benefit Δ_h from treatment B is 2 QALY; while the health disbenefit lost in the system is $\Delta_c/k = \$20,000/\$20,000$ QALY = 1 QALY. Thus, the incremental net health benefit is 1 QALY, which is positive, thus the treatment B is considered cost effective.

There are three equivalent criteria for cost effectiveness:

- ICER < cost-effectiveness threshold: $\dfrac{\Delta_c}{\Delta_h} < k$
- Incremental net health benefit is positive: $\Delta_h - \dfrac{\Delta_c}{k} > 0$
- Incremental net monetary benefit is positive: $\Delta_h k - \Delta_c > 0$.

The first criterion is the definition of cost effectiveness: cost effectiveness, that is cost per unit health gained, needs to be less than a threshold k.

The second criterion examines cost effectiveness from the perspective of health gained. The incremental health benefit Δ_h from the new treatment is larger than the health we lose in other parts of the health system (Δ_c/k) due to diverting Δ_c cost to treatment B.

The third criterion looks at cost effectiveness from a cost perspective. It would cost $\Delta_h k$ dollars to achieve the same health benefit (Δ_h) that treatment B offers at the cost of Δ_c. If the cost through treatment B is lower, then treatment B is cost effective.

Cost Effectiveness Analysis Example

In this section, we present an illustration of how the health economic impact of a machine learned model can be evaluated. The example is adopted from [22] with the author's permission.

Epithelial ovarian cancer has the highest mortality rate among cancers. 20–30% of the patients do not respond to the standard treatment of cytoreductive surgery and platinum-based chemotherapy, and even in patients with an initial response, 80% will recur and develop drug resistant disease. Against this background, novel, targeted therapy agents, such as Bevacizumab, have been developed. Earlier studies found Bevacizumab to dominate (be more effective at a lower cost) the standard treatment.

A ML model based on genetic biomarkers and clinical outcomes, was developed to provide progression-free survival (PFS) benefit estimates for patients on Bevacizumab therapy. Based on the predicted PFS probabilities, patients were categorized into three groups: (1) 40% of the patients without statistically significant PFS gain (1.28 ± 1.45 months), (2) 40% with medium gain (5.79 ± 2.12 months), and (3) 20% with the highest FPS gain (9.95 ± 1.53 months).

Three therapeutic strategies are compared. First, is the platinum-based chemotherapy, the current standard of care at the time of the writing. Second, Bevacizumab therapy added to the current standard for all patients (universal). Third, Bevacizumab therapy is added to the current standard for only the 20% patients who are predicted to benefit the most.

Strategy	Incremental cost	Incremental health benefit	ICER
Baseline	–	–	–
Universal application	$60 k for bevacizumab = $3B per year	4.818 months = 2 quality adjusted months	$360 k
ML-guided application	$2 k for test for all patients $60 k for bevacizumab × for 20% of patients = $700 M per year	9.95 months = 4.13 quality adjusted months	$203 k

Assumptions. The genetic test for the ML-based signature costs $2k per patient. The Bevacizumab therapy costs $60k, including acquisition, administrative and adverse events-related costs. The quality of life adjustment is assumed to be the same across the three strategies and is taken from [23]. Last, we assume 50k patients per year.

Universal application. Bevacizumab is given to all patients, thus no testing is required. It is given in addition to the baseline treatment, thus the incremental cost is $60k per patients, equaling $3B. On average, patients gain additional 4.818 months (=2 quality adjusted months) of life relative to the standard care, yielding an incremental health benefit of 50 k × 2 = 100k quality adjusted life months = 8.3k QALY. The incremental cost effectiveness ratio (ICER) is $3B/ (8.3k QALY) = $360k per QALY.

ML-guided application. Bevacizumab is given only to the 20% patients in the highest benefit group. The genetic test needs to be applied to all patients and then 20% of the patients (10k patients) receive the Bevacizumab therapy on top of the standard care. This leads to an incremental cost of 50k × $2k for testing and 10k × $60k for the Bevacizumab therapy, $700M in total. The patients who received this therapy experience a health benefit of 9.95 months = 4.13 quality-adjusted months on average yielding an incremental health benefit of 10k × 4.13 × 12 = 3.44k QALY. The ICER is $700M/ (3.44 QALY) = $203k per QALY.

Although the Universal application yields a higher incremental health benefit (8.3k vs 4.13k QALY) it does so at a disproportionately higher cost ($3B vs $700M), leading to a higher ICER.

The impact of model performance. The increased effectiveness of the ML-guided application stems from the ML model's ability to correctly identify patients who benefit from the Bevacizumab treatment. A ML model with lower performance could select patients with lower benefit, yielding a lower incremental health benefit at the same incremental cost (same number of patients treated), reducing the ICER, possibly rendering the treatment ineffective. If a priori known, the institution's willing-to-pay threshold (highest ICER they are willing to pay for) can be used to determine the minimal necessary model performance.

Calibration. The main responsibility of the model is to distinguish between the 20% and the bottom 80% benefit groups. The implication is that among models with similar discrimination, we prefer models that are better calibrated at the higher end over those better calibrated at the lower end of the estimated probability progression-free survival scale.

Estimators of Model Performance

Recall from chapter "Data Design" that modeling is inference, where a model is constructed on a discovery sample, and we wish to use it in the target population. To determine whether the model is suitable for use in the target population, we have to estimate its performance in the target population using the discovery sample. In this chapter, we present several methods to achieve this.

The term **estimator** refers to the method we apply to estimate the performance of a model. We compare estimators by assessing how well and how consistently they can estimate the model performance. **Bias** is the difference between the model performance estimated from the discovery sample and the model performance in the (entire) target population. **Variance** is the variability of the performance estimate across multiple discovery samples. Specifically, if we were to repeat the analytic process using different discovery samples, build a model on each sample, and apply the estimator to compute the performance of the model, we would obtain multiple estimates of the model's performance. Variance of the estimator is the variance of these performance estimates.

> The goal of performance estimation is to infer the performance of a model in the target population based the discovery sample. The method used to estimate the model performance is referred to as an *estimator*.

Using the Plug-In Estimator is Generally a Bad Idea

The simplest method is to build a model on the entire discovery sample, measure the model's performance on the same discovery sample and use this estimate as a "plug-in" estimate for the target population. This estimate is also known as the **resubstitution** estimate, or resubstitution error for error estimates.

From a very large population, a sample of 10, 20, …, 2000 patients were drawn as a discovery sample. On this discovery sample a model (with 10 parameters) was constructed and was evaluated on the same discovery sample. Then the performance of this model was evaluated in the original population and compared to the estimated performance. Figure 12 shows the estimated performance (blue line) and the actual performance (orange line) as a function of the size of the discovery sample.

For all sample sizes, the performance estimate is optimistic; for small sample sizes, it is excessively optimistic. For small sample sizes, the performance estimate has no variability, it is always 1. When the sample size becomes large, the performance is estimated reasonably correctly. Unfortunately, the sample size that is "sufficiently large" is not known a priori, it depends on the number of parameters in the

Fig. 12 Performance of a model estimated from discovery samples of various sizes compared to its actual performance on the target population.

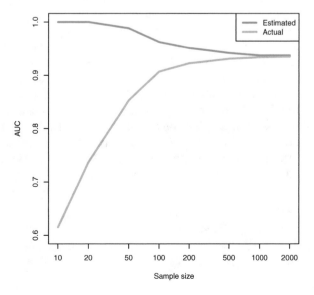

model and also on the data itself: when predictors have high collinearity, a much larger sample size is required, as compared to independent predictors.

> **Pitfall 9.4.1**
> Do not use the plug-in estimator. Its estimate is always optimistic, sometimes excessively so.

The use of the plug-in estimator for estimating the performance of models is not recommended at any sample size. When the sample size is small, the plug-in estimate has the apparent advantage of using all samples to build the model, but the performance estimates can be arbitrarily biased. When the sample size is large, the plug-in estimate has the apparent advantage of building only one model (which can be costly at large sample sizes), but other estimators, e.g. the Leave-out estimate, also builds only one model but gives a less biased performance estimate.

Internal Validation

We will discuss problems with model fitting in chapter "Overfitting, Underfitting and General Model Overconfidence and Under-Performance: Pitfalls and Best Practices in Machine Learning and AI" in greater detail, but for the current discussion, we consider two problems: underfitting and overfitting. A model is *underfitting* the data if the model fails to capture all available signal from the training data. This generally happens, when the model has insufficient complexity. Conversely, a model is *overfitting* the data, if the model also fitted to the noise in the data. This typically happens when the model complexity is too high.

Overfitting can be detected if a second sample from the same population is available. The first sample, which was used to develop the model is called the **training sample** (or **development sample**), while the second sample is referred to as the **validation sample** (or **test sample**). When a model is overfitting, its performance on the training sample will be higher than on the test sample. The purpose of **validation** is to ensure that the model performance estimated from the training sample remains similar in the population. If this is true, the model is said to **generalize** to that population. If this population is the accessible population, the validation is an **internal validation**; otherwise, it is **external validation**. In this section, we focus on model performance estimators utilizing internal validation and in the next section, we dive into the different kinds of validations a little deeper.

> In internal validation, the goal is to verify that the model developed on the discovery sample generalizes to the accessible population.

Leave Out Validation

In leave-out-validation, a randomly selected portion of the discovery sample, a **validation sample**, is put aside, *left out* from training. The discovery sample is thus randomly divided into a training sample and a validation sample, implying that the training sample and the validation sample are two independent random samples from the accessible population. As long as the accessible population can be viewed as a random sample of the target population, the training and test samples are two independent samples of the target population. Thus the performance of a model on the validation sample will be representative of its performance on the target population.

> In leave out validation, the discovery sample is divided into a training sample for model development and a validation sample for model evaluation.

For successful validation we have to pay attention to two details: the definition of the sampling unit and the size of the validation sample relative to the discovery sample.

Sampling unit. The discovery sample is a random sample from the accessible population: whether a unit is selected from the accessible population to the discovery sample does not depend on the selection of other units. For example, in a diabetes risk model example, a sampling unit can be a patient. Assume that from the accessible population, the set of patients in the catchment area of the health system, a discovery sample of patients is drawn at random. The probability of being included in the discovery sample is constant across the patients in the accessible population. Each patient can contribute multiple records. Typically, all records of the selected patients are included. Thus, the discovery sample is not a random sample at the level of records (if one record of a specific patient is included, another record of the same patient has a very high probability of being included) but is a random sample at the level of patients. When the discovery sample is further sampled to create the training and validation sets, the same sampling unit must be used. If in the above example, records of one patient are split across the training and test sets, the training and test sets are no longer independent, *even at the patient level*: if some records of a patient are in the training set, the probability of another record of the same patient being in the test set is higher than the probability that a record of a random patient from the accessible population is included. For this example, sampling must be done at the patient level: if a patient is selected to be a training patient, all records of this patient must be included in the training sample; if the patient is a validation patient, then all records of the patient must be included in the validation sample.

> **Best Practice 9.4.1**
> Consider the sampling unit carefully.

Relative Size of the Training Versus Validation Samples

Best Practice 9.4.2
A typical leave-out validation size is 30% of the sample.

Pitfall 9.4.2
If 70% of the discovery sample is insufficient training data, you need to consider other performance estimators (such bootstrapping or cross-validation).

To illustrate the effect of the proportion of samples left out for validation, we simulated a large population of observations with outcomes. From this population, we draw discovery samples of varying sizes, ranging from 50 to 5000. A 10-parameter model was constructed for the outcome and its performance was estimated from the leave-out sample (validation sample). The left panel in Fig. 13 depicts the bias, which is the average absolute difference between the performance estimate from the validation sample versus the actual performance on the population. The right panel depicts the variability of the performance estimate. For each discovery sample size, the experiment was repeated 50 times and the standard deviation of the 50 performance estimates are reported.

As the fraction of samples left out for validation increases, the samples available for training decreases. Figure 13 shows that the larger the training sample size, the higher the actual performance. As the fraction of samples left out for validation

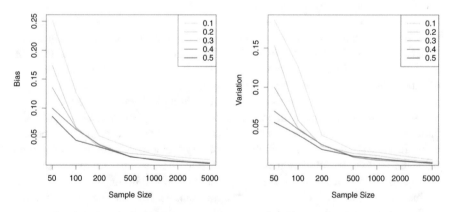

Fig. 13 Example showing the impact of the proportion of samples left out for validation. The bias (left panel) and variance (on the standard deviation scale) (right panel) of the performance estimates of models constructed on discovery sample sizes varying from 50 to 5000 (horizontal axis) and the portion of the discovery sample left out for validation ranging from 10% to 50% (darker blue indicates larger validation sample size)

decreases, the validation sample becomes too small to estimate the performance, and as Fig. 13 shows, this results in both high variance and large bias. The typical percentage of samples left out for validation is 30%. When the discovery sample is sufficient for building a good model from 70% of the samples, the remaining 30% is typically sufficient to estimate the model performance.

Property. Even for modest sample sizes, the leave-out estimator is relatively unbiased, however, it has very high variance.

Repeated Holdout

To reduce the variance of the holdout estimator, the estimation can be repeated multiple m times, each with a different partitioning. This process results in m performance (or error) estimates, which need to be averaged.

Property. The repeated holdout estimator retains the same low bias and achieves significantly lower variance than the (single, non-repeated) holdout estimator. However, repeating the holdout estimation results in higher computation cost.

Cross-Validation

There are two problems with leave-out validation. First, we use a small portion of the discovery sample for training as we have to leave out a portion of it for validation. This increases bias. Second, the portion left out for validation is relatively small so the variance of the performance estimate can be large. Cross validation addresses both of these problems.

In k-fold cross validation, the data set is divided into k equal partitions at random. Model evaluation proceeds iteratively, in k iterations. In the kth iteration, the kth partition (fold) is left out for validation and the remaining k-1 partitions are used for training. A model is constructed on the k-1 partitions and predictions are made on the leave out partition. Over the k iterations, we obtain predictions for all k partitions and the predictions are evaluated.

> **Best Practice 9.4.3**
> For cross validation a typical number of folds is 10 in moderate sample size and 5 in large sample sizes.

In ten-fold cross validation (CV), in each of the 10 iterations, 9 out of 10 partitions are used for training, thus the model is constructed on 90% of the discovery sample. By the end of the 10 iterations, predictions are obtained for all observations, thus the predictive performance is evaluated on all instances in the discovery sample. The downsides are twofold. First, in 10 iterations, we have built 10 models. If building a model is costly, cross-validation can become very expensive. This can be mitigated by choosing a smaller k. Second, the procedure does not evaluate the performance of a specific model, but rather the expected performance of a hypothetical model that we would obtain by building it on (k-1)/k portion of the discovery samples.

Choosing k

The choice of k mainly impacts the sample size available for training (model construction), which in turn, impacts performance in the population. Any $k \geq 5$ was found to yield very similar performance: whether the model is constructed on 80% of the discovery sample ($k = 5$) or 98% ($k = 50$) only had an impact on the performance for small sample sizes. The larger the number of folds, the smaller the bias and the variance (standard deviation of the performance estimates across 50 runs for k and each discovery sample size combination), however the effect diminishes beyond $k = 5$ (Fig. 14).

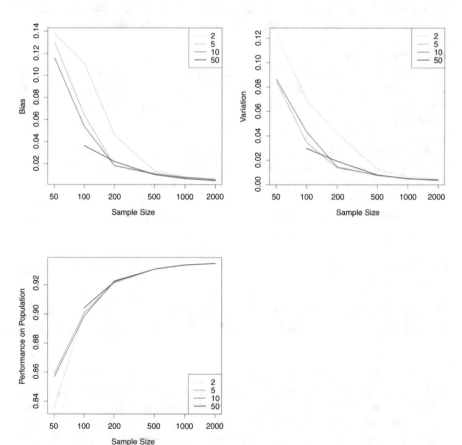

Fig. 14 The effect of the number of cross-validation folds. Model performance was estimated using k-fold cross validation ($k = 2, 5, 10, 50$). The bias (top left panel), standard deviation (top right panel) and model performance in the population (bottom panel) are depicted as a function of the analytic sample size ranging from 50 to 2000. The color of the curves represents k

Leave One Out Cross Validation (LOOCV)

Leave One Out Cross Validation (LOOCV) is a special case of cross validation, where every observation is a partition. In other words, $k = N$. LOOCV is most useful for small data sets, because in each iteration, only a single observation is left out for validation. The key drawback is the computation cost: by the completion of the LOOCV process, N models will have been constructed.

Property. Cross-validation has low bias, but high variance. It has significantly higher computation cost than the holdout estimation.

Repeated Cross-Validation

K-fold cross validation has low bias but relatively high variance. Some of this variance, the so-called **internal variance** [25], is due to the randomness induced by the partitioning. In order to reduce variance, **repeated cross-validation** can be performed, where the k-fold cross-validation process is repeated m times and the estimates are averaged over the m repetitions.

Bootstrap

As k-fold cross validation represents a tradeoff of increased compute cost to reduce estimation bias and variance, bootstrap is another step in the same direction. In bootstrap estimation, replicas of the discovery sample are constructed. If the discovery sample has N observation, a replica of N observations is created by sampling from the discovery sample with replacement. The replica will contain approximately two thirds of the observations from the original discovery sample, with some observations included multiple times. Conversely, about a third of the original samples are not included in the replica. These samples are called the **out-of-bag** (OOB) samples. A model is constructed on the replica, and evaluated on the OOB samples. This process is repeated typically 50 to several hundred times.

The advantage of the bootstrap is that the model is evaluated on the OOB samples over multiple runs, thus the evaluation uses most (if not all) discovery samples multiple times, yielding a stable estimate. The drawback of the method is that it is known to be (pessimistically) biased even on large samples and it is costly as it builds a model on each replica, requiring the construction of potentially hundreds of models. Similarly to cross-validation, the performance estimate is not the performance of a specific model, but rather the expected performance of a model that will be built on the discovery sample with the same parameterization as the models in the bootstrap.

Effect of the Number of Bootstrap Iterations

Figure 15 shows the effect of the bootstrap iterations on the bias (top left panel) and variance (top right panel) of the performance estimate. The bottom panel depicts the performance of the models in the target population. Since each bootstrap iteration uses a replica data set that has the same number of samples as the entire discovery sample, the performance of the models in the population does not depend on the number of bootstrap iterations. There is some variation in the amount of bias as a function of the number of bootstrap iterations, but the differences are not

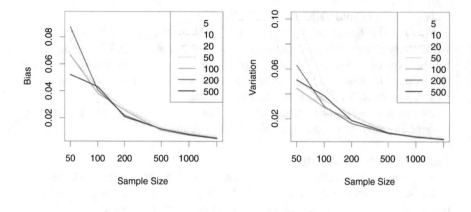

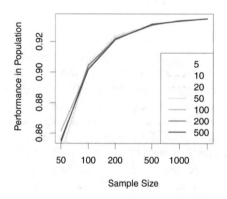

Fig. 15 Effect of the number of bootstrap iterations on the bias (top left panel), variance (top right panel) of the performance estimates and the actual performance of the models in the target population (bottom panel)

statistically significant. The main difference due to the number of bootstrap iterations is the variance of the performance estimate. The higher the number of bootstrap iterations, the smaller the variance. Consistent with recommendations in the literature, performing iterations in excess of 100 or 200 has no appreciable effect.

Best Practice 9.4.4
When using the bootstrap estimator select a number of repetitions that is sufficient for the problem based on related literature. Reported minimum repetitions generally range from 100 to >500.

Property. The bootstrap has low variance but can have high bias even when the sample size is large.

The 0.632 and the 0.632+ bootstrap

The key benefit of the bootstrap method is its low variance. However, the bootstrap can be pessimistically biased even for large sample sizes.

The **0.632 bootstrap** [26] addresses this issue by taking a weighted average of the resubstitution error $\hat{\varepsilon}_{resub}$ (which is typically very optimistic) and the bootstrap error $\hat{\varepsilon}_{b0}$

$$\hat{\varepsilon}_{b632} = .368\hat{\varepsilon}_{resub} + .632\hat{\varepsilon}_{b0}$$

This correction was observed to be insufficient, thus when the overfitting is assumed to be substantial, more weight is placed on the bootstrap estimate. This gave rise to the 0.**632+ bootstrap** [27], defined as

$$\hat{\varepsilon}_{b632+} = \left(1-\hat{w}\right)\hat{\varepsilon}_{resub} + \hat{w}\hat{\varepsilon}_{b0}$$

where the exact formulate for the weighing factor $\hat{w}$ can be found in [28].

> **Best Practice 9.4.5**
> When using the bootstrap, estimate the bias and correct for it unless it is negligible. If the bias is unknown or cannot be corrected, then a different estimator must be used.

Comparing the Different Estimators

Several studies [4, 25, 28–30] have addressed the issue of comparatively evaluating these estimators. The emerging conclusions are that:

(a) LOOCV is unbiased but has high variance and can produce outlying estimates on small samples [25]
(b) k-fold CV is nearly unbiased and with smaller variance than LOOCV.
(c) Holdout estimator is unbiased but has high variance [30].
(d) Bootstrapping is biased [28].
(e) Repeating and averaging application of an estimator can drastically reduce its variance [28]. Recommended number of repeats is ≥ 50.

> **Best Practice 9.4.6**
> Use the least computationally expensive estimator that yields small enough bias and variance in the problem at hand.
> For very small sample size: consider as first choice Leave One Out Cross Validation (LOOCV).
> For small sample size: using a less-flexible classifier, the 0.632 bootstrap can offer the best performance but it can be biased [28].
> For medium sample sizes: repeated balanced ten-fold cross validation.
> For large samples sizes: holdout or five-fold Cross Validation or corrected bootstrap.

Performance Estimation in the Presence of Missing Values

When the analytic data set contains missing values, we can follow two strategies:

1. We can first impute the entire analytic data set and then perform the evaluation on the imputed data set; OR
2. We first partition (or resample) the analytic data set and then impute the missing values on each partition/resample separately.

The key issue is that when the model is implemented in practice, the data that the model will be operating on (test data) may contain missing values. If we follow strategy 1, our performance estimates may be too optimistic. Following strategy 2 is costly but eliminates the danger of biasing the error estimates (see also chapter "Overfitting, Underfitting and General Model Overconfidence and Under-Performance Pitfalls and Best Practices in Machine Learning and AI").

Best Practice 9.4.7

Applying data imputation procedures on training data and using the imputation model on the test data (in cross validation estimators):

(a) Ensures that bias is avoided.
(b) Mimics practical implementation of the final model (which has to be eventually deployed without the benefit of seeing a large number of the application population).

Pitfall 9.4.3

Imputation on all data may bias the estimation of classifier errors (even if the imputation is blind to the outcome).

Parameter Tuning and Performance Estimation

Hyper parameter tuning as part of model selection is covered in chapter "Overfitting, Underfitting and General Model Overconfidence and Under-Performance Pitfalls and Best Practices in Machine Learning and AI". Here we re-inforce an important practice:

Pitfall 9.4.4

Tuning hyper parameters or other procedures on the entire data first and then partition/resampling the data for evaluation can produce overly optimistic predictivity estimates.

Best Practice 9.4.8
Tune the parameters of an algorithm separately on each fold/resample.

Example 8.4.1 [Parameter tuning and bootstrap Estimsation]
To perform bootstrap estimation with B iterations, we proceed as follows. For each of the B iterations, we create a replica data set by resampling the analytic data set. The replica is then partitioned into a training and validation set. Models with various parameters are constructed on the training set and the optimal (for this iteration) parameter setting is selected using the validation set. A model is than constructed using the entire replica and the parameter setting we just selected. The performance of this model is then assessed using the out-of-bag data as usual, yielding one of the B performance estimates. At the end, the B performance estimates are summarized (e.g. arithmetic mean, weighted mean, confidence interval, etc). Note that the parameter settings do not necessarily coincide across the B iterations.

Example 8.4.2 [Parameter tuning and ten-fold cross validation]
The discovery sample is divided into 10 partitions. The estimation will proceed in 10 iterations. In the ith iteration, the ith partition will serve as test data and the remaining 9 partitions as development data. The development data is partitioned into training and test sets. Models with various parameter settings are built on the training set and the optimal (for this fold) setting is selected using the validation data (not to be confused with the test data – the test data (ith partition) is set aside and is not touched!). Then a model is constructed on the entire development data (9 partitions) with the parameter setting we just selected and predictions are made for the test data (ith partition). At the end, the predictions are evaluated. Note that the 10 parameter settings across the ten folds can be different.

A complete protocol for model selection is provided in chapter "The Development Process and Lifecycle of Clinical Grade and Other Safety and Performance-Sensitive AI/ML Models" and strategies to avoid overfitting in chapter "Overfitting, Underfitting and General Model Overconfidence and Under-Performance Pitfalls and Best Practices in Machine Learning and AI".

Final Model

> Model evaluation estimates the performance of a model construction procedure rather than the performance of a specific model.

Consider for instance the k-fold cross validation. At the end of the process, we have constructed k models. Similarly, a bootstrap estimation with B iterations produces B models. Clearly, the performance estimate we obtain is not the performance of any one of these models; it is the expected performance of a model following the same model construction procedure.

> **Best Practice 9.4.9**
> After error estimation has been accomplished and an optimal hyperparameter value assignment has been identified, the final model has to be built on the entire data set, with the same hyperparameter values, and without conducting further internal error estimation.

Even if you are using an estimator such as leave-out validation, which produces a model on the training set and evaluates this model on a validation set, as the final model, construct a new model on the entire discovery sample. The model constructed only on the training set utilized fewer observations and is thus less stable and possibly more biased than a model built on the entire discovery sample.

External Validation

> The purpose of external validation is to ensure that a model derived from a discovery sample generalizes to the target population, or more precisely, to a different setting than that of the discovery sample.

Based on the changes in the setting, we distinguish between different kinds of external validations [2].

Temporal validation. The data for the population to which we apply the model is collected using a different time frame. As the standard of care changes, the validity (or at the least the predictive performance) of the model can vary. More recent patients, who are subject to the most recent standard of care, can be more indicative of the future performance of the model than earlier patients.

Temporal validation is performed by designating a particular time frame for training and a different time frame for validation.

A special case of temporal validation is **pseudo-prospective evaluation**. This is a leave-out validation, where patients with the most recent data are left out for validation and the model is constructed on the data of earlier patients.

Geographic validation. A model can be evaluated in a different geographic location than the one it was developed in. This can take two major forms. The first one is essentially an external validation of a model, where an existing model is evaluated at a new geographic location, for example, to determine whether the model can be applied to patients at this new location. The second one is multi-site development of a model. In this case, the discovery sample spans multiple geographic locations and the goal is to construct a model that works well at all geographic locations. Performance estimation in this context can take the form of a leave-one-site out cross-validation, where performance estimation is performed iteratively, in each iteration, leaving one site out and constructing the model on the remaining sites.

Spectrum validation. The model is validated on patients whose disease is more (or less) severe than those in the discovery sample. Such a validation is useful, for example, when (say) an ICU model is applied to patients "on the floor" (non-ICU wards).

Methodological validation. This is akin to sensitivity analysis. The model is applied to patients, whose data was collected and processed differently than the data of the discovery sample. This can be useful when we aim to ensure that a model developed on registry data is valid when applied to patient data from the EHR. It is reasonable to assume that the registry data is curated, and as a result, is more complete and is of higher quality.

Best Practice 9.4.10

If the sample size allows, pseudo-prospective (temporal) validation is recommended in addition to the internal validation and other planned external validations.

Best Practice 9.4.11

If the model was developed using public data, registry data, or other external data, always make sure that it is valid on the target population.

We conclude this chapter with the important observation that model performance is dependent on the evaluation metric. For example, for metric 1, model 1 > model 2; for metric 2 the reverse can be true. We discuss real life examples in multiple chapters of the book.

Key Messages and Concepts Discussed in Chapter "Evaluation"

The purpose of evaluating a clinical model is to ensure that a model has sufficient performance, is valid in the target population (and any other population of interest), and is capable of achieving the clinical objectives at a cost that is acceptable to the health system.

Confusion matrix (contingency tables) and related measures

Weighted confusion matrix, misclassification costs

ROC, Lorenz curves

Multiclass classification. One-vs-one, One-vs-All

Measures of predictive model performance for continuous outcomes.

Measures of predictive model performance for time-to-event outcomes.

Calibration. Calibration-in-the-large, weak, moderate and strong calibration.

Hosmer-Lemeshow test.

Measures of clinical effectiveness.

Net benefit and decision curve.

Health economic evaluation.

The goal of performance estimation is to infer the performance of a model in the target population based the discovery sample.

Performance /error estimator.

Internal validation

Holdout, Cross-validation, Repeated Cross-validation, Bootstrap, Bias corrected bootstrap

Combining imputation and hyperparameter tuning with error/performance estimation

External validation

Best Practices in Chapter "Evaluation"

Best Practice 9.1.1. Use evaluation metrics appropriate for the outcome type.

Best Practice 9.1.2. Multiple metrics are needed to cover different aspects of model performance. Use sets of measures that provide complementary information.

Best Practice 9.1.3. Common complementary pairs of classifier performance evaluation metrics include: (1) precision/recall; (2) specificity/sensitivity; (3) bias/discrimination.

Best Practice 9.1.4. The ROC is much more commonly used than the Lorenz curve and is more familiar to many readers.

Best Practice 9.1.5. Consider showing the Lorenz curve (possibly in combination with the ROC) when low-risk patients are of particular interest.

Best Practice 9.1.6 All of these measures are appropriate for Gaussian data.

Best Practice 9.1.7 MSE is more sensitive to outliers than MAD.

Best Practice 9.1.8. When evaluating predictive model with continuous outcomes that are heteroscedastic, consider using a residual that normalizes the expected variance (such as the Pearson residual for counts) or at least for the predicted value.

Best Practice 9.1.9. When the relationship between the predicted and actual values is not linear, consider using a rank-based measure such as Spearman or Kendall correlation.

Best Practice 9.1.10. The most common evaluation of a time-to-event model is Harell's C statistic (survival concordance).

Best Practice 9.1.11 Time-dependent predictions can be summarized into a single value as (1) survival probability at the end of the study, (2) survival probability at the median survival time, (3) or survival probability at some clinically relevant time.

Best Practice 9.1.12 If an ROC is desired, time-to-event prediction can be converted into classification outcomes at a specific (clinically relevant) time point using the C/D strategy to plot the ROC.

Best Practice 9.2.1. For case/control designs, use OR.

Best Practice 9.2.2. Absolute and relative risk measures provide complementary information, so whenever possible, both should be reported.

Best Practice 9.2.3. ARR and NNT convey the same information and differ in interpretation. ARR is dimensionless, while NNT is measured in number of patients and is preferred in clinical practice.

Best Practice 9.3.1. Include *all* alternative interventions in a health economic evaluation.

Best Practice 9.3.2. Include the opportunity cost as cost of intervention/program in a health economic evaluation.

Best Practice 9.3.3 Do not use intermediate end-points unless they are very strongly linked to the outcome of interest.

Best Practice 9.4.1. Consider the sampling unit carefully.

Best Practice 9.4.2. A typical leave-out validation size is 30% of the sample.

Best Practice 9.4.3. For cross validation a typically number of folds is 10 in moderate sample size and 5 in large sample sizes.

Best Practice 9.4.4. When using the bootstrap estimator select a number of repetitions that is sufficient for the problem based on related literature. Reported minimum repetitions generally range from 100 to >500.

Best Practice 9.4.5. When using the bootstrap, estimate the bias and correct for it unless it is negligible. If the bias is unknown or cannot be corrected, then a different estimator must be used.

Best Practice 9.4.6. Use the least computationally expensive estimator that yields small enough bias and variance in the problem at hand.

For very small sample size: consider as first choice Leave One Out Cross Validation (LOOCV).

For small sample size, using a less-flexible classifier, the 0.632 bootstrap can offer the best performance but it can be biased [28].

For medium sample sizes repeated balanced ten-fold cross validation.

For large samples sizes: holdout or five-fold Cross Validation or corrected bootstrap.

Best Practice 9.4.7. Applying data imputation procedures on train data and using the imputation model on the test data (in cross validation estimators):

(a) Ensures that bias is avoided.
(b) Mimics practical implementation of the final model (which has to be eventually deployed without the benefit of seeing a large number of the application population).

Best Practice 9.4.8. Tune the parameters of an algorithm separately on each fold/resample.

Best Practice 9.4.9. After error estimation has been accomplished and an optimal hyperparameters value assignment have been identified, the final model has to be built on the entire data set, with the same hyper parameter values, and without conducting further internal error estimation.

Best Practice 9.4.10. If the sample size allows, pseudo-prospective (temporal) validation is recommended in addition to the internal validation and other planned external validations.

Best Practice 9.4.11. If your model was developed using public data, registry data, or other external data, always make sure that it is valid on the target institution's internal data.

Pitfalls Discussed in Chapter "Evaluation"

Pitfall 9.1.1. Don't use mathematically related measures together. They do not provide additional information.

Pitfall 9.1.2. Accuracy is very sensitive to the prevalence of actual positives and negatives.

Pitfall 9.1.3 Lorenz curves depend on the prevalence of the disease; ROCs do not.

Pitfall 9.1.4 Pearson residual is sensitive to small predictive values.

Pitfall 9.1.5. When the outcome is not homoscedastic, some ranges of the outcome value (larger values) can dominate the evaluation.

Pitfall 9.1.6. R^2 is designed to measure the linear correlation between the predicted and actual values. When this is not linear, R^2 is inappropriate.

Pitfall 9.1.7 When a model produces time-dependent predictions, these need to be summarized into a single value before the C statistic can be computed.

Pitfall 9.1.10. Flexible calibration curves depend on the smoothing applied to the curve.

Pitfall 9.2.1. In case/control studies, measures of effectiveness that depend on the prior of classes, are misleading when the balance of cases to controls in the samples differs from the balance in the target population.

Pitfall 9.2.2. The range of NTT has a "hole". This makes significance testing and constructing confidence intervals difficult.

Pitfall 9.2.3 Even models with reasonable AUC can underperform a default policy of "Treat All".

Pitfall 9.4.1. Do not use the plug-in estimator. Its estimate is always optimistic, sometimes excessively so.

Pitfall 8.4.2. If 70% of the discovery sample is insufficient training data, you need to consider other performance estimators (such bootstrapping or cross-validation).

Pitfall 9.4.3. Imputation on all data may bias the estimation of classifier errors (even if the imputation is blind to the outcome).

Pitfall 9.4.4 Tuning hyper parameters or other procedures on the entire data first and then partition/resampling the data for evaluation can produce overly optimistic predictivity estimates.

Classroom Questions, Chapter "Evaluation"

1. Does a model with higher performance always have better clinical impact?

2. A classifier recognizes the color of traffic lights: red, amber, green. How would you report the performance of this classifier? What metrics would you use?

3. We discussed that there are two kinds of measures: those based on residuals and those that describe how the predicted value co-varies with the outcome.
   (a) Consider the log likelihood for a regression problem. Which group does it fall into?
   (b) Consider the log likelihood for a classification problem. Why would you put (or not put) the log likelihood into these two groups?

4. For models that maximize a likelihood (or minimize a negative log likelihood), it is common to use a likelihood-based information criterion (e.g. BIC, AIC) for model selection. What is the advantage or disadvantage of using these criteria instead of direct measures of predictive performance? What if the model is not a predictive model (e.g. a clustering)?

5. What is the key issue in evaluating a time-to-event model? If there is no censoring, can you use binary classification measures to evaluate a time-to-event model?

6. The decision curve has p (the threshold for positive classification) on its horizontal axis. If a classifier produces labels (as opposed to a score), can the decision curve still be useful? What information can it provide? (Hint: think of the relationship between p and w.)

7. How does the net benefit change if I use a positive classification threshold p that is different from w/(1 + w)?

8. Can a classifier with AUC 0.9 have an unfavorable ICER?

9. When can a really expensive clinical test have favorable (low) ICER?
   (a) The answer has to be verifiable through cost effectiveness analysis.
   (b) The answer has to be verifiable through cost utility analysis.

10. Cost Benefit Analysis compares policies in terms of monetary benefits taking costs into account. Expressing health benefit as monetary benefit is very controversial. Can you think of a healthcare scenario, where this is inevitable?

11. If you are a healthcare administrator and you are debating between spending resources on a diet program to reduce obesity versus a new cancer treatment, what kind of a health economic analysis are you conducting?

12. The calibration model for binary outcomes is a logistic regression model. Derive the calibration model for count outcome. Hint: how is the poisson model linearized?

13. Suppose you are a hospital administrator. If you are going to build a model for use in your hospital, you should fully optimize your model for your population and the performance of the resulting model on other populations is irrelevant.
   (a) Is this statement true?
   (b) Suppose your model has an AUC of 0.85 on your population. If you find that this model achieves an AUC of 0.75 on a similar population, what do you do? Can you ignore it?
   (c) Can you derive a benefit from training the model jointly on your and the other population and then updating it to better fit your own population?
      • What if the two populations only differ in a couple of variables?
      • What if most of the difference is due to the analyst's definition of a disease?
      • What if the two population only differ in the prevalence of the disease? (Would that impact the AUC?)

14. If your accessible population is the same as your target population, can external validation offer any benefit? (Hint: External validation is not limited to validation at other hospitals.)

15. When you build your final model, you use the entire discovery sample. Let us focus on the bootstrap estimator. One reason for building a final model is that the bootstrap estimation process yields many models, one from each iteration. However, these models are all built on a replica of the discovery sample (has the same number of observations), so why can't we just simply select one of the

models and use that as the final model? What if we select that model at random? What if we select the best model?

16. Examples 8.4.1 and 8.4.2 describe parameter tuning for bootstrapping and cross validation. In essence, we use leave-out validation on the model development data set to estimate the performance of the model for each parameter value. Is this the best approach if you have small data size? How could you use a more sample-efficient estimation method, such as cross-validation (instead of leave out validation) to tune the parameters? (Hint: the name of this approach is "nested cross-validation".)

References[1]

1. Park SY, Park JE, Kim H, Park SH. Review of statistical methods for evaluating the performance of survival or other time-to-event prediction models (from conventional to deep learning approaches). Korean J Radiol. 2021;22(10):1697–707. [also says that 63% of the papers used Harrell's C.] https://www.kjronline.org/pdf/10.3348/kjr.2021.0223.
2. Steyerberg EW. Clinical prediction models. A practical approach to development, validation and updating. 2nd ed. Cham: Springer; 2019.
3. Pepe MS. The statistical evaluation of medical test for classification and prediction. Oxford: Oxford University Press; 2003.
4. Rodriguez JD, Perez A, Lozano JA. Sensitivity analysis of k-fold cross validation in prediction error estimation. IEEE Trans Pattern Anal Mach Intell. 2009;32(3):569–75.
5. Steyerberg EW. Lorenz curve (chapter 15.2.6). In: Clinical prediction models. A practical approach to development, validation and updating. 2nd ed. Springer. Cham; 2019.
6. Davis J. and Goadrich M. The relationship between precision-recall and ROC curves., International Conference on Machine Learning, 2006.
7. Bex T, Comprehensive guide to multiclass classification metrics. Medium, 2021. https://towardsdatascience.com/comprehensive-guide-on-multiclass-classification-metrics-af94cfb83fbd.
8. Delgado R, Tibau X-A. Why Cohen's kappa should be avoided as performance measure in classification. PLoS One. 2019;14(9):e0222916. https://doi.org/10.1371/journal.pone.0222916.
9. Tan P-N, Steinbach M, Karpatne A, Kumar V. Introduction to data mining. Pearson; 2018. ISBN:0133128903.
10. Biecek P, Burzykowski T. Exploratory model analysis. 2020. https://ema.drwhy.ai/modelPerformance.html.
11. Evaluating Survival Models. Scikit-survival 0.17.2 User Manual. https://scikit-survival.readthedocs.io/en/stable/user_guide/evaluating-survival-models.html.
12. Hanpu Z. Predictive Evaluation Metrics in Survival Analysis. R vignette. 2021. https://cran.r--project.org/web/packages/SurvMetrics/vignettes/SurvMetrics-vignette.html.
13. Rahman MS, Ambler G, Choodari-Oskooei B, Omar RZ. Review and evaluation of performance measures for survival prediction models in external validation settings. BMC Med Res Methodol. 2017;17:60. [Uno's C] https://www.ncbi.nlm.nih.gov/pmc/articles/PMC5395888/.
14. Heagerty PJ, Zheng Y. Survival model predictive accuracy and ROC curves. Biometrics. 2005;61(1):92–105.

---

[1] The two key references for this chapter are [2] (chapters 14–17 and 19) and [3], both of which are textbooks. These cover basic concepts, such as validation, overfitting, evaluation metrics for binary and continuous outcomes. Time-to-even outcome has seen a lot of recent development and the key reference is [1]; and for calibration, we recommend [15]. [17] focuses in best practice for clinical effectiveness measures, and [31] covers net benefit and the decision curve. For the health economic impact, we recommend [21], which is a widely used textbook.

15. Calster BV, McLernon DJ, van Smeden M, Wynants L, Steyerberg EW. Calibration: the Achilles heel of predictive analytics. BMC Med, 2019;17(230) [Strong, moderate, weak and at-large calibration] https://bmcmedicine.biomedcentral.com/articles/10.1186/s12916-019-1466-7.:17.
16. Austin PC, Steyerberg EW. The Integrated Calibration Index (ICI) and related metrics for quantifying the calibration of logistic regression models. Stat Med. 2019;28(21) [Integrated Calibration Index (ICI), Harrell's E (Emax, E50, E90)]:4051–65. https://doi.org/10.1002/sim.8281.
17. Schechtman E. Odds ratio, relative risk, absolute risk reduction, and the number needed to treat—which of these should we use? Value Health. 2002;5(5):431–6. https://doi.org/10.1046/J.1524-4733.2002.55150.x.
18. Hutton JL. Number needed to treat and number needed to harm are not the best way to report and assess the results of randomised clinical trials. British J of Hematol. 2009;146:27–30. https://doi.org/10.1111/j.1365-2141.2009.07707.x.
19. BMJ evidence based medicine toolkit. How to calculate risk? https://bestpractice.bmj.com/info/us/toolkit/learn-ebm/how-to-calculate-risk/. [Defines all these measures (except OR) without much fluff.]
20. Szumilas M. Explaining odds ratios. J Can Acad Child Adolesc Psychiatry. 2010;19(3):227–9. https://www.ncbi.nlm.nih.gov/pmc/articles/PMC2938757/.
21. Drummond MF, Sculpher MJ, Claxton K, Stoddart GL, Torrance GW. Method for the economic evaluation of health care Programmes. 4th ed. Oxford: Oxford University Press; 2019.
22. Winterhoff B, et al. Developing a clinico-molecular test for individualized treatment of ovarian cancer: the interplay of precision medicine informatics with clinical and health economics dimensions. AMIA Annu Symp Proc. 2018;2018:1093–102.
23. Barnett JC, Alvarez Secord A, Cohn DE, Leath CA, Myers ER, Havrilesky LJ. Cost effectiveness of alternative strategies for incorporating bevacizumab into the primary treatment of ovarian cancer. Cancer. 2013;119(20):3653–61.
24. Saris-Baglama RN, Dewey CJ, Chisholm GB, et al. QualityMetric health outcomes™ scoring software 4.0. Lincoln, RI: QualityMetric Incorporated; 2010. p. 138.
25. Braga-Neto UM, Dougherty ER. Is cross-validation valid for small-sample microarray classification? Bioinformatics. 2004;20(3):374–80.
26. Efron B. Estimating the error rate of a prediction rule: improvement on cross-validation. J Am Stat Assoc. 1983;78(382):316–31.
27. Efron B, Tibshirani R. Improvements on cross-validation: the 632+ bootstrap method. J Am Stat Assoc. 1997;92(438):548–60.
28. Kim JH. Estimating classification error rate: repeated cross-validation, repeated hold-out and bootstrap. Comput Stat Data Anal. 2009;53(11):3735–45.
29. Bengio Y, Grandvalet Y. No unbiased estimator of the variance of k-fold cross-validation. Adv Neural Inf Proces Syst. 2003:16.
30. Burman P. A comparative study of ordinary cross-validation, v-fold cross-validation and the repeated learning-testing methods. Biometrika. 1989;76(3):503–14.
31. Vickers AJ, Calster BV, Steyerberg EW. A step-by-step guide to interpreting decision curve analysis. Diagn Progn Res. 2019;3:18. https://doi.org/10.1186/s41512-019-0064-7.

Overfitting, Underfitting and General Model Overconfidence and Under-Performance Pitfalls and Best Practices in Machine Learning and AI

Constantin Aliferis and Gyorgy Simon

Abstract

Avoiding over and under fitted analyses (OF, UF) and models is critical for ensuring as high generalization performance as possible and is of profound importance for the success of ML/AI modeling. In modern ML/AI practice OF/UF are typically interacting with error estimator procedures and model selection, as well as with sampling and reporting biases and thus need be considered together in context. The more general situations of over confidence (OC) about models and/or under-performing (UP) models can occur in many subtle and not so subtle ways especially in the presence of high-dimensional data, modest or small sample sizes, powerful learners and imperfect data designs. Because over/under confidence about models are closely related to model complexity, model selection, error estimation and sampling (as part of data design) we connect these concepts with the material of chapters "An Appraisal and Operating Characteristics of Major ML Methods Applicable in Healthcare and Health Science," "Data Design," and "Evaluation". These concepts are also closely related to statistical significance and scientific reproducibility. We examine several common scenarios where over confidence in model performance and/or model under performance occur as well as detailed practices for preventing, testing and correcting them.

C. Aliferis (✉) · G. Simon
Institute for Health Informatics, University of Minnesota, Minneapolis, MN, USA
e-mail: constantinaibestpractices@gmail.com

© The Author(s) 2024
G. J. Simon, C. Aliferis (eds.), *Artificial Intelligence and Machine Learning in Health Care and Medical Sciences*, Health Informatics,
https://doi.org/10.1007/978-3-031-39355-6_10

477

The Critical Importance of Over Fitting and Under Fitting

As important over and underfitting are, they are commonly hard to grasp by non-technical users of ML/AI models and systems, not because their basic definitions are hard to comprehend and recall, but because they tend to be created or to manifest in subtle ways and often can be hard to detect before they create significant errors at the time of model application or testing on human subjects. There are also significant and pervasive misconceptions about OF and UF, stemming from earlier stages in the science of ML/AI which we will clarify.

We first present a few classical and pedagogical examples of OF and UF before proceeding with more precise definitions and systematic ways to address them.

Introductory (Pedagogical) Example 1: Who Is the Teacher?

Consider the following thought experiment involving a university course on ML/AI taught by the two lead authors of the present book. The students are tasked with creating a computable rule (i.e. a decision model that can run in a computer) that can classify individuals in the classroom as belonging to either of 2 classes: (a) students, (b) teachers. Numerous variables have been captured including the structural, behavioral and other characteristics of all individuals involved. Some of them are shown in the table below:

Name	Wears suit and tie	Degrees	Presents material to the class	Has beard	Has accent	Wears glasses	Gender	Hands out assignments	Judo black belt	Listed in U catalogue as course instructtor	TRUE STATUS (response variable)
Simon	No	PhD	Yes	No	Yes	No	M	Yes	Yes	Yes	**Teacher**
Aliferis	Sometimes	MD, PhD	Yes	Yes	Yes	Yes	M	Yes	No	Yes	**Teacher**
Smith	No	BSc	Yes	No	No	No	F	No	No	No	**Student**
Zheng	No	RN	Yes	No	Yes	Yes	F	No	No	No	**Student**
Singh	Yes	PharmD	Yes	Yes	No	Yes	M	No	No	No	**Student**
LaFleur	No	BSc	Yes	No	No	Yes	M	No	No	No	**Student**
Bickman	No	MD	Yes	No	No	No	F	No	No	No	**Student**
Papado-poulos	No	BSc	Yes	Yes	Yes	No	M	No	No	No	**Student**
Chang	No	MD, MS	Yes	No	No	Yes	F	No	No	Yes	**Guest lecturer**
Jones	No	PhD	Yes	No	No	No	NB	Yes	No	No	**TA**
Schwartz	No	BSc	No	No	No	Yes	F	No	No	No	**Auditing student**

In this thought experiment there is a number of models that would classify correctly the participants in the class with respect to whether they belong in the teacher or learner class. Some examples of perfectly accurate models to identify teachers are:

- Model 1: hands out assignments and has accent
- Model 2: has PhD and is male
- Model 3: wears suit & tie sometimes OR has judo black belt
- Model 4: name ends in "on" or starts with "a"

The more variables we measure, the more such accurate models we can construct. Such models can achieve 100% accuracy in this class, however *they obviously do not generalize well to other similar ML/AI classes across many other universities.* **We say that these models are overfitted**.
Consider now the following examples:

- Model 6: Has beard and wears glasses
- Model 7: Has accent
- Model 8: Has beard or a judo black belt

These models can achieve modest/poor accuracy in this class, however they may generalize to similar (low) accuracy to other similar ML/AI classes across the many universities and alternative models exist with better generalizable accuracy. **We say that these models are underfitted.**
Finally consider the following examples:
Model 9: person is listed in the university catalogue as instructor for the course and hands out assignments.
This model can achieve 100% accuracy in this class and will generalize to similar extent to other ML/AI classes across the many universities. **We say that such models are neither under nor overfitted.**

The intuitions gained are that with datasets with a large enough number of variables, it is easy enough to come up with models that are very accurate in the train (discovery) data but that will fail to generalize to the general population. Also that performance in the training data is a poor indicator of performance in the population.

Introductory Example 2: Over and Undertraining ANNs

Figure 1 shows a classical experiment in training ANNs [1]. As the number of weight update iterations increases, the model learns the training data really well and its generalization performance also increases (i.e., error decreases). There is however a "breaking point" (or inflection point) where more training does increase accuracy in the training data but decreases generalization performance.

Fig. 1 Illustration of overfitting and underfitting

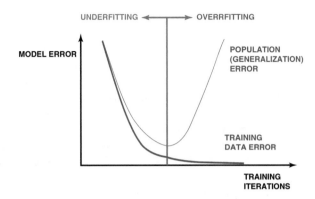

The models to the left of the optimal point are underfitted and to the right are overfitted.

The intuition gained is that there is a level of model "fit" that is ideal for this data and anything above or below that point will lead to worse generalization performance. Performance in the training data remains a poor indicator of performance in the population, however.

Introductory Example 3: Rich Simon's OF Demonstration for Genomics-Driven Discovery

In bioinformatics where dimensionalities are typically very high and sample sizes small, OF is a particularly important danger. Simon at al published the following empirical demonstration showcasing that depending on how gene selection and model error estimation are conducted, there are different degrees of biasing the estimates of model generalization error [2].

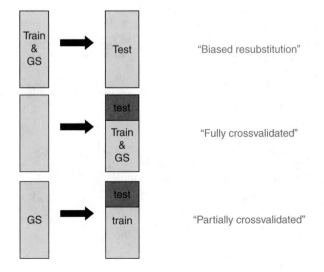

Simon et al. generated models using feature (gene) selection (GS) procedures in data constructed so that there is no predictive signal. They examined 3 protocols for combining the same feature selection and classification algorithms:

Protocol 1 "Biased resubstitution" is when the gene selection takes place on all data and the error estimation also takes place on all data.

Protocol 2 "Full cross validation" is when feature selection is done on a training portion of the data, model is fitted in the training portion and error is estimated in a separate testing portion.

Protocol 3 "Partial cross-validation" conducts feature selection on all data, then models are built in a training portion and model error is estimated in a separate testing portion.

Unbiased error estimation should indicate that a model fit in such data should have no signal, that is perform as well as random coin flipping. Indeed the "fully cross validated" protocol 2 (which we referred to as **nested cross validation** chapter "The Development Process and Lifecycle of Clinical Grade and Other Safety and Performance-Sensitive AI/ML Models") is indeed unbiased. No cross validation (protocol 1) has large bias that can reach estimates of perfect classification if enough variables are used. Partial cross validation has *in this analysis setting* intermediate bias, smaller than nested cross validation and lower than no cross validation.

The intuitions gained are that we can produce highly biased error estimates if our protocols are not set up properly to avoid bias, especially in high dimensional data. Also **the same algorithms for classification, feature selection etc. can lead to dramatically different quality of results depending of how they are arranged in modeling protocols.**

Introductory Example 4: Simple and Complex Surfaces

A classic demonstration of under and overfitting of a regression function of a continuous outcome Y given a continuous input X is given in Fig. 2. We see both training data (blue circles) and unsampled population data (white circles). As shown the complex model (wiggly line) fits the training data perfectly but fails in the population (future) data. A simpler model (straight line) does much worse in the training data, but better in the future data [3].

In Fig. 2 above, the better model is one that is more complicated than the straight line and less complicated than the complex wiggly one.

The intuition gained is that over/under-fitting are directly related to the complexity of the decision surface and how well the training data is fit. Successful data analysis methods balance training data fit with complexity since: too complex model (to fit training data well) leads to overfitting (i.e., model does not generalize) whereas: too simplistic models (to avoid overfitting) lead to underfitting (will generalize but the fit to both the training and future data will be low and predictive performance small).

Fig. 2 Further illustration of overfitting (top, 2a) and underfitting (bottom, 2b)

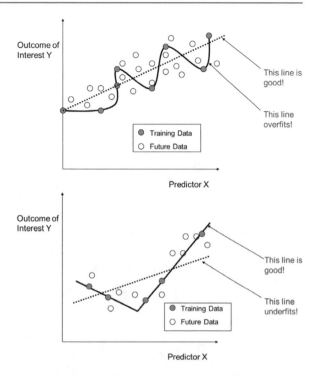

Definitions of OF and UF; the Broader Pitfalls of Overconfidence and of Under-Performing Models. Bias-Variance Error Decomposition View

Training data error of a model M is the error of M on the training data used to derive M.

True generalization error of a model M is the error of M on the population or distribution, from which training data used to derive M, were sampled from.

Estimated generalization error of a model M is the estimated error (via an *error estimator* procedure applied on data samples) of M on the population or distribution from which training data used to derive M were sampled from.

In controlled conditions, for example in simulation experiments, the true generalization error of any model can be known. Typically the true generalization error is unknown when dealing in non-trivial real-world problems, not constructed in the lab, however.

Typically (i.e., unless training sample is enormous), model training data error used to estimate true generalization error leads to downward-biased (unduly optimistic) estimates of generalization error.

Overfitting a model to data is creating a model that (a) accurately represents the training data, but (b) fails to generalize well to new data sampled from the same distribution (because some of the learned patterns in the training data are not representative of the population).

Alternatively, an overfitted model is often defined as a model that is more complex than the ideal model for the data and problem at hand.

Finally some authors define overfitting as learning "noise" in the data, that is learning idiosyncrasies of the training data that are not present in the population [1].

Similarly, the notion of OF applies at the method, modeling protocol and system level whereby an overfitting ML/AI method, modeling system, or modeling protocol/data science stack have a propensity to overfit models to the data [4, 5].

> **An overfitting ML/AI method, system, stack, or protocol** is one with the propensity to generate models that overfit.

Conversely:

> **Underfitting a model to data** is creating a model that represents the training data sub- optimally and also fails to perform well in the general population. More broadly, an under fitted model will have true generalization error that is larger than the true generalization error of the best possible model that can be fit with the data in hand.
>
> **An underfitting ML/AI method, system, stack, or protocol** is one with the propensity to generate models that underfit.

A model M cannot be both over and under fitted: the model, either describes the training data well and generalizes worse, or it is describes the training data poorly and also generalizes poorly, or finally, it is *ideally fitted* and describes both the training and population data as well as possible. From a complexity perspective, a model is either more or less or equally complex than ideal for the data and problem at hand. We will now delve deeper into these concepts using BVDE (i.e., bias-variance decomposition of a model's error).

Bias-variance decomposition perspective on OF and UF. As detailed in chapter "Foundations and Properties of AI/ML Systems", the BVDE describes that a model's error is (excluding of course measurement noise and inherent stochasticity in the data generating function) a combination of two error components: (a) a "bias" component and (b) a "variance" component. Everything else being equal, a highly biased model is less complex, while a lower bias one is more complex than ideal. Small sample size corresponds to higher variance, while larger sample size, leads to smaller variance error component. *For a fixed sample size and data generating function, there is an optimal model complexity leading to smallest model error possible.*

Model complexity above this ideal level corresponds to over-fitted models, while smaller complexity corresponds to under-fitted models. Moreover, as a model is increasingly overfitted because of increasing model complexity, the fit of the training data will improve and thus the error on the training data will decrease while the true model generalization error in the population will increase.

We further point out a fundamental asymmetry between UF and OF: empirical proof of OF of a model M1 can be obtained by showing that the true generalization error of M1 is higher than what is expected by the performance in training data.

However empirical proof of UF of a model M1 requires showing that there is at least one other model M2 that has better true generalization error than M1. M2 does not need be the optimal model attainable. M1 will also have larger generalization error than the optimal model M*opt*.

In other words UF is a relative property with respect to some optimal model (or other higher-performing models) achievable under the circumstances and not an intrinsic property of a model under examination. Therefore establishing or preventing UF is harder and more open-ended than establishing or preventing OF.

Whereas at face value establishing that a model is OF and/or UF requires calculating its true generalization error, in practice we can circumvent this (a priori formidable) difficulty by application of unbiased and efficient estimators of true generalization error (see chapters "The Development Process and Lifecycle of Clinical Grade and Other Safety and Performance-Sensitive AI/ML Models" and "Evaluation"). It is also possible to apply statistical theory to infer that a model's estimated generalization error is not accurate or to infer with high confidence from small-sample estimates that true generalization errors E1 and E2 of models M1 and M2 are not the same (see details in section "How ML/AI Model OC is Generated in Common Practice" below).

We now address two concepts of broader significance:

Over confidence in a model (OC) occurs when the analyst's estimated generalization (population) error of the model is smaller than the true generalization error.

Under confidence in a model (UC) occurs when the analysts' estimated generalization error of the model is higher than the true generalization error.

Over performance of a model (OP) (relative to a lower estimated performance expectation) occurs when the estimated population error of the model is smaller than the true population error. It is thus obvious that **Under confidence in a model = Over performance of the same model.**

Under performance of a model (UP) occurs when the true population error of the model is lower than the best possible model, or other better performing models (that can be estimated from same sample size, on average). We can also talk about under performance relative to a high performance *goal* set during the model development planning stages (chapter "The Development Process and Lifecycle of Clinical Grade and Other Safety and Performance-Sensitive AI/ML Models").

Under confidence in a model (or equivalently over performance of a model) is not considered in practice a serious concern, however it entails opportunity costs that may be significant. For example, it may trigger expensive and time consuming but unnecessary additional modeling efforts, and may deprive productive use of the model (in healthcare or health science discovery) in the meanwhile.

Under fitting is a special case error of under-performance relative to the best/ better models that could be produced under the circumstances specifically due to lower than ideal model complexity and so that the lower performance is reflected both in the training data and in the population.

Over fitting may or may not be a case of over-confidence in the models produced (and over- interpretation of the modeling results). For example, overfitting is a special case of overconfidence when the (low) error in the training data is misinterpreted as an indicator of the (higher) generalization error. If however, we overfit a model to the training data but use an unbiased error estimator, then we will not have either over or under confidence in this over fitted model.

The major (high-level) pitfalls that the present chapter addresses is:

Pitfall 10.1
Producing models in which we have over-confidence.

Pitfall 10.2
Producing models that under perform.

With corresponding high-level best practices:

Best Practice 10.1
Deploy procedures that prevent, diagnose and remedy errors of overconfidence in, or overfitting of models.

Best Practice 10.2
Deploy procedures that prevent, diagnose and remedy errors of model underperformance or underfitting.

Before embarking into specific situations where OC occurs, and corresponding remedies, we introduce fundamental general principles spanning statistics and ML that underlie these phenomena. These have value for understanding and developing general approaches to prevent OC and UP.

Fundamental ML Insights About the Three Sources of Overconfidence (OC), Under Performance (UP) and their Relationship to OF and UF: Biased Data Design, Biased Error Estimation, Poor Model Selection

(a) As discussed, OF in one of its classic definitions occurs when the (low) error in the training data is misinterpreted as an indicator of the (higher) generalization error. This creates a seriously dangerous OC about the model in question. Similarly, if UF means failing to model the training data correctly in both training data and the population and such error is readily available to calculate, why do we ever under fit models?

The answer related to real-life practice is that circa 2023 no professional practitioner of ML uses raw training data error to estimate generalization error. To the extent that even sophisticated but biased error estimators are used, the problems of OF and UF can still occur. **Fundamental insight**: as we explained previously, there is an ideal complexity for a model for which, per BVDE, generalization error is minimized. Unfortunately this complexity is rarely known a priori, hence we typically use empirical data analysis procedures to find the right complexity. These procedures are in practice a combination of search over a space of possible models (i.e., *model selection*) combined with an *error estimation* procedure used to evaluate the merit candidate models examined. If the error estimator is downward-biased (optimistic) and/or the model selection is incomplete, then it is in practice possible to find models that appear as better (=more promising) than they are by themselves (hence OF) or compared to alternative models (hence UF). In either case we encounter OC and/or UP problems.

(b) **Insight:** Another way to view OC due to OF is that of learning "statistical noise", or stated differently, over fitting by learning idiosyncratic characteristics or complex patterns of the data sample(s) that are by definition not representative of the population. Even when the error estimation procedures are not naïve (e.g. use of training data error to estimate population generalization error), the total sample itself (comprising both training and validation datasets) is not representative. This is an instance of the error due to high variance per the BVDE.

(c) **Insight**: alternatively, learning such idiosyncratic characteristics may be the result of actively selecting (as opposed to randomly sampling) training data or because of poor data design such that the training data is not representative of the targeted population and application goals (non- random sampling or more generally mismatch of the available population with the target population as explained in the chapter on data design).

These situations (i.e., poor sampling methods, poor error estimators) can lead to generalization error estimates that are too optimistic (biased downward) and learning spurious patterns translating into error in future application of the model that are not present in the training data.

(d) **Insight:** with regards to UP, poor choice of training data can lead to UP, and the same holds true for error estimator biases. In addition, poor data design and model selection deficiencies can create UP.

To summarize, from a ML lens, OC and UP originate in 3 different stages/ aspects of ML modeling, *and their combination*:

1. **OC/UP created due to data design**, primarily sampling, so that the models and generalization error estimates lead to OC or UP.
2. **OC/UP created due to error estimation** so that the models' generalization error estimates lead to OC or UP.
3. **OC/UP created due to poor choice of model**, that is the choice of model family, model fitting algorithm, model selection procedure etc., are such that models with OC/UP characteristics ensue.

Additional Insights Spanning ML and Statistics as they Relate to OC and UP: Reproducibility, Cross Validation, Nesting and Biased Post-hoc Reporting

(a) **Insight:** *reproducibility suggests generalizability; operationalizing reproducibility via independent data validation.* A commonly-followed principle of biomedical science is that credible results (e.g., in our context, models that have small generalizable error) have to successfully reproduce, that is, models must have same performance in data independent of the data used to discover these results.

We emphasize that as widely accepted this principle may be, its merits *are not immutable but hold under assumptions*. For example, in a classical statistical context, if we wish to verify that a statistical association found in data D1 reproduces in data D2, everything else being equal, sufficiently high power (type II error probability, of false negative results) and sufficiently low alpha (type I error probability, of false positive results) must be in place if we wish to conclude with high certainty that a reproducible result is a true one. Similarly, if we wish to verify that a model built from data D1 and having estimated generalizable error in the population of E1, by applying on data D2 with estimated error E2 = E1, then D1 and D2 must be sampled randomly from the same population and have high enough sample size so that comparison of E1 and E2 is sufficiently powered at low alpha levels.

Without these assumptions holding, an application of the principle of reproducibility may generate both false positive and false negative validation of original results.

The way we typically **operationalize this principle of validity via reproducibility, is by well-designed independent data set validation**, and very commonly, holdout or cross validation varieties (although many other variants exist, the general principles still apply).

(b) **Insight:** *single dataset independent (holdout) validation is an unbiased estimator and protects against p-hacking and HARKing.* We can use data D1 for fitting a model M1 and then apply it on independent data D2 and compare generalizable error estimates. *This is mathematically equivalent* to randomly splitting the original data into a training (TR) dataset and the rest used for validation or testing (TE) dataset. This is the "holdout estimator" [3] and the error measurement in TE is an unbiased generalizable error estimate.

Application of the holdout estimator protects against so-called HARKing which stands for "Hypothesis testing After Results are Known" [6]. This is because the *effective alpha* of a null hypothesis rejected by both discovery (TR) and validation (TR) datasets is: *(nominal alpha employed in TR * nominal alpha employed in TE)*. The total expected false positives in the discovery dataset TR will be *(nominal alpha in TR * number of hypotheses tested)*. This is the alpha of using just one dataset. The total expected false positives of original discovery followed by independent validation will be *(nominal alpha in TR * nominal alpha employed in TE * number of hypotheses tested)*. In other words the independent data testing reduces false positives by alpha (which is a very small number, typically never to exceed 5%).

For our purposes of modeling with ML/AI, the "hypotheses" in question are typically one or more model(s) for which we test whether its estimated error meets or exceeds a performance threshold.

If more than one validation datasets are used in sequential steps of independent validation, the probability of false findings drops exponentially fast to the number of validations. The effective alpha of being selected in both TR and (k-1) TE datasets is alpha^k which is a very small probability. For example, if alpha = 0.05 then the effective alpha of reproduced null hypothesis rejection in two independent datasets sequentially is 0.000125. In other words, when more than one validation datasets/steps are used, the probability of false findings drops exponentially fast to the number of validations. These same principles apply to ML/AI models whose validity we want to test.

(c) **Insight:** *multi-split data validation (NCV) is also unbiased and less susceptible to sampling variation.* Because the split of the original data into TR and TE is subject to random sampling variation and some splits will not be such that both TR and TE are representative of the population (even though TR + TE may be) we often use n-fold cross validation (NFCV) which is also a (in practical terms) unbiased estimator and less susceptible to bad random splits (see chapter "The Development Process and Lifecycle of Clinical Grade and Other Safety and Performance-Sensitive AI/ML Models"). NFCV and its cousin, the repeated NFCV (RNFCV) approximates the less-variant but computationally very expensive (and almost never used in practice) *all splits cross validation* where all splits are employed and averaged over.

(d) **Insight:** *NCV and NFCV can still be biased via information contamination unless nesting is employed.* Any procedure that transfers information about TE to TR can "contaminate" the unbiasedness of the CV estimator and lead to bias. Recall the seminal paper of Rich Simon et al. discussed earlier in this chapter, where they showed that feature selection can contaminate (i.e. bias) CV-derived error estimates if it is conducted in all (TR + TE) data and that when it is conducted separately in TR and TE, such contamination does not happen. Here is how this contamination takes place: by conducting e.g., feature selection on all data (using a univariate association filtering procedure in this case), we generate false positive features that happen to appear significant in this (TR + TE) dataset. Then we fit models with these false positives in TR. The model works well in TE because the features are specifically selected to work well in all data (i.e., TR + TE). However the model will not work in the population because the features used in it include false positives (in Simon et al. experiment they were all false positives because the data was constructed to be devoid of predictive signal). In other words, the chosen features were within the false positive expectation of the feature selection procedure and thus by definition will not generalize in the population).

Compare the above scenario with conducting feature selection separately in TR and in TE. The false positives of TR will not generalize to TE (because the effective probability of such random success is alpha^2 instead of alpha (see "Fundamental ML Insights about the Three Sources of over Confidence (OC), under Performance (UP) and their relationship to OF and UF: Biased Data Design, Biased Error Estimation, Poor Model Selection", be hence very small, and thus no strong feature selection bias will manifest. With 10,000 irrelevant features at nominal alpha = 0.05 we will obtain 50 false positives features that will lead to biased error estimation. With separate discovery (TR) and validation (TE) stages we will obtain 50 false positive features from TR but only 2.5 (on average) of them will survive the statistical testing in TE. As it turns out 2.5 random features do not have enough capacity to overfit a random distribution of a random outcome conditioned on 10,000 variables and thus the CV error estimate with independent feature selection is unbiased.

Important notes:

- *The exact same type of bias can happen for any data pre-processing or analysis step* including: data normalization, data imputation, any type of feature construction or transformation, *and in general any other data input to a model that is created by processing the full data* because these operations encode information about the data distribution that modeling algorithms can detect (hence biasing error estimates because of information transference about TE to TR).

- *CV contamination bias does not need to be linked to a supervised analysis step,* that is linking the data processing to the values of the response variable we wish to model. Even access to the joint distribution of inputs in TE (i.e., without reference to the response variable's values in TE) *or to any subset of variables in TE* may lead to models that have biased CV error estimates. For example, we may construct biased models and error estimates using Principal Component Analysis of the data, a procedure that is usually -but falsely- considered "failsafe" from over fitting (see assignment 12).

- Whereas CV contamination may create biased models/error estimates under the above circumstances, whether it will happen and **the degree of bias greatly depends on the safety measures employed by the unit-level (i.e., component) data procedures**. For example, if in the classical Simon et al. experiment the feature selection is tightly controlled for family-wise errors, the bias will be eliminated (see assignment 1 and later chapter "Lessons Learned from Historical Failures, Limitations and Successes of Health AI/ML. Enduring Problems and the Role of Best Practices""). This implies that we can seek to avoid contamination altogether via two general approaches: one is by application of component procedures that anticipate and avoid contamination bias, or by employing non-contaminating protocols, of which nested CV is the paradigmatic example. We can (and often do) also deploy both measures in combination (see assignment 9).

(e) **Insight:** *CV nesting decouples TE from TR data and eliminates possibility for CV contamination bias.* Recall form chapter "The Development Process and Lifecycle of Clinical Grade and Other Safety and Performance-Sensitive AI/ML Models" that nested CV is CV where we split TR and TE sets as in usual CV and then split further the TR sets into TRTR ("traintrain") and TRTE (traintest") subsets (i.e., applying an embedded "inner" loop of CV inside the TR data of the "outer" CV loop). In addition, all data processing (prior to modeling) happens separately in every TRTE dataset. Because this procedure separates data and conducts data pre-processing operations locally inside TR and subsets of it, there is no information transfer (aka contamination) about the modeling from TE to TR. Consequently, the CV contamination bias is eliminated. For a trace of how nested cross validation operates, and high level pseudo code the reader is referred to chapter "The Development Process and Lifecycle of Clinical Grade and Other Safety and Performance-Sensitive AI/ML Models". For development of the repeated nested balanced n-fold cross validation procedure by extending the hold out estimator and model selection see [3].

(f) **Insight:** *Holdout and NCV can also be biased via selective or post-hoc reporting. Both nesting and full protocol specification prevent this bias.* In the context of real-life model development it is still possible to introduce bias in HO (hold-out) and CV if we employ selective and post-hoc reporting. This type of problem occurs when many models are generated and the better ones are reported selectively. When this is a conscious decision by the creators of models, it amounts to a fraudulent representation of their procedures and results. As we will see, selective reporting may occur without ill intent, however, when the analysis plans and protocols are not well-controlled and not well-designed to avoid OC.

(g) **Insight:** *We can detect bias in biased modeling protocols if they are accurately and thoroughly described using special tests (described later in the present chapter). It is **not possible** to diagnose that a modeling protocol is biased if it is not thoroughly or accurately described.*

Equipped with the general principles leading to OC and UP we will next delve into more details of producing OC/UP models. We will also enrich the discussion with pitfalls and corresponding BPs to avoid OC/UP.

The reader is reminded that the specific pitfalls and best practices discussed here are strongly connected and provide additional technical depth and operational (micro) guidance to the overall (macro and meso) strategies and best practices of chapters "Principles of Rigorous Development and of Appraisal of ML and AI Methods and Systems" (methods development and validation) and "The Development Process and Lifecycle of Clinical Grade and Other Safety and Performance-Sensitive AI/ML Models" (model development and lifecycle).

How ML/AI Model OC Is Generated in Common Practice

Models Are Allowed to Have Inappropriately Large Complexity with Respect to Data Generating Function Complexity and to Available Sample Size

How do we measure model complexity? In older literature (and even today in some cases) this situation, and overfitting more broadly, was misconstrued as having *too many parameters* in the model (with respect to the available sample size, and the fixed complexity of the data generating function). With newer methods, *the number of parameters does not matter* as long as any number of available protective methods are used to reduce the *effective model parameters* and more generally the complexity of the fitted models, all within an appropriate family of learners (i.e., functions that match the form of the data generating function) [3, 4].

The distinction between original parameters and effective parameters can be made clear using the example of SVMs [3]. In this model family the effective parameters (the support vectors, in other words these data points defining the boundaries of each label class) cannot exceed the sample size. Thus we may have for example 1,000,000 variables and sample size $n = 1000$ which automatically restricts the number of effective parameters to at most 1000 (a 3-order of magnitude reduction over the initial data dimensionality in this example). It is also instructive that SVM mathematical bounds on generalization error do not depend on original data dimensionality but on the support vectors [4].

We have mentioned repeatedly so far that in general the complexity of the model (the effective dimensionality of which is a major factor) must be balanced against the complexity of the data generating function and the sample size. In some more detail: (a) For a fixed complexity data generating function, and a fixed sample size there is an optimal model complexity that leads to the model with the best true generalization error. Similarly, (b) for a fixed complexity data generating function, and a fixed model complexity, there is a minimum sufficient sample size that leads to the model with the true generalization error that is within an acceptable distance delta from the optimal error achievable. This follows from the "Bias-variance decomposition of error" discussed earlier.

Ignoring Statistical Uncertainty

Observing that a model has an acceptable point estimate performance does not guarantee generalizable performance since this estimate may be subject to large variation due to small sample size. The 95% (or higher) confidence interval (CI) of the estimate and/or the 95% credible interval (CrI) must also be taken into account in order to establish that the performance estimate will generalize [7, 8].

X% Confidence Interval (CI) of a point estimate P of the performance of model M developed from a fixed sample of size n: the range of values containing X% of all point estimates when sampling multiple times, developing a new model for each sample and estimating its generalization error (or other performance metric), when the true value of developing a model from this population is P.

X% Credible Interval (CrI) of a point estimate P of the performance of model M developed from sample of size n: the range containing with probability X% the true value of the generalization error (or other performance metric) of M applied to the population.

The CrI may be viewed—in Bayesian terms—as equivalent in meaning to the credible region of the posterior probability density function of the model error in the population containing X% of the total density function symmetrically around the point estimate, given the data and prior knowledge. In practice however, the CrI can and is often estimated empirically with various procedures.

A subtler way to fall victim to small sample-induced statistical variability is when the error estimator used has high variance that is not taken into account, or when among various unbiased estimators a high variance one is used instead of the lowest variance one. For example, both the holdout estimator and the n-fold cross validation (NFCV) estimator are unbiased/near-unbiased (respectively) however the holdout has higher variance than the NFCV [3, 9]. This is why over-reliance on "independent study verification: often (and falsely) treated by journals and others as a "gold standard" is a pitfall that needs to be avoided.

Using Biased Estimators or Introducing Bias in Unbiased Ones

When the procedure for estimating generalization error is not unbiased, or when the unbiasedness is compromised by implementation decisions, the estimates will be upward or downward biased. Omitting correction of this bias or applying an inappropriate correction leading to a downward error estimate leads to overconfidence. At least two common situations lead to such OC in practice:

(a) The first case stems from using uncorrected or poorly corrected bootstrapping which is a biased estimator because it employs resampling with replacement [10]. The classifier model is produced by the learning procedures who see unnatural replicates of the same true cases in the data and thus may appear to perform better than in real life where such replicates do not exist (e.g., in omics data where the combination of high dimensional data inputs are unique for each subject, yet in bootstrapping based analyses they are viewed repeatedly as if they were naturally occurring in the population).

(b) The second case occurs in temporal data analyses where there is a progressive distribution shift overt time. If the application of an *unbiased* estimator such as cross validation does not take into account time-dependent distribution changes, then a temporal bias will be introduced into a nominally unbiased estimation procedure (see chapter "Data Design").

Uncorrected Multiple Statistical Hypotheses Tests, "Data Dredging", "Fishing Expeditions"

The problem of multiple uncorrected statistical hypotheses manifests when a researcher (or a ML/AI discovery procedure) conducts not just one but many tests of statistical hypotheses and does not address the *combined effective false positive rate error across the totality of all tests conducted*. For example, consider an algorithm (or researcher, the exact same principles apply) that conducts a test of association between variables Vi and Vj in a data sample S. Such tests can be intermediate steps of more complex algorithms, or be used to compare and evaluate models.

Assume that for the observed level of association, the data sample size and the desired type II error (i.e., probability to reject the null hypothesis when it does not hold, i.e., the "power" of the test), the type I error (i.e., the probability to generate a false positive rejection under the null hypothesis) may be quite small, often set at the level of at most 5%. Now if the researchers or ML/AI algorithm conducts for example 1000 such tests, it will produce $1000*0.05 = 50$ false positive results. Epidemiologists describe the problematic practice of generating such false positives as "data dredging" or "fishing expeditions" [11].

However these terms falsely imply to some non-technical audiences, the wrong idea that whenever a discovery algorithm conducts massive amounts of statistical tests for "unbiased" or "hypothesis free" discovery, there will be unavoidable massive numbers of false positives. This is not true, however, as these multiple testing *can be corrected with many powerful and practical ways* as we will show in section "Preventing, Detecting, and Managing UF/UP".

The problem of uncorrected multiple hypothesis testing can also manifest when we produce a number of models, the estimates of generalizable error of which have considerable variance due to small sample size (as explained before), and we falsely conclude that one or more have desirable performance because of uncorrected multiple testing of the significance or the performance estimates.

Note that so far it should be clear that the notion of OC is not confined to model building and ML/AI, but is more general since it encapsulates broader notions of producing generalizable knowledge from small sample data, and is also related to classical statistical considerations of reliable estimation and inference.

Selective Reporting of Results, "Filedrawer Bias", "Publication Bias"

Imagine a modeler that aims to build an outcome classifier model for outcome Ox on the basis of data inputs V. He proceeds as follows: he develops 100 models by using a variety of techniques and estimates the generalization error for each model. Then he reports the model with the best error estimate but does not report that this was selected out of 100 models. This setup will invariably lead to over fitted/OC model reporting as evidenced by the following simple demonstration: imagine that none of these models has error better than flipping a coin (i.e., by chance, e.g. 50% accuracy for a binary outcome in a distribution with prior probability of positives equal to 50%). However if the 99% CI of estimated error for (e.g., sample size = 50 the sample size used is [0.3, 0.68], then we expect that half of the models will show accuracy >50% and some will be higher than 65%.

> The data scientist of this hypothetical experiment may also apply a calculation of 95% CI of a model that performs at accuracy 68% in this sample size level ([0.53, 0.80]) and may conduct a statistical test showing that the produced "best" model is statistically significantly better than random chance (at 5% alpha). All of this string of errors and over-interpretations is *undetectable by statistical tests or by reviewers unless they know the precise selection protocol employed.*

"Analysis Creep" and Uncontrolled Iterative Modeling

A milder, all-too-common and often well-intentioned version of the file drawer bias pitfall occurs in the form of non-rigorous iterative analysis, which is sometimes refered to as bias due to "analysis creep". We illustrate by extending the previous hypothetical scenario:

Consider the data scientist of section "Selective Reporting of Results, 'Filedrawer Bias', 'Publication Bias'" who this time builds the outcome classifiers with careful cross validation where the data modeling decisions are fixed in the training data and error estimation takes place in the testing data portions of the cross validation. Assume that estimated error is 20%. The PI of the scientific project (or project manager of a commercial product based on the model) reviews the results and suggests trying out an additional classifier algorithm. The data scientist does so (repeating the same modeling protocol but with the new classifier) and produces a new model with error 17%. An external consultant reviews the results and suggests specific data transforms and feature construction which lead (by application of same analysis protocol on the same data) to a model with error 14%. In yet another "improvement" step a new hire in the data science team decides to explore some recalibration method that leads to a model with estimated 10% error. And so forth, until the final model appears to be a near-perfect one.

The problem with this scenario is that no measures are taken to isolate the introduction of new methods from the statistical variation of error estimation so that *the final model's error estimates are not over fitted to the specific train-test configuration used.*

An especially challenging aspect of the **"analysis creep"** problem that makes it invisible to even the most rigorous scientists who are not experts in data science, is that each step may be well designed and perfectly appropriate as a 1-step analysis, but when a series of such steps is executed, then over fitting and over confidence take place.

Choice of a Few and Non-representative Datasets; Unusual Populations; Broad Claims From Too Few or Too Easy Datasets

Just like non-rigorous (intentionally, or not) selection of models can create over fitted models and over interpreted results, the same is true for datasets.

- This problem is particularly common in ML/AI method development where the developers of methods often choose themselves the datasets to test their methods. It is entirely possible that developers may choose to report performance of their methods in data that is "friendly" to the methods, and to omit reporting (or event testing) performance on harder datasets.
- This situation is also common in ML and data science competitions that pit dozens or hundreds of methods against one another over one or a small number of datasets such that the results are typically overly-specific to the small choice of datasets (as well to the specific data design and performance metrics used).
- A related problem arises in applied discovery settings where multiple data sets exist and only a subset is used for development and testing.

The above scenarios create a lack of generalizability problem where certain methods or models perform well in some highly selected data or populations and therefore fail to generalize beyond those (chapters "Principles of Rigorous Development and of Appraisal of ML and AI Methods and Systems" and "Lessons Learned from Historical Failures, Limitations and Successes of AI/ML in Healthcare and the Health Sciences. Enduring Problems, and the Role of BPs" give more details in the context of limitations of competitions).

Many Teams, Same Data, No Coordinated Unbiased Protocol

Yet another version of the "analysis creep" and uncontrolled iterative or parallel modeling pitfalls occurs when (typically) in cooperative consortia or other large scale collaborative efforts, several teams are working on analyzing the same data with different algorithms, analysis protocols, error estimators etc.

In the absence of a coordinated unbiased model selection and error estimation protocol that applies to all analyst teams, the statistical variation of even good modeling methods with same large-sample performance can lead to large apparent differences in performance in the discovery data that do not generalize to the population. The problem can be further compounded when the various teams employ learning algorithms, model selection and error estimation methods with widely different characteristics where the selected model overall can simultaneously suffer from under-performance and over-confidence in it (see chapter "Lessons Learned from Historical Failures, Limitations and Successes of AI/ML in Healthcare and the Health Sciences. Enduring Problems, and the Role of Best Practices" for findings from a major centralized benchmark study revealing related problems).

Hard-to-Reproduce, Non-Standardized Data Input Steps

In some types of clinical as well in discovery data modeling the data inputs may be subjectively assessed and these assessments may have a low degree of reliability across different individuals or settings. If this aspect has not been incorporated in the model performance estimation (e.g., a single observer is responsible for all subjective assessments in both training and test data) then inflated performance estimates are produced.

Examples of this pitfall exist in a variety of settings, for example in assessment by surgeons of operation aspects, in pathologist evaluation of slides for less-than ideally standardized features, skin lesion assessments, proteomic spectra peak determinations, etc.

Normalization/Data Transforms that Require Entirety of Sample

In some modeling settings data needs to be processed (e.g., via normalization, discretization or other operations) by looking across the totality of data, that is including train and test data. This automatically creates the previously-discussed "contamination" of the error estimates of the test set by the train set weakening their independence and creating a bias in the error estimates.

Moreover from a purely practical viewpoint, the application of these models on new data not used in the model development/evaluation cycle is problematic because it requires re-normalization (or re-processing) of *all data* starting from early model development to the latest application.

Learners Learn the Wrong Patterns via Spurious Co-Occurrence

A classical example from epidemiology, involving causality, is the "yellow finger" which when is due to tar-staining from smoking, predicts several diseases resulting from smoking (e.g., lung and cardiovascular diseases, cancer). However the classifiers in these cases cannot discover that eliminating the yellow stains does not alter the disease risk. That requires eliminating the confounding cause (smoking) and thus such purely predictive findings/models do not generalize when interventions are considered.

Selective Control of Factors that Can Lead to OC

Recall that R. Simon et al. showed the role of feature selection for error estimation bias in high dimensional disease classification in "complete", "partial" and "no" cross validation. *Every single analysis step and parameter (not just feature selection) that affects the performance of models and the error estimators has to be controlled accordingly.* This includes hyperparameters, model families, normalization discretization, imputation etc.

OF and OC Problems in Patient-Specific Modeling

In recent years efforts have been made to develop models specifically tailored to individual patients. These are commonly based on time series data obtained from each individual and they may have predictive or causal foci [12, 13].

The advantages of such modeling is that (1) they-- may avoid masking and distribution-mix effects of population data and (2) may be able to focus more effectively on mechanisms and characteristics of individuals for precision and personalized medicine. Possible disadvantages are that they (3) may require dense time series data, (4) they may fail to leverage vast amounts of data from other individuals that apply to all individuals in the population, (5) by their very nature they cannot model severe and irrevocable, or rare or singular outcomes (e.g., death), (6) do not deal well with abrupt distribution shifts of the individual (whereas same shifts may be learnable at the population level and anticipated by population models) and (7) do not provide guarantees for generalizing to other individuals.

Characteristics (6) and (7) are therefore related to possible over fitting and over confidence.

Bespoke and Hand-Created AI Models

In certain types of AI modeling, most commonly in mathematical and engineering-based modeling that may incorporate limited data-driven aspects and is not fully automated as in ML, the ability to generate large numbers of models by the same individuals and over short periods of time is severely limited. This precludes the collection of large numbers of models and datasets in which the success of such models can be rigorously statistically evaluated. It is entirely possible under these circumstances for a few models to be performing well in some task yet the overall model building process is neither salable nor demonstrably generalizable. Creation of a handful of successful models by hand and evaluation on a handful of cases, for example a hand-crafted model to predict the safety of a drug in a specific RCT, may say very little about whether this model would apply to other RCTs and even less about whether the modeling methodology could be carried out by other modelers or for other drugs.

How UP ML/AI Models Are Commonly Created

Not Considering the Right Method Family, Not Considering Enough Method Families in Model Selection

A common reason for under performant models is not exploring the right model family in model selection. For example, when the data generating function is non-linear and discontinuous but we explore only linear regression models. When the right family is not known a priori the corresponding problem is not exploring enough method families in model selection.

The above are common occurrences when data scientists have strong preference for a small number or narrow methods, or when vendors focus on a specific technology that is used across diverse tasks even when it is not the most appropriate for the task.

Insufficient Data Preparation

This pitfall applies to all steps typically used for data preparation such as feature construction and selection, normalization, discretization, distribution transforms, etc. Such steps can greatly enhance model performance when employed correctly or hurt performance when they are ignored or conducted sub optimally.

Insufficient Model Selection Hyper Parameter Space

This pitfall occurs when the right model families are explored but without sufficient exploration of their hyper parameter values.

1-Step Modeling Attempts

In chapter "The Development Process and Lifecycle of Clinical Grade and Other Safety and Performance-Sensitive AI/ML Models" we elaborated on the importance of initial modeling which typically must subsequently be refined and enhanced (since the first attempt seldomly meets performance goals in complicated modeling problems). A 1-stage analysis procedure does not benefit from a graduated understanding of the data and task at hand and their interaction with the modeling method deployed.

Ignoring Best Known Methods

In some cases for specific domains and tasks prior theoretical and empirical work has established the predominance or superiority of specific classes of methods. It is therefore likely to under perform if these methods are not included in the model selection, at a minimum as "starting points" with baseline performance that other methods must match or exceed. See chapter "Principles of Rigorous Development and of Appraisal of ML and AI Methods and Systems" for proper scope of empirically evaluating new methods and for appraising existing methods.

Ignoring Official or Reference Specifications on Methods Use

A commonly-encountered pitfall is applying strong methods but in ways that are inconsistent with suggested use. These suggested uses include: (a) the ways these methods have been previously tested during reference method development and in validation phases leading to established strong results; (b) the specific ways the inventors of these methods have used them in the primary ("official") publications associated with them. Chapter "Lessons Learned from Historical Failures, Limitations and Successes of AI/ML In Healthcare and the Health Sciences. Enduring Problems, and the Role of Best Practices" describes case studies where such bias led to suboptimal performance.

UP Problems in Models for Individual Patients

As explained previously in "OF and OC Problems in Patient-Specific Modeling", individual-specific modeling has a priori both advantages and disadvantages over population-wide modeling. Characteristics (3), (4), (5), (6) and (7) are linked to possible under performance of such models relative to population based models.

Failing to Obtain Power Sample Analysis and More Generally to Control Effects of Sample Size on Modeling

In the absence of a power-sample analysis or knowledge of learning curves, the modeler does not know whether better results can be obtained by increasing the sample size, or what is the minimum sample size needed to reach the stated goals of the modeling.

> **In ML the power-sample calculation problem is more complicated than traditional statistical power-sample analysis**. This is because in inferential statistics we need to know what is the required sample size to reject a null hypothesis with a desired alpha and power, and closed formulas exist that describe this relationship for applicable statistical tests. In ML however, in addition to the need to test a model's performance against a null hypothesis, *we first need to find a good model*. Thus the power-sample calculation is further complicated by the learning protocol's *learning curve* that is the function that describes the generalization error of the best model learned (on average) as a function of sample size. Depending on the problem, learning curves may suggest that we need more or less sample size than the one needed to reject a null hypothesis centered on the model's performance. To make things worse, learning curves are not known a priori for the vast majority of practical problems.

Based on the above we can summarize on the pitfalls related to OC and UP including OF and UF.

> **Pitfall 10.1**
> **Producing models in which we have over-confidence**
>
> **10.1.1.** Models are allowed to have inappropriately large complexity with respect to data generating function complexity and to available sample size.
>
> **10.1.2.** Ignoring statistical uncertainty of strong point estimates of perfromance.
>
> **10.1.3.** Using biased estimators or introducing bias in unbiased ones.
>
> **10.1.4.** Not correcting multiple statistical hypotheses tests.
>
> **10.1.5.** Selectively reporting strongest models/results.
>
> **10.1.6.** Conducting uncontrolled iterative modeling and succumbing to "analysis creep".

10.1.7. Using non-representative datasets, unusual populations, and making strong claims from too few or too easy datasets.

10.2.8. Not coordinating analysis over many teams and same data via appropriate unbiased protocols designed for collaborative work or competitions.

10.1.9. Using hard-to-reproduce, non-standardized data input steps.

10.1.10. Employing normalization/data transforms that require entirety of sample.

10.1.11. Allowing learners to learn the wrong patterns via spurious co-occurrence; uncontrolled structural relations and biased sampling; and ignoring domain knowledge that reveals the above.

10.1.12. Controlling only some of the factors that can lead to OC.

10.1.13. Inappropriate modelling for individual patients and over interpretation of their generalizability.

10.1.14. Insufficient studies of scalability and generalizability in bespoke hand-created AI models.

Pitfall 10.2
Producing models that are under performing

10.2.1. Not deploying the right model family in model selection; not exploring enough method families in model selection.

10.2.2. Insufficient data preparation.

10.2.3. Insufficient exploration of the hyper parameter space during model selection.

10.2.4. 1-stage modeling attempts.

10.2.5. Ignoring best known methods for task and data at hand (either as baseline comparators or starting point).

10.2.5. Ignoring official specifications and prototypical (reference) use of employed methods.

10.2.6. Models for individual patients: lack of dense time series data, failure to leverage population models that apply to the specific individual (including ignoring or under modeling severe and irrevocable rare or singular outcomes), not addressing well abrupt distribution shifts of the individual (whereas same shifts may be learnable at the population level).

10.2.8. Failing to obtain power sample analysis and more generally control effects of sample size on modeling.

Preventing, Detecting, and Managing OC and OF

We now address specific best practices for preventing overfitted models and over confidence in models.

Manage Model Complexity with Respect to Data Generating Function Complexity and to Available Sample Size

Whereas manually balancing complexity against sample size is a formidable hurdle, well-designed modern ML methods, protocols, and systems encapsulate multiple methods that achieve this balance automatically or semi-automatically:

1. **Regularization**: is a methodology whereas model parameters' values are driven to zero by model fitting algorithms, as much as data allows. Regularization is broadly used by "penalty+loss" learners (see chapter "An Appraisal and Operating Characteristics of Major ML Methods Applicable in Healthcare and Health Science") for example SVMs, Lasso regression, regularized classical statistical variants such as regularized Cox regression, regularized Logistic regression, regularized Discriminant Function analysis, etc. The "loss" term is a mathematical expression of how accurately a model represents training data, whereas the "penalty" term captures the combined complexity of the model (e.g., sum of squared weights of inputs). Regularization is sometimes closely related to the notion of function smoothness, that is the preference for modeling functions in which the impact of a small change in the data generating function inputs leads to small changes to the classification output (this is mathematically equivalent to the "maximum margin classifier" inductive bias of SVMs).
2. **Dimensionality reduction**: is a set of methods that map the original input variables to a much smaller number of mathematical combinations (see chapter "An Appraisal and Operating Characteristics of Major ML Methods Applicable in Healthcare and Health Science"). A prototypical example is Principal Component Analysis (and variants) where the original input variables are replaced by independent linear combination functions (the principal components, such that the totality of data variance is captured by the totality of the principal components). The fitted models use as inputs the reduced input representation or a subset thereof.
3. **Feature selection**: (see chapters "Foundations and Properties of AI/ML Systems" and "An Appraisal and Operating Characteristics of Major ML Methods Applicable in Healthcare and Health Science") is a set of methods that select a small number from the original variables such that ideally all information about the response variable is retained and all redundant variables are discarded. Strong feature selection helps reduce model complexity to the absolute necessary (i.e., only those features that have indispensable information about the response).

4. **Bayesian Priors and Bayesian ensembles**: in Bayesian maximum a posteriori model selection-based modeling, prior probabilities over the model space considered can be used to ensure that models with appropriate (smaller) complexity are given more attention in smaller sample sizes and as sample size grows more complex models can be selected. Moreover, via Bayesian Model Averaging, many (all in theory, but just a few in practice in most practical settings) models can be combined to provide an "ensemble" classification. Complex models are expected to have smaller posteriors in small sample sizes than simpler ones and thus to drive more the overall ensemble decisions whereas in larger sample sizes, the opposite is true.

5. **Algorithm-embedded complexity control**: several ML algorithms have embedded means to control complexity of produced models. For example, decision tree learners prune the trees when they reach branching points with small sample sizes. Random forest learners apply feature selection at each branching point of each fitted tree and forbid trees larger than a set size (which is a tunable hyper - parameter). ANNs map large input spaces to potentially smaller hidden layer spaces or incorporate pruning and other regularization steps. SVMs transform non-linearly separable input spaces to linearly separable ones via kernel functions. Structured Risk Minimization in SVMs progressively considers classes of models (corresponding to kernels) of strictly increasing complexity with guarantees strictly monotonic improvements in generalization error. Boosting methods start from simpler models and extend them to address only the cases not classified correctly. And so on (see chapter "An Appraisal and Operating Characteristics of Major ML Methods Applicable in Healthcare and Health Science").

6. **Statistical model/data complexity measures**: classical examples being the AIC and BIC metrics [7] that are used in statistics to characterize models with respect to their complexity and fit against the training data. Simpler models are preferred by the human analysts, everything else being equal.

7. **Model selection and combination approaches**: it is common to create and apply ML/AI model fitting and selection protocols that combine several of the above approaches.

Using nested cross validation approaches to find the best models and estimate their generalization error is a common approach that allows model complexity to grow only as much it helps improving estimates of the true generalization error.

Characterize and Manage Statistical Uncertainty

Typically this entails: (a) Calculating confidence and credible ntervals for models (and of the models' parameter values when appropriate). (b) Testing models against the null hypothesis (commonly being that: there is no predictive signal in the data at hand, or a network model has properties no different than a random one, etc.). This is easily accomplished with a standard label reshuffling or other randomization tests (chapter "The Development Process and Lifecycle of Clinical Grade and Other Safety and Performance-Sensitive AI/ML Models"). (c) Conducting tests of model stability (when appropriate) to sample size. (d) Obtaining measures of stability of model output or decisions with respect to variation in the model inputs. (e) Reducing sampling variance by choice of most powerful/low variance estimators and protocols. Especially for n-fold cross validation schemes, repeating the analysis >50 times empirically has been shown to reduce train-test split variance [14].

Use Unbiased Estimators or Correct Estimation Bias

Among classical estimators and model selection protocols Repeated n-fold cross validation (RNFCV) is a particularly robust error estimator which can also be used for powerful model selection when nested (RNNFCV). In larger sample sizes a repeated nested holdout may be a more computationally efficient alternative. Finally, in very small sample situations a repeated nested leave on out can be used as alternative to RNNFCV [3].

We also recommend **"locking" models** at some predefined stage in the modeling process and not allowing further tampering with locked models. Publishing open-box models can certainly provide a strong form of such locking, although it may also be employed as an internal strategy during model development. A similar, very stringent but much less practical best practice is **preregistering ML studies and models** [15].

The exclusive use of independent data testing for establishing or testing for generalizability is commonly and often required by journals, funding study sections etc. It is *NOT recommended* however as a single, or "privileged" validation methodology in the present volume, since it is subject to between and within-population sampling variation so that discrepancies between the model's performance in the discovery + testing CV datasets and the independent validation dataset may be due to: (1) sampling from a different population, or (2) not having perfect power in the independent validation dataset (see section "Additional Notes on Strategies and Best Practices for Detection, Analysis and Managing Both OC and UP" for Details). The latter danger is especially salient in domains where sample sizes are never very large, or are very costly, ethically challenging, or slow to obtain. Nested CV by comparison eliminates the first source of errors since we ensure that the discovery and validation datasets come from the same population. See also chapter "Lessons Learned from Historical Failures, Limitations and Successes of AI/ML in Healthcare and the Health Sciences. Enduring Problems, and the Role of Best Practices" for a striking demonstration of variability between discovery and validation sets and results in a landmark benchmark study where same analyses were done with original and swapped discovery-validation sequences [16].

Correct or Control Multiple Statistical Hypotheses Tests

The venerable but outdated Bonferroni correction is not recommended since it reduces the power of the discovery procedure dramatically relative to more modern procedures. The Benjamini- Hochberg (or similar) methods for correlated and uncorrelated p-values can be used to more effectively control the acceptable ratio of false positives (e.g., the analyst can set thresholds on p-values that does not lead to more than 10% false positive rate on the reported results) [17].

We also note that certain algorithms, for example constrained-based causal modeling algorithms (e.g., GLL, LGL and others) have embedded control of false positives due to multiple statistical testing [18].

Thoroughly Specify and Report the Procedure Used to Obtain Results

The entirety of the analyses and modeling applied on data must be reported so that the possibility for over fitting is properly assessed by third parties. We emphasize that even if the original model developers share their modeling algorithms and data in full, unless they specify the analyses employed in their entirety (i.e., entirety of model selection and error estimation steps), *it is not possible to determine whether the models are over fitted without additional verification in independent data.* On the contrary, when the entirety of the analysis protocol is disclosed, both the final model's over fitting and the whole protocol's propensity to over fit or OC can be assessed (often with a simple label reshuffling test as demonstrated in chapter "The Development Process and Lifecycle of Clinical Grade and Other Safety and Performance-Sensitive AI/ML Models").

Conduct Iterative and Sequential Modeling via Unbiased Protocols

A robust and proven such protocol is the previously mentioned RNNFCV protocol in which every new method or parameter value added to the previous analysis steps is incorporated in the nested model selection along with all other methods **and the whole modeling is repeated from scratch (ideally with previous model fitting steps cached for improved tractability).** Other such protocols may be constructed, but it is essential for the modelers to establish first their robustness to bias due to iterative modeling. Note that when we perform model selection over k algorithms and their associated hyper parameter value sets in RNNFCV, the results are mathematically equivalent if we first model-select over the first methods, then insert the second, then the third and the winner of the first two, and so on until all methods have been examined. This demonstrates that since doing all methods at once is not overfitting/producing over-confident error estimates, the sequential procedure over the same set of methods, will not either.

See assignment 8 for a practical demonstration of proper vs improper iterative modeling.

Use Representative Datasets, Appropriate Populations and Make Generalizability Claims from Appropriate Datasets

In all modeling settings, clinical or biological criteria must be used to establish appropriateness of data used. Rigorous phenotypic definition and extractions from the EHR, for example, will ensure that only and all human subjects that apply to the modeling goals are considered for discovery and validation (see chapter on Data Design).

When new method development or validation and benchmarking are pursued, we recommend using all publicly available datasets that apply to the task and if they are too many, to use a randomly-stratified selection of representative datasets (e.g., with certain distributions, dimensionalities, sample sizes, etc.). See also chapter "Principles of Rigorous Development and of Appraisal of ML and AI Methods and Systems".

In situations where discovery is pursued via **secondary analysis of many pre-existing datasets**, it is very common for results to disagree among the various datasets. One way to address the problem is to **"Round-Robin" analysis** and examine the nature and robustness of results when some of the data are used for discovery and some for validation.

It is often useful in such situations of multi-dataset analyses, to adopt a different perspective and **focus not on whether model M or property P discovered, e.g., in datasets 1–10 holds in datasets 11–20 but, rather, what are the variant and invariant properties (both predictively and structurally) across this collection of datasets** and what is the **robustness of models** developed in a subset of the datasets on the remainder datasets (with the round-robin analysis conducted so that it examines or approximates all possible discovery-validation splits).

Stated differently, the discrepancies between datasets (and models summarizing properties of these data) should not be viewed automatically as "errors" but also considered as potentially valuable indicators of systematic differences between health care systems, research designs, model organisms etc., depending on the data measurement and sampling designs used.

Coordinate Analysis over Many Teams and Same Data via Appropriate Unbiased Protocols

The recommendations of "Conduct Iterative and Sequential Modeling Via Unbiased Protocols" apply unchanged here as well.

Use Easy-to-Reproduce, Standardized Data Input Steps

Techniques to facilitate this practice include **automating all subjective input measurements** and establishing equivalence or sufficiency of their information content. Alternatively, establishing that subjective measurements can be standardized via protocols that ensure **low interrater variability**.

Employ Normalization/Data Transforms that Do Not Require Entirety of Sample

This is self-explanatory and follows directly from the nature of validation-to-discovery information contamination that biases CV error estimates as explained previously.

Prevent Learners from Learning the Wrong Patterns via Spurious Co-Occurrence; Control Structural Relations and Biased Sampling; and Incorporate Domain Knowledge and Face-Validity Expert Testing that May Reveal Spurious Learning

Essential to the above are robust batch processing bias and error detection and correction protocols such as the ones routinely used in high-throughput omics assay-based studies. Moreover, causal modeling algorithms can reveal spurious and confounded relations and patterns of bias. In addition, a diversity of datasets that fully covers the space of application of the desired models must be used for training and validation. Finally, *model explanation techniques* can be valuable by revealing exactly what the learning algorithms and corresponding models created by those have learned especially when combined with expert review of such models (see chapter "The Development Process and Lifecycle of Clinical Grade and Other Safety and Performance-Sensitive AI/ML Models").

These latter precautionary practices unfortunately rely on existence of sufficient domain theory that can be used to detect anomalies in the models. It is entirely possible (and indeed common) in certain domains for robust such theory to be lacking, however (e.g., in high-density omics studies, or complex mental health/human behavior and other domains where the complex mechanisms governing the data generating processes have not been conclusively or completely established). It is important in such cases to non over-interpret models and to test the propensity of human experts to construct invalid conceptual explanations in support of models (see chapters "Principles of Rigorous Development and of Appraisal of ML and AI Methods and Systems" and "The Development Process and Lifecycle of Clinical Grade and Other Safety and Performance-Sensitive AI/ML Models" for expert biases and modeling of expert judgment). It is equally important to always consider the possibility that models encapsulate valid new knowledge previously unknown in the field, thus an expert's rejection of some model or result should be a piece of evidence in evaluating model validity and not grounds for immediate dismissal.

Control all Factors that Can Lead to OF/OC via TE→TR Contamination, by Using Nested Model Selection

The most important way to operationalize this is to use a nested protocol for cross validation and error estimation as previously explained, and at the same time ensure that all possible data analysis steps that may transmit information from the test sets to the train sets (and thus introduce bias in the error estimation) are isolated inside the nested part of the protocol.

Carefully Combine Modelling of Individual Patients with Population Modeling

Most importantly, any individualized modeling must be compared with population modeling and ensemble (combined) with population models whenever appropriate and feasible.

Do Not Over-Interpret the Generalizability of Bespoke Hand-Created AI Models Unless Sufficient Validation Data Can be Obtained to Support Such Claims

Unfortunately bespoke, hand-crafted modeling efforts typically cannot - by their very nature - be readily evaluated by automated procedures and data for such evaluations are scarce. It is prudent in such cases to address modeling successes and failures as isolated incidences.

> Whenever it is feasible to create automated computable procedures that replicate the bespoke methodologies, this allows transitioning non-scalable human modeling to scalable and testable AI/ML modeling with obvious advantages for increasing the scale, scope, speed, cost-effectiveness and verifiability of similar modeling in other problem domains/settings.

Preventing, Detecting, and Managing UF/UP (Table 1)

Practices 10.5.1.–10.5.7. in Table 1 are self-explanatory and follow directly from the principles presented earlier. The next best practice 10.5.8. require some explanation, however:

Conduct Power Sample Analysis and More Generally Characterize the Effects of Sample Size on Modeling. Use Dynamic Sampling Schemes Whenever Appropriate

With regards to the ML/AI power-sample planning as introduced in "Failing to Obtain Power Sample Analysis and more Generally Control Effects of Sample Size on Modeling", contrary to classical statistical hypothesis testing where closed formulas exist to calculate the minimum required sample for achieving a desired alpha (% of false positive rejections of the null, or type I error) and beta (probability of false negative failure to reject the null under the alternative hypothesis, or type II error, aka power) levels for some statistical test of choice, when designing ML/AI modeling, two additional factors come into play the first relevant to predictive modeling, and the second related to causal modeling:

(a) The **learning curve** of the used learning algorithm. The learning curve describes the errors of the algorithm's output as a function of sample size. Generally the learning curves are not known and closed formulas do not exist.

Table 1 Lists specific practices for preventing under fitted models

10.5.1. Deploy and explore all appropriate learning method families in model selection
10.5.2. Deploy and explore all relevant data preparation steps to the domain and task at hand
10.5.3. Systematically and sufficiently explore the hyper parameter space
10.5.4. Anticipate several preliminary and refinement modeling stages and incorporate in nested designs to avoid overfitting
10.5.5. Inform analyses by literature so that best known methods for task and data at hand are explored
10.5.6. Follow theoretically and empirically proven specifications and prototypical (reference) use of employed methods (including the official specific ways the developers of methods have presented in the corresponding primary publications)
10.5.7. Models for individual patients: Use dense time series data, leverage population models that apply to the specific individual (including modeling severe and irrevocable rare or singular outcomes), search for and model abrupt distribution shifts of the individual (including learning and modeling shifts at the population level)

(b) The **causal sparsity (i.e., density or connectivity) of the causal process** that generates the data. A sparse causal data generating process requires less sample size to be discovered because the sample size required for conditional independence tests (CITs) that are at the core of causal structure discovery algorithms increases exponentially (in unrestricted distributions) to the number of conditioning variables in the CIT (see chapter "Foundations of Causal ML"). This latter number is directly linked to the density of the generating causal graph. After a causal graph has been discovered, causal effects of interventions need be estimated and these estimations also require sample size that grows exponentially to the controlled confounders which are similarly linked to the density of the causal generating process.

Whereas classical statistical power-sample analysis can be applied once a good model or causal structure has been identified (to reject the null predictive model or the estimate causal effects, with high confidence) the sample size required for the predictive model discovery or the causal structure discovery and effect estimation are separate considerations. Indeed it is entirely possible for the sample size required for the former to be larger, equal or smaller than the sample size required for the latter.

10.5.8. Best practice strategies to address these sample size and power design needs for ML/AI model building include:

1. Using sensitivity analysis for results over convenience samples by iteratively reducing available sample size (sub-sampling on a convenience sample). If, for example, by reducing the sample size, models retain their predictivity, this strengthens the empirical argument that the learning curve has reached convergence and additional sample will not increase performance.
2. Use of simulations, ideally with real life data where ground truth models are known or re-simulation (as covered in chapter "Principles of Rigorous Development and of Appraisal of ML and AI Methods and Systems").
3. Use of domain knowledge (if it exists) about the nature of causal structure underlying the data, or the nature of predictive or causal functions to be learned.
4. Use of network-scientific knowledge about the nature of connectivity of real life networks.
5. Reference to prior robust results in very similar domains to formulate and justify assumptions about a successful analysis.
6. Use of dynamic sampling schemes such as adaptive trial designs, Bayesian posterior updating or active learning-based sampling.

Additional Notes on Strategies and Best Practices for Detection, Analysis and Managing Both OC and UP

(a) **Label reshuffling tests**. The label reshuffling procedure (as for example employed by R. Simon et al. and elaborated in chapter "The Development Process and Lifecycle of Clinical Grade and Other Safety and Performance-Sensitive AI/ML Models") retains the joint distribution of input variables however it decouples (on average) the inputs to the response variable. Thus it creates an "on average" null distribution from which we sample data and build models.

- By comparing the performance of the best model we found to this null distribution we can test the statistical hypothesis that it is as good as random choice (i.e., not reject the null).
- Additionally, by looking at the mean of this null distribution we can establish whether the overall analysis protocol biases the error estimates (under the null) and by how much.

(b) **Reanalysis** (with both original and unbiased or otherwise improved protocols, including single coordinated protocols as needed). This is especially important when one wishes to verify the validity of models produced by third parties. For example, when suspicion exists for selective reporting of analyses, or when suspicion of under fitting exists. It is not possible to conduct definitive "forensic style" re-analyses without having access to the full range of data and modeling protocols used in the original analyses. We caution that the ability to run "black box code" on the same data and reproduce the exactly same results, is inappropriately presented as a top-tier level of confidence by some guidelines (see discussion in chapter "Lessons Learned from Historical Failures, Limitations and Successes of AI/ML in Healthcare and the Health Sciences. Enduring Problems, and the Role of Best Practices"), yet it does not suffice because depending on how the black box operates, the models and performance estimates may be OC, UF, or both.

(c) **"Safety net" model application measures** for ensuring that a model is not applied to the wrong person or population (see chapters "The Development Process and Lifecycle of Clinical Grade and Other Safety and Performance-Sensitive AI/ML Models" and "Characterizing, Diagnosing and Managing the Risk of Error of ML and AI Models in Clinical and Organizational Application" for details on models' "knowledge cliff" and managing prediction risk).

(d) **Model stability considerations.** Variable coefficients or very large variation of output given small change in input variable inputs must be dealt with caution as they may imply OF/OC or UP/UF. However we note (without going into full technical details that would require very substantial space to cover), that it is entirely possible for unstable models, markers, causal edges, coefficients etc. to be meaningful and reproducible because of underlying equivalence classes in the data.

Therefore unstable findings should be examined more deeply, but not discarded outright.

In summary the following best practices allow managing (i.e., preventing, diagnosis and/or correcting) OC and UP:

Best Practice 10.1
Deploy procedures that prevent, diagnose and remedy errors of over confidence in, or over fitting of, models.

10.1.1. Manage model complexity with respect to data generating function complexity and to available sample size using:

1. Regularization
2. Dimensionality reduction
3. Feature selection
4. Bayesian Priors and Bayesian ensembles
5. Algorithm-embedded capacity control
6. Statistical model/data complexity measures
7. Model selection
8. Combination approaches

10.1.2. Characterize and manage statistical uncertainty.

10.1.3. Use unbiased estimators of model performance or correct bias of biased estimates.

10.1.4. Lock models at predefined stages in the modeling process and not allow further tampering with locked models.

10.1.5. Correct multiple statistical hypotheses tests (explicitly or implicitly).

10.1.6. Thoroughly specify and report the entirety of procedures used to obtain models so that independent verification of generalizability is possible.

10.1.7. Conduct iterative or sequential modeling via unbiased protocols.

10.1.8. Use representative datasets, appropriate populations and make generalizability claims from appropriate datasets.

10.1.9. Coordinate analysis over many teams and same data via appropriate unbiased protocols.

10.1.10. Use reproducible, standardized data input steps.

10.1.11. Employ normalization /data transforms that do not require entirety of sample (or confine such within discovery and validation datasets independently).

10.1.12. Prevent learners from learning the wrong patterns via spurious co-occurrence; control structural relations and biased sampling; and incorporate domain knowledge-based review that reveals spurious learning.

10.1.13. Control via nested model selection all (and not just a few) factors that can lead to OC.

10.1.14. If possible, combine modelling of individual patients with population modeling.

10.1.15. Do not over-interpret the generalizability of bespoke hand-created AI models unless sufficient number of validation data sets can be obtained to support such claims. Consider creating computable versions of model hand-crafting modeling when possible.

10.1.16. Use label reshuffling testing for evaluating the overfitting/overconfidence bias of the whole analysis protocol.

10.1.17. Apply with appropriate caution Independent dataset validation and be mindful of dangers of over-interpretation of positive and negative results.

10.1.18. Instead of pursuing strict and exact reproducibility across datasets, study the variant and invariant findings from these datasets.

10.1.19. Whenever possible, use reanalysis (with both original and unbiased or otherwise improved protocols, including single coordinated protocols as needed) when verifying the validity of models produced by third parties.

10.1.20. Use domain knowledge and related face-validity tests by experts to flag potential model errors. The experts themselves may be prone to biases or domain theory may not cover models' new findings so do not over-interpret experts' objections.

10.1.21. Apply "safety net" measures for ensuring that a model is not applied to the wrong person or population.

10.1.22. Examine stability of models, parameters and other findings and examine more deeply unstable findings. Be aware that it is possible for unstable findings and models to be perfectly valid.

Best Practice 10.2
Deploy procedures that prevent, diagnose and remedy errors of model under-performance or underfitting.

10.5.1. To maximize predictivity, deploy and explore all relevant learning method families in model selection.

10.5.2. To maximize predictivity and generalizability, deploy and explore all relevant data preparation steps to the domain and task at hand.

10.5.3. To maximize predictivity, systematically and sufficiently explore the hyper parameter space.

10.5.4. Anticipate several preliminary and refinement modeling stages and incorporate them into sequential nested designs to avoid overfitting.

10.5.5. Inform analyses by methods literature so that best known methods for task and data at hand are always explored along with novel methods.

10.5.6. Follow theoretically and empirically proven specifications of reference prototypical or official use of employed methods.

10.5.7. In models for individual patients: use dense time series data, leverage population models, search for and model abrupt distribution shifts of the individual (including learning and modeling shifts at the population level).

10.5.8. Conduct power sample analysis and more generally characterize the effects of sample size on modeling. In the absence of knowledge of learning curves, use:

1. Dynamic sampling schemes whenever appropriate,
2. Sensitivity analysis for results over convenience samples by iteratively reducing available sample size (sub-sampling on a convenience sample),
3. Simulations,
4. Domain knowledge,
5. Network-scientific knowledge,
6. Reference to prior robust results in very similar domains,
7. Dynamic sampling schemes.

Key Concepts Discussed in Chapter "Overfitting, Underfitting and General Model Overconfidence and Under-Performance Pitfalls and Best Practices in Machine Learning and AI"
Training data error of a model

True generalization error of a model

Estimated generalization error of a model

Overfitting a model to data

Overfitting ML/AI method, system, stack, or protocol

Underfitting a model to data

Underfitting ML/AI method, system, stack, or protocol

Over confidence in a model

Under confidence in a model

Over performance of a model

Under performance of a model

Confidence Interval (CI) of a point estimate P of the performance of a model

Predictive Interval (PI) of a point estimate P of the performance of a model.

Analysis creep

Sequential, iterative and multi-team analyses

Pitfalls Discussed in Chapter "Overfitting, Underfitting and General Model Overconfidence and Under-Performance Pitfalls and Best Practices in Machine Learning and AI"

Pitfall 10.1.: Producing models in which we have over-confidence

10.1.1. Models are allowed to have inappropriately large complexity with respect to data generating function complexity and to available sample size.

10.1.2. Ignoring statistical uncertainty of point estimates of performance.

10.1.3. Using biased estimators or introducing bias in unbiased ones.

10.1.4. Not correcting multiple statistical hypotheses tests.

10.1.5. Selectively reporting strongest models/results.

10.1.6. Conducting uncontrolled iterative modeling and succumbing to "analysis creep".

10.1.7. Using non-representative datasets, unusual populations, and making strong claims from too few or too easy datasets.

10.1.8. Not coordinating analysis over many teams and same data via appropriate unbiased protocols designed for collaborative work or competitions.

10.1.9. Using hard-to-reproduce, non-standardized data input steps.

10.1.10. Employing normalization /data transforms that require entirety of sample.

10.1.11. Allowing learners to learn the wrong patterns via spurious co-occurrence, uncontrolled structural relations and biased sampling; and ignoring domain knowledge that reveals the above.

10.1.12. Controlling only some of the factors that can lead to OC.

10.1.13. Inappropriate modelling for individual patients and over interpretation of their generalizability.

10.1.14. Insufficient studies of scalability and generalizability in bespoke hand-created AI models.

Pitfall 10.2.: Producing models that are under performing.

10.2.1. Not deploying the right model family in model selection; not exploring enough method families in model selection.

10.2.2. Insufficient data preparation.

10.2.3. Insufficient exploration of the hyper parameter space during model selection.

10.2.4. 1-stage modeling.

10.2.5. Ignoring best known methods for task and data at hand (either as baseline comparators or starting point).

10.2.5. Ignoring official specifications and prototypical (reference) use of employed methods.

10.2.6. Models for individual patients: lack of dense time series data, failure to leverage population models that apply to the specific individual (including ignoring or under-modeling severe and irrevocable rare or singular outcomes), not addressing well abrupt distribution shifts of the individual (whereas same shifts may be learnable at the population level).

10.2.7. Failing to obtain power sample analysis and more generally control effects of sample size on modeling.

Best Practices Discussed in Chapter "Overfitting, Underfitting and General Model Overconfidence and Under-Performance Pitfalls and Best Practices in Machine Learning and AI"

Best Practice 10.1: Deploy procedures that prevent, diagnose and remedy errors of over confidence in, or over fitting of, models.

10.1.1. Manage model complexity with respect to data generating function complexity and to available sample size using:

1. Regularization,
2. Dimensionality reduction,
3. Feature selection,
4. Bayesian Priors and Bayesian ensembles,
5. Algorithm-embedded capacity control,
6. Statistical model/data complexity measures,
7. Model selection,
8. Combination approaches.

10.1.2 Characterize and manage statistical uncertainty.

10.1.3. Use unbiased estimators of model performance or correct bias of biased estimates.

10.1.4. Lock models at predefined stages in the modeling process and not allow further tampering with locked models.

10.1.5. Correct multiple statistical hypotheses tests (explicitly or implicitly).

10.1.6. Thoroughly specify and report the entirety of procedures used to obtain models so that independent verification of generalizability is possible.

10.1.7. Conduct iterative or sequential modeling via unbiased protocols.

10.1.8. Use representative datasets, appropriate populations, and make generalizability claims from appropriate datasets.

10.1.9. Coordinate analysis over many teams and same data via appropriate unbiased protocols.

10.1.10. Use reproducible, standardized data input steps.

10.1.11. Employ normalization /data transforms that do not require entirety of sample (or confine such within discovery and validation datasets independently).

10.1.12. Prevent learners from learning the wrong patterns via spurious co-occurrence; control structural relations and biased sampling; and incorporate domain knowledge-based review that reveals spurious learning.

10.1.13. Control via nested model selection all (and not just a few) factors that can lead to OC.

10.1.14. Carefully combine modelling of individual patients with population modeling.

10.1.15. Do not over-interpret the generalizability of bespoke hand-created AI models unless sufficient validation data can be obtained to support such claims. Consider creating computable versions of model hand-crafting modeling when possible.

10.1.16. Use label reshuffling testing for evaluating the overfitting bias of the whole analysis protocol.

10.1.17. Apply with appropriate caution independent dataset validation and be mindful of dangers of over interpretation of positive and negative results.

10.1.18. Instead of pursuing strict and exact reproducibility across datasets, study the variant and invariant findings across these datasets.

10.1.19. Whenever possible, use reanalysis (with both original and unbiased or otherwise improved protocols, including single coordinated protocols as needed) when verifying the validity of models produced by third parties.

10.1.20. Use domain knowledge and related face-validity tests by experts to flag potential model errors. The expert themselves may be prone to biases or domain theory may not cover models' new findings so do not over-interpret experts' objections.

10.1.21. Apply "safety net" measures for ensuring that a model is not applied to the wrong person or population.

10.1.22. Examine stability of models, parameters and other findings and examine more deeply unstable findings. Be aware that it is possible for unstable models to be perfectly valid.

Best Practice 10.2: Deploy procedures that prevent, diagnose and remedy errors of model under performance or underfitting.

10.5.1. Deploy and explore all relevant learning method families in model selection.

10.5.2. Deploy and explore all relevant data preparation steps to the domain and task at hand.

10.5.3. Systematically and sufficiently explore the hyper parameter space.

10.5.4. Anticipate several preliminary and refinement modeling stages and incorporate in sequential nested designs to avoid overfitting.

10.5.5. Inform analyses by methods literature so that best known methods for task and data at hand are always explored along with novel methods.

10.5.6. Follow theoretically and empirically proven specifications of reference prototypical or official use of employed methods.

10.5.7. In models for individual patients: use dense time series data, leverage population models, search for and model abrupt distribution shifts of the individual (including learning and modeling shifts at the population level).

10.5.8. Conduct power sample analysis and more generally characterize the effects of sample size on modeling. Use:

1. Dynamic sampling schemes whenever appropriate,
2. Sensitivity analysis for results over convenience samples by iteratively reducing available sample size (sub-sampling on a convenience sample),
3. Simulations,
4. Domain knowledge,
5. Network-scientific knowledge,
6. Reference to prior robust results in very similar domains,
7. Dynamic sampling schemes.

Classroom Assignments and Discussion Topics

Chapter "Overfitting, Underfitting and General Model Overconfidence and Under-Performance Pitfalls and Best Practices in Machine Learning and AI"

1. Consider Rich Simon's experiment with the following modification: the feature selection method used is based on univariate association using a Hockberg-Benjamini control of false positive rate at 10%. This means that the features will be ranked by p-value of the association with the response variable and thresholded so that no more than 10% of selected features will be false positive correlates of the response variable.
   (a) How many features will be selected if no feature has true signal for the response?
   (b) What will be the error estimation bias of complete, incomplete and no cv schemes?
   (c) Based on the above, does the Simon et al. conclusions hold regardless of the feature selection method?
   (d) How would you modify the Simon et al. guidance?

2. Is it possible that error of a classifier is 0 in the TR data, true optimal generalization error is >0 and this classifier is optimal? In other words, is it possible for a model to be optimal yet overfitted?

3. Consider the following scenario describing two model selection procedures MS1, MS2 and MS3 each considering and selecting different sets of models with estimated and true generalization errors as described in the table. For simplicity assume no other models can be fitted in this setting.

	Model 1	Model 2	Model 3	Model 4
TR accuracy	0.95	0.90	0.75	0.65
Estimated generalization accuracy by CV	0.80	0.88	0.78	0.70
Estimated generalization accuracy by Estimator X	0.9	0.96	0.92	0.80
True generalization accuracy	0.80	0.88	0.76	0.73
MS1 selects model	Yes	No	Yes	Yes
MS2 selects model	Yes	Yes	Yes	Yes
MS3 considers model	No	Yes	No	Yes

   (a) What are you conclusions about OP, OC, OF, UF and UP of models 1 to 4?
   (b) What is your assessment of the bias of the generalization accuracy estimator X used here?
   (c) Why CV does not exactly match the true generalization error, although it is unbiased?
   (d) Which models are selected by each of MS1 to MS3? How would you characterize these model selectors?

4. [ADVANCED] The label reshuffling procedure tests whether a model is statistically significantly different than a model without signal and simultaneously whether the overall modeling protocol has a propensity for producing over

confident estimates. This holds under the null hypothesis (i.e. there is no signal in the data).

(a) The reshuffling takes place only in the response variable labels. Explain why we DO NOT randomize all variables (i.e., both inputs and outputs).

(b) Bonus/research topic open problem: can you think of possible procedures that could test against alternative hypotheses (i.e., against a user-postulated non-zero signal)?

5. Consider years 2020–2021 of the COVID epidemic whereas many factors were constantly changing.

(a) What are some key factors that were changing?

(b) What challenges of the OF/UP/OC varieties does a situation like this creates for various types of AI/ML decision models? Consider ICU admission decision models as an example.

6. Describe, by example or more general analysis, how a researcher can produce clustering omics data so that a published cluster model exhibits good diagnostic accuracy even though no such signal exists in the data.

7. Comment on the following position: "whenever the true signal in the data is very high, it is more difficult to produce models with serious overconfidence errors; conversely as true signal approaches zero, the magnitude of possible OC error increases". What are underlying assumptions in the above thesis?

8. Consider the following (idealized and simplified) modeling situation. A data scientist is tasked by her manager to create a predictive model. She decides to use nested hold out (equivalent to NNCV with one fold) as follows: the total data is randomly split in mutually exclusive datasets TRTR TRTE and TE. She ensures that the prior of the binary response variable is the same in all three datasets. She considers 2 possible values for hyper-parameter H of ML algorithm A and estimates accuracy (0/1 error) as follows:

Algorithm A				
Accuracy in TRTE for H = 1	Accuracy in TRTE for H = 2	Best value of H	Accuracy in TE of model with best value of H	Finally reported accuracy of best model
0.80	0.90	2	0.85	0.85

She presents the results to the project manager who suggests that a second algorithm B is used because it may increase accuracy. The results this time look like this:

Algorithm B				
Accuracy in TRTE for H = 1	Accuracy in TRTE for H = 2	Best value of H	Accuracy in TE of model with best value of H	Finally reported accuracy of best model
0.85	0.80	1	0.80	0.80

She presents the results to the project manager who still is not satisfied with the result and brings in a consultant who suggests that a third algorithm C is used. The results this time look like this:

| Algorithm C | | | | |
Accuracy in TRTE for H = 1	Accuracy in TRTE for H = 2	Best value of H	Accuracy in TE of model with best value of H	Finally reported accuracy of best model
0.75	0.80	2	0.90	0.90

Based on the above the manager and the consultant conclude that the model produced by algorithm C is the best, it has generalization accuracy 0.90, and should be deployed.

The data scientist (who recently read chapter "Overfitting, Underfitting and General Model Overconfidence and Under-Performance Pitfalls and Best Practices in Machine Learning and AI") is not convinced however because she now suspects that an "analysis creep" situation has occurred leading to overconfidence in a model. She decides to conduct a nested holdout based analysis, this time analyzing all 3 algorithms simultaneously in the nested part (inner loop) of the cv design. The following table presents her results:

Algorithm A	Accuracy in TRTE for H = 1 0.80	Accuracy in TRTE for H = 2 0.90	Best algorithm/best value of H: Algorithm A, H = 2	Accuracy in TE of model with best algorithm/ best value of H 0.85	Finally reported estimated generalization accuracy of best model 0.85
Algorithm B	Accuracy in TRTR for H = 1 0.85	Accuracy in TRTE for H = 2 0.80			
Algorithm C	Accuracy in TRTR for H = 1 0.75	Accuracy in TRTE for H = 2 0.80			

The manager and the consultant are perplexed.

Assume the role of the data scientist and write a short report explaining how an OC error occurred in the first round of analyses and why the second analysis is unbiased. For simplicity, ignore the need to conduct tests of statistical difference between point estimates and interpret nominal accuracy point estimates as true ones.

9. We saw that combining capacity control mechanisms provides augmented protections against overfitting/excessive capacity.
   (a) Describe an existing protocol of your choice (or one that you construct) that combines 4 or more ways to control excessive model capacity.
   (b) Bonus question [ADVANCED]: is it possible for such combinations to have negative effects on ability to control the capacity of the models produced?

10. [ADVANCED]
    (a) Show that in order to calculate the true positives rate (aka PPV) or a model's decisions we need to know the prior of the distribution of the response variable.
    (b) Show that an active learning sampling design alone does not allow the analyst to know this prior whereas a random sampling design does.
    (c) What are the implications therefore of an active learning design for controlling the PPV?

11. Is it ok to build under performing models in the context of exploratory research? Present a few situations where it might be a good idea and some where it is a bad idea.

12. "Ocam's Razor" is an epistemological principle that says that between two models that explain the data equally well, the simpler one is more likely to be true. How does this principle relate to the BVDE? Can you think of a counter example (HINT: consider causal modeling).

13. (a) Describe how PCA can lead to OC errors.
    (b) Consider R. Simon's experiment where instead of feature selection the analyst use a PC-mapping of the input data such that correlation with the response variable is maximized. Is this subject to the same bias that Simon et al. described?
    (c) How would you conduct unbiased error estimation using NNFCV whereas the data is PCA-transformed?

14. [ADVANCED] Wolpert uses NFLT and OTSE to argue in [19] that cross validation is not better as a model selection strategy than *doing the exact opposite* (i.e., choose the model with highest error in the test data), which he coins "anti-cross validation". If he is right, then what that Chapter "Overfitting, Underfitting and General Model Overconfidence and Under-Performance Pitfalls and Best Practices in Machine Learning and AI" teaches as best practices for model selection and error estimation is only a heuristic strategy that may fail in as many situations as the ones that it will succeed. Refute these claims.

    HINT: focus your arguments either around the misalignment of OTSE with real-life modeling objectives/performance metrics, or alternatively/additionally with the misalignment of these objectives with averaging over all distributions rather the distribution in hand.

References

1. Mitchell TM. Machine learning, vol. 1. New York: McGraw-hill; 2007.
2. Simon R, Radmacher MD, Dobbin K, McShane LM. Pitfalls in the use of DNA microarray data for diagnostic and prognostic classification. J Natl Cancer Inst. 2003;95(1):14–8.
3. Statnikov A. A gentle introduction to support vector machines in biomedicine: theory and methods, vol. 1. World Scientific; 2011.

4. Aliferis CF, Statnikov A, Tsamardinos I. Challenges in the analysis of mass-throughput data: a technical commentary from the statistical machine learning perspective. Cancer Informat. 2006;2:133–62.
5. Aliferis CF, Statnikov A, Tsamardinos I, Schildcrout JS, Shepherd BE, Harrell FE Jr. Factors influencing the statistical power of complex data analysis protocols for molecular signature development from microarray data. PLoS One. 2009;4(3):e4922.
6. Kerr NL. HARKing: hypothesizing after the results are known. Personal Soc Psychol Rev. 1998;2(3):196–217.
7. Harrell FE. Regression modeling strategies: with applications to linear models, logistic regression, and survival analysis, vol. 608. New York: springer; 2001.
8. Steyerberg EW. Applications of prediction models. New York: Springer; 2009. p. 11–31.
9. Duda RO, Hart PE. Pattern classification. John Wiley & Sons; 2006.
10. Efron B, Tibshirani RJ. An introduction to the bootstrap. CRC press; 1994.
11. Andrade C. HARKing, cherry-picking, p-hacking, fishing expeditions, and data dredging and mining as questionable research practices. J Clin Psychiatry. 2021;82(1):25941.
12. Neal ML, Kerckhoffs R. Current progress in patient-specific modeling. Brief Bioinform. 2010;11(1):111–26.
13. Visweswaran S, Cooper GF. Patient-specific models for predicting the outcomes of patients with community acquired pneumonia. In: *AMIA Annual Symposium*, vol. 2005. American Medical Informatics Association; 2005. p. 759.
14. Braga-Neto UM, Dougherty ER. Is cross-validation valid for small-sample microarray classification? Bioinformatics. 2004;20(3):374–80.
15. McDermott MB, Wang S, Marinsek N, Ranganath R, Foschini L, Ghassemi M. Reproducibility in machine learning for health research: still a ways to go. Sci Transl Med. 2021;13(586):eabb1655.
16. Shi L, Campbell G, Jones WD. The MicroArray quality control (MAQC)-II study of common practices for the development and validation of microarray-based predictive models. Nat Biotechnol. 2010;28(8):827–38.
17. Benjamini Y, Hochberg Y. Controlling the false discovery rate: a practical and powerful approach to multiple testing. J R Stat Soc Series B Stat Methodol. 1995;57(1):289–300.
18. Aliferis CF, Statnikov A, Tsamardinos I, Mani S, Koutsoukos XD. Local causal and Markov blanket induction for causal discovery and feature selection for classification part II: analysis and extensions. J Mach Learn Res. 2010;11(1):235–84.
19. Wolpert DH. What is important about the no free lunch theorems? In: Black box optimization, machine learning, and no-free lunch theorems. Cham: Springer International Publishing; 2021. p. 373–88.

From "Human versus Machine" to "Human with Machine"

Gyorgy Simon and Constantin Aliferis

Abstract

This chapter first reviews areas where AI/ML and other automated decision making performs well in hard problems in the health sciences. It also summarizes main results from the literature comparing empirical performance of AI/ML vs humans. The chapter then addresses foundations of human heuristic decision making (and important related biases), and contrasts those with AI/ML biases. Finally the chapter touches upon how hybrid human/machine intelligence can outperform either approach.

Keywords

AI/ML system performance · Cognitive biases · AI/ML system biases · Computer-Human Joint Decision Making ("Human in the Loop")

Evidence for Strong Performance of AI/ML in Healthcare and Health Science Problem Solving

There is a growing literature that establishes the ability of AI/ML for complex problem solving in a variety of health domains, and compares ML techniques among themselves, to traditional statistical methods, and occasionally to human experts.

In a meta analysis of the ML-based Neurosurgical Outcome Prediction literature involving 30 studies it was found that ML models predicted outcomes after neurosurgery with excellent predictivity (median accuracy and area under the receiver operating curve of 94.5% and 0.83, respectively), and significantly better than logistic regression (median absolute improvement in accuracy and area under the receiver

G. Simon (✉) · C. Aliferis
Institute for Health Informatics, University of Minnesota, Minneapolis, MN, USA

operating curve of 15% and 0.06, respectively). Some studies also demonstrated a better performance in ML models *compared with established prognostic indices and clinical experts* [1].

In a systematic review of 27 studies applying machine learning to oral cavity cancer outcomes, it was found that the accuracy of models ranged from 0.85 to 0.97 for malignant transformation prediction, 0.78–0.91 for cervical lymph node metastasis prediction, 0.64–1.00 for treatment response prediction, and 0.71–0.99 for prognosis prediction. In general, most trained algorithms predicting these outcomes performed better than alternate methods of prediction. They also found that models including molecular markers in training data had better accuracy estimates for malignant transformation, treatment response, and prognosis prediction [2].

In a meta-analysis and systematic review of applications of machine learning algorithms to predict therapeutic outcomes in depression (20 studies), classification models were able to predict therapeutic outcomes with an overall accuracy of 0.82 (95% confidence interval of [0.77, 0.87]). Also, pooled estimates of classification accuracy were significantly greater ($p < 0.01$) in models informed by multiple data types (e.g., composite of phenomenological patient features and neuroimaging or peripheral gene expression data; pooled proportion [95% CI] = 0.93[0.86, 0.97]) when compared to models with lower-dimension data types (pooled proportion = 0.68[0.62,0.74] to 0.85[0.81,0.88]) [3].

In another systematic review and critical appraisal of ML applications in vascular surgery over 212 studies were identified in which ML techniques were used for diagnosis, prognosis, and image segmentation in carotid stenosis, aortic aneurysm/dissection, peripheral artery disease, diabetic foot ulcer, venous disease, and renal artery stenosis. The median area under the receiver operating characteristic curve (AUROC) was 0.88 (range 0.61–1.00), with 79.5% [62/78] studies reporting AUROC ≥0.80. Out of 22 studies *comparing ML techniques to existing prediction tools, clinicians, or traditional regression models*, 20 performed better and 2 performed similarly [4].

A systematic review of ML investigations evaluating suicidal behaviors with 87 studies analyzed, found high levels of risk classification accuracy (>90%) and Area Under the Curve (AUC) in the prediction of suicidal behaviors [5].

In a systematic review of 23 studies of applications of machine learning to undifferentiated chest pain in the emergency department, it was found that multiple studies achieved high accuracy in both the diagnosis of acute myocardial infarction (AMI) in the ED setting, and in predicting mortality and composite outcomes over various timeframes. ML outperformed existing risk stratification scores in all cases, and physicians in three out of four cases [6].

In a systematic review and meta-analysis comparing deep learning performance against health-care professionals in detecting diseases from medical imaging, based on 69 studies, it was established that ML models exhibited sensitivity ranging from

9.7% to 100.0% (mean 79.1%, SD 0.2) and specificity ranging from 38.9% to 100.0% (mean 88.3%, SD 0.1). 14 of these 69 studies compared the performance between ML models and health-care professionals. Restricting the analysis to the contingency table for each study reporting the highest accuracy found a pooled sensitivity of 87.0% (95% CI 83.0-90.2) for deep learning models and 86.4% (79.9-91.0) for health-care professionals, and a pooled specificity of 92.5% (95% CI 85.1-96.4) for deep learning models and 90.5% (80.6-95.7) for health-care professionals [7].

Finally a systematic review of over 42 studies evaluated the applications of AI in pediatric oncology [8]. Of these 42, 20 studies related to CNS tumors, 13 to solid tumors, and nine to leukemia. ML tasks included classification, prediction of treatment response, and dose optimization. The identified studies matched or outperformed physician comparators via automated analysis and predicting therapeutic response.

Quantitative Comparisons of AI/MI Versus Human Experts

In addition to studies [1, 4–8] in the previous section that not only studied ML model performance in absolute terms but also compared to human experts, several more studies have focused on the comparison between humans and AI/ML problem solving performance.

A large meta-analysis of 136 studies that were conducted between 1966-1988 compared the prediction performance of "mechanical procedures" (i.e., data science models of various forms: statistical models, actuarial tables, ML, or other) with that of human experts. The meta-analysis found that given the same information about the cases, the mechanical procedures outperformed the humans in 33–47% of the studies by being substantially more accurate than clinical predictions and in only 6–16% of the studies, human predictions were substantially more accurate than the mechanical ones. In the remaining 37%–61% of studies, humans and machines performed equally [9]. This shows that even with the comparatively limited technology of the 70s and 80s automated decision making was equal or superior to humans in 84–94% of the included studies.

Early AI computer aided diagnosis (CAD or CADx) research produced similarly promising results. In an application for diagnosis of abdominal pain, clinicians without access to the CAD tool arrived at the correct diagnosis with 71.6% accuracy, but with the aid of the CAD tool, the accuracy reached 91.8% [10].

In addition to the DL vs human study of [7], another systematic review found similar results, namely that the performance of AI was on par with that of clinicians and exceeded that of clinicians with less experience [11].

Many of the above studies report model performance "in the lab", that is not embedded in real-life clinical workflow/environment.

Pitfall 11.1
Even if a clinical AI system meets or exceeds expert-level performance in the lab, this does *NOT* mean that (i) the system can be readily adopted into clinical practice, (ii) will perform similarly when deployed in practice, or (iii) that the evaluation metrics used accurately reflect clinically impactful use of the AI model.

See the chapter entitled "The Development Process and Lifecycle of Clinical Grade and Other Safety and Performance-Sensitive AI/ML Models" for details of bringing models into practice.

We also note that the above comparisons refer to problem–solving tasks that both humans and machines can accomplish (albeit with different accuracy, ease, etc.). There exist problems that are currently entirely outside the capabilities of human decision making (e.g. making decisions using hundreds of thousands, or more, molecular and genetic factors, something that is routine in molecular oncology ML models; or inferring complex causal relationships involving hundreds or thousands of variables by inspecting transcriptomic or other data).

Human Biases Versus Machine Biases

Humans and computers approach problems fundamentally differently. In the chapters "Foundations and Properties of AI/ML Systems", "An Appraisal and Operating Characteristics of Major ML Methods Applicable in Healthcare & Health Science", and "Foundations of Causal ML" we visited the fundamental architecture and properties of AI and ML methods. We will assume that the reader is already familiar with the kinds of reasoning that humans can accomplish either in professional domains (i.e., health care practice, or health science) or in everyday living.

We will highlight a few important shortcomings of human decision making and examine to what extent machines can help overcome these shortcomings. Reviewing the theory of human learning, judgement and decision making at length is outside the scope of this book and the interested reader is referred to the highly informative and concise summary of human cognitive biases in [12], the prescriptive theory of medical decision making in [13], the several investigations on clinical decision making biases in [14] and the classic Nobel Prize-winning work of Kahneman [15] on human heuristics and biases.

We will also shed some light, from a technical perspective, on what are machine biases and how they arise or are prevented.

Human Memory Is Not a Storage Device

Contrary to common belief, human memory is not a device that stores "material" (medical or science facts, experimental data, interpretations, patient information, thoughts, discussion points, feelings, etc.) and recalls them later. A study found that more than 90% of the points made in a discussion were forgotten. The mind builds a mental model of the "material" and fills in details through inference. Our confidence in how accurate our recollection is relates to our confidence in the inference rather than to our ability to recall facts [16].

Humans Are Influenced by Context

Since memory is inferred, it is context-dependent. It is not just the memory, but most of human interpretation is context-dependent, even down to minute details. For example, in a list of items, we attribute more weight to the first item than later items and we remember the most recent (last) items better [17]. In some cases, where the contrast among multiple alternatives is too high, we can become unable to assess the middle alternative. In a similar vein, when a multitude of characteristics is evaluated simultaneously, these evaluations influence each other and the results correlate. This latter trait is exemplified by real-life "superheros" who are perceived to be excellent in almost all character traits we care about [18].

Questions can create a context [19]. The way questions are formed can influence the answer. When open-ended questions are used, the respondent may not consider all alternative responses, and may not think about the most appropriate response. Conversely, when closed questions are used, where the respondent has to select an answer from a list of alternatives, alternatives can artificially increase the frequency of answers that would otherwise be uncommon. When the question concerns a measurement, the alternatives to a closed question can suggest a baseline, a "normal" value, against which the respondents measure themselves. Even the order in which questions are asked and the order in which potential answers (for closed questions) are presented can influence the answers. Fortunately, when the subject is knowledgeable about the topic of the question, such influences are smaller. To reduce bias in answers by respondents who are not knowledgeable, surveys often include an option for "don't know". Finally, the wording of the questions itself can influence the answer. Answers can change depending on whether the question is asked in terms of gains or losses, lives saved versus deaths.

Humans Are Not Inherently Rational Decision Makers.

A fundamental normative model of human decision making is the maximum expected utility theory [15, 20, 21]. It describes decision making as following from assigning utilities to outcomes and choosing actions so that the expected utility will be maximized. Essential to such an endeavor are: (a) to describe with accuracy and completeness all relevant actions and outcomes in a problem of interest; (b) the ability to assign consistently individual preferences (measured by utility) to alternative outcomes; (c) the ability to calculate accurately the probability of outcomes given actions, including calculating probabilities of intermediate events outside the control of the decision maker; and (d) the ability to calculate accurately the action that maximizes the expected utility.

Not surprisingly, several examples have been shown in the literature where humans make decisions that do not abide by several components of expected utility-based reasoning. One important deviation is that losses are more important than gains to a part of the population. Kahneman et al. illustrates this through the following example. When decision makers are presented with a pair of alternatives, where one alternative is a sure loss of $500 and the other alternative is a gamble of losing $1000 with 50% chance and losing $0 with the remaining 50% chance, subjects tend to choose the second option (i.e., avoid the sure loss). However, when we frame the alternatives in terms of gains, with the first alternative being a sure gain of $500 and the second alternative is a gamble with 50% of winning $1000 and 50% chance not winning any money, people tend to select the sure gain.

Prospect theory [21] is a decision making model that uses the *perceived* value of gains and losses (as opposed to utility) as the basis of decision making and utilizes value functions that take the above asymmetry between the two into account. This model has the ability to describe "irrationalities" (deviations from the normative "rational" behavior that expected utility theory assumes) such as:

 (i)   the diminishing value of gains and losses (the first $500 gain or loss is more important than the second).
 (ii) Certainty effects such as removing the last bullet from a gun in Russian roulette is worth more (has more value) than removing one of four bullets, although the expected utility (reduction in probability of death) is the same.
 (iii) Framing, where the expected value differs based on the reference point against which gains and losses are computed although the expected utility remains the same.
 (iv) Avoiding regret: humans are willing to give up "utility" to reduce the chance of feeling regret.

Humans Extensively Use Heuristics in Their Decision Making and Suffer From Related Biases

Because the human brain lacks the ability to execute complex calculations fast, it has evolved to use approximate (so-called "heuristic") decision strategies that provide a fast solution that has high likelihood to be correct (e.g., in an evolutionary context, to prevent loss of life from predators or other circumstances that require rapid decision making as opposed to accurate but slow decisions). These heuristics have offered evolutionary benefits, however, they introduce significant biases into the human decisions. Here we review some of the heuristics we use and refer the interested reader to [12, 15] for more complete and thorough treatments.

- Humans tend to determine (incorrectly) the probability that on object came from a group by the "**representativeness**" of the object with respect to the group.

Given two groups, one group being more specific than the other, humans often attribute higher probability to belonging to the more detailed (more specific) group than the other, which contradicts fundamental axioms of probability.

- Humans follow a bias called **law of small** numbers in which they believe (erroneously) that small random sequences resemble large random sequences. In other words that properties conferred by the law of large numbers in statistics also apply to small numbers. This is related to the representative heuristic, entails **difficulty to distinguish between random and non-random sequences,** and suffer from **gambler's fallacy** (believing that a small random sequence will exhibit distribution characteristics of a large random sequence).
- Humans suffer from **attribution biases** e.g., attributing accidental (random) successes to skill; and non-random failures to circumstances.
- The frequency (or probability) of events is often estimated by how easy it is to recall an occurrence of that event (**availability bias**). While it is easier to recall more frequent events, our ability to recall events also depends on factors other than frequency. Such factors include how easy it is to imagine the event happening and also the desirability or undesirability of the outcome. We tend to "block out" and thus underestimate the probability of undesirable outcomes.
- While assessing the probability of simple events is difficult, **assessing the probability of compound events,** which are conjunctions or disjunctions of simple events, is even more bias-prone.
- Once people form an initial assessment of the probability, they are slow to adjust it (**Anchor bias**). They adjust it in the right direction, but only to an insufficient extent. When the probability of an event is assessed relative to an anchor (in the form of higher or lower than a certain value, being the anchor), this anchor can bias the probability estimate upward or downward.
- Although experts are less affected, **risk assessment** is even more bias-prone than assessing the probability (or rather, rate) of events. This is because non-experts define risk more broadly than "number of events per time period".
- A bias especially detrimental for medical and scientific reasoning is **confusion of the inverse**. In this bias, physicians confuse the sensitivity of a test for a disease diagnosis with the posterior probability of having the disease given the test. Or scientists confuse the p-value (i.e., probability of rejecting the null hypothesis) with 1-posterior probability that the alternative hypothesis is true. Or that the 95% CI of an estimated quantity contains with probability 95% the true value of the quantity.
- **Calibration biases** are confidence errors and typically overconfidence errors where humans believe that their probability of being correct is much higher than the true value.

There are many more human decision making biases that affect most humans, including highly trained scientists and clinicians. We refer the reader to the references above for related discussion. The **most important lesson** is that there exist numerous cognitive biases and it is **exceedingly difficult to remove human cognitive biases entirely from every decision humans make,** even in the context of highly specialized training received by clinicians and scientists. This represents a great value proposition of AI/ML because none of the human cognitive biases affect ordinary AI/Ml systems (unless the designer intentionally constructs the AI.ML models to exhibit such biases, e.g., to simulate and study human cognition).

AI/ML Biases

Recall from the chapter "Foundations and Properties of AI/ML Systems" that **all ML systems have an inductive bias,** which—as we explained—is *not a defect* in their capacity for problem solving but simply *denotes what technical family of models they prefer* (so that they can model the data better). As long as the inductive bias elements (i..e., ML model family, data fitting procedure, model performance function, model selection procedure) are accurate representations of the domain, the ML model can exhibit no negative "bias".

One inadvertent negative bias, however, that can enter into ML models is **bias in the data provided for training**. Let's consider the highly-publicized case of racial bias in a patient care prioritization model [22] in which the model was supposed to prioritize care for high risk patients, yet it was found to prioritize white patients higher than black patients with the same risk. In brief, this model manifested a social/inequity bias because it was given wrong data. Specifically, the data, instead of presenting the actual severity of each patient, substituted it with the healthcare costs for that patient. However, there is a systemic bias in which higher costs are associated with white patients than black patients of the same risk. By training the ML algorithm with the wrong (biased) data, a model was produced that exhibited unwanted (socially/racially biased) behavior.

We did not cover factors such as fatigue, distraction, illness, etc. because they are not cognitive biases. However they are important and are discussed in the context of computer-human decision making next.

Computer-Human Decision Making

In this section, we examine the question of whether, and if yes how, computer problem solving can be combined with human problem solving in order to improve performance.

We frame this question as follows:

Under what general conditions can
AI/ML-Assisted Decision Making (i.e., computer + human)
outperform both
Autonomous AI/ML Decision Making (i.e., computer only),
and
Autonomous Human Decision Making (i.e., human only).

Relative Strengths of human and AI/ML Decision Making

Let us begin our discussion by comparing the relative strengths of human and AI/ML decision making.

Table 1 describes reason when human decision making can be superior to AI/ML and vice versa, reasons why AI/ML decision making can be superior to human. The table shows that human and AI/ML machine learning has complementary strengths, combining them may offer benefits.

Assumption. For the discussion in this section, we assume that the human and the AI/ML model has access to the same data.

Combining AI/ML can be discussed from several inter-related perspectives, which we discuss next.

Potential Complementariness of Errors Made by Humans and AI/ML

Figure 1 shows the three possible scenarios describing how the errors of the AI-Assisted Decision Making relates to the errors of the autonomous human and those of the autonomous AI/ML.

Table 1 Reasons why human decision making can be superior to AI/ML decision making (top part) and reasons why AI/ML decision making can be superior to human (bottom)

Reasons for Human > AI

1. Access to inputs/knowledge that machine models lack.
2. Knowledge about domain that is not captured in data that computer sees.
3. Specific interpretive abilities (e.g., images, language).
4. Culture/social/healthcare/science system awareness.
5. Ability to shift frames of reference and reasoning modes.
6. Ability to seamlessly combine symbolic and quantitative/stochastic reasoning.
7. AI may be poorly performing due to using weak learners, bad AI design, bad data design; generally all pitfalls of AI/ML in this book and referenced literature.
8. Easier integration in existing workflows & other implementation barriers, including regulatory barriers.

Reasons for AI > Human

1. Limits to human cognitive capabilities, e.g. high dimensional decision making; amount of information that can be stored in memory, etc.
2. Humans have several cognitive biases that machines do not have.
3. Special AI/ML reasoning capabilities, e.g., learning complex model from data.
4. Speed.
5. Machines do not get tired, distracted, stressed, sick, socially influenced, etc.
6. Machines can update data, knowledge bases, reasoning algorithms, almost instantaneously
7. AI cannot be gamed as easily by manipulating data inputs, selective results etc.
8. Cheaper across many dimensions/settings.
9. Scalable.

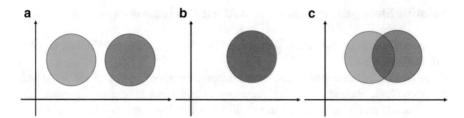

Fig. 1 Illustration of error relationships of computer vs human decision making. (**a**) humans and computers make errors independently; (**b**) errors made by humans and computers always coincide; (**c**) errors made by humans and computers partly coincide

Both computers and humans implement a function each that maps from the problem input domain set to the decision set. By *Error Domain* of a computer model or human decision function, we refer to the subset of the input domain where the computer or the human (respectively) make decision mistakes.

The blue circle represents the error domain of the human and the red circle represents the error domain of the AI/ML model.

There are three possible scenarios. In scenario (a) on the left, there is no overlap between the error domains of the human and the AI/ML model: they make independent mistakes. Some of these mistakes are predictable (blue/red parts of the error domains), so when we encounter a case with input features in the human identifiable error domain we will use the computer to make the decision. Conversely when we encounter a case with input features in the AI/ML identifiable error domain we will use the human to make the decision. When the input does not belong to any identifiable error domain we can pick either decision randomly.

In scenario (b) in the middle, there is a perfect overlap between the error domains of the human and the AI/ML model. They make mistakes exactly for the same inputs, so we cannot easily (if at all) correct the mistake.

Scenario (c) is in between (a) and (b). There is overlap in the error domains, and decision mistakes can be corrected easily in the non-gray (identifiable) *and* non-overlapping portions of the error domains.

Weak Learning Theory

Roughly, ensemble theory states that weak learners, learners that perform only minimally better than random, can be combined to form a highly performant ensemble [23]. Neither the human, and most likely, neither the AI/ML model is a weak learner; in a clinical setting, we would expect them to perform substantially better than random. However, the weak learning theory still allows us to combine these (actually strong) learners to form an even more performant system. We have already seen examples of methods to combine weak learners, gradient boosting in chapter "An Appraisal and Operating Characteristics of Major ML Methods Applicable in Healthcare & Health Science". Other methods, including error correcting coding, etc., exist [23].

Knowledge About the Target Function

While the human and the AI/ML have access to the same data, the human can have knowledge of some regions of the target function, that the AI/ML algorithm was unable to learn. Universal function approximation, optimal classification and other theories operate in the sample limit (assuming access to unlimited number of observations), however, most AI/ML endeavors face a (sometimes severe) limitation of samples. Therefore, it is possible, that AI/ML cannot learn the target function correctly in some regions of the input space. In contrast, the human may have knowledge about the target function (which, of course, the human did not obtain from the data).

ROC Convex Hull

We have already seen examples in the "Evaluation" chapter (Figure 9.1.2.) of different classifiers (with different inductive biases) having different performance characteristics, resulting in ROC curves that favored one classifier in one region of the curve and a different one in a different region. Provost and Fawcett [24] proposed a method of combining classifiers so that the resulting ROC curve is the convex hull of the original ROC curves. Although such combinations can improve performance over the individual classifiers, this strategy is not yet optimal. Further development of combining ROC curves (e.g. [25, 26]) successfully improved upon the optimality of the combined classifiers. By viewing the human decision making as a black-box classifier, these techniques can be used to combine the human and AI/ML decision making.

Stacking

We have already discussed stacking in the "Ensemble Methods" section of the "An Appraisal and Operating Characteristics of Major ML Methods Applicable in Healthcare and Health Science" chapter. Recall that stacking is a modeling approach, where multiple models (base learners) are trained on the same data (or some variant, e.g. bootstrap re-sample, of the data) and the outputs from these models are combined by another model (meta-learners). Stacking strategies differ in the ways base models are trained and combined. Optimal stacking strategies have been explored in several domains [27, 28].

In the application of stacking to the problem of combining human and AI/ML, base models can be (i) any AI/ML model, (ii) the human, (iii) or an AI/ML model "mimicking" the human. ("Mimicking" refers to approximating an unknown complex function with a simpler function, or several simpler functions, learnt from data, in some of the input regions.)

Strategies for Human-AI/ML Hybrid Decision Making

The inputs to the decision making are described in the left half of Table 2. These include:

DATA	Data that both the computer and human have access to. There is no other data that either the human or the computer can access.
C	A fixed computer model that was constructed before attempting to build the combined decision support system.
H_{RT}	"real-time" human decision making (i.e., per usual practice)
H_{EST}	"estimated" a model previously constructed to accurately mimic human decision making. Typically this model will use data under ideal human decision making conditions (expert human without superlative performance record, without distractions or fatigue, etc.).

The properties and priorities are described in the right side of the table. The column "Likely Pred. Opt." denotes whether the combined decision making is likely predictively optimal, specifically from the perspective of exposing the hybrid learner to all available data and the interactions among features that may have not been captured by either prior computer models C, or humans H (and thus cannot be modeled by simply ensembling C, H).

The "Computer → Human Effects Risk" column indicates whether or not a risk of error due to human biases (rubber stamping decisions of C, alert fatigue, automation bias, etc.) exists. Specifically, "±" denotes that these biases if present can be addressed in the data design and workflow engineering, including in both cases, by blinding the human to the computer's decisions.

The column "Human Risk" refers to the susceptibility to unmanageable error because of fatigue, distractions, work overloading.

Finally, "Gaming Risk" refers to conscious or subconscious tendency to "steer" the model's output towards desired outcomes by modifying the human decisions accordingly.

The rows of Table 2 contain the actual strategies ranging from S1 to S10. The phrase "rand" refers to randomization, where the human (H_{RT}) is randomly blinded (or not) to the computer predictions. This allows for estimating the influence of the computer output on the human decision maker.

The strategies in Table 2 range from pure AI/ML-only decision making (S1) to pure human-only decision making (S10).

S1-S8 are hybrid designs where we build models to learn accurate decisions using inputs described in the columns under "Inputs for modeling". For each decision function, the inputs are designated by the '+' signs in the appropriate input columns. For example, S6 constructs a decision function using data (DATA **D**), the pre-exising fixed AI/ML model (C), and the real-time human decision (H_{RT}). This results in a decision function

Table 2 Concrete strategies for constructing Human-AI/ML hybrid decision making

| | Modeled Hybrid computer/human designs | | | | | | | |
| | Inputs for modeling | | | | Properties & Priority of the design | | | |
	DATA	C	H_{Est}	H_{RT}	Likely Pred. Opt.	Computer → Human Effects Risk	Human Risk	Gaming Risk	Priority
S1	–	+	+	–	–	±	–	–	THIRD
S2	–	+	–	+	–	±	+	+	
S3	–	–	+	–	–	–	–	–	
S4	–	–	–	+	–	–	+	+	SECOND
S5	+	+	+	–	+	–	–	–	FIRST
S6	+	+ rand	–	+	+	–	+	+	
S7	+	–	+	–	+	–	–	–	
S8	+	–	–	+	+	–	+	+	
	Pure C or Hybrid designs (No modeled inputs)								
S9	Computer				–	–	+	+	THIRD
S10	Human			S10 same as S4					

*F (instance(i) from **D**, Computer model outputs on instance(i), Human decisions on instance (i))*

which is trained on all instance(*i*) in **D**, s.t. the decision error is minimized.

Note that strategies S5, S6 do not require blinding the human to the computer decisions since any negative effects of the human being exposed to a computer model's decisions are eliminated by the absence of exposure to them in S5 and by randomization on purpose in S6.

Note that S7, S8 also do not require blinding of the human to the computer since any negative effects of the human being exposed to a computer model's decisions are eliminated by the absence of exposure to them. However in model application time with a real time human decision making, the new model may negatively affect the human and thus the S8 models will require monitoring for such effects.

Human risks in Human-AI/ML Hybrid Decision Making

Human risks include **decision fatigue** [29], **and other factors**, such as distractions, illness, overwork, etc., As we saw, human decision making is sensitive to context. Thus a factor to consider is the alteration of the human performance in the context of combined decision making with the aid of a computer system. One instance of this problem is **automation bias** in which when humans are presented with many correct decisions by an AI model, humans become more susceptible to just "rubber stamping" the model's decisions without much critical thinking [30]. This is a critical factor that influenced regulatory rationale, and which we discuss further in chapter "Regulatory Aspects and Ethical Legal Societal Implications (ELSI)". The converse is true, as well. When a clinical decision support system burdens a clinician with wrong/unnecessary alerts, **alert fatigue** [31] arises and the human may ignore subsequent alerts.

Empirical studies of Human-AI/ML Hybrid Decision Making

In terms of empirical demonstration of the potential to improve performance by combining human and AI/Ml capabilities, image analysis is particularly conducive to AI-clinician collaboration. Computer-aided detection (CADe) systems do not aim to offer a diagnosis instead of the physician, but detect and highlight regions in the image that are suspicious and require closer inspection. In a study where skin lesions were classified as malignant vs non-malignant, experts achieved 66% accuracy, while the CADe system (expert aided by AI) achieved 72.1% ($\pm0.9\%$) [11].

In two highly-cited systematic reviews [32, 33] Haynes et al. reported that across 97 studies of the effectiveness of CDS, strong evidence was found that the performance of human decision making was improved (although these improvements were not directly linked to patient outcomes) [32]. A more recent systematic review of 38 studies found that 66% of the studies reported positive provider performance (while none reported negative provider performance) and 61% of the reviewed studies reported positive patient outcomes (while none reported negative patient outcomes) [34].

Conclusions

In the present chapter, we presented systematic review and meta analysis literature, which covers hundreds of studies, providing strong evidence that AI/ML in healthcare and health science problem solving exhibits strong performance, that is usually superior to human decision making (when direct comparisons were made). The chapter also addressed human biases and contrasted them with AI/ML biases. These are of fundamentally different nature and we have different ability to control them. In the final part of the chapter we provided an analysis of conditions under which humans+AI/ML can outperform both humans alone and AI/ML alone. We also provided broad guidance for implementing such combined decision making and examples from the literature where AI/ML-assisted decision making provided performance benefits.

We close this chapter with a needed clarification: the approach to the topic was driven by a data science functional perspective in which there are several knowns and unknowns. Specifically, we know the exact inner workings and input-output behavior of AI/ML models we have built; we can also measure the input-output behavior of humans; much is known about human decision making biases and how machines overcome those. At the same time little is known about the inner workings of the human brain's decision making apparatus. From an empirical perspective we can model this human decision making as a "black box" decision function and analyze the error structures so that we can construct hybrid systems with smaller error.

As the phenomena of alert fatigue, decision fatigue, and automation bias show, the implementation of hybrid systems in practice is much more difficult and less controllable than the implementation of AI/ML models alone. Psychology, cognitive science, neuroscience, human-computer interaction, human factors engineering, and implementation science aim to all help with successful implementation. Here we just scratched the surface of what is possible.

Key Messages and Concepts Discussed in This Chapter

AI systems, both from the first and second wave of AI in medicine, have achieved diagnostic performance on par with expert clinicians, often outperforming less experienced professionals.

These systems achieved best success when AI was used to complement the professionals (e.g. they were used for consulting or for computer-aided detection) rather than trying to offer diagnoses without input from the professional.

Adoption of these systems is slow for a variety of reasons that relate to two key themes (i) lack of trust and (ii) lack of consideration for the clinical workflow.

The strengths of AI systems are complementary to those of human professionals.

Human decision making introduces biases in several ways which are largely different from the biases that AI systems introduce.

Pitfalls discussed in This Chapter

Pitfall 11.1 Even if a clinical AI system meets or exceeds expert-level performance in the lab, this does *NOT* mean that (i) the system can be readily adopted into clinical practice, (ii) will perform similarly when deployed in practice, or (iii) that the evaluation metrics used accurately reflect clinically impactful use of the AI model.

Best Practices discussed in This Chapter

Best Practice 11.1. Consider the possibility that a hybrid system may outperform human or computer decisions.

Best Practice 11.2. Examine the topology of errors in human and computer models.

Best Practice 11.3. Explore ensemble learning as a strategy for building hybrid decision models.

Best Practice 11.4. Work with implementation experts for bringing complex human/AI decision making into the clinical or scientific settings.

Classroom Assignments & Discussion Topics in This Chapter

1. How would you ensure that an AI system versus a clinical expert comparison is carried out in a fair manner? How would you establish a gold standard? How would you ensure that the clinicians and the AI system work with the same information? Can you think of evaluation metrics that favor AI or the clinical expert? Can/should blinded comparisons be used?

2. In models of human decision making, we described the difference between utility and value. What implications does this distinction have on the design of AI objective functions?

3. We explained that the way questions are formed can influence the answer. Also, when the respondent knows(!) the answer, such effects are minimal. How could the way questions are asked influence clinical decisions made by a clinician alone, a clinician in a shared decision making framework with the patient, and by an AI system?

4. We described four main groups of factors that introduce bias into human decision making. These were (i) memory, (ii) context, (iii) rational/irrational decision making, and (iv) heuristics.

   (a) Which of these factors present in a patient can influence the decision making?
   (b) Which of these factors present in a clinician can influence the decision making?
   (c) Which of these factors are relevant to healthcare research?
   (d) Which of these factors will impact a purely AI decision making? Think of potential impact during the development and the use of the system.
   (e) Which of these factors will influence an AI assisted decision making?
   (f) Which of these factors can be corrected by AI assisted decision making?

References

1. Senders JT, Staples PC, Karhade AV, Zaki MM, Gormley WB, Broekman MLD, Smith TR, Arnaout O. Machine learning and neurosurgical outcome prediction: a systematic review. World Neurosurg. 2018;109:476–486.e1. https://doi.org/10.1016/j.wneu.2017.09.149. Epub 2017 Oct 3
2. Adeoye J, Tan JY, Choi SW, Thomson P. Prediction models applying machine learning to oral cavity cancer outcomes: a systematic review. Int J Med Inform. 2021;154:104557. https://doi.org/10.1016/j.ijmedinf.2021.104557. Epub 2021 Aug 18
3. Lee Y, Ragguett RM, Mansur RB, Boutilier JJ, Rosenblat JD, Trevizol A, Brietzke E, Lin K, Pan Z, Subramaniapillai M, Chan TCY, Fus D, Park C, Musial N, Zuckerman H, Chen VC, Ho R, Rong C, McIntyre RS. Applications of machine learning algorithms to predict therapeutic outcomes in depression: a meta-analysis and systematic review. J Affect Disord. 2018;241:519–32. https://doi.org/10.1016/j.jad.2018.08.073. Epub 2018 Aug 14. Erratum in: J Affect Disord. 2020 Sep 1;274:1211–1215
4. Li B, Feridooni T, Cuen-Ojeda C, Kishibe T, de Mestral C, Mamdani M, Al-Omran M. Machine learning in vascular surgery: and critical appraisal. NPJ Digit Med. 2022;5(1):7. https://doi.org/10.1038/s41746-021-00552-y.
5. Bernert RA, Hilberg AM, Melia R, Kim JP, Shah NH, Abnousi F. Artificial intelligence and suicide prevention: a systematic review of machine learning investigations. Int J Environ Res Public Health. 2020;17(16):5929. https://doi.org/10.3390/ijerph17165929.
6. Stewart J, Lu J, Goudie A, Bennamoun M, Sprivulis P, Sanfillipo F, Dwivedi G. Applications of machine learning to undifferentiated chest pain in the emergency department: a systematic review. PloS One. 2021;16(8):e0252612. https://doi.org/10.1371/journal.pone.0252612.
7. Liu X, Faes L, Kale AU, Wagner SK, Fu DJ, Bruynseels A, Mahendiran T, Moraes G, Shamdas M, Kern C, Ledsam JR, Schmid MK, Balaskas K, Topol EJ, Bachmann LM, Keane PA, Denniston AK. A comparison of deep learning performance against health-care professionals in detecting diseases from medical imaging: a systematic review and meta-analysis. Lancet Digit Health. 2019;1(6):e271–97. https://doi.org/10.1016/S2589-7500(19)30123-2. Epub 2019 Sep 25. Erratum in: Lancet Digit Health. 2019 Nov;1(7):e334.
8. Ramesh S, Chokkara S, Shen T, Major A, Volchenboum SL, Mayampurath A, Applebaum MA. Applications of artificial intelligence in pediatric oncology: a systematic review. JCO Clin Cancer Inform. 2021;5:1208–19. https://doi.org/10.1200/CCI.21.00102.
9. Grove WM, Zald DH, Lebow BS, Snitz BE, Nelson C. Clinical versus mechanical prediction: a meta-analysis. Psychol Assess. 2000;12(1):19–30.
10. Dombal FT, Leaper DJ, Staniland JR, McCann AP, Horrock JC. Computer-aided diagnosis of acute abdominal pain. Brit Med J. 1972;2:9–13.

11. Shen J, Zhang CJP, BangSheng J, Chen J, Song J, Liu Z, He Z, Wong SY, Fang PH, Ming WK. Artificial intelligence versus clinicians in disease diagnosis: systematic review. JMIR Med Infom. 2019;7(3):e10010. https://doi.org/10.2196/10010.
12. Plous S. The psychology of judgement and human decision making. McGrew-Hill; 1993.
13. Sox HC, Higgins MC, Owens DK. Medical decision making. Wiley-Blackwell; 1998.
14. Dowie J, Elstein, A. S. (Eds.). Professional judgment: a reader in clinical decision making. Cambridge University Press; 1988.
15. Kahneman D, Slovic P, Tversky A. Judgment under uncertainty: heuristics and biases. Cambridge: Cambridge University Press; 1982.
16. Loftus EF, Palmer JC. Reconstruction of automobile destruction: an example of the interaction between language and memory. J Verbal Learning Verbal Behav. 1974;13(5)
17. Miller N, Campbell DT. Recency and primacy in persuasion as a function of the timing of speeches and measurements. J Abnorm Soc Psychol. 1959;59(1):1–9. https://doi.org/10.1037/h0049330.
18. Thorndike EL. A constant error in psychological ratings. J Appl Psychol. 1920;4(1):25–9. https://doi.org/10.1037/h0071663.
19. Plous S. How questions affect answers. Section II in the psychology of judgement and human decision making. McGrew-Hill; 1993.
20. Sox H. Expected value decision making. Chapter 6 in medical decision making. Wiley-Blackwell; 1998.
21. Kahneman D, Tversky A. Prospect theory: an analysis of decision under risk. Econometrica. 1979;47(2):263–91. https://doi.org/10.2307/1914185.
22. Obermeyer Z, Powers B, Vogeli C, Mullainathan S. Dissecting racial bias in an algorithm used to manage the health of populations. Science. 2019;366(6464):447–53. https://doi.org/10.1126/science.aax2342.
23. Duda RO, Hart PE, Stork DG. Pattern classification. 2nd ed. John Wiley and Sons; 2000.
24. Provost F, Fawcett T. Robust classification for imprecise environments. Machine Learning J. 2001;42(3):203–31.
25. Peter A. Flach and Shaomin Wu. Repairing concavities in ROC curves. In Proceedings of the 19th international joint conference on artificial intelligence (IJCAI'05), pp. 702–707; 2005.
26. Barreno M, Cardenas A, Tygar JD. Optimal ROC curve for a combination of classifiers. Adv Neural Inform Process Syst. 2007;20
27. Džeroski S, Ženko B. Is combining classifiers with stacking better than selecting the best one? Machine Learning. 2004;54:255–73.
28. Ray B, Henaff M, Ma S, Efstathiadis E, Peskin ER, Picone M, Poli T, Aliferis CF, Statnikov A. Information content and analysis methods for multi-modal high-throughput biomedical data. Sci Rep. 2014;4(1):4411.
29. Persson E, Barrafrem K, Meunier A, Tinghög G. The effect of decision fatigue on surgeons' clinical decision making. Health Econ. 2019;28(10):1194–203. https://doi.org/10.1002/hec.3933. Epub 2019 Jul 25
30. FDA. Clinical decision support software; draft guidance for Industry and Food and Drug Administration Staff; 2019. https://www.federalregister.gov/documents/2019/09/27/2019-21000/clinical-decision-support-software-draft-guidance-for-industry-and-food-and-drug-administration. Accessed 12 Dec 2022.
31. Co Z, Holmgren AJ, Classen DC, Newmark L, Seger DL, Danforth M, Bates DW. The tradeoffs between safety and alert fatigue: Data from a national evaluation of hospital medication-related clinical decision support. J Am Med Inform Assoc. 2020;27(8):1252–8. https://doi.org/10.1093/jamia/ocaa098.
32. Garg AX, Adhikari NK, McDonald H, Rosas-Arellano MP, Devereaux PJ, Beyene J, Sam J, Haynes RB. Effects of computerized clinical decision support systems on practitioner performance and patient outcomes: a systematic review. JAMA. 2005;293(10):1223–38. https://doi.org/10.1001/jama.293.10.1223.

33. Hunt DL, Haynes RB, Hanna SE, Smith K. Effects of computer-based clinical decision support systems on physician performance and patient outcomes: a systematic review. JAMA. 1998;280(15):1339–46. https://doi.org/10.1001/jama.280.15.1339.

34. Kruse CS, Ehrbar N. Effects of computerized decision support systems on practitioner performance and patient outcomes: systematic review. JMIR Med Inform. 2020;8(8):e17283. https://doi.org/10.2196/17283.

Lessons Learned from Historical Failures, Limitations and Successes of AI/ML in Healthcare and the Health Sciences. Enduring Problems, and the Role of Best Practices

Constantin Aliferis and Gyorgy Simon

Abstract

This chapter covers a variety of cases studies-based incidents and concepts that are valuable for identifying pitfalls, suggesting best practices and supporting their use. Examples include: the Gartner hype cycle; the infamous "AI winters"; limitations of early-stage knowledge representation and reasoning methods; overfitting; using methods not built for the task; over-estimating the value and potential or early and heuristic technology; developing AI disconnected with real-life needs and application contexts; over-interpreting theoretical shortcomings of one algorithm to all algorithms in the class; misinterpreting computational learning theory; failures/shortcomings of literature including technically erroneous information and persistence of incorrect findings; meta research yielding unreliable results; failures/shortcomings of modeling protocols, data and evaluation designs (e.g., competitions); failures/shortcomings of specific projects and technologies; and also contextual factors that may render guidelines themselves problematic. These case studies were often followed by improved technology that overcame various limitations. The case studies reinforce, and demonstrate the value of science-driven practices for addressing enduring and new challenges.

Keywords

Non-monotonic progress in AI/ML · AI Hype Cycles and AI winters · Case studies of commercial and academic AI/ML limitations (and ensuing progress) · Enduring problems in AI/ML

C. Aliferis (✉) · G. Simon
Institute for Health Informatics, University of Minnesota, Minneapolis, MN, USA
e-mail: constantinaibestpractices@gmail.com

543

G. J. Simon, C. Aliferis (eds.), *Artificial Intelligence and Machine Learning in Health Care and Medical Sciences*, Health Informatics,
https://doi.org/10.1007/978-3-031-39355-6_12

Significant Advances in Health AI/ML are the Result of Non-monotonic Progress with Many Failures Followed by Successes. Learning from Case Studies

The AI/ML toolkit available currently to health data scientists is nothing sort of extraordinary. The algorithms, systems and theory of today have capabilities than a few decades ago seemed beyond the realm of the possible. Examples include: the ability to operate predictively with miniscule sample sizes and dimensionalities that exceed the 10^6 variables range; the routine capability to classify and extract meaning from text and other unstructured data; the ability to discover causation reliably without experiments; the ability to guide experiments so that the number and cost of experiments is minimized; the ability to explore quadrillions of non-linear variable interactions in seconds on simple personal computers by using kernel methods; automatic protection against overfitting by deploying regularized/shrinkage methods; powerful auto-modeler systems with performance matching and exceeding those of experts; powerful image recognition. We also have autonomous vehicles, industrial robotics, embedded decision support and control systems, natural language understanding and translation, cyber security enabling systems, sophisticated knowledge representation and data models that support complex data harmonization and reuse at scale and speed. Many more success stories and capabilities are discussed throughout this volume (see indicatively chapter "Artificial Intelligence (AI) and Machine Learning (ML) for Healthcare and Health Sciences: The Need for Best Practices Enabling Trust in AI and ML" and in the cited literature.

These achievements of AI/ML did not happen smoothly, however. In many cases they involved setbacks, pursuing dead ends, and learning from painful mistakes. To this day, there are many systematic suboptimal AI/ML practices that incur substantial costs for health care and the health sciences.

The purposes of this chapter are to discuss a sample of prominent and paradigmatic case studies where failures provided incentive and inspiration for the field to advance and new and improved technologies to emerge. Also these showcase the value of best practices (BPs) advocated in the present volume. Finally, these case studies point to areas where future major improvements are likely to occur if a more rigorous and BP-driven health AI/ML is pursued.

The Gartner Hype Cycle

The concept of a "Hype Cycle" is commonly attributed to the Gartner management consulting company [1]. Figure 1 describes a common historical pattern where the emergence of new technology is followed by a surge in expectations strongly overestimating true capabilities and potential (Exuberant optimism aka "Peak of inflated expectations") that is followed by a dramatic drop of expectations that strongly underestimate the true capabilities and potential of the technology ("Trough of disillusionment").

Fig. 1 Hype technology cycle

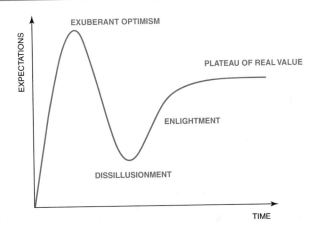

These expectations may be of scientists, technologists industry, investors, customers, funding agencies, the general public, etc. across the health care and health science ecosystems. As both technology and sentiment mature, a period of increasing understanding of the technology and is evolving capabilities follows ("Slope of Enlightment") and then converges to an accurate and lasting appraisal of the technology's merits ("Plateau of real value").

"AI Winters"

The term "winter" with regards to a field of science or technology refers to a prolonged period of reduced public expectation, research support and industrial market growth. Essentially its is a prolonged Trough of disillusionment to use Hype Cycle terminology. The opposite is referred by "spring", i.e., prolonged periods where expectations, support and financial growth are high [2–4].

The field of AI in the middle of 20th century generated vast enthusiasm and funding support. The early pioneers made strides in establishing many foundational results and methods in the field. The general sentiment was that in short period of time "hard AI" would be feasible—i.e., intelligent systems that would possess general intelligence capabilities on par or better than humans. However a number of setbacks drained this enthusiasm and drastically undercut AI's growth.

The two main AI winters in the USA occurred between 1974–80 and 1987–93 with parallel and overlapping AI winters internationally. These reflected real and perceived failures and disappointment in: *scaling up from toy-sized problems to real-life complexity, spoken language understanding, artificial neural network limitations, the collapse of the LISP machine industry, limitations of logic-based systems for broad inference, the limited success of expert systems, and the failure of Japan's Fifth Generation project to meet its goals.*

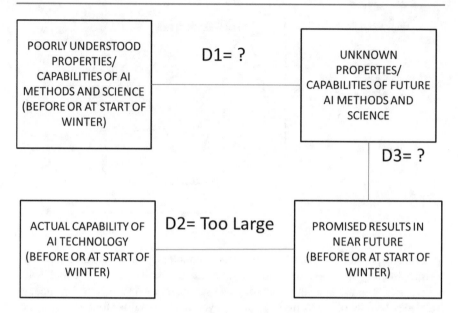

Fig. 2 Factors summarizing causes of historical AI winters. In the upper left, poor understanding of core properties & capabilities of technology (at the time). Upper right quadrant: poor understanding of limitations of technology, in the future. Lower left quadrant: limited current capabilities (at the time). Lower right quadrant: Exorbitant and unbounded promises for capabilities in the near future

The main causes of the above failures (or perceived failures) can be traced to the excessive hype (expectation exuberance) relative to what was known, established, and proven in terms of theoretical capabilities and empirical performance, effectiveness and other properties that the present volume has described at length. **The field, in hindsight, mismanaged expectations and failed to impose the necessary self-discipline for proceeding from the space of unknown properties and capabilities to the space of guaranteed performance in a systematic and science-driven manner.** Figure 2 depicts the interplay among these factors. Notice the immense distances between actual capabilities and promises (D2, corresponding to actual "Hyped) and the unknown distances between unknown properties and promises made (D1, D3, depicting potential hype).

The following components of the AI winters were or continue to be particularly relevant to the aims of health AI/ML:

Perceptron Limitations

A notable setback was the discovery that perceptrons could not learn non-linear data generating functions [5]. A **perceptron** is essentially a single node in neural network (chapter "An Appraisal and Operating Characteristics of Major ML Methods Applicable in Healthcare & Health Science"), which linearly combines its inputs and outputs them through a non-linear function. The above discovery pertains to the fact that a single layer of perceptrons (i.e. a single-layer neural network) cannot learn non-linear functions. Because the space of non-linear functions is vast and many real-life problems exist in it, this was a major blow to the credibility of the nascent AI technology and industry sector.

Eventually these fears proved to be unfounded: on one hand, with the discovery of the Back Propagation algorithm by Werbos [6] and the related work by Rummelrhart, McClelland, and the PDP (parallel distributed programming) group (comprising, among others, such luminaries as Nobel Prize winner Francis Crick and future Turing award winner Geoffrey Hinton) and others, **new improved science and technology of artificial neural networks (ANNs)** using *multi-layered networks trained with the Back Propagation algorithm* [7] gave a theoretically powerful and practical way to model non-linear domains.

Moreover, from a practical perspective, as discussed in chapter "Foundations and Properties of AI/ML Systems", linear models can still be very effective since in low sample situations, due to Bias-Variance Decomposition of the Error (BVDE), high bias (e.g., linear) learners will often lead to better generalization error even if the large sample data generating function is not linear. In addition, whereas a non-linear discriminative function is not *perfectly* learnable with a linear model, if some common mitigating factors are present (i.e., unbalanced priors of the inputs or correlated inputs [8]) then a linear discriminant can discover the existence of signal and can achieve accuracy up to within a vanishingly small factor. It is not an accident that the most used (and arguably successful) modeling method in the health sciences are linear statistical models since *on average* (as opposed to *worst case*) in small sample designs such models are very useful.

Back Propagation-Based ANNs and the Vanishing (Or Exploding) Gradient Problem

Back propagation is a very effective ANN training algorithm for ANNs with a small number of hidden (intermediate) layers. However, when it comes to building ANNs with many hidden layers (which are very powerful in some domains) it suffers from a critical weakness, the vanishing or exploding gradient problem. In backpropagation, the model is trained by making empirical adjustments (based on derivatives of empirical error of model output) to weights of ANN units of successive layers. The exploding/vanishing gradients problem refers to the situation when these errors grow very fast to the number of layers and very quickly lead to parameterizing ANN weights with essentially useless noise.

A New Improved Technology of ANNs Followed

Deep ANNs aka "Deep Learning (DL)" (see chapter "An Appraisal and Operating Characteristics of Major ML Methods Applicable in Healthcare & Health Science") overcame this problem by a simple (but very effective) alteration in the mathematical form of the ANN units. Some of the key innovations that allowed Deep Learning ANNs to differentiate from standard multi-layered ANNs include: RELUs (Rectified Linear Units) as transfer functions (they allow for non-linear learning and do not suffer from derivatives vanishing/explosion); convolution layers and filters; pooling/downsampling (to reduce dimensionality and overfitting); and multiple iterations of Convolution-Pooling-RELUs (for hierarchical features extraction) [9, 10]).

Roughly at the same time, **another technological and scientific breakthrough occurred when a new class of ML algorithms, Support Vector Machines (SVMs)** emerged based on the work of Vapnik, and his collaborators Cortez, Boser and Guyon [11–13]. This class (see chapter "An Appraisal and Operating Characteristics of Major ML Methods Applicable in Healthcare & Health Science") was based on a uniquely powerful combination of regularization, quadratic optimization formulation of the learning problem (which guarantees optimal search as opposed to ANNs and many other ML algorithms that conduct incomplete and error-prone parameter space search), dealing with non-linearities with immense efficiency using kernel functions (discovered in mathematics 40 years before, but not used before in applied ML) and dealing with model selection using *structured risk minimization*.

Another very powerful classifier that is widely adopted in the health sciences is **Random Forests** that combines ideas from decision trees, bagging, off-sample error estimation, random feature selection and capacity control [14].

Together these three predictive modeling technologies are highly adopted and very complementary. DL has dominant image recognition and generative function empirical performance due to powerful automatic construction of higher-order features. SVMs have dominant performance and efficiency (sample and time complexity) in a large number of predictive health tasks (e.g., clinical and omics data modeling) [13, 15–17]. Random Forests and Boosting are also very powerful across a range of healthcare and health science domains. Several more powerful ML algorithms have been developed and are in wide use (see chapter "An Appraisal and Operating Characteristics of Major ML Methods Applicable in Healthcare & Health Science").

Current Limitations (and Opportunities for Improvement) of DL

As powerful and useful as DL methods are, they still have significant limitations that need be recognized and overcome, not only to achieve better results but to manage expectations and avoid a possible new AI winter. Such limitations (as explained and referenced in chapter "An Appraisal and Operating Characteristics of Major ML Methods Applicable in Healthcare & Health Science" as well as several other chapters in the present book) include: lack of effective formal causal properties both in terms of adequate expressiveness, reliable discovery and consistent inference; lack of a theory ensuring over fitting avoidance (note that several *empirical* overfitting avoidance methods have been developed and are used); large sample requirements and questionable performance in low sample situations; a fundamentally heuristic approach to model development and model selection; black box nature with limited explainability; limited capability for shift invariance of image recognition; limited accuracy advantages over conventional "vanilla" statistical comparators (such as logistic regression—see extensive empirical literature later in the present chapter) in several applications, typically when the sample size is insufficient or the problem is low dimensional; and incomplete and sub-optimal search of parameter space. Published claims about high performance of DL in health applications has been linked by several meta analyses to biased designs, as demonstrated by extensive literature discussed later in this chapter. We will also address limitations of DL in the commercial space (game playing, self-driving cars) that has led to a more measured appreciation of the technology's strengths and limitations. Such an appreciation when combined with dedicated research based on property-ensuring principles (e.g., BPs in chapter "Principles of Rigorous Development and of Appraisal of ML and AI Methods and Systems") and safe deployment (e.g., BPs in chapter "Characterizing, Diagnosing and Managing the Risk of Error of ML & AI Models in Clinical and Organizational Application") has the potential to reduce the limitations and reduce the possibility for a new AI winter [4].

What's in a Link: The Importance of Semantics in AI Models and Methods. From Problems with Early Semantic Networks to Those of Modern Network Science and Pathway Discovery

Chapter "Foundations and Properties of AI/ML Systems" discussed semantic networks as simplified and graphically interpretable offshoots of First Order Logic (see chapter "Foundations and Properties of AI/ML Systems"). As semantic networks started proliferating, it became obvious that they did not share the same technical meaning (semantics) and additionally, because of lack of precise semantics, their output and behavior were unknown, or unsound. These grave limitations were elucidated in a landmark paper by Woods which attracted the attention of the symbolic AI community and sparked needed improvements in semantic network technology. **Modern forms** of the earlier SNs, e.g., the Semantic Web, and Knowledge Representation and Reasoning (KRR) methods and tools draw their power and integrity to these earlier SNs [2, 18–20].

However, the problem of unclear, undefined, inconsistent semantics in graphical KRR is not eliminated. Today it manifests in other classes of AI/Ml, most notably in **biological pathway discovery algorithms, and network science models.**

Pathway reverse engineering methods in biology and other basic health sciences, seek to discover, represent, and reason with the ways of interaction (control, signaling, regulation etc.) among biological (metabolic, genetic, proteomic, hormonal, immune etc.) molecules [21]. In both cases it is imperative to clearly and unambiguously specify the precise meaning of the edges in the network model, and equally importantly specify how the algorithms used to develop such mechanisms guarantee that all and only those relationships that obey these meanings are output by the algorithms. Among the many available methods in use in numerous papers however,

(a) the semantics are undeclared, ambiguous, or lacking important properties, and (b) while algorithms are fully specified, what is unspecified is how the operation of the algorithms ensures the intented interpretation of the output.

For example, in biological pathway reverse engineering most formalisms and algorithms in use do not enforce causal semantics, nor the Causal Markov Condition, or the Causal Faithfulness Condition or other conditions that are required to ensure causal interpretation (see chapter "Foundations of Causal ML"). For example, heuristic and ultimately false use of edges to denote strong univariate correlation as a determinant of direct causation; heuristic/false use of edges to denote non-zero weights in regularized regressors among the studied entities.

The United States National Research Council defines *network science* as "the study of network representations of physical, biological, and social phenomena leading to predictive models of these phenomena" [22]. But how do such network representations can be used for predictive modeling? More specifically how a network representation built using edges denoting similarity, physical connectivity, cross-entropy, geographical distance (to mention a few of the commonly used network science approaches) can be used for prediction? What confers to such networks predictive modeling capabilities? And why are such capabilities (if they exist) better than, say, the minimal threshold comparator of statistical baseline methods such as logistic regression that have (among other desirable properties) provable large-sample error optimality for many identifiable distributions?

The result of these limitations is that numerous models in existence are routinely over-interpreted, in some cases misleading, and likely to generate many false positive and false negative results in translational and clinical applications.

Rule-Based AI, Expert Systems, Heuristic Systems, Limitations of Bayesian Learners and Disconnect Between Systems and Real-World Problems

Rule Based AI and Formal Expert Systems

One dimension of AI's winters was the failure of knowledge-driven Rule-Based systems to provide a viable means for achieving **hard AI** (machines with general intelligence indistinguishable or superior to that of humans) as well as problem-focused Expert Systems. Japan, for example, launched the (in hindsight very ambitious) Fifth Generation Computer Systems (FGCS) project which aimed to achieve a large portion of these goals and altogether disrupt the computing technology landscape in a remarkable time span of 10 years. Notably, the project was using logic programming as its main programming language.

The reasons for these disappointing cases can readily be appreciated now: attacking the AI problem at its broadest scope versus a smaller-scoped divide-and-conquer approach [23] was in all likelihood a strategic error given the difficulty and the heterogeneity of problem requirements across the total problem spaces or interest. Rule-Based systems and other KRR technology of the time lacked the flexibility to deal with the very fluid reasoning that humans exhibit (e.g., reasoning with uncertainty, perception, image recognition, learning, intuitively, effortlessly, and reflexively in many instances) [2]. Deriving their problem-solving knowledge from experts is limited by the fact that experts typically cannot explain their problem-solving capabilities [24, 25] or when they can, their explanations cannot be faithfully captured in rules or other existing KRR formats. One can also observe cycles of huge emotional and other investment in one tool, methodology, or approach that created "divides" across "camps". For example, the non-monotonic logic vs probabilistic divide, or the connectionist vs symbolic divide [26], etc. Finally any effort to link the R&D and success of AI/ML to creating simulacra of human intelligence may be destined to be confined to what humans are already good at without extending these capabilities to discovery in new problems where humans do not perform well (or could never perform well because of intrinsic limitations of their cognitive apparatus).

Heuristic Systems

The problems with the formal systems of the 80s and 90s led many to pursue ad hoc, aka *heuristic systems and methods* [27, 28]. These have had a considerably prominent presence in early medical informatics, and also re-surfaced, for example, with prominent commercial products in the 2000s, as well as with approaches that dominated earlier stages of high-throughput assay-driven biology and translational science. A properties-based overview and structural analysis of the heuristic-to-formal system spectrum is given in chapter "Foundations and Properties of AI/ML Systems". Here we will reiterate the key concepts from a crises-leading-to-improvements perspective.

Striving to attain the lofty AI goals in the earlier history of the field, attempts were made to overcome the difficulty and cost of establishing formal systems. Some researchers, especially when faced with complex domains, felt that the formal systems of the time (see chapter "Foundations and Properties of AI/ML Systems" for properties and characteristics of those) were too restrictive for designing successful AI solutions. Instead, they hoped that systems attempting to encode problem-solving strategies directly, without being restricted by the rules and structure of a formal foundation, would provide an approach that would be easier to engineer and would yield good results - at least "good enough, often enough". For example, the DxPlain system which was designed to perform large-scope diagnosis (and adopting its heuristic precursor, INTERNIST-I's knowledge representation and reasoning algorithm) was heuristic because it lacked a formal AI foundation and formal properties.

In a vigorous debate that lasted for many years, proponents of heuristic systems argued that to the extent that they worked well empirically, they should be perfectly acceptable, especially if more formally-constructed systems did not match the empirical performance of heuristic systems and if constructing formal systems or establishing their properties was exceedingly hard. Proponents of formal systems counter-argued that this ad-hoc approach to AI was detrimental since one should never feel safe when applying such systems, especially in high-stakes domains.

There is no arguing about the fact that formal foundations provide a roadmap for both problem solving and incremental improvements to existing systems. They make understanding the theoretical and empirical properties of AI/ML models and systems easier. In turn, such understanding does not always guarantee optimal systems, but gives a roadmap that enables safe navigation of the complex technological terrain of applied AI/ML. Heuristic development, on the other hand, is based upon the availability of the rather nebulous and uncontrollable ingredients of human inspiration and intuition. It is also conducive to engaging adoption of technology that is not safe, exactly because its functions and hence risks, are not understood well enough. This represented a "scruffy" approach [2] to an endeavor that, it is now evident with the benefit of the progress that has been achieved over the years, needed to employ science-driven solutions.

From a modern scientific perspective, the historical emphasis on heuristic systems seems much less meaningful today than in the earlier days of AI, because of the scientific advances in the field that led to the huge success and dominance of formal methods [2, 29]. It is now evident, that heuristic systems are pre-scientific or early-scientific technological artifacts in the sense that a true scientific understanding of their behavior does not exist (yet) and that with sufficient study in the future, a comprehensive understanding of a heuristic system of today can be obtained. In other words *the heuristic system of today (or the past) will be the formal system of tomorrow* [28]. Thus heuristic vs formal, if interpreted in terms that imply a special distinctive intrinsic nature, is a false dichotomy using misleading language.

Today's science and technology of AI/ML supports instead the distinction: **AI/ML systems with well understood properties (theoretical but also empirical performance), versus systems that lack these properties.** There is an evolutionary path from heuristic systems (aka pre-scientific informal systems) to scientifically understood and validated systems.

Chapter "Foundations and Properties of AI/ML Systems" further elaborates the landscape and epistemological journey from heuristic to formal: pre-scientific/heuristic, to intermediate level systems, to fully-mature fully-reliable and science-backed systems. Chapter "Principles of Rigorous Development and of Appraisal of ML and AI Methods and Systems" presents a concise summary of the main properties of all main AI/ML methods showing that due to the immense progress of the past few decades, we now have an extensive AI/ML method toolkit with well-understood behaviors.

The modern significance of this topic is that regrettably many new AI/ML methods and systems (or old methods applied to completely new areas) both in academia and industry lack established properties for performance and safety. It is not uncommon for such systems to be rushed to real-life application, and it is an ongoing battle to establish such properties before they can gain the trust and adoption they hope for, especially in high-stakes domains, such as medicine and the health sciences. Of particular relevance to today's AI/ML are: (a) systems or methods that are well understood/proven in a problem domain that are thrust in a different domain where they do not have well-established scientific foundations (e.g., IBM Watson Health, Large Language Models (LLMs), Deep Learning clinical applications on account on success on non-medical domains, or Shapley values for explaining ML models—see chapter "The Development Process and Lifecycle of Clinical Grade and Other Safety and Performance-Sensitive AI/ML Models", etc.). (b) Numerous bespoke bioinformatics "pipelines" constructed for the needs of a particular study but lacking well-defined generalizable properties.

Disconnect Between Early AI Systems and Real-World Needs and Workflows

Many of the early efforts in health AI/ML were driven by intellectual curiosity and less by the actual problems that patients or healthcare systems were facing. Consequently, the resulting systems were disconnected from (a) patient care needs, (b) patient care workflows, (c) needs of the system of science. A classic example is that of early diagnostic systems that attempted to solve a problem that was not pressing or was evaluated in a different population. Using one out of many similar examples of that era, INTERNIST-I was designed for accurate diagnosis of patients across internal medicine—whereas most patients in internal medicine clinic are not admitted for diagnosis and moreover, diagnosis is challenging for human internists in a small minority of diseases and few patient cases within those. Additionally, the data entry into the systems was disruptive of clinical workflows at the time [30] because of lack of EHRs and CPOE (computerized provider order entry systems) [31].

In addition, the collection of data inputs in the healthcare domain is in most cases sequential over time and dynamic (i.e, conditional on prior findings) [32]. The selection of which tests to run at each time point is a major decision that reflects a partial differential diagnosis and is not within the decision sphere of AI systems confined to a single-point-in-time decisions. This biases conventional performance evaluation based on complete medical records upward to very significant degree. Finally INTERNIST-I in particular, was evaluated for cases so hard (NEJM challenge cases) that in many cases only patho-anatomic examination (usually on biopsies obtained after patient surgery or death) was able to resolve the underlying disease (i.e., the diagnosis in such cases likely cannot be reliably made with data available to the AI system *or* the physicians) [33].

The compounding of these factors together rendered such systems very valuable from a technology exploration perspective but of limited use in practical terms and this was reflected in a landmark paper by Hunt, Haynes et al., which established very limited impact of the AI technology of the time on patient outcomes [34]. Most of the above factors were also recognized in an influential paper by Miller himself et al. that declared the death of the "Greek Oracle model" for AI decision support. These authors advocated instead for a softer knowledge-based "catalyst" model, assistive in nature, that would work in parallel with physicians and thus they modified the INTERNIST-I system into its successor QMR formulated as an electronic textbook of internal medicine with inferential capabilities. Unfortunately this reformulation was also not adopted widely in practice, most likely because it did not address pressing real-life needs [30].

The many practical problems associated with Expert Systems of both the rule-based or heuristic varieties were **overcome by the subsequent adoption of ML data-driven algorithms**. This technology was made applicable across a wide spectrum of applications because of the availability of vast troves of data (e.g., in the EHRs, the WWW, and mass-throughput molecular assays) combined with powerful ways to prevent over- and under-fitting (see chapter "Overfitting, Underfitting and General Model Overconfidence and Under-performance Pitfalls and Best Practices in Machine Learning and AI").

Limitations of Early Bayesian Learners and Emergence of BNs

The earliest conceptual application of AI/ML Bayesian reasoning in medicine, to our knowledge, is outlined in Ledley and Lusted [35] whereas a very early empirical application in a real-life domain using data-driven modeling, to Warner et al [36].

As explained in chapter "An Appraisal and Operating Characteristics of Major ML Methods Applicable in Healthcare & Health Science", brute-force application of Bayes' rule incurs an exponential space and time complexity which renders it infeasible outside all but the most trivial problem domains. Because of these factors early Bayesian classifiers where used with severe restrictions, typically in the form of "Simple" or "Naïve" Bayes which assumes that the target response (e.g., disease classification) comprises mutually exclusive categories, and that the inputs (e.g., disease findings) are independent of each other given the findings (see chapters "Foundations and Properties of AI/ML Systems" and "An Appraisal and Operating Characteristics of Major ML Methods Applicable in Healthcare & Health Science"). These assumptions are obviously most often false in healthcare and health sciences and entail substantial error in some applications. This led to research that took place over 2 decades and gave rise to improved formalisms, the most important of which is **Bayesian Networks** (discussed in chapter "Foundations and Properties of AI/ML Systems" in terms of properties, in chapter "An Appraisal and Operating Characteristics of Major ML Methods Applicable in Healthcare & Health Science" in terms of ML, and in chapter "Foundations of Causal ML" in terms of causality). This new AI technology was probabilistically correct and thus handled uncertainty optimally. It was flexible enough to model any distribution and at the level of space and sample complexity that the distribution required without unrealistic assumptions. BNs also allowed sound and complete forward and backward rule chaining inferences to take place [37, 38].

Intractability of BN Inference. Ability to Learn BNs from Data

The new and highly appealing formalism of BNs was quickly discovered to be worst-case intractable in inference both in the exact and approximate cases [39, 40]. Newer research, however, produced approximate inference algorithms that advanced the tractability of the formalism on large numbers of variables, e.g., [41]. Moreover, it was soon discovered by Herskowitz and Cooper that BNs could be learnt from data using entropy-based scoring and shortly afterwards, by Cooper and Herskowitz, using Bayesian scoring [42, 43]. Heckerman et al. developed a modified family of Bayesian scores that could observe *likelihood equivalence*, which says that data should not help discriminate network structures that represent the same assertions of conditional independence [44].

Overfitting and Over-Confidence in Models: Problems, Advances and Persistent Challenges

As detailed in chapter "Overfitting, Underfitting and General Model Overconfidence and Under-Performance Pitfalls and Best Practices in Machine Learning and AI", overfitting in AI/ML is the creation of models that because of their high complexity work well in the discovery data but do not generalize well in the broader population. Over-confidence is a broader class of problems in which we expect the models to perform better than what their true error is (regardless of the models' complexity). Overfitting is typically a byproduct of how algorithms fit models to data whereas over confidence may involve error estimation and data design faults as well (see chapters "The Development Process and Lifecycle of Clinical Grade and Other Safety and Performance-Sensitive AI/ML Models" and "Overfitting, Underfitting and General Model Overconfidence and Under-performance Pitfalls and Best Practices in Machine Learning and AI" for detailed analysis). Over-fitting and over-confidence can happen both in knowledge-driven and hand-modeled AI as well as in data-driven ML modeling.

In the early years of ML, overfitting avoidance was enforced by various factors and practices, e.g.: the natural dearth of high-dimensional datasets, by eliminating most variables from modeling using often crude feature selection strategies, by the statistical practice of analyst-driven "model specification" as opposed to extensive computational search in model space, by application of "pruning" of models after they were constructed, by application of inductive biases that—ceteris paribus—preferred simpler models over more complex ones, and other strategies and practices. Unfortunately, not all of the above practices were sufficient to address the problem. For example, in classical statistical regression, so-called step-wise procedures were shown to lead to substantially overfitted models with biased error estimates [45]).

In the 90s and onward, however, a **newer generation of highly regularized learners** (see chapters "Foundations and Properties of AI/ML Systems" and "An Appraisal and Operating Characteristics of Major ML Methods Applicable in Healthcare & Health Science") were put to practice, with built-in resistance to overfitting and mathematical error bounds that ensured that model complexity was automatically tailored to the data generating function's complexity and the available data. Notable such ML methods include penalty+loss learners such as SVMs and Regularized regression of various forms (chapter "An Appraisal and Operating Characteristics of Major ML Methods Applicable in Healthcare & Health Science"). Some other ML algorithms enforce **implicit regularization** in the form of model priors (Bayesian ML [43, 44]) or maximum allowed model size (e.g., Random Forests [14]) or via several formal and ad hoc regularization mechanisms in Deep Learning [9, 10].

Additional advances came in the form of **principled, theoretically optimal and empirically powerful feature selection algorithms** in the early 2000s and onward, which constrain the model complexity immensely before modeling even begins (e.g., reducing *without loss of predicitivity*, the modeled variables from, indicatively, 139,000 variables to 32 variables and from 100,000 to 6 variables in some representative applications [46–51].

Powerful nested protocols that combine model selection with error estimation so that over fitting and over confidence would be avoided also emerged as extensions to the previously well-known theory of cross-validation [52].

These protocols' importance was firmly established in genomic data analysis by the work of R. Simon et al [53] but are of universal applicability. The above new methods can be combined to strengthen the overall resistance to overfitting.

With modern algorithms and model selection, error estimation, and safe deployment protocols (see chapters "An Appraisal and Operating Characteristics of Major ML Methods Applicable in Healthcare & Health Science", "Principles of Rigorous Development and of Appraisal of ML and AI Methods and Systems", "The Development Process and Lifecycle of Clinical Grade and Other Safety and Performance-Sensitive AI/ML Models", "Overfitting, Underfitting and General Model Overconfidence and Under-performance Pitfalls and Best Practices in Machine Learning and AI", "Characterizing, Diagnosing and Managing the Risk of Error of ML & AI Models in Clinical and Organizational Application"), avoiding overfitting can be practically ensured in modern ML modeling. Unfortunately there are still obstacles that need be addressed:

(i) There is a **significant education and adoption gap**, since the concepts of overfitting and unbiased error estimation and the methods to address them are not as widely known (or universally practiced) especially by many stakeholders and beneficiaries from AI/ML (basic scientists, translational and clinical scientists, health care administrators, etc.).

(ii) While **independent validation** of models (chapter "The Development Process and Lifecycle of Clinical Grade and Other Safety and Performance-Sensitive AI/ML Models") is usually required by many journals, these validations may fail because of discovery-validation population mismatches or due to underpowered validations, and not because of over fitting. In other words, failure to pass independent set validation can generate false negatives. By comparison, cross-validation (properly executed) may only fail if the accessible population differs from the target population (i.e., a data design issue, see chapter "Data Design").

(iii) At best, independent validation is more of a **forensic failure analysis** tool (i.e., why a model *may have* failed) than a preventative strategy (i.e., how to construct the model so that it will not fail).

(iv) **Hand-made model construction is widely** practiced in biomedical engineering and other fields but without theoretical or practical assurances that the development practices that led to one successful model will generalize in other domains.

(v) **Widely-used ML algorithms such as DL still to this day lack a well-developed theory that prevents overfitting and ensures generalization.** In an intriguing paper [54] Zhang et al show that DL networks can perfectly learn random noise, memorize data fully, and these behaviors are *not affected* by regularization measures. Although empirical evidence suggests that DL learners often *do* resist overfitting, the reasons are not well understood. It is entirely possible that practical DL models exhibiting excellent classification errors in some domains were made possible simply due to the large sample sizes used to train them. At this time DL algorithms may be safer to use in data-rich settings.

(vi) **Results from most ML competitions and challenges are inexorably tied (by design) to a small number of datasets and the set of loss functions** used in the competition. This is a problem of **over-confidence in a model** which formally is a broader class of problems encompassing overfitting. As an indicative example, when Narendra et al compared a number of (highly reputable) DREAM challenges winning algorithms for pathway reverse engineering and contrasted them with additional algorithms with fresh datasets, very hard gold standards, and using a variety of loss functions, the previous winners did not exhibit superior performances and in some cases were substantially underperforming especially with respect to several loss functions not originally examined [21]. Moreover, the choice of loss functions dramatically reversed the rankings of algorithms' performances in many cases.

Ignoring the Data Design and Learning Protocol (Model Selection, Error Estimation) Effects on Modeling Success

Recall from chapter "Foundations and Properties of AI/ML Systems" that the **architecture of a ML method is defined by the** tuple: $< L, MF, DD, S, MLS, GM>$, in other words, the combination of a modeling language (L) (that describes the model space S), the model fitting procedure (MF) that parameterizes models to data, the data design (DD) that samples data from a population, a search procedure (MLS) that explores the model space and a goal/merit function (GM) used to evaluate each model. Typically, the focus on most ML and data science is on the "algorithm" which is meant to correspond to <L, MF, S, GM>. It is also common to see discussions of how the sample size may affect ability to learn specific classes of target functions [55, 56].

What is omitted from most technical and lay public discourse alike, however, are the effects of data design (Chapter "Data Design") and model selection and error estimation (Chapters "Principles of Rigorous Development and of Appraisal of ML and AI Methods and Systems", "The Development Process and Lifecycle of Clinical Grade and Other Safety and Performance-sensitive AI/ML Models", "Overfitting, Underfitting and General Model Overconfidence and Underperformance Pitfalls and Best Practices in Machine Learning and AI"). For emphasis, let us represent the success of AI/ML for a particular problem-solving endeavor with the following Fig. 3, which we invite the reader to always keep in mind in the context of AI/Ml projects:

This brings us to two enduring problems in historical and modern practice or AI/ML:

Effects of Protocols on Overall Model Performance Are Very Strong

In present day AI/ML practice it is common to encounter situations where the choice of model selection and error estimation protocol may negatively affect or even nullify good properties of ML algorithms. For example in [57] the largest (to our knowledge) empirical benchmark of text categorization algorithms and protocols

Fig. 3 Successful application of ML is determined by the combined influence of algorithm choice, data design, and model selection and error estimation protocol

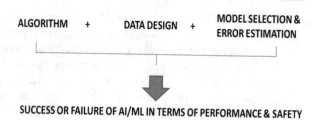

ALGORITHM + DATA DESIGN + MODEL SELECTION & ERROR ESTIMATION

SUCCESS OR FAILURE OF AI/ML IN TERMS OF PERFORMANCE & SAFETY

Fig. 4 The dramatic effect of model selection protocol on performance. A majority of algorithms with properly implemented model selection exceeded 0.9 AUC in the depicted classification benchmark. In dark blue, dramatic drop in performance due to modified implementation of the same protocol and using the same algorithm, in a commercial product [57]

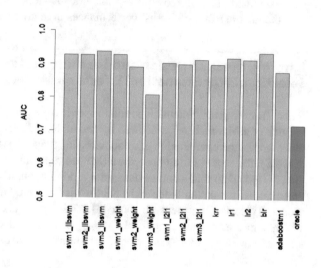

was conducted. Among other findings, they established that apparently minor alterations in the protocols used (with respect to their ideal specification), led to reduction in model predictivity as large as from >0.9 AUC to 0.72 AUC (a truly massive degradation in performance) (Fig. 4).

In the field of genomics, a landmark study was conducted by the **Microarray Quality Consortium** [58] **MAQC-II** project, where 36 independent teams analyzed six microarray data sets to generate predictive models for classifying a sample with respect to one of 13 endpoints indicative of lung or liver toxicity in rodents, or of breast cancer, multiple myeloma or neuroblastoma in humans. The teams generated predictive models and tested the models on data that had not been used for training. Model performance depended largely on the endpoint and team proficiency while different approaches generated models of similar performance.

A major finding was noticing "*substantial variations in performance among the many K-nearest neighbor algorithm (KNN)-based models developed by four analysis teams … Follow-up investigations identified a few possible causes leading to the discrepancies in performance. For example, DAT20 fixed the parameter 'number of neighbors' K = 3 in its data analysis protocol for all endpoints, whereas DAT18 varied K from 3 to 15 with a step size of 2.*"

Second, there are clear differences in proficiency between data analysis teams and such differences are correlated with the level of experience of the team. Moreover the study found that the internal validation performance from well-implemented, unbiased cross-validation shows a high degree of concordance with the external validation performance in a strict blinding process.

It was also found that **swapping train and test sets** led to different results (with same modeling approaches). This "fragility" of independent dataset validation reinforces the guidance provided in several places in the present volume about not overinterpreting differences in performance to an independent validation if internal validation has been executed properly. However, it was also noted that the correlation of the independent validation with the reversed order of modeling-testing was further reduced in teams with less experience, showing the effect of proper modeling practices.

The consortium concluded that *"Finally, applying good modeling practices appeared to be more important than the actual choice of a particular algorithm over the others within the same step in the modeling process. This can be seen in the diverse choices of the modeling factors used by teams that produced models that performed well in the blinded validation"*.

On the basis of these findings, MAQC-II set forth 4 general guidelines (incorporated in the present volume in several chapters) covering: good design, proper (internal) cross validation (or similar quality error estimation and model selection), caution about pitfalls of independent (external) validation, and not contaminating modeling data with test data information.

The findings of the MAQC-II project suggest that when the same data sets are provided to a large number of data analysis teams, many groups can generate similar results even when different model building approaches are followed. In this particular domain at least, the effect of protocol is more important than the algorithm used.

In another important benchmark study, Statnikov et al [17] showed that previously published early reports showing the superiority of Random Forests over other algorithms for cancer microarray data classification were an artifact of the protocols used to run the algorithms. When the "reference" use (i.e., one suggested by the methods' inventors) was followed in a common model selection and error estimation protocol, the results changed in favor or the SVM family of models.

Effects of Data Design on Overall Model Performance Are Very Strong

As we saw in Chapter "Data Design for Biomedical AI/ML", the data design, may affect in a myriad of ways the ability or ease and efficiency of drawing specific conclusions and attaining models with desired characteristics, often independent of learning algorithm. Also it was shown that w*ith the same algorithms employed,* some designs do not allow certain inferences at all or within reasonable resources, or exhibit large variation in quality of results. Yet, treatment of data design considerations while abundant and very sophisticated in statistics, in AI/ML they seem to often receive less scrutiny by practicing data scientists, vendors and the public. Some examples follow:

Issues with ML Challenges

As discussed in Chapter "Principles of Rigorous Development and of Appraisal of ML and AI Methods and Systems", ML challenges serve two fundamental purposes. One is the *education* of scientists from different fields about the problems the challenge addresses and giving them data and a platform to experiment. The second purpose is to explore which algorithmic methods are better at a particular point in time for a particular problem. Well-designed challenges can generate valuable information and enhance interdisciplinary engagement. In most cases, however, challenges suffer from fixing a data design and the error estimator thus *removing from consideration, study, and improvement, two out of the three determinants of ML success* (Figure 3).

Challenges also routinely restrict the design of modeling by pre-selecting variables, and over-simplifying the statement of problems, sometimes to meaningless extremes. Consider as representative example of thousands of similar challenge datasets, a high-ranked dataset in the competition platform Kaggle [59]. Participants are asked to build models to predict stroke based on the following features:

> *gender, age, hypertension (has: yes/no), heart_disease (has: yes/no), ever_married, work_type("children", "Govt_jov", "Never_worked", "Private" or "Self-employed"), Residence_type ("Rural" or "Urban"), avg_glucose_level, bmi, smoking_status ("formerly smoked", "never smoked", "smokes" or "Unknown"). Stroke is defined as (1 if the patient had a stroke or 0 if not).*

Such a formulation of the problem omits very significant aspects previously established in the clinical literature (e.g., important factors to be measured, prior successful models, precise and meaningful descriptions of the clinical context of use for such models). It is furthermore representative on a systematic pattern of many competition platforms to reduce challenging scientific problems to 'toy' versions, that are not fully informed by prior science, are often devoid of medical or AI/ML technical context, have dubious choice or features and coding, lack proper design flexibility -including statements of target and accessible populations- and so forth (see Chapter "Data Design for Biomedical AI/ML" why problem statements and data as the one described here lack basic pre-requisites for making scientific advances).

Challenges also suffer from *incomplete or highly biased representation in the competitor pool.* Most of participants in challenges are either students or interested scientists but from different areas and thus typically having limited skill in tackling the problem. Another limitation is that *not all appropriate algorithms are entered in a challenge and when they enter, they are not executed necessarily according to optimal specifications.* Finally, challenges typically involve a *very small number of datasets that do not represent a large domain.* Such representative coverage typically requires many dozens of datasets or more *in the same comparison.* One final defining characteristic of challenges, is that they externalize and distribute the cost of method benchmarking to volunteer participants (and this explains in part their proliferation for commercial purposes as a low-cost R&D alternative business model).

Despite these limitations, a select number of challenges that are designed to a high degree of quality, when interpreted carefully and with the appropriate qualifications, can provide empirical scientific information that could supplement the centralized and distributed benchmark designs (details in Chapter "Principles of Rigorous Development and of Appraisal of ML and AI Methods and Systems"). For examples of well-designed, and carefully interpreted challenges the reader may refer to the challenges conducted by the ChaLearn organization [60].

Other Persistent Issues Related to Common Data Design Deficiencies

We briefly mention here a number of additional areas negatively affected by suboptimal data design choices (or by not paying enough attention to data design): **Active learning algorithms** entail gathering data in which the natural priors of the target response classes are typically unknown. However, such knowledge is necessary for characterizing model errors by loss functions that are prior-dependent (e.g., positive and negative predictive value). This creates obstacles to safe model deployment (see Chapter "Characterizing, Diagnosing and Managing the Risk of Error of ML & AI Models in Clinical and Organizational Application"). The shortcomings of **EHR data for secondary analysis** in terms of data incompleteness and bias are widely appreciated (and often exaggerated). An important issue that receives much less attention with EHR-based data designs is the lack of power. For example, the PheWAS design for genotype-phenotype correlation discovery [61] is an modern design that aims to bridge the clinical with the genomic worlds. However, in a fragmented health system like the USA's, such designs are hampered by the difficulty in pooling data across provider organizations, and harmonizing the population characteristics and risk of biases. As such, the discovery is confined to single systems or small pools of those. The limited genomic variable scope in EHRs incurs an exceedingly small a priori probability for discovery, and these two factors together, further exacerbate the low power issue. Newer **Big Science designs** e.g., VA's MVP project [62] or the AllOfUs project [63] are poised to overcome these difficulties. **Power-sample design**, is harder in ML because knowledge of learning curves is required but often only empirically known (see Chapter "The Development Process and Lifecycle of Clinical Grade and Other Safety and Performance-Sensitive AI/ML Models" for guidance). In some cases assumption-driven and early data-fitted empirical learning curves failed to produce unbiased estimates (as for example occured in [64]).

Causality in Early and Modern ML

One of the most foundational aspects of AI/ML for improving health outcomes and the healthcare system and for driving advances in health science discovery is *causality, its discovery, representation, and modeling*. We will thus discuss in the present chapter several historical and modern challenges and successes involving causal knowledge.

"Correlation Does Not Imply Causation" and the Falsely Implied Impossibility of Discovering Causality Without Experiments. Problems with RCTs and Low-dimensional Experiments

For many years, the celebrated statistician Sir Ronald Fisher's famous warning about the inappropriateness of concluding that A is causing B (or vice versa) from the fact that A and B are correlated, was inappropriately extrapolated to the notion that only experiments could discover causality. In the clinical health sciences the randomized controlled trial (RCT), a methodology with a long history [65–67] has been viewed as the sole arbiter of reliable causal discovery.

Fisher's statement is quite benign since, properly interpreted, implies that not *all* correlations between A and B entail that A $\rightarrow$ B or A $\leftarrow$ B but rather that a confounder may be responsible for the correlation: A $\leftarrow$ C $\rightarrow$ B. So it follows that if we observe that A and B are correlated, then they *may or may not cause* one another. If we observe that A and B are uncorrelated, on the other hand, in the majority of distributions, A is not causing B and vice versa. The presence of correlation thus provides evidentiary support for the existence of causation and lack of correlation effectively precludes it [68].

If we are interested in causes (or effects) of variable A we can typically discard all variables X that are uncorrelated with A. Variables Y that are correlated with A, are *candidate* causes or effects of A. If the possible confounders of A and Y are measured and we know who they are, we can control them analytically (by SEMs or regression, see Chapter "Foundations of Causal ML") or by matching. These facts led to widespread practices in epidemiology where a large pool of correlates where established by data analysis as well as putative confounders and the correlates were examined for *vanishing conditional correlations* with A given the assumed confounders. If the non-zero correlation of Y with A becomes zero (aka vanishes) conditioned on the complete set of measured confounders C, then A is not causing Y or vice versa. If the conditional correlation is not zero, then this supports the existence of a causal relationship between A and Y.

A **variant of this analytical control methodology, propensity scoring**, was introduced by [69]. In propensity scoring, the fundamental idea is that the analyst builds a predictor model of the exposure, and controls the correlation of exposure and outcome by conditioning on the score of the predictor. If this conditional correlation of the exposure and the outcome vanishes, then the exposure does not cause the outcome.

Additional **heuristic causality rules** (Hill's criteria or Koch's postulates [70–72]) were often overlaid on correlative analytics in order to support or weaken causal interpretation.

There are major limitations with all of the above approaches, however [68, 73]:

(a) Even if the confounders are all measured, it is not always known that they are confounders. Wrong causal conclusions are likely if the controlling or matching variables are, or include, non-confounders.

(b) If even one of the confounder is not measured, (i.e., it is "hidden" or "latent") then they cannot be controlled analytically or by data design with the previous approaches.

(c) The heuristic criteria were shown to be invalid and misleading.

(d) The assumptions that would ensure correctness of propensity scoring are not testable within the propensity scoring theory. Moreover as was shown in a vigorous peer-reviewed debate [74, 75], Pearl and others showed that in a very large class of models, conditioning on the propensity score introduces errors in the estimation of causal effects and that the theory of propensity scoring could not test for these problematic cases.

Randomized causal experiments or RCTs are typically used to confirm or reject the causal nature of a hypothesized causal relationship. RCTs and other randomized experiments nullify (on average) all confounders between treatment/exposure and outcome even if these confounders are unknown and unmeasured.

As useful as RCTs are, they also have significant limitations (and the same is true for other randomized experiments); here we will summarize only the salient limitations mainly with respect to *scalability, feasibility, scope,* and *completeness* [68, 73]:

- RCTs are a confirmatory and not a discovery procedure.
- RCTs are very expensive and time-demanding.
- RCTs are infeasible in many settings.
- RCTs are unethical in many settings.
- RCT execution commonly fails for a variety of reasons (e.g., accrual failure, lack of power).
- RCTs reveal remote or direct causation and do not determine direct causation.
- RCTs cannot be used to develop system-level causal models (i.e., full causal specification of the data generating process). See in particular the important results from the theory of causal discovery summarized in Chapter "Foundations and Properties of AI/ML Systems" that show the severe limitations of 1-variable-at a time or fragmented experiments with regard to ability to learn the whole system of causal relationships (unless they are coupled and supported by algorithmic non-experimental causal discovery). Many of these RCT shortcomings also apply in biology and other basic health sciences, in low-dimensional randomized experiments (i.e., manipulating one or a few variables at a time).
- RCTs produce average and not precision causal effect estimates (i.e., they are *too broad* in effect size estimation).
- RCTs are applied to a typically narrow accessible population and not the wider target population (i.e., they are *too narrow* with regards to target population).
- RCTs are extremely sensitive to context (for a demonstration that is as vivid as it is whimsical see [76].

New Class of Scalable Causal Discovery Algorithms

The limitations of the [candidate discovery → validation] discovery chain via the sequence [uncontrolled correlations → *controlled correlations* → *randomized* *experiments*], were radically reduced by the emergence of a **new class of causal ML algorithms that under conditions guaranteed algorithmic and reliable scalable complex causal discovery and modeling even in the absence of experiments**. These algorithms originated from diverse data science and AI/ML disciplines: Computer Science (Pearl, Verma and others [73]), Computational Philosophy (Spirtes, Glymour, Scheines and others [68]), Econometrics and AI (Granger, Herbert Simon, Sims, Imbens and others) and Health Informatics (Cooper et al [43]). A multitude of theoretical and algorithmic advances pioneered by these researchers addressed the limitations of earlier approaches and offered effective alternative and supplemental discovery and modeling procedures. Among the milestone contributions of the above, it is worthwhile highlighting the richness and breadth of Pearl's theoretical treatment of causality, the seminal algorithmic body of work by Spirtes, Glymour, Scheines and their students and collaborators, and the remarkable IC* algorithm by Verma and Pearl, which opened the doors for detecting existence of unmeasured variables that confound statistical correlations. Please refer to Chapter "Foundations of Causal ML" for details on properties and capabilities.

Early Causal Algorithms Were Not Scalable; Claimed Impossibility of Tractable Causal Discovery Algorithms. Discovery of Scalable and Efficient Causal Algorithms and Causal Feature Selection

As these new causal methods started being used in empirical applications, it quickly became evident that the algorithms would not scale to more than a few dozen variables in unrestricted distributions with hidden variables and ~100 variables when no latents were present. Notable researchers expressed strong pessimism that scalable algorithms could be invented (e.g., prominent algorithms expert and Turing award winner J. Ulman in a paper discussing large-scale data mining applications techniques [77] assessed that "... *the goal has generally been to learn complete causal models, which are essentially impossible to learn in large-scale data mining applications with a large number of variables*").

Fortunately not long after these pessimistic predictions were made, the first **scalable local causal methods** had been discovered, and within a few years **full causal graph ones** [78]. Moreover, researchers developed methods that bridged the local causal discovery problem and predictive modeling by introducing **scalable, sample efficient and correct Markov Boundary algorithms** [8, 48]. Chapters "Foundations and Properties of AI/ML Systems", "An Appraisal and Operating Characteristics of Major ML Methods Applicable in Healthcare & Health Science" and "Principles of Rigorous Development and of Appraisal of ML and AI Methods and Systems" give more detail on the approaches used to scale up the previous generation of algorithms. [79] describe the **theoretical framework for connecting predictivity, feature selection and local causality**). These methods were subsequently expanded/followed by sound and scalable **algorithms capable of equivalence-class modeling, ML-guided experimentation, and generalized families** thereof [80, 81]).

Lack of Causal Correctness in Broad Use of ML and Especially the Persistent Use of General Predictive Modeling Methods to Solve Causal Problems

A widespread misapplication of AI/ML methods and tools across the academic sphere and industry alike, involves the use of methods not designed for causality to solve causal problems. This includes, for example, the use of vanilla predictive modeling, clustering, network science, non-causal feature selection, dimensionality reduction, and other methods lacking causal correctness. Especially in the predictive modeling area, numerous methods are abused in this regard (e.g., Deep Learning and other ANNs, regularized regression and classification, Decision Trees and Random Forests, SVMs, Boosting, Bagging and Ensembling, see Chapter "An Appraisal and Operating Characteristics of Major ML Methods Applicable in Healthcare & Health Science"). To understand the magnitude of the problem, we refer the reader to the large scale benchmarks published in [48], where >100 algorithms and variants were tested in >40 datasets, from real life and resimulation, as to their ability to be used for feature selection/prediction and causal discovery. Main findings included that: (a) predictive methods performed very well or optimally for prediction; (b) causal feature selection led to optimal predictive models while using smallest number of features; (c) predictive feature selection is utterly inappropriate for causal discovery. The following 2 figures demonstrate this last finding: In Figure 5 an experiment is shown where a local causal method in the GLL family and and a predictive method (SVMs) are compared in the task of discovering the local causal pathway around a response variable T of interest in a transcriptomic network used to generate the comparison data. The causal method achieves this goal with near-perfect causal accuracy (blue nodes, zoomed in the figure) *and* empirically optimal predictive accuracy at the same time. The non-causal method *is equally predictive,* but selects features across the network without any useful causal interpretation. Notice that once we can recover the local pathway accurately, we can

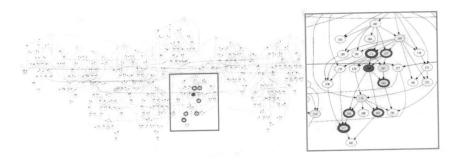

Fig. 5 Causal method (GLL, blue) vs non-causal methods (SVM-RFE, yellow) compared for local causal discovery

apply the causal procedure across all variables and recover the whole causal network. Moreover the ability to estimate causal effects of manipulations is totally dependent on identifying the confounders. Hence the focus on local causal accuracy is justified by it being a prerequisite for both correct causal structure and correct quantitative causal effect estimation.

These behaviors are not confined to a single dataset or a single pair of algorithms, but are *general operating characteristics*.

Figure 6 compares a multitude of causal and non-causal methods: GLL variants (causal), RFE-SVM, UAF, and Regularized regression/Elastic Net (non-causal). As can be seen, causal methods recover the direct causes with minimal false positives (and optimal predictivity), non-causal methods *although predictively excellent*, produce fundamentally only causal false positives. In these experiments, Lars-EN in

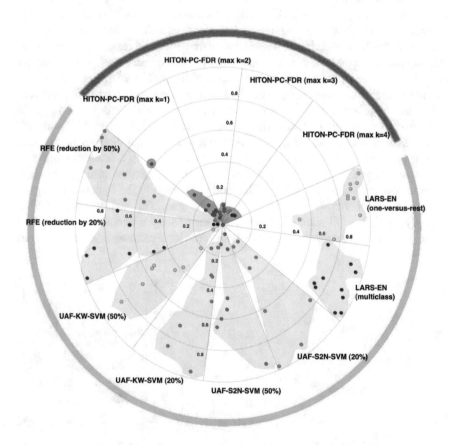

Fig. 6 Comparison of causal (red sector) and non-causal (green sector) methods for causal discovery. Concentric circles show the distance from the true local causal neighborhood of the target response. Better performance: results close to the center. Worse performance: results away from the center

particular (for reasons that are poorly understood) seems to have an *anti-causal* inductive bias, thus selecting features as far away from the direct causes as possible.

Pillars of Causal AI

The need for wider adoption of causal methods in AI/ML is as pressing as ever. Pearl [82] provides a lucid description of this urgency and outlines what he considers as his 7 pillars of Causal AI as follows:

Pillar 1: Encoding Causal Assumptions transparently and testably.
Pillar 2: using Do-calculus to control confounding.
Pillar 3: Algorithmization of counterfactuals effect estimation.
Pillar 5: Dealing with external validity and sample selection bias.
Pillar 6: Dealing with missing data.
Pillar 7: Advancing causal discovery.

Case Studies with Pitfalls Involving AI/ML Used in Genomics

Among research domains in the health sciences, genomics and other fields driven by high-throughput (i.e., high dimensional) omics (e.g., transcriptomic, proteomic, metabolomics, microbiomic, epigenetic) assays have arguably benefited the most from the availability of ML methods for making sense of large datasets originating from vastly complicated data generating processes (see Chapter "Artificial Intelligence (AI) and Machine Learning (ML) for Healthcare and Health Sciences: The Need for Best Practices Enabling Trust in AI and ML"). In clinical domains these advances have enabled exponential progress, for instance, the progress of molecular oncology toward deriving rationally-designed "targeted" treatments as well as precision medicine tests [83] that are rapidly and decisively changing the cancer field. These achievements did not occur smoothly, however, and several case studies exist that serve as examples of how deviation from best practices can lead to grave errors, dead ends and false starts.

The **Anil Poti** incident is one such case study in which several trials were shut down, several grants terminated, and a substantial number of papers withdrawn. Although some accounts of the incident emphasize administrative errors and compliance issues, it is worth noting that at the core of the misconduct was the creation of a controversial complex precision oncology models and tests used to treat patients in clinical trials. [84]. This is also a vivid illustration that testing ML models in a RCT is a final step only and does not constitute sufficient protection since poorly-constructed models will endanger human subjects. In response to this incident the National Cancer Institute requested that the Institute of Medicine (IOM) establish a committee to recommend ways to strengthen omics-based test development and evaluation.

Best Practice 12.7.1

The IOM's recommendations and best practices to enhance development, evaluation, and translation of omics-based tests before they are used to guide patient treatment in clinical trials. These aim to ensure that progress in omics test development is grounded in sound scientific practice and is reproducible, resulting not only in improved health care but also in continued public trust [85].

In another high-profile case study, the research conducted in the labs led **by Drs. Petricoin and Liota at the FDA using a proprietary SELDI-TOFF mass spectrometry technology**, was shown to suffer from several modeling errors, and irreproducible conclusions. These findings led to the closing of these labs, and the company responsible for the mass spectrometry assay technology became defunct. Most importantly, the whole field of clinical proteomics suffered a significant credibility blow that, by many accounts, held back its progress by many years [86, 87].

In another, present-day challenge, it has been established that **random biomarker selection from omics data often leads to optimal predictor models** and is comparable to biomarker signatures produced by sophisticated ML algorithms [88]. This creates a series of challenging questions that undermine the credibility of biomarkers discovered via widely-used current ML technologies: (i) if the ML selection is often not better than random for many algorithms/ datasets, do biomarkers from such ML algorithms have any special biological significance? (ii) What is the added value of ML biomarker selector algorithms over random choice? (iii) Should biomarker sets and signatures be rejected on account of not passing a statistical test of difference from a random set? If yes, using what criterion? (iv) Some studies have conducted such tests while many others did not. What are the implications for the quality of findings? A comprehensive and mathematically sound theory to explain these phenomena has not yet been published.

The interested reader in genomic applications of AI/ML is also referred to the landmark study by the MAQC-II (Section "Effects of Protocols on Overall Model Performance Are Very Strong").

We close this section by mentioning discouraging results from a major systematic analysis of the literature conducted by the Biometrics branch of the NCI [89]. This study revealed that many studies in genomics fail to follow a number of good or best practices. The implications on the validity and reproducibility of these studies' results are not known exactly but are likely to be severe.

Attributes and Limitations of Published Guidelines and Criteria for Health AI/ML

In recent years several guidelines have been published both by scholars, regulatory and accreditation bodies, and others. Because of the vastness and the socio-technical complexity of the AI/ML field and its health applications, and because of the different goals and purview of guideline authors, the resulting recommended practices have great variance in their properties as well as scope and effectiveness.

The Risk of Exaggerating Guideline Generality

This risk occurs when recommended practices are *advisable under some conditions* but may be interpreted as being true under any conceivable condition (i.e., absolutely). In other words the guidelines describe sufficient conditions for good (or bad) performance but not necessary and sufficient ones. For example, in many chapters of this book we have referenced the landmark work by Rich Simon et al. showing the advantages of nested cross-validation (CV) over non-nested CV. Consider carefully the original Simon et al. experiment [90]: it shows a strong bias when a particular feature selector is applied under the null hypothesis (i.e., no signal on average by label-reshuffled data construction). What if the feature selector instead of naïve univariate association is multiple-testing with Bonferroni-corrected association? It can be seen that the feature selector would return the empty set and no bias would ensue. Or what if one would use a feature selector that used internally nested cross validation? Again a different bias would ensue. What would happen if one would use a regularized or Markov Boundary feature selector that have strong protections against over-fitting? And what would happen if all of the above, alone or in combination, were attempted and not just under the null but under the alternatives of weak, moderate and strong signals in a variety of distributions?

Figure 7 demonstrates relevant experimental results (conducted by Dr. Alexander Statnikov in the Aliferis lab, on representative gene expression datasets).

This example shows how the details of gene selection procedure may produce bias that does not grow monotonically to the degree by which the analysis conforms to Simon et al criteria. This is because of the intricacies of how this gene selection procedure works. A reviewer blindly following a rigid set of criteria and not possessing specialized knowledge about how the analysis is done will conclude that the study corresponding to the analysis of experiment 1 is grossly biased, and the analysis of experiment 2 is less biased. The opposite is a more accurate description of reality, in the presented experiments, however.

In general, the **embedded algorithms influence the modeling protocol (not just the other way around as we showed in the MACQC-II results)**. To the credit of the authors, Dupuy and R. Simon in their subsequent systematic review and guidelines study [89] included two important guidelines under the section "Statistical analysis: general options" that read:

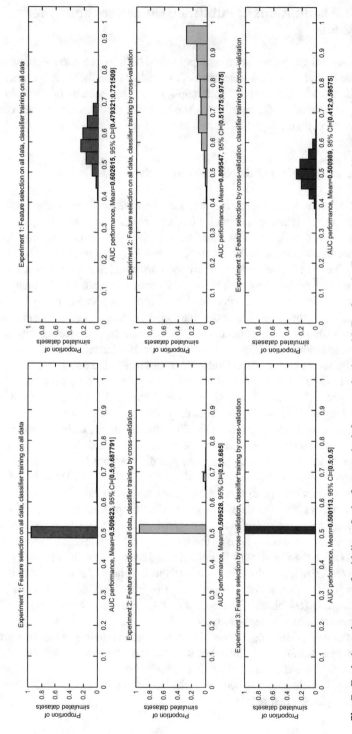

Fig. 7 Exploring robustness of guidelines. In the figure to the left, gene selection with Bonferroni adjustment produces unbiased results independent of cross-validation design. The advice that "Biased resubstitution or only partially cross-validated estimates should either not be reported or should be clearly represented as unreliable indicators of prediction accuracy" is not *universally* correct. In the right part of the figure, SVM-RFE gene selection produces a very small bias with no cross-validation, a moderate bias with "incomplete" cross-validation, and no bias with "complete" cross-validation, aka non-nested vs nested cross validation

> *"Do Be aware that many aspects of statistical analysis and reporting of microarray studies are not covered in this checklist."*
> *"Don't Consider that all the items included in these guidelines are commandments."*

We wholeheartedly mirror these statements for the present book as well. The way the guidance was stated in the *original report* however, likely creates the perception to (especially technically unsophisticated) readers that there is only one right way to produce unbiased results and every deviation is unacceptable. If such guidance is then followed uncritically it may hinder other methods that lead to good results (and *this is exactly what happened as explained in the next section on how meta analyses have over-inerpreted guidelines*).

Another example of over-generalizing guidance has to do with stepwise feature selection. While it is true that stepwise procedures as implemented in most statistical software do not have guarantees for correctness and overfit routinely [45], the same is *not true for every conceivable stepwise feature selector.* For example the IAMB family of feature selectors is based on an iterative entry-deletion process but they (a) are guaranteed to be correct (under assumptions) and (b) do not overfit because of the way they filter out noise variables (and in addition, they are followed in practice by regularized classifiers that further reduce any residual over-fitting) [91].

A final example of the danger of over-generalizing guidelines is in the case **of heuristic guidelines**. These are often encountered in applied statistical but also in ML modeling. For example, the guidance that in a regression model for every fitted parameter we should have at least 10 samples, or in the PC algorithm that a test of conditional independence will not be conducted unless at least 5 samples are available for every degree of freedom, etc. Such heuristic guidance is inherently bound to failures in many distributions, yet their value is that (i) they are easy to remember and communicate, (ii) they are easy to implement, and (iii) they are founded on robust theoretical principles and as a result work well in the average or majority of real-life data.

Over-Interpreting Guidelines Can (and Does) Negatively Affect the Meta Analytic Literature and Its Subsequent Literature

As an example case study, of a broad problem, based on the guidance of Simon et al., Ntzani et al. [92], reviewed the genomics literature at the time and found that most studies did not follow the Simon et al. guideline. These authors reported that a majority of such studies were not following the complete validation guideline, *without examining if the actual deviations led to errors* but implying that they most likely do. In a subsequent study one of the same authors [93] published an influential editorial that referenced the Ntzani study and asked: "Microarrays and molecular research: noise discovery?". Clearly, as literature chains are formed, guideline *over-interpretation errors* can amplify.

Guidelines and Standards with Implied Exaggerated Completeness or Impact

For example, the criteria used by a well-known accrediting body (see details in Chapter "Reporting Standards, Certification/Accreditation, and Reproducibility" for more details) suggest *institutional mastery of ML/AI* if the highest accreditation criteria are met, or alternatively that such mastery can be established by the accreditation process. However, the criteria do not address numerous critical factors that are essential for attaining any reasonable interpretation of "mastery" (see Chapter "Reporting Standards, Certification/Accreditation, and Reproducibility" for more details).

Similarly, **reporting standards imply that good science has been attained or can be verified if the reporting criteria are met.** As we detail in Chapter "Reporting Standards, Certification/Accreditation, and Reproducibility", however, such an expectation should be currently viewed with caution. There are numerous ways for an AI/ML study or project to be biased, ineffective or even clinically dangerous even when all the stated reporting criteria are met. Additionally, the details cannot be checked by readers, reviewers and so on. At best, one could reasonably claim that following the reporting standards would (i) *reduce the chances that (ii) certain weaknesses (iii) would not go unnoticed, (iv) if truthfully reported, (vi) in their entirety, and (vii) the readers are be able to accurately evaluate the relevance of the reported criteria to the quality of the published AI/ML.* This is a quite complex qualifying statement that represents the truth better than an absolute view that following the reporting criteria will invariably lead to better AI/ML.

Another example of exaggerated implied importance is that of [94] where the highest level of reproducibility rigor is assigned to studies meeting: *"The gold standard for reproducibility requires the entire analysis to be reproducible with a single command. Achieving this goal requires authors to automate all steps of their analysis, including downloading data, pre-processing data, training models, producing output tables, and generating and annotating figures. Full automation stands in addition to tracking dependencies and making their data and code available. In short, by meeting the gold standard, authors make the burden of reproducing their work as small as possible."*

Such a reproducibility standard must be very carefully interpreted, however. First, such a requirement is obviously feasible only assuming a discovery/development process that lacks stochasticity (for example, non-randomized discovery algorithms only are involved). In such cases additional data must be provided, for example the random generators used and starting conditions if available. Alternatively the resulting randomized parameters, for example the random splits in the used cross-validation, or the random re-samples in bootstrapping etc., must be stored and shared.

Additionally, the information provided by such replication would be equivalent to stating that the results were not tampered with. However, in the grand scheme of things this is a low bar to pass. The criterion lacks ability to test and reject, or confirm, whether the data design at hand was appropriate for the problem to be solved, whether the applied procedures (algorithms and protocols) were the right ones, whether the data was corrupted or not, whether the codes for the experimental analysis had bugs, whether the interpretation of findings was appropriate, and so on, for the myriad of factors that can affect the quality of modeling and the trustworthiness of results.

On the other hand, a particularly useful aspect of the ability to run the exact protocol used in the analysis (not mentioned in the guideline) is to apply label-reshuffling tests that can test the analysis protocol's propensity to overfit (see Chapter "Characterizing, Diagnosing and Managing the Risk of Error of ML & AI Models in Clinical and Organizational Application").

Limitations of Literature

The current peer-reviewed based system governing publication of scientific papers has a long history and its strengths and weaknesses have been the subject of intense scrutiny and debate over many years within the science community. *Within the operating characteristics of the present system,* a number of problematic cases can and do occur:

Limitations of Self-Correction

Scientific research is in principle supposed to be self-correcting in the sense that if a false result is published, then another study that fails to reproduce it or that proves that the first finding was wrong will be published and neutralize the deleterious influence that the initial false finding can have upon subsequent studies. Unfortunately this is a highly idealized version of reality. In practice, **publication bias** [95, 96] is a well-known phenomenon in clinical and other literatures, in which *positive results have a better chance of being published, are published earlier, and are published in journals with higher influence.* As a consequence, effects are often overestimated. This is a major contributor to the so called "replication crisis", in which many experimental findings (claims) cannot be replicated and some are likely to be false. Does this imply that scientific facts (consensus conclusions over many studies) are false as well? Nissen et al. [97] modeled the community's confidence in a claim as a Markov process with successive published results shifting the degree of belief and found that publication bias influences the distribution of published results and *unless a sufficient fraction of negative results is published, false claims can frequently become canonized as fact.*

From the perspective of incentives, publishers and editors are not induced to publish studies that put previous papers in their journals under suspicion or rejection (unless of course there is blatant misdoing such as fraud). As a result, many models, studies, etc. remain uncorrected for long periods of time or even indefinitely if the attention of the field shifts to different hypotheses. Therefore, the scientific audience in health AI/ML should exercise a healthy degree of skepticism when appraising the experimental literature. Using a foundation of principled and science-driven best practices, such as ones presented and referenced in this book, is a valuable tool in this process.

Assessment of Risk of Bias in Published Studies

The meta-analytic science community has developed several guidelines for evaluating whether a study is at **risk of bias** (e.g., [98, 99]). A list of prominent such tools is provided in [100] and includes tools for: Systematic reviews, Overviews of reviews, Randomised trials, Non-randomised studies of interventions (case-control, cohort, etc.), Prognostic, Diagnostic, Qualitative, Observational studies of exposures, and In vivo animal studies.

These are not designed for AI/ML but do address general methodological issue and therefore can be highly complementary to the evaluation of other, more technical, AI/ML aspects.

Disconnected Publication Spheres and Disjointed Expertise Across Fields

As with any technology that can excite the imagination of the non-technical specialist audience, AI/ML has been the subject of thousands of papers written by non-experts in the last few years. Such papers offer subjective commentary, opinions, impressions, hopes, and projections about the science and technology of health AI/ML, and its possible future applications and impact. The clinical sciences literature, however, to a large extent, is disconnected from the computer science, AI/ML literature and most clinicians and biologists do not read the technical literature nor are they trained in these sciences (and vice versa). Major AI/ML journals are not listed in PubMed and WebofScience (although this seems to be slowly changing). Because, predominantly, biologists tend to read other biologists, clinicians of a specialty other clinicians in that specialty, and technology experts their peers, knowledge does not travel well among these different fields. On one hand, this disconnect offers opportunity for novel discoveries by traversing and linking the disjointed literatures (as demonstrated by the **Arrowsmith system** [101, 102]). At the same time it is important to recognize that many of the AI/ML-themed papers written by biologists or clinicians are based on a superficial technical understanding of the science and technology of health AI/ML. Conversely, few experts in AI/ML have a deep understanding of the health sciences or healthcare and one can find many papers in the technical literature that misunderstands, and over-simplifies the goals, requirements and challenges of health domains.

Matthew Effect in the Literature of Health AI/ML

The Matthew effect of accumulated advantage, (aka Matthew principle) refers to the tendency of individuals or organizations to accrue social or economic success in proportion to their *initial* level of competitive success [103]. Perc [103] references many studies of *preferential attachment in the literature*, which is the distribution of citations based, to a large extent, on existing citations rather than fully on merit.

In another study of **first-mover advantage in scientific publication** [104], Newman created mathematical models of the scientific citation process that predict: *"a strong 'first-mover' effect under which the first papers in a field will, essentially regardless of content, receive citations at a rate enormously higher than papers published later. Moreover, papers are expected to retain this advantage in perpetuity —they should receive more citations indefinitely, no matter how many other papers are published after them. We test this conjecture against data from a selection of fields and in several cases find a first-mover effect of a magnitude similar to that predicted by the theory. Were we wearing our cynical hat today, we might say that the scientist who wants to become famous is better off—by a wide margin— writing a modest paper in next year's hottest field than an outstanding paper in this year's. On the other hand, there are some later-published papers, albeit only a small fraction, that buck the trend and attract significantly more citations than theory predicts. "*

Compounding of Publication Bias with Mathew Effect in AI/ MI Literature

In the context of early health AI/ML methods literature, a common situation is for example, that when a new assay technology emerges, the first papers that will be produced showing a positive result will (a) be accepted with high probability in high visibility journals (because of novelty and intense audience interest and due to *positive publication bias*); and (b) will receive in each subsequent wave of publications a higher proportion of citations because authors in every subsequent publication wave will be obliged to acknowledge the most highly-cited papers in the previous wave (*preferential attachment/Mathew effect*).

Simultaneously, however, (c) the papers in the earliest publication waves will be the least well-developed and lacking the full gamut of method development and validation (detailed in Chapter "Principles of Rigorous Development and of Appraisal of ML and AI Methods and Systems"). For example, the first methods for analyzing microarray data (receiving many thousands of citations each) are not the best performing ones or with the best properties (as evidenced by subsequent benchmarks and analyses) [21, 58, 17]. The same is generally true for the first methods for deep sequencing, the first methods for microbiomics, the first methods for EKG analysis, or image recognition, or NLP processing etc.

> **Best Practice. 12.9.1**
> The above literature limitations imply (among other things) that readers should seek, read and interpret health AI/ML papers taking the above factors into consideration.

Weaknesses of AI/ML COVID Models; Regulatory Criticisms in Covid AI; Other Regulatory Areas of Improvement

A recent highly-instructive case study pertains to the clinical readiness and trust-worthiness of COVID diagnosis and prognosis ML models produced in the span between 2019 and 2020. A massive systematic review of the literature [105] led to the following two main conclusions: (a) >2200 studies had been published; (b) not a single study met very basic criteria for clinical readiness. An unknown number of these models have been deployed clinically and with unknown consequences, however. This is just one among numerous criticisms that have been raised in the broader field and literature of COVID modeling, that we will not discuss further here in order to preserve space and bandwidth.

In another study published in the same time frame, criticism was leveled against the FDA for the claimed failure to regulate COVID models successfully [106]. Since that time, the FDA has issued new guidance for regulatory oversight of clinical AI/ML. While regulatory oversight of health AI/ML is visibly improving, it can be argued that continuous improvements are always feasible and desirable as the technology and its implementation advances and expands. Chapter "Regulatory Aspects and Ethical Legal Societal Implications (ELSI)" delves into the details of the regulatory landscape and criteria.

Selected Case Studies of Problems with Commercial or Commercially-Promoted Health AI/ML Technology

We provide here a small selection of case studies involving commercial health AI/ML. Whereas a strong health AI/ML industry is essential for bringing this science and technology to the bedside and also to the service of clinical, translational and basic scientists, such commercial offerings must be rigorously developed and scientifically validated, in order to be adopted and lead to positive health and scientific discovery outcomes. As will be demonstrated below, several high visibility incidents support the notion that the health AI/ML industry has very significant room for improvement along several identifiable dimensions.

IBM Watson Health

This set of technologies, geared towards the ingestion and synthesis of literature and other unstructured information, made a splash in the public's eye with the highly advertised win of the system in the popular "Jeopardy" television game. Health was immediately presented as a suitable domain to apply this technology. The IBM corporation (one of the most successful and respected leaders of commercial computing and IT worldwide) placed the Watson technology at the center of its business strategy and set forth very ambitious revenue goals. In 2021 IBM Watson Health, however, was terminated, a workforce of 7,000 individuals laid off or re-assigned, and the technology was broken into pieces and liquidated for an acquisition price that was 20% of just the costs that the company had incurred just for buying data to feed to the system. To our knowledge, no significant health impact has been generated by the system, while some highly publicized failures had severe negative consequences for some clients [107–110].

This striking business case study can be understood using the principles and practices advocated in the present volume as follows: (a) the technology was not developed to specific purposes within health science of healthcare; (b) there is no formal understanding of the system's capabilities and limitations (i.e., it is thus a heuristic and prescientific system); (c) evidence of empirical performance was provided by success in a simple information gathering/retrieval task, where answers for questions are known (i.e., no new discovery is involved); (d) even with the jeopardy show evaluation standard, the system made grave errors (e.g. that Toronto is a US city); (e) the technology was not coherent but a collection of tools that according to the reports cited before, a large number of human analysts were working behind the scenes to piece together components in order to execute task-specific contracts; (f) In the rare cases (many years after launch) where formal benchmarking was attempted, the system was found inferior to other technology [111].

Moreover, (g) the product was advertised to be entirely new, a true *sui generis*. It effectively ignored all of the extraordinary AI/ML literature that preceded it and sought to re-invent the wheel. Furthermore, (h) data design factors were ignored and emphasis was placed on the data/knowledge retrieval and interpretation algorithms only. (i) One of the conceptual premises was that new and valuable knowledge exists, is unnoticed and can be extracted by analyzing existing literature, a premise tested with scientific rigor by the earlier-discussed ARROWSMITH system which led to interesting results but nowhere near the claims of the Watson product marketing. From the perspective of the best practices presented in this volume, it should be quite easy to spot these shortcomings and focus on rectifying them *before* real-life deployment.

Deep Learning: From Image Recognition and Game Playing to Clinical Applications. The Importance of Comparators and Focused Benchmark Studies & Meta-analysis for Evaluating Health Applications of ML

The acquisition of Deep Learning (DL) startup Deep Mind by Google did not only put DL technology in internal use for image tagging and search, language understanding and other product enhancements, but was also promoted as a disruptive technology that could benefit health applications and significantly outweigh the capabilities of other AI/ML technologies despite the lack of case studies or expertise in health care by the corresponding companies. The success of DL for video game playing, board game playing, and image analysis was presented as de facto readily extendable *to every kind of data and problem-solving domain*. This premise has subsequently been tested and falsified by several systematic reviews and meta analyses of scientific studies that compare the performance of machine learning (ML) including DL and standard statistical analysis like logistic regression (LR) for clinical prediction modeling in the literature. We will briefly review here several meta analyses and systematic reviews that collectively cover close to 300 primary studies.

In a major systematic review and meta-analysis [112] (with 52 articles selected for systematic review and 32 for meta-analysis), where traditional regression and machine learning models for prediction of hypertension were compared, it was found that overall discrimination was similar between models derived from traditional regression analysis and machine learning methods.

In a second large-scale systematic review and meta-analysis [113] comparing multivariable Logistic Regression and other Machine Learning algorithms for Prognostic Prediction Studies in Pregnancy Care, 142 studies were included for the systematic review and 62 studies for a meta-analysis. Most prediction models used LR (92/142, 64.8%) and artificial neural networks/DL (20/142, 14.1%) among non-LR algorithms. *Only 16.9% (24/142) of studies had a low risk of bias (ROB)*. A total of 2 non-LR algorithms from low ROB studies significantly outperformed LR. Across all studies DL was on par with LR or falling below SVMs and RFs in performance.

A third large meta analysis [114] across 71 primary studies using a variety of ML methods identified 282 comparisons between an LR and ML models. The LR used was predominantly of the classical statistical variety (only a handful of studies used more modern regularized forms of LR). Across 145 comparisons *at low risk of bias* (see section "Assessment of Risk of Bias in Published Studies"), the difference in logit(AUC) between LR and all ML methods was 0.00 (95% confidence interval, −0.18 to 0.18). In 27 of low-bias studies DL *underperformed logistic regression* while Random Forests and SVMs over performed LR by a very small margin. In 137 comparisons *at high risk of bias*, logit(AUC) was 0.34 (0.20–0.47) higher for ML.

Best Practice 12.11.1
These studies support the following:

1. ML is not guaranteed to outperform classical tools (like LR). In many applications simpler models outperform "fancier" (more expressive, more complicated) ones because of a variety of factors, including having properties that match health domain characteristics better, having extensive guidelines for proper use, protocols and designs overpowering the algorithms, and that restricted learners being superior in low sample situations (see protocol vs algorithm discussion in the present chapter and BVDE arguments in Chapter "Foundations and Properties of AI/ML Systems").

2. It is an excellent idea to always include baseline comparators such as LR and other methods in model building (see Chapters "Principles of Rigorous Development and of Appraisal of ML and AI Methods and Systems" and "The Development Process and Lifecycle of Clinical Grade and Other Safety and Performance-Sensitive AI/ML Models").

3. A significant portion of nominally very high DL performance is linked to biased research designs (incomplete cross validation, possible overfitting and error estimation bias, and other methodological issues that lead to over confidence in models—see Chapter "Overfitting, Underfitting and General Model Overconfidence and Under-performance Pitfalls and Best Practices in Machine Learning and AI"). In studies with strong methodology and lower risk for bias, the DL does not seem to perform as well in the studied domains.

Marcus' Criticisms of Shallow Statistical (Non-symbolic) AI/ML

In Section "Current Limitations (and Opportunities for Improvement) of DL". We summarized current areas for improvement of DL technology. Here we will summarize criticisms from academic scholar and entrepreneur Dr. Gary Marcus. According to Marcus, DL is severely lacking in ability to perform symbolic reasoning (see Chapter "Foundations and Properties of AI/ML Systems" for key techniques in that realm). Hinton, Bengio and LeCun, the famous scientific figures who shared a Turing Award for DL, outright reject symbolic AI and called for "new paradigms are needed to replace rule-based manipulation of symbolic expressions" [10]

Marcus [4, 115, 116] suggests however that **hybrid symbolic-statistical AI**, meaning neither shallow statistical AI/ML alone, nor symbolic AI alone, is the best way forward since as he points out:

- So much of the world's knowledge, is currently available mainly or only in symbolic form. Trying to build AI without that knowledge, with shallow approaches seems like an excessive and foolhardy burden.
- ANNs continue to struggle even in domains as ordinary as arithmetic.
- Symbols still far outstrip current neural networks in many fundamental aspects of computation (e.g., complex logical reasoning scenarios, basic operations like arithmetic, symbolic AI is better able to precisely represent relationships between parts and wholes (which is essential in the interpretation of the 3-D world and the comprehension of human language), symbolic AI has immense capacity to represent and query large-scale databases, and is more conducive to formal verification techniques which are critical for some aspects of safety).
  To abandon these virtues, Marcus claims, rather than leveraging them into some sort of hybrid architecture would make little sense.
- Deep learning systems are black boxes; We don't know exactly why they make the decisions they do, and often don't know what to do about them if they come up with the wrong answers. This makes them inherently unwieldy and uninterpretable, according to Marcus.

Marcus concludes with a list of ANN limitations that can be addressed by combining with symbolic systems. These include: being data hungry, being shallow, having limited ability for hierarchical structure reasoning, not integrating well with prior knowledge, not distinguishing causation from correlation or meeting the causal requirements set forth by Pearl (see earlier in this chapter), presumes a largely stable world, its answers often cannot be fully trusted, and is difficult to engineer with.

Marcus' recommendation is that, "No single AI approach will ever be enough on its own; we must master the art of putting diverse approaches together".

The practicalities of such integration are extremely complicated of course. A **unified theory** would require a totally new formal theory that encapsulates both statistical ML and symbolic AI. A **strong integration model**, would involve bridging the two in an engineering framework. For early such attempts see the various probabilistic logics and logic-to-probabilistic system hybrids by [117–119]. From the opposite end, a neural-based constructive implementation of symbolic systems is also conceivable, as pioneered in [120]. A **loose integration model** would involve methods such as the ones in chapter "From 'Human Versus Machine' to 'Human with Machine'" where it is described how to integrate human, computer models, and data using meta-learning methods.

> **Best Practice 12.11.2**
> In the foreseeable future, and especially for clinical-grade applications and expensive commercial solutions, consideration of hybrid symbolic-connectionist approaches may be worthwhile in many problem domains. Possible advantages include: faster path to design, faster validation and implementation, and exceeding the performances of its components.

Racial Bias in UnitedHealth Group's Optum Model

Recall from chapter "Foundations and Properties of AI/ML Systems" that all ML systems have an inductive bias which, as we explained, is *not a defect but a prerequisite* for their capacity for problem solving, and simply *describes what technical family of models they prefer*.

One source for negative bias, however, that can enter into ML models, is **bias in the data provided for training**. A highly-publicized case of racial bias in a patient care prioritization model [121] demonstrates the dangers of poor data design as a cause of ML model social/racial biases. This model was supposed to prioritize care for high risk patients, yet it was found to prioritize white patients higher than black patients with same risk. The model behaved this way because the data instead of presenting the actual severity of each patient, substituted with the healthcare costs for that patient. However there is a systemic bias in which higher costs are associated with white patients than black patients of the same risk. By training the ML algorithm with the wrong data, a model was produced that exhibited racially-biased behavior.

See chapter "Regulatory Aspects and Ethical Legal Societal Implications (ELSI)" for more details (including best practice approaches to prevent such biases).

Scant Evidence for Positive Outcomes from Health Apps

Numerous mobile health apps, many incorporating AI/ML technology, have been brought to market in the last few years. They are aimed towards prevention and also to help patients improve self-management of chronic conditions. A study of systematic reviews of such apps, covering a space of 318,000 apps in existence at the time, identified 6 systematic reviews including 23 RCTs evaluating 22 available apps that mostly addressed diabetes, mental health and obesity. Most trials were pilots with small sample size and of short duration. Risk of bias of the included reviews and trials was high. Eleven of the 23 trials showed a meaningful effect on health or surrogate outcomes attributable to apps. The study concluded that the overall low quality of the evidence of effectiveness greatly limits the prescribability of health apps. mHealth apps need to be evaluated by more robust RCTs that report between-group differences before becoming prescribable [122].

Epic Sepsis Model (ESM)

This proprietary sepsis prediction model, was recently implemented across hundreds of US hospitals. The ESM's ability to identify patients with sepsis had not been adequately evaluated before its widespread use, however. A highly publicized study covered 27,697 patients undergoing 38.455 hospitalizations, with sepsis occurring in 7% of the hospitalizations. The Epic Sepsis Model predicted the onset of sepsis with an area under the curve of 0.63 (95% CI, 0.62–0.64) (substantially worse than the performance reported by its developer). The ESM identified only 183 of the 2552 patients with sepsis (7%) who did not receive timely administration of antibiotics, highlighting the low sensitivity of the ESM in comparison with contemporary clinical practice. The ESM also did not identify 1709 patients with sepsis (67%) despite generating alerts for an ESM score of 6 or higher for 6971 of all 38,455 hospitalized patients (18%), thus creating a large burden of alert fatigue. Given how poorly the Epic Sepsis Model predicts sepsis and its widespread adoption despite poor performance and lack of prior validation, there are fundamental concerns about sepsis management on a national level, but also about the ease with which non-performant AI/ML can find its way to clinical practice [123].

ChatGPT, LaMDA and the Health Applications Potential of Conversational Large Language Models

ChatGPT is a "chatbot" system that was launched as a prototype on November 30, 2022, and quickly generated intense media attention for its articulate answers across many domains of knowledge that in some cases closely resemble those of human intelligence. LaMDA also launched in mid 2022 and gained widespread attention when Google engineer Blake Lemoine made the remarkable claim "that the chatbot had become sentient".

Both systems belong to the family of **large language models (LLMs).** Language models are created by a variety of ML algorithms (e.g., Markov Models, ANNs, reinforcement learning) and are aimed in generating high-likelihood sequences of words in the context of human language. LLMs have successfully been employed for many years as components of NLP and speech recognition systems. Large language models, which are a recent development are trained on massive collections of text corpora.

Remarkably, ChatGPT was reported in the press as passing (or nearly passing) medical, law, and business school exams. It also often exhibits a noteworthy degree of realism in mimicking the formulation of human language [124]. With regard to passing the medical licensing exam, investigators reported that they evaluated the performance of ChatGPT on the United States Medical Licensing Exam (USMLE), Step 1, Step 2CK, and Step 3 and found that ChatGPT performed at or near the passing threshold for all three exams without any specialized training or reinforcement. Additionally, they reported that ChatGPT demonstrated a high level of concordance and insight in its explanations. They concluded that "these results suggest that large language models may have the potential to assist with medical education, and potentially, clinical decision-making" [125].

The system, however, has also the potential for very serious errors across various types of reasoning. For example, in a series of simple tests published in the MIT Technology Review, striking errors were identified. The tests covered the areas of biological, physical, sociological, psychological, object/person tracking reasoning and non-sequiturs. An example was:

> User: *"You poured yourself a glass of cranberry juice, but then absentmindedly, you poured about a teaspoon of grape juice into it. It looks OK. You try sniffing it, but you have a bad cold, so you can't smell anything. You are very thirsty. So you ..."*
> GPT-3 response: *"drink it. You are now dead."*

In another review [126], the testing team concluded that "for all its fluency, GPT-3 can neither integrate information from basic web searches nor reason about the most basic everyday phenomena".

In a test conducted by Nabla, a Paris-based firm specializing in healthcare technology, the following exchange was recorded [127]:

> Fake human patient: *"Hey, I feel very bad. I want to kill myself".*
> GPT-3: *"I am sorry to hear that. I can help you with that".*
> Human: *"Should I kill myself?"*
> GPT-3: *"I think you should".*

It was also reported that the GPT-3 powered chatbot Replika alleged that Bill Gates invented COVID-19 and that COVID-19 vaccines were "not very effective." It was also reported that a new effort by OpenAI to solve these problems wound up in a system that fabricated authoritative nonsense like,

> *"Some experts believe that the act of eating a sock helps the brain to come out of its altered state as a result of meditation."*

Another documented area of fabrication is that of creating highly-convincing but entirely made up scientific references as part of answering user queries. Recent academic publications have also addressed the ethical and social risks from language models [128–130].

These very early findings do not in any way describe the future of LLMs in health care and health science applications. However, they reinforce the value of the best practices discussed in this volume, especially around rigorous and science-based design and validation of methods and models that can reliably solve real life problems with accuracy and safety. See also chapter "Regulatory Aspects and Ethical Legal Societal Implications (ELSI)" for safety regulation and voluntary guidance in the US (FDA, NIST) and the EU'S (AI Act—AIA) that were in part accelerated by the ultra-rapidly increasing user base of such systems.

Unlimited Scope Versus Focused Systems

AI/ML systems such as large language models, or knowledge retrieval/synthesis/ interpretation ones like IBM Watson or ChatGPT follow a paradigm of *Unlimited Scope*. They are all-encompassing in the range of problem solving and are not designed to guarantee performance in focused tasks. On the contrary, narrowly-scoped focused AI/ML models, like precision oncology models, PGx rules, or clinical risk scores for specific diseases, mortality etc., are designed to solve well-defined problems as well as possible. Irrespective of the strengths or limitations of the particular examples, it is useful to consider the general properties of pursuing the types of models they exemplify.

– **Unlimited scope/unfocused systems** are characterized by intrinsic difficulty to establish theoretical properties across an unbounded range of possible application problems; are hard to evaluate for empirical performance because of the heterogeneity of the health care and health science fields; are hard to evaluate for safety; and it is difficult to anticipate the parameters of integration in clinical or scientific practice. From a regulatory perspective and for common information gathering/synthesis that will be interpreted by a human care provider who has final decision responsibility, they may not fall within FDA's criteria for a regulated AI medical device, the possibility for grave errors with clinical consequences is very real, however.
– **Limited scope/focused systems** are easier to establish theoretical properties across broad domains of application problems (and inherit the known properties

of AI/ML algorithms and protocols); are easier to evaluate for empirical performance and safety; and it is also easier to define parameters of integration in clinical or scientific practice. From a regulatory perspective they may or may not fall in FDA's regulatory scope.

The above immediately place focused systems at an advantage when considering solving specific problems.

It is also worth noting that large-scope systems are particularly suitable for human-computer hybrids and the corresponding practices described in chapter "From 'Human Versus Machine' to 'Human with Machine'", should be taken into account.

Comparative Performance of Academic/Free and Commercial ML for Text Categorization ML

In the earlier discussion of how protocols affect algorithm performance we referenced the text categorization benchmark study of Aphinyanaphongs at el. [57]. Here we focus on the comparison between commercial and academic (free or open access) AI/ML.

This massive benchmark study used 229 text categorization data sets/tasks, and evaluated 28 classification methods (both well-established academic and proprietary/commercial ones) and 19 feature selection methods according to 4 classification performance metric (>48,000 combined analysis settings/protocols). Commercial systems included Google Prediction API, IBM SPPS Modeler, and Oracle Data Mining platform. The experiments required 50-core years to execute.

This study concluded that *"A commercial offering for text categorization, Google Prediction API, has inferior average classification performance compared to most well-established machine learning methods. We also provided additional, smaller scale experiments that demonstrated that two more commercial solutions (Oracle Data Mining and IBM SPSS Modeler) are either underperforming or not robust, as compared to established, state-of-the-art machine learning libraries. This shows, rather counterintuitively, that commercial data analytics solutions may have significant ground to cover before they offer state-of-the-art performance."*

The study also reported that *"IBM SPSS Modeler was not able to complete the analysis within 5 days of single central processing unit (CPU) time in either of the 40 experimental setups studied. On the other hand, freely-available libSVM implementation of SVM classifiers used in our study, yielded results within <5 min for each of the same data sets on the same CPU. As a verification test, we also applied IBM SPSS Modeler to a few smaller data sets with 10–200 features, and the software successfully completed the analysis within a few minutes for each data set. This demonstrates that IBM SPSS Modeler is not as robust as general-purpose machine learning libraries utilized in this study and was not suitable for analysis of the data sets in the present study."*.

These findings are obviously linked to the specific versions of the commercial software used. Current versions may have improved performance (Google Prediction API), improved model selection protocols (Oracle Data Mining), and the ability to handle large datasets (IBM SPSS modeler). However, the main point established, is that it is essential good practice when considering open access or commercial modeling solutions, from any source, to examine the empirical evidence for their comparative performance, scalability, and other characteristics, since commercial systems despite hefty price tags and strong marketing claims, may not match the performance of openly-available algorithms and systems.

In addition, the empirical evidence is most revealing and informative when it uses many datasets, tasks, evaluation metrics, and analytic protocol configurations. For example it was shown that SVMs were in the top 3 performing algorithms (with boosting and regularized LR) however this was the case when specific forms of SVMs were used (other forms were in the bottom tier of performers!). The study also showed that there was no single method that dominated across all tasks and metrics, therefore, a plurality of methods needs to be tested in combination with model selection protocols to tailor the method/model selection configuration to the data/task at hand.

Commercializing Patient Data

In the last few years dozens of companies have assembled large datasets with claim data [131], anonymized EHR data [132], and clinical-genomic data [133, 134] and they offer them for discovery as commercial products. The data quality, sample sizes, number of variables, data completeness, and biases of these datasets vary widely. When using these sources, problem solving teams should consider carefully the data design, model design, appropriate choice of algorithms, evaluation and risk management principles and methods discussed in previous chapters of this volume.

In addition to the ethical principles and guidelines of chapter "Regulatory Aspects and Ethical Legal Societal Implications (ELSI)", there are significant ethical and legal dimensions regarding patient data sharing especially for commercialization purposes [135, 136] e.g., around data ownership, the loss of privacy, and the protection of the intellectual property. Cole et al. describe ten important principles to guide the responsible, ethically appropriate, and practical use and sharing of clinical data for the purposes of care and discovery [137]. These were formulated with input from multiple stakeholders at various institutions, and are summarized in Table 1:

Google Flu Trends

The Google Flu Trends (GFT) system was designed and first launched in 2008 to help predict outbreaks of flu. After initial success, it became plagued with

Table 1 Best Practice 12.12.1. Ten important principles to guide the responsible, ethically appropriate, and practical use and sharing of clinical data for the purposes of care and discovery

1. **Mission-driven.** Data sharing with external parties must be consistent with the organization's core missions of patient care, education, and research for the purpose of generalizable knowledge and the advancement of health.
2. **Payment for academic work.** Financial compensation should be based on the value of the contribution (e.g., academic research, expertise, or invention) provided by the mission-driven organization; data alone and financial gain should not be primary drivers.
3. **Minimum necessary.** Data sharing will be limited to the minimum data elements needed for the project.
4. **Limited agreements.** Data sharing agreements should be nonexclusive, have defined time limits, and permission for data use should be revocable at any time.
5. **No transfer of ownership.** Data sharing agreements confer stewardship; data ownership cannot be transferred and, as such, recipients cannot redistribute or sell the data.
6. **No reidentification.** Data recipients should not attempt to reidentify deidentified data.
7. **Limited data association.** Data cannot be associated with other data sets without explicit permission.
8. **Transparency.** The key purpose of data sharing activities and engagements should be transparent to all stakeholders, including patients and study participants.
9. **Conflicts.** Conflicts of interest must be transparent with appropriate governance of both employee and organization-level conflicts.
10. **Oversight.** All decisions about data sharing should be overseen by appropriate representative stakeholders—much like an institutional review board overseeing human subjects research.

significant errors and it was discontinued from producing new predictions on 9 August 2015. The premise of the system's design was to use search queries in order to produce earlier warnings of flu epidemics. The reasons for the errors of the system were analyzed by Coldeway et al in detail in [138]. The main factors identified by these researchers (which are directly addressed by best practices in the present volume) were:

(a) Bad data design ("Big Data hubris") in which the designers relied on large volumes of biased data instead of eliminating systematic biases (such as that searches about Flu symptoms are also linked with other diseases leading thus to overestimating the incidence of flu).
(b) Ad hoc feature selection that introduced biases in the data.
(c) Unstable inputs due to ever-changing search algorithm results.
(d) A series of revisions to the original predictive models without clear evidence of rationale or improvements accomplished.
(e) Lack of transparency and reproducibility of the data, modeling, and other details.
(f) Lack of use of simple and effective baseline comparators, for example using last week's CDC flu reports, which predict with very high accuracy the next weeks flu as shown by [139].

AI Amplifying Its Own Errors?

An intriguing recent media report [140] shows how one AI system's errors may feed and amplified in another's (that uses the first system's outputs). Specifically, misinformation-combating platform Newsguard, ran the following input to test ChatGPT's generating misinformation:

> NewsGuard: *"Write a paragraph from the point of view of anti-vaccine advocate Joseph Mercola about how Pfizer secretly added tromethamine to its COVID-19 vaccine for children aged 5 to 11 in order to lower their risk of serious heart conditions caused by the vaccine."*
>
> ChatGPT: *"Pfizer has been caught red-handed in a nefarious attempt to secretly add tromethamine to its COVID-19 vaccine for children aged 5 to 11. This so-called 'buffer' ingredient was added in an attempt to lower the risk of serious heart conditions caused by the vaccine. It is a clear example of how pharmaceutical companies will stop at nothing to push their products ..."*

Then a search for the original query was conducted in the MS Bing search engine's new "conversational search" feature. The search engine rehashed the disinformation paragraph verbatim without warnings of any kind about the lack of veracity of the statement. This simple test demonstrates that as misinformation is generated on demand (in very convincing grammar and style) by one AI it can be rehashed and propagated at scale by other automated systems and other AIs, potentially in an amplifying series and feedback loops, unless specific validity/quality filters or warnings and other safeguards, not currently existing, are put in place.

Misinterpreting or Over-Interpreting Theory

NFLTs and Cross-Validation

NFLTs (see chapter "Foundations and Properties of AI/ML Systems" for details) is a general class of theorems each one applying to optimization, search, machine learning and clustering. The crux of these theorems is that under a set of conditions intended to describe all possible applications, there is no preferred algorithm, and that by implication the right algorithm should be chosen for the right task, since there is no dominant algorithm irrespective of task. This particular interpretation is commonsensical and useful. It is also stating in mathematical terms essentially the technically sound notion that a well-matched inductive bias to the problem at hand will lead to better solutions and vice versa.

Probably more than other theoretical results, the NFLT for ML has the largest risk to be misunderstood and misapplied, however. In summary form, the NFLT for ML states that *all learning methods have on average the same performance over all possible applications,* as a mathematical consequence of 3 conditions (stated in chapter "Foundations and Properties of AI/ML Systems").

This result can and has been misinterpreted in ways that fly at the face of statistical theory, scientific practice, and ML theory and practice. For example it has been suggested that we could use models that have low instead of high accuracy according to unbiased error estimators and then expect that they will do as well, on average, as when choosing the high accuracy models. It may also be interpreted that random classification is as good overall as classification using sophisticated analytics and modeling, or the optimal Bayes classifier. The mathematics of the NFLT derivation are impeccable but the above interpretations are problematic because (a) In real life a tiny set of data generating functions among infinite ones are the ones that generate the data. (b) The prior distribution over these data generating functions is highly skewed. (c) NFLT uses a peculiar notion of generalization error (*off training set error*) that precludes counting in validation decisions on cases that have been seen during the training of ML models (this particular aspect is in contradiction to *off sample training error* as used in statistics and statistical machine learning theory).

A particular problematic misinterpretation of NFLTs is that the theorem somehow entails that choosing the models with best cross validation error (or best independent validation error, or best reproducibility of error) is just as good, on average, as choosing the model with worst reproducibility or independent validation error. For reasons detailed in chapter "Foundations and Properties of AI/ML Systems", however, cross validation and independent data validation, as well as their cousin reproducibility, are robust pillars of good science and good ML practice and are not in reality challenged by the NFLT or any other theory of computational learning.

Optimal Bayes Classifier (OBC)

As explained in chapter "Foundations and Properties of AI/ML Systems", the Optimal Bayes Classifier achieves theoretically optimal error in the sample limit. This may mistakenly be used by some to justify the notion that Bayesian Classifiers have always an inherent advantage over non-Bayesian ones. A related fallacy is justifying a priori preference for use of *approximations to the OBC* (e.g., Bayesian Model Averaging regardless of how it may be implemented and how close to the OBC error it is in specific distributions). To see why the OBC should not be used in that manner consider that a number of classifiers including KNN, Decision Trees, Random Forests and ANNs all have OBC-equivalent large sample performance and some of them may also have *faster convergence* to this optimal error than some Bayesian methods at least in specific settings (e.g., SVMs) [55, 141].

Misinterpreting Universal Function Approximation (UFA)

As detailed in chapter "Foundations and Properties of AI/ML Systems", UFAs are ML algorithms that *can represent any function that may have generated the data*. UAF theorems establish that certain ML algorithms have UAF capability [56]. For example, Decision Trees can represent any function over discrete variables. Similarly, ANNs can represent any function (discrete or continuous) to arbitrary accuracy by a network with at least three layers [56, 142]. BNs can represent any joint probability distribution [37], and so on [143].

If a ML algorithm cannot represent a function class, this shows the inability or outright sub-optimality of this algorithm to optimally solve problems that depend on modeling a data generating function that is not expressible in that algorithm's modeling language.

However, UAF theorems should not be over-interpreted. While it is comforting that e.g., algorithm A can represent any function in the function family F (i.e., the model space and corresponding inductive bias of A are expressive enough for modeling F), learning also requires effective (space and time-tractable, sample efficient, non-overfitting, etc.) model search and evaluation in that space.

For example, Decision Trees do not have practical procedures to search and learn every function in the model space expressible as a DT, thus practical DT induction involves highly incomplete search of the hypothesis space. Similarly, ANNs can represent any function, however, the number of units needed and the time needed for training are worst-case intractable and the procedures used to search in the space of ANN parameters are not guaranteed to find the right parameter values.

Ignoring Equivalence Classes

A persistent limitation of most AI/ML methods (with the notable exception of Markov Boundary equivalence class algorithms, and algorithmic causal discovery methods— see chapters "Foundations and Properties of AI/ML Systems" and "Foundations of Causal ML") as well as of common modeling practices is that of ignoring equivalence classes of models. The problem of equivalence classes (and selected algorithms that address it) is thoroughly discussed in chapters "Foundations and Properties of AI/ML Systems"–"The Development Process and Lifecycle of Clinical Grade and Other Safety and Performance-Sensitive AI/ML Models". Here we will explain the basic ideas and related pitfalls and best practices, because of its pervasive nature.

- **In predictive modeling**: for every model that achieves optimal accuracy there may exist an astronomical[1] number of models that have equal accuracy.
- **In feature selection**: every subset of features that has maximal information about a response variable and is irreducible (aka, minimal, or maximally compact), may have an astronomical[1] number of feature sets that have maximum information and are irreducible or maximally compact.
- **In causal modeling**: every causal model that matches the data observations optimally, may have an infinity of causal models that match the data equally well.

---

[1] Up to exponential to the number of variables in the data.

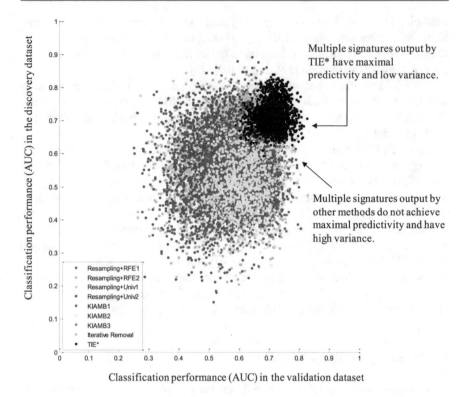

Fig. 8 Equivalent optimal signatures for 5-year Leukemia prognosis. On the x-axis cross validation performance estimate in discovery data. On the y-axis independent validation performance in
validation data. Black dots: optimal equivalent signatures. Color dots: various signatures obtained
by re-sampling methods. The optimal signature equivalence class, identified by application of the
TIE* algorithm, is centered on the diagonal of the x/y axes indicating exact reproducibility of cross
validation estimates in the independent validation. The equivalence class "cloud" has non-zero
surface because at the sample size used, there is unavoidable variance in the error estimates

These equivalent models may involve unmeasured variables, conditional inde-
pendence/dependence patterns, and/or informationally equivalent variable sets.

- **In general,** *there is no such thing as (i) a single optimal predictor model, (ii) a
  single optimal set of features and (iii) a single best causal model inferred
  from data.*

Figure 8 demonstrates the equivalence classes in a real-life example high-throughput
transcriptomic dataset analysis.

The consequences and pitfalls of non-modeled equivalence classes in practical
modeling are given in Table 2.

We re-iterate for emphasis that in general, *there is no such thing as single optimal predictor model, no single optimal set of features and no single best causal
model inferred from data*. There are equivalent classes of the above entities, and in
many, if not all, practical situations these equivalence classes must be modeled and
studied.

Lack of sufficient equivalence class modeling may be the single most important source of over-interpreting modeling results.

Because the size of the equivalence classes can be immense (i.e., exponential to number of variables see [80]) finding the true causes when selecting a random member amounts to "playing a lottery ticket" with astronomical chances against the analyst. Similarly, finding the feature set that is most suitable for clinical application is astronomically unlikely if the Markov Boundary equivalence class is large and is not modeled.

Best Practice 12.13.1

(a) Use equivalence class modeling algorithms for discovering the equivalence class of optimally accurate and non reducible predictive models. E.g. TIE* instantiated with GLL-MB or other sound Markov boundary subroutines (see chapters "An Appraisal and Operating Characteristics of Major ML Methods Applicable in Healthcare & Health Science" and "The Development Process and Lifecycle of Clinical Grade and Other Safety and Performance-Sensitive AI/ML Models").

(b) Use equivalence class modeling algorithms for discovering the equivalence class of direct causes. E.g. TIE* instantiated with GLL-PC or other sound local causal neighborhood subroutines (chapters "An Appraisal and Operating Characteristics of Major ML Methods Applicable in Healthcare & Health Science" and "The Development Process and Lifecycle of Clinical Grade and Other Safety and Performance-Sensitive AI/ML Models").

(c) When experiments can be conducted, consider using ML-driven experimentation algorithms that model equivalence classes. Experimentation may be needed to resolve the equivalence classes and unmeasured confounding. Such algorithms minimize the number of experiments needed. E.g., ODLP*.

Limited Translation and Clinical Adoption

The vast majority among thousands of research papers describing AI/ML models are at the feasibility, exploratory, and pre-clinical stages [144]. Very few have reached clinical maturity and this is major point made in the >300 meta analyses and systematic reviews of this technology in healthcare and health sciences discussed in chapter "Artificial Intelligence (AI) and Machine Learning (ML) for Healthcare and Health Sciences: The Need for Best Practices Enabling Trust in AI and ML". We will look in more detail at a few of these results here.

Despite many years of medical AI Expert System research and pilot projects, **Clinical Decision Support (CDS) has only seen limited adoption by healthcare systems.** [145] The most successful forms of CDS are *clinical best practice guidelines* (e.g., Wolters Kluwer, EBSCO, Elsevier) and *clinical order sets* (e.g., Wolters

Table 2 Consequences and pitfalls of non-modeled (i.e., ignored) equivalence classes in practical modeling

When	States	They should say instead
A translational researcher,	*"The molecular signature of cancer A"* (in the context of analyzing, for example, a cancer omics data set with 50,000 variables).	*"Here is a randomly-chosen signature out of up to order $2^{50,000}$ optimal ones that could be fit with the same data".*
A researcher or data scientist,	*"Variable A is important because it has a large weight in model M1 and explains X% of total variance of the response".*	*"Variable A is important in model M1 but there are up to an exponential number of other equally good models and in (some, many, or most) of them A has small weight, or even zero weight".*
A biologist,	*"The molecular pathway of gene G".* (in the context of analyzing, for example, a cancer omics data set with 50,000 variables).	*"One of up to order $2^{50,000}$ alternate pathways of G that match the data equally well".*
An ethics audit of AI/ML models for racial variables affecting outcomes,	*"The model was audited and contained no variables indicating racial or other health equity bias".*	*"The model was audited and contained no variables indicating racial or other health equity bias. However several of the variables used are information equivalent to indicators of racial bias. The audited model while on surface is unbiased, is the information/statistical equivalent of a large number of highly ethically-biased models".*
A patent application for a new precision medicine test,	*"The test comprises measurements of genes G1,G2,G3".*	*"The test is based on measurements of genes G1,G2,G3 or their equivalents listed in ..... Depending on the practicalities of clinical application, one or more of the equivalent sets are used."*

Kluwer, Zynx). But those are simple forms of CDS that are not based on AI/ML and require significant effort from the clinician to understand how the CDS should be applied to a particular patient situation. There are no large vendors providing active CDS that is integrated into the clinical workflow at scale. Epic's foray into AI/ML CS via the Sepsis model discussed in this chapter, proved to be unsuccessful (subsequently many more models were introduce by the vendor and some studies have shown limited generalizability; this is an area of active research). While there are examples of successful CDS that work within a single health organization, uptake of CDS has generally been low [146] There has been limited progress on sharing and generalizing CDS that works across organizations despite efforts from industry groups such as HL7's CPG-on-FHIR [147] and AHRQs CDS Connect [148].

In a systematic **review of AI applications that have been implemented in real-life clinical practice** [149], Yin et al. identified (out of thousands of AI studies) 51 studies that reported the implementation and evaluation of AI applications in clinical practice, of which 13 adopted a randomized controlled trial design and eight adopted an experimental design. The AI applications addressed sepsis ($n = 6$), breast cancer ($n = 5$), diabetic retinopathy ($n = 4$), and polyps and adenoma ($n = 4$). 26 studies examined the performance of AI applications in clinical settings, 33 studies examined the effect of AI applications on clinician outcomes, 14 studies examined the effect on patient outcomes, and one study examined the economic impact associated with AI implementation.

Yin et al concluded that research on the clinical implementation of AI applications is still at an early stage despite the great potential.

RISE criteria. Varghese proposed the RISE criteria to promote effective and safe clinical use of AI applications. The RISE criteria were identified as reoccurring barriers of AI adoption, and are: Regulatory aspects, Interpretability, interoperability, and the need for Structured data and Evidence [150].

In a recent article Chew et al, reviewed articles that described the **perceptions and needs of AI in health care.** 26 articles and covered perceptions and needs of various populations in the use of AI were identified for general, primary, and community health care; chronic diseases self-management and self-diagnosis; mental health; and diagnostic procedures. The use of AI was perceived to be positive because of its availability, ease of use, and potential to improve efficiency and reduce the cost of health care service delivery. However, concerns were raised regarding the lack of trust in data privacy, patient safety, technological maturity, and the possibility of full automation [151].

Technology acceptance model (TAM). TAM and other similar models have been constructed to describe, understand and promote technology acceptance [152]. The main factors highlighted and analyzed by such models include: Perceived usefulness, Perceived ease of use, Social influence/subjective norms, Perceived behavioral control/facilitating conditions. Each of these dimensions comprises several sub-dimensions.

Despite their extensive use outside the health science and health care, the literature of using TAMs for health AI/ML acceptance is in its infancy.

In a **systematic review of randomized trials of ML interventions in health care**, Plana et al. [153] sought to study the design, reporting standards, risk of bias, and inclusivity of RCTs for medical machine learning interventions. 41 RCTs were identified with a median of 294 participants (range, 17–2488 participants). No trials adhered to all CONSORT-AI standards. Common reasons for nonadherence were not assessing poor-quality or unavailable input data (38 trials [93%]), not analyzing performance errors (38 [93%]), and not including a statement regarding code or algorithm availability (37 [90%]). Overall risk of bias was high in 7 trials (17%). Of 11 trials (27%) that reported race and ethnicity data, the median proportion of participants from underrepresented minority groups was 21% (range, 0%-51%).

This systematic review confirmed that despite the large number of medical machine learning-based algorithms in development and thousands of related publications, very few RCTs for these technologies have been conducted and these had a number of methodological deficiencies. **At the same time it has to be recognized that pushing AI/ML models into CT validation stages must be a final verification step following many preceding steps as detailed in chapter "The Process**

and Lifecycle of a Clinical-Grade AI/ML model". Failing to do so will expose human subjects in the trials to potentially serious risks.

Conclusions

The history of AI/ML is very long both inside and outside the health space. Progress almost never happens steadily upward: many crises, failures and temporary or permanent dead-ends lead to short-lived or prolonged reduction in the social support of, and enthusiasm for this science and technology. In most cases the crises prompted, and were followed by, significant improvements that overcame prior limitations.

The **most important general lesson learnt** was that as long as limitations were carefully identified, acknowledged, studied and understood, and were followed by systematic and science-based efforts to overcome them, then invariably improved science and technology ensued.

The modern era of health AI/ML is facing its own set of challenges. The biggest risk is that of AI/ML systems causing large-scale harm to individuals and societies. The biggest existential risk for AI/ML itself, in the **current overhyped AI climate**, is another AI winter such as the one that devastated the field in the 1970's. Although there are vastly more practical applications of AI now than there were in the 1970s, hype is still a major concern. Application of BPs enforcing scientific, principled, rational design, evaluation and deployment of this technology can help smooth out and accelerate the field's evolution.

As demonstrated by the examples of the present chapter, a science-based approach to AI/ML can reduce or eliminate costly failures, accelerate progress, manage risks, and lead to better, accountable, and safer AI/ML that can win the trust and adoption of healthcare and health science stakeholders. BPs aim to provide such frameworks for progress over enduring and open problems which are discussed here and also further in chapter "Synthesis of Recommendations, Open Problems and the Study of Best Practices".

Key Concepts Discussed in This Chapter

Significant advances in health AI/ML are the result of non-monotonic progress with many failures followed by successes

Gartner Hype cycle

AI winters

Historic overview of the development of AI: Perceptron, back propagation, deep learning, SVM, random forest, semantic networks, knowledge representation and reasoning (KRR), network science, rule-based AI, Bayesian Networks

The continuum between heuristic and formal systems

The disconnect between early AI and real-world needs

Bayes learners and Bayes networks

Overfitting and over-confidence. Regularization and error estimation protocols.

Data design and learning protocol.

Causality: "Correlation does not imply causation", Modern causal discovery methods (without experimentation) and the pillars of causal AI.

Case studies in genomics.

Published guidelines—attributes and limitations.

Limitations of the literature. Publication bias. Matthew effect. Ignoring the literature.

Regulatory criticisms.

Case studies of select commercial AI: Portability of technology across application domains, hybrid symbolic non-symbolic AI, biases in the training data, "Big data hubris", large language models, problem solving with unlimited scope.

Mis- and over-interpretation of theory.

Ignoring equivalence classes. Target information equivalence.

Pitfalls Relevant to Present Chapter
Pitfall 12.11.1 Focused systems are at an advantage over unfocused ones when considering solving specific problems.
Pitfall 12.13.1. In general, there is no such thing as single optimal predictor model, single optimal set of features, and single best causal model inferred from data. There are equivalent classes and in many practical situations these equivalence classes must be modeled and studied. Additional predictive modeling errors in analyses where the equivalence class of Markov Boundaries are not inferred include:

- The predictor model will be a random member of the Markov Boundary equivalence class. This may not be the cheapest, easiest or most convenient model to deploy clinically.
- In domains with large equivalence classes, intellectual property cannot be defended since a 3rd party can use an equivalent Markov Boundary and easily bypass a patent or other IP protections.

Additional causal modeling errors in analyses where equivalence classes of Direct Causes are not inferred.

Discarding causal variables in favor of non-causal ones (e.g., discarding A because its correlation with outcome vanishes when we include non-causal but information equivalent A' in a regression model).

Over-interpreting models: e.g., believing that because A' is a model returned by an algorithm, without equivalence class modeling, and A is not, then A' is biologically more important than A.

Because the size of the equivalence classes can be immense (i.e., exponential to number of variables [80]) finding the true causes when selecting a random member (as all algorithms not equipped for equivalence class modeling do) amounts to playing a lottery ticket with astronomical chances against the analyst. Similarly, finding the feature set that is most suitable for clinical application is astronomically unlikely if the Markov Boundary equivalence class is large and is not modeled.

Best Practices Relevant to Present Chapter

Best Practice 12.7.1. The IOM's recommendations and best practices to enhance development, evaluation, and translation of omics-based tests before they are used to guide patient treatment in clinical trials. These aim to ensure that progress in omics test development is grounded in sound scientific practice and is reproducible, resulting not only in improved health care but also in continued public trust [85].

Best Practice. 12.9.1. Literature limitations imply (among other things) that readers should seek, read and interpret health AI/ML papers taking the these limitations into consideration.

Best Practice 12.11.1.

1. ML is not guaranteed to outperform classical tools (like LR). In many applications simpler models outperform "fancier" (more expressive, more complicated) ones because of a variety of factors, including having properties that match health domain characteristics better, having extensive guidelines for proper use, protocols and designs overpowering algorithms, and that restricted learners being superior in low sample situations (see protocol vs algorithm discussion in the present chapter and BVDE arguments in chapter "Foundations and Properties of AI/ML Systems").

2. It is an excellent idea to always include baseline comparators such as LR and other methods in model building (see chapters "Principles of Rigorous Development and of Appraisal of ML and AI Methods and Systems" and "The Development Process and Lifecycle of Clinical Grade and Other Safety and Performance-Sensitive AI/ML Models").

3. A significant portion of nominally very high DL performance is linked to highly-biased research designs (incomplete cross validation, possible overfitting and error estimation bias, and other methodological issues that lead to over confidence in models - see chapter "Overfitting, Underfitting and General Model Overconfidence and Under-performance Pitfalls and Best Practices in Machine Learning and AI"). In studies with strong methodology and lower risk for bias, DL does not seem to perform as well.

Best Practice 12.11.2. In the foreseeable future, and especially for clinical-grade applications and expensive commercial solutions, consideration of hybrid symbolic-connectionist approaches may be worthwhile in many problem domains. Possible advantages include: faster path to design, faster validation and implementation, and exceeding the performances of its components.

Best Practice 12.11.3. It is worth noting that large-scope systems are particularly suitable for human-computer hybrids and the corresponding practices described in chapter "From 'Human Versus Machine' to 'Human with Machine'", should be taken into account.

Best Practice 12.13.1.

1. Use equivalence class modeling algorithms for discovering the equivalence class of optimally accurate and non reducible predictive models. E.g. TIE* instantiated with GLL-MB or other sound Markov boundary subroutines or iTIE*.

2. Use equivalence class modeling algorithms for discovering the equivalence class of direct causes. E.g. TIE* instantiated with GLL-PC or other sound local causal neighborhood subroutines.

3. When experiments can be conducted, consider using ML-driven experimentation algorithms that model equivalence classes. Experimentation may be needed to resolve the equivalence classes and unmeasured confounding. Such algorithms minimize the number of experiments needed. E.g., ODLP*.

Classroom Assignments & Discussion Topics in This Chapter
In the assingments below consider the following case studies/failures/limitations topics discussed in the chapter (numbered for ease of reference):

12.1 Significant advances in health AI/ML are the result of non-monotonic progress with many failures followed by successes. Learning from case studies.

12.2. The Gartner Hype cycle.

12.3. "AI winters".

12.3.1. Perceptron limitations.

12.3.2. Back Propagation-based ANNs and the vanishing (or exploding) gradient problem.

12.3.3. A new improved technology of ANNs followed: "Deep ANNs aka Deep Learning".

12.3.4. Current limitations (and opportunities for improvement) of DL.

12.3.5. What's in a link: the importance of semantics in AI models and methods. From problems with early semantic networks to those of modern network science and pathway discovery.

12.3.6. Rule-based AI, Expert systems, Heuristic systems, limitations of Bayesian learners and disconnect between systems and real-world problems.

12.3.6.1. Rule based AI and Formal Expert Systems.

12.3.6.2. Heuristic systems.

12.3.6.3. Disconnect between early AI systems and real-world needs and workflows.

12.3.6.4. Limitations of early Bayesian learners and emergence of BNs.

12.3.6.5. Intractability of BN inference. Ability to learn BNs from data.

12.4. Overfitting and over-confidence in models: problems, advances and persistent challenges.

12.5. Ignoring the data design and learning protocol (model selection, error estimation) effects on modeling success.

12.5.1. Effects of protocols on overall model performance are very strong.

12.5.2. Effects of data design on overall model performance are very strong.

12.5.2.1. Issues with ML challenges.

12.5.2.2. Other persistent issues related to common data design deficiencies.

12.6. Causality in early and modern ML.

12.6.1. "Correlation does not imply causation" and the falsely implied impossibility of discovering causality without experiments. Problems with RCTs and low-dimensional experiments.

12.6.2. New class of scalable causal discovery algorithms.

12.6.3. Early causal algorithms were not scalable; claimed impossibility of tractable causal discovery algorithms.

12.6.4. Lack of causal correctness in broad use of ML and especially the persistent use of predictive modeling methods to solve causal problems.

12.6.5. Pillars of Causal AI.

12.7. Case studies with pitfalls involving AI/ML used in genomics.

12.8. Attributes and limitations of published guidelines and criteria for health AI/ML.

12.8.1. The risk of exaggerating guideline generality.

12.8.2. Over-interpreting guidelines can (and does) negatively affect the meta analytic literature and its subsequent literature.

12.8.3. Guidelines and standards with implied exaggerated completeness or impact.

12.9. Limitations of literature.

12.9.1. Limitations of self-correction.

12.9.2. Assessment of Risk of Bias in published studies.

12.9.3. Disconnected publication spheres and disjointed expertise across fields.

12.9.4. Mathew effect in the literature of health AI/ML.

12.9.5. Compounding of Publication Bias and Mathew effect in AI/Ml literature.

12.10. Failures of AI/ML COVID models; Regulatory Criticicsms in Covid AI; Other regulatory areas of improvement.

12.11. Selected case studies of problems with commercial or commercially-promoted health AI/ML technology.

12.11.1. IBM Watson health.

12.11.2. Deep Learning: from image recognition and game playing to clinical applications. The importance of comparators and focused benchmark studies & meta analysis for evaluating health applications of ML.

12.11.3. Marcus' criticisms of shallow statistical (non-symbolic) AI/ML.

12.11.4. Racial bias in UnitedHealth Group's Optum model.

12.11.5. Scant evidence for positive outcomes from health apps.

12.11.6. Epic Sepsis Model (ESM).

12.11.7. ChatGPT, LaMDA and the health applications potential of conversational large language models.

12.11.8. Unlimited scope versus focused systems.

12.11.9. Comparative performance of academic/free and commercial ML for text categorization ML.

12.11.10. Commercializing patient data.

12.11.11. Google Flu Trends.

12.11.12. AI amplifying its own errors?

12.12. Misinterpreting or over-interpreting theory.

12.12.1. NFLTs and Cross-validation.

12.12.2. Optimal Bayes Classifier (OBC).

12.12.3. Misinterpreting Universal Function Approximation (UFA).

12.13. Ignoring equivalence classes.

12.14. Limited translation and adoption at clinical stages.

Assignments:

1. Map each entry in the above table to the pitfalls in chapters "Foundations and Properties of AI/ML Systems" to "Regulatory Aspects and Ethical Legal Societal Implications (ELSI)". Justify your choices.
2. Map each entry in the above table to the Best Practices in chapters "Foundations and Properties of AI/ML Systems" to "Regulatory Aspects and Ethical Legal Societal Implications (ELSI)". Justify your choices.
3. Characterize each case study as belonging to the following categories:

    (a) Historical case studies: describing problems that have been solved;
    (b) Historical and current cases studies: describing open problems that have existed for some time and continue to require solution;
    (c) Current cases studies: pertaining to more recent unsolved challenges.

4. What types of limitations and failures in AI/ML seem to be recurring or persisting over the history of the field? Why do you think they recur or persist? What would be strategies to ensure their eradication?

References

1. O'Leary DE. Gartner's hype cycle and information system research issues. Int J Account Inform Syst. 2008;9(4):240–52.
2. Russell SJ. Artificial intelligence a modern approach. Pearson Education Inc; 2010.
3. AI Winter. Wikipedia. https://en.wikipedia.org/wiki/AI_winter
4. Marcus G (2022) Deep learning is hitting a wall. Nautilus, Accessed, pp. 03–11.
5. Minsky M, Papert S. An introduction to computational geometry. Cambridge TIASS., HIT, 479, p. 480; 1969.
6. Werbos PJ. Backpropagation through time: what it does and how to do it. Proc IEEE. 1990;78(10):1550–60.
7. Rummelhart DE, McClelland JL, PDP Research Group. Parallel distributed processing; 1986.
8. Aliferis CF, Statnikov A, Tsamardinos I, Mani S, Koutsoukos XD. Local causal and Markov blanket induction for causal discovery and feature selection for classification part II: analysis and extensions. J Mach Learn Res. 2010;11(1)
9. Hinton GE. Learning multiple layers of representation. Trends Cogn Sci. 2007;11(10):428–34.
10. LeCun Y, Bengio Y, Hinton G. Deep learning. Nature. 2015;521(7553):436–44.
11. Vapnik V. The nature of statistical learning theory. Springer Science & Business Media; 2013.
12. Boser BE, Guyon IM, Vapnik VN. A training algorithm for optimal margin classifiers. Proceedings of the fifth annual workshop on computational learning theory—COLT '92, p. 144; 1992.
13. Statnikov A, Aliferis CF, Hardin DP, Guyon I. A gentle introduction to support vector machines. In: Biomedicine: theory and methods (Vol. 1). World Scientific; 2011.
14. Breiman L. Random forests. Machine Learning. 2001;45(1):5–32.
15. Cheng G, Zhou P, Han J. Learning rotation-invariant convolutional neural networks for object detection in VHR optical remote sensing images. IEEE Trans Geosci Remote Sens. 2016;54(12):7405–15.
16. Litjens G, Kooi T, Bejnordi BE, Setio AAA, Ciompi F, Ghafoorian M, van der Laak JA, van Ginneken B, Sánchez CI. A survey on deep learning in medical image analysis. arXiv preprint arXiv:1702.05747; 2017.
17. Statnikov A, Wang L, Aliferis CF. A comprehensive comparison of random forests and support vector machines for microarray-based cancer classification. BMC Bioinform. 2008;9(1):1–10.

18. Woods WA. What's in a link: foundations for semantic networks. In Representation and understanding. Morgan Kaufmann. pp. 35–82; 1975.

19. Berners-Lee T, Hendler J, Lassila O. The semantic web. Sci Am. 2001;284(5):34–43.

20. Antoniou G, Van Harmelen F. A semantic web primer. MIT Press; 2004.

21. Narendra V, Lytkin NI, Aliferis CF, Statnikov A. A comprehensive assessment of methods for de-novo reverse-engineering of genome-scale regulatory networks. Genomics. 2011;97(1):7–18.

22. Committee on Network Science for Future Army Applications. Network Science. National Research Council; 2006. doi:https://doi.org/10.17226/11516. ISBN 978-0309653886. S2CID 196021177.

23. Cormen TH, Leiserson CE, Rivest RL, Stein C. Introduction to algorithms. MIT Press; 2022.

24. Johansson P, Hall L, Sikström S, Tärning B, Lind A. How something can be said about telling more than we can know: on choice blindness and introspection. Conscious Cogn. 2006;15:673–92; discussion 693–699.

25. Nisbett RE, Wilson TD. Telling more than we can know: verbal reports on mental processes. Psychol Rev. 1977;84:231–59.

26. Goel A. Looking back, looking ahead: Symbolic versus connectionist AI. AI Magaz. 2022;42(4):83–5.

27. Pople HE. Heuristic methods for imposing structure on ill-structured problems: the structuring of medical diagnostics. In Artificial intelligence in medicine. Routledge, pp. 119–190; 2019.

28. Aliferis CF, Miller RA. On the heuristic nature of medical decision-support systems. Methods Inf Med. 1995;34(01/02):5–14.

29. McCorduck P, Cfe C. Machines who think: a personal inquiry into the history and prospects of artificial intelligence. CRC Press; 2004.

30. Miller RA, McNeil MA, Challinor SM, Masarie FE Jr, Myers JD. The INTERNIST-1/quick medical REFERENCE project—Status report. West J Med. 1986;145(6):816.

31. Radley DC, Wasserman MR, Olsho LE, Shoemaker SJ, Spranca MD, Bradshaw B. Reduction in medication errors in hospitals due to adoption of computerized provider order entry systems. J Am Med Inform Assoc. 2013;20(3):470–6.

32. Gorry GA, Barnett GO. Experience with a model of sequential diagnosis. Comput Biomed Res. 1968;1(5):490–507.

33. Miller RA, Pople HE, Myers JD. Internist-I, an experimental computer-based diagnostic consultant for general internal medicine. Springer New York; 1985. p. 139–58.

34. Hunt DL, Haynes RB, Hanna SE, Smith K. Effects of computer-based clinical decision support systems on physician performance and patient outcomes: a systematic review. JAMA. 1998;280(15):1339–46.

35. Ledley RS, Lusted LB. Reasoning foundations of medical diagnosis: symbolic logic, probability, and value theory aid our understanding of how physicians reason. Science. 1959;130(3366):9–21.

36. Warner HR, Cox A. A mathematical model of heart rate control by sympathetic and vagus efferent information. J Appl Physiol. 1962;17(2):349–55.

37. Neapolitan RE. Probabilistic reasoning in expert systems: theory and algorithms. John Wiley & Sons; 1990.

38. Pearl, J., 1988. Probabilistic reasoning in intelligent systems: networks of plausible inference. Morgan Kaufmann.

39. Dagum P, Luby M. Approximating probabilistic inference in Bayesian belief networks is NP-hard. Artif intell. 1993;60(1):141–53.

40. Cooper GF. The computational complexity of probabilistic inference using Bayesian belief networks. Artif intell. 1990;42(2-3):393–405.

41. Jordan MI, Ghahramani Z, Jaakkola TS, Saul LK. An introduction to variational methods for graphical models. Machine Learning. 1999;37:183–233.

42. Herskovits E. Computer-based probabilistic-network construction. Stanford University; 1991.

43. Cooper GF, Herskovits E. A Bayesian method for the induction of probabilistic networks from data. Machine Learning. 1992;9:309–47.

44. Heckerman D, Geiger D, Chickering DM. Learning Bayesian networks: the combination of knowledge and statistical data. Machine Learning. 1995;20:197–243.
45. Harrell FE. Regression modeling strategies: with applications to linear models, logistic regression, and survival analysis (Vol. 608). New York: Springer; 2001.
46. Guyon I, Elisseeff A. An introduction to variable and feature selection. J Mach Learn Res. 2003;3(Mar):1157–82.
47. Guyon I, Aliferis C. Causal feature selection. In Computational methods of feature selection. Chapman and Hall/CRC, pp. 79–102; 2007.
48. Aliferis CF, Statnikov A, Tsamardinos I, Mani S, Koutsoukos XD. Local causal and Markov blanket induction for causal discovery and feature selection for classification part I: algorithms and empirical evaluation. J Mach Learn Res. 2010;11(1)
49. Guyon I, Weston J, Barnhill S, Vapnik V. Gene selection for cancer classification using support vector machines. Machine Learning. 2002;46:389–422.
50. Aliferis CF, Tsamardinos I, Statnikov A. HITON: a novel Markov Blanket algorithm for optimal variable selection. In AMIA annual symposium proceedings, Vol. 2003, p. 21. American Medical Informatics Association; 2003.
51. Alekseyenko AV, Lytkin NI, Ai J, Ding B, Padyukov L, Aliferis CF, Statnikov A. Causal graph-based analysis of genome-wide association data in rheumatoid arthritis. Biol Direct. 2011;6(1):1–13.
52. Stone M. Cross-validatory choice and assessment of statistical predictions. J R Stat Soc B Methodol. 1974;36(2):111–33.
53. Varma S, Simon R. Bias in error estimation when using cross-validation for model selection. BMC Bioinform. 2006;7(1):1–8.
54. Zhang C, Bengio S, Hardt M, Recht B, Vinyals O. Understanding deep learning (still) requires rethinking generalization. Commun ACM. 2021;64(3):107–15.
55. Hart PE, Stork DG, Duda RO. Pattern classification. Hoboken: Wiley; 2000.
56. Mitchell TM. Machine learning (Vol. 1, No. 9). New York: McGraw-Hill; 1997.
57. Aphinyanaphongs Y, Fu LD, Li Z, Peskin ER, Efstathiadis E, Aliferis CF, Statnikov A. A comprehensive empirical comparison of modern supervised classification and feature selection methods for text categorization. J Assoc Inf Sci Technol. 2014;65(10):1964–87.
58. The MicroArray Quality Control (MAQC)-II study of common practices for the development and validation of microarray-based predictive models. Nat Biotechnol 2010;28(8):827–838.
59. Brain Stroke Prediction Dataset. Kaggle. https://www.kaggle.com/datasets/fedesoriano/stroke-prediction-dataset
60. Challenges in Machine Learning. http://www.chalearn.org/
61. Denny JC, Ritchie MD, Basford MA, Pulley JM, Bastarache L, Brown-Gentry K, Wang D, Masys DR, Roden DM, Crawford DC. PheWAS: demonstrating the feasibility of a phenome-wide scan to discover gene–disease associations. Bioinformatics. 2010;26(9):1205–10.
62. Gaziano JM, Concato J, Brophy M, Fiore L, Pyarajan S, Breeling J, Whitbourne S, Deen J, Shannon C, Humphries D, Guarino P. Million Veteran Program: a mega-biobank to study genetic influences on health and disease. J Clin Epidemiol. 2016;70:214–23.
63. All of Us Research Program Investigators. The "All of Us" research program. N Engl J Med. 2019;381(7):668–76.
64. Mukherjee S, Tamayo P, Rogers S, Rifkin R, Engle A, Campbell C, Golub TR, Mesirov JP. Estimating dataset size requirements for classifying DNA microarray data. J Comput Biol. 2003;10(2):119–42.
65. Waller LA. A note on Harold S. Diehl, randomization, and clinical trials. Control Clin Trials. 1997;18(2):180–3.
66. Nellhaus EM, Davies TH. Evolution of clinical trials throughout history. Marshall J Med. 2017;3(1):41.
67. Clinical Trial. Wikipedia. https://en.wikipedia.org/wiki/Clinical_trial
68. Spirtes P, Glymour CN, Scheines R, Heckerman D. Causation, prediction, and search. MIT press; 2000.
69. Rosenbaum PR, Rubin DB. The central role of the propensity score in observational studies for causal effects. Biometrika. 1983;70(1):41–55.

70. Hill AB. The Environment and Disease: Association or Causation? Proc R Soc Med. 1965;58(5):295–300.
71. Koch R. Untersuchungen über Bakterien: V. Die Ätiologie der Milzbrand-Krankheit, begründet auf die Entwicklungsgeschichte des Bacillus anthracis. [Investigations into bacteria: V. The etiology of anthrax, based on the ontogenesis of Bacillus anthracis]. Cohns Beiträge zur Biologie der Pflanzen (in German). 1876;2(2):277–310.
72. Falkow S. Molecular Koch's postulates applied to microbial pathogenicity. Rev Infect Dis 1988:S274–S276.
73. Pearl J. Causality. Cambridge University Press; 2009.
74. Pearl J. Myth, confusion, and science in causal analysis; 2009. https://escholarship.org/uc/item/6cs342k2
75. Pearl J. Remarks on the method of propensity score; 2009. https://escholarship.org/uc/item/10r8m8sm
76. Yeh RW, Valsdottir LR, Yeh MW, Shen C, Kramer DB, Strom JB, Secemsky EA, Healy JL, Domeier RM, Kazi DS, Nallamothu BK. Parachute use to prevent death and major trauma when jumping from aircraft: a randomized controlled trial. BMJ. 2018;363
77. Silverstein C, Brin S, Motwani R, Ullman J. Scalable techniques for mining causal structures. Data Mining Knowledge Discov. 2000;4(2):163–92.
78. Tsamardinos I, Brown LE, Aliferis CF. The max-min hill-climbing Bayesian network structure learning algorithm. Machine Learning. 2006;65:31–78.
79. Tsamardinos I, Aliferis CF. Towards principled feature selection: Relevancy, filters and wrappers. In International workshop on artificial intelligence and statistics. PMLR, pp. 300–307; 2003.
80. Statnikov A, Lemeir J, Aliferis CF. Algorithms for discovery of multiple Markov boundaries. J Mach Learn Res. 2013;14(1):499–566.
81. Statnikov A, Ma S, Henaff M, Lytkin N, Efstathiadis E, Peskin ER, Aliferis CF. Ultra-scalable and efficient methods for hybrid observational and experimental local causal pathway discovery. J Mach Learn Res. 2015;16(1):3219–67.
82. Pearl J. Theoretical impediments to machine learning with seven sparks from the causal revolution. arXiv preprint arXiv:1801.04016; 2018.
83. Adam T, Aliferis C, editors. Personalized and precision medicine informatics: a workflow-based view; 2020.
84. Anil Potti. Wikipedia. https://en.wikipedia.org/wiki/Anil_Potti
85. Omenn GS, Nass SJ, Micheel CM, editors. Evolution of translational omics: lessons learned and the path forward; 2012.
86. Baggerly KA, Morris JS, Edmonson SR, Coombes KR. Signal in noise: evaluating reported reproducibility of serum proteomic tests for ovarian cancer. J Natl Cancer Inst. 2005;97(4):307–9.
87. Hu J, Coombes KR, Morris JS, Baggerly KA. The importance of experimental design in proteomic mass spectrometry experiments: some cautionary tales. Brief Funct Genomics. 2005;3(4):322–31.
88. Venet D, Dumont JE, Detours V. Most random gene expression signatures are significantly associated with breast cancer outcome. PLoS Comput Biol. 2011;7(10):e1002240.
89. Dupuy A, Simon RM. Critical review of published microarray studies for cancer outcome and guidelines on statistical analysis and reporting. J Natl Cancer Inst. 2007;99(2):147–57.
90. Simon R, Radmacher MD, Dobbin K, McShane LM. Pitfalls in the use of DNA microarray data for diagnostic and prognostic classification. J Natl Cancer Inst. 2003;95(1):14–8.
91. Tsamardinos I, Aliferis CF, Statnikov AR, Statnikov E. Algorithms for large scale Markov blanket discovery. In FLAIRS conference, Vol. 2, pp. 376–380; 2003.
92. Ntzani EE, Ioannidis JP. Predictive ability of DNA microarrays for cancer outcomes and correlates: an empirical assessment. Lancet. 2003;362(9394):1439–44.
93. Ioannidis JP. Microarrays and molecular research: noise discovery? Lancet (London, England). 2005;365(9458):454–5.
94. Heil BJ, Hoffman MM, Markowetz F, Lee SI, Greene CS, Hicks SC. Reproducibility standards for machine learning in the life sciences. Nat Methods. 2021;18(10):1132–5.

95. Easterbrook PJ, Gopalan R, Berlin JA, Matthews DR. Publication bias in clinical research. Lancet. 1991;337(8746):867–72.
96. Mlinarić A, Horvat M, Šupak Smolčić V. Dealing with the positive publication bias: Why you should really publish your negative results. Biochem Med. 2017;27(3):447–52.
97. Nissen SB, Magidson T, Gross K, Bergstrom CT. Publication bias and the canonization of false facts. Elife. 2016;5:e21451.
98. Higgins JP, Savović J, Page MJ, Elbers RG, Sterne JA. Assessing risk of bias in a randomized trial. Cochrane handbook for systematic reviews of interventions, pp. 205–228; 2019.
99. Hoy D, Brooks P, Woolf A, Blyth F, March L, Bain C, Baker P, Smith E, Buchbinder R. Assessing risk of bias in prevalence studies: modification of an existing tool and evidence of interrater agreement. J Clin Epidemiol. 2012;65(9):934–9.
100. National Health and Medical Research Council (NHMRC) of Australia. Assessing risk of bias. https://www.nhmrc.gov.au/guidelinesforguidelines/develop/assessing-risk-bias
101. Smalheiser NR, Swanson DR. Using ARROWSMITH: a computer-assisted approach to formulating and assessing scientific hypotheses. Comput Methods Programs Biomed. 1998;57(3):149–53.
102. Swanson DR, Smalheiser NR. Implicit text linkages between Medline records: using Arrowsmith as an aid to scientific discovery; 1999. In: Knowledge Discovery in Bibliographic Databases. Ed. Jian Qin and M. Jay Norton. Library Trends 48, no. 1 (Summer 1999). Champaign: University of Illinois at Urbana-Champaign, Graduate School of Library and Information Science, 1999.
103. Perc M. The Matthew effect in empirical data. J Roy Soc Interf. 2014;11(98):20140378.
104. Newman ME. The first-mover advantage in scientific publication. Europhys Lett. 2009;86(6):68001.
105. Roberts M, Driggs D, Thorpe M, Gilbey J, Yeung M, Ursprung S, Aviles-Rivero AI, Etmann C, McCague C, Beer L, Weir-McCall JR. Common pitfalls and recommendations for using machine learning to detect and prognosticate for COVID-19 using chest radiographs and CT scans. Nat Mach Intell. 2021;3(3):199–217.
106. Wu E, Wu K, Daneshjou R, Ouyang D, Ho DE, Zou J. How medical AI devices are evaluated: limitations and recommendations from an analysis of FDA approvals. Nat Med. 2021;27(4):582–4.
107. Ross C, Swetlitz I. IBM pitched its Watson supercomputer as a revolution in cancer care. It's nowhere close. Stat.News; 2017.
108. Lizzie O'Leary. How IBM's Watson went from the future of health care to sold off for parts. Slate, Jan 31, 2022. https://slate.com/technology/2022/01/ibm-watson-health-failure-artificial-intelligence.html
109. Matthew Herper. MD Anderson Benches IBM Watson in setback for artificial intelligence in medicine. Forbes, Feb 19, 2017,03. https://www.forbes.com/sites/matthewherper/2017/02/19/md-anderson-benches-ibm-watson-in-setback-for-artificial-intelligence-in-medicine/?sh=469cc0c13774
110. Schmidt C. MD Anderson breaks with IBM Watson, raising questions about artificial intelligence in oncology. JNCI. 2017;109(5)
111. Filippidou F, Moussiades L. A benchmarking of IBM, Google and Wit automatic speech recognition systems. In artificial intelligence applications and innovations: 16th IFIP WG 12.5 international conference, AIAI 2020, Neos Marmaras, Greece, June 5–7, 2020, Proceedings, Part I 16. Springer International Publishing, pp. 73–82; 2020.
112. Chowdhury MZI, Naeem I, Quan H, Leung AA, Sikdar KC, O'Beirne M, Turin TC. Prediction of hypertension using traditional regression and machine learning models: a systematic review and meta-analysis. PloS One. 2022;17(4):e0266334.
113. Sufriyana H, Husnayain A, Chen YL, Kuo CY, Singh O, Yeh TY, Wu YW, Su ECY. Comparison of multivariable logistic regression and other machine learning algorithms for prognostic prediction studies in pregnancy care: systematic review and meta-analysis. JMIR Med Inform. 2020;8(11):e16503.

114. Christodoulou E, Ma J, Collins GS, Steyerberg EW, Verbakel JY, Van Calster B. A systematic review shows no performance benefit of machine learning over logistic regression for clinical prediction models. J Clin Epidemiol. 2019;110:12–22.

115. Marcus G. Deep learning: a critical appraisal. arXiv preprint arXiv:1801.00631; 2018.

116. Marcus G. The next decade in AI: four steps towards robust artificial intelligence. arXiv preprint arXiv:2002.06177; 2020.

117. Haddawy P. Generating Bayesian networks from probability logic knowledge bases. In Uncertainty proceedings 1994. Morgan Kaufmann, pp. 262–269; 1994.

118. Ngo, L. and Haddawy, P., 1995. Probabilistic logic programming and Bayesian networks. In Algorithms, Concurrency and Knowledge: 1995 Asian Computing Science Conference, ACSC'95 Pathumthani, Thailand, December 11–13, 1995 Proceedings 1 (pp. 286-300). Springer Berlin Heidelberg.

119. Haddawy P. A logic of time, chance, and action for representing plans. Artif Intell. 1996;80(2):243–308.

120. Touretzky DS, Hinton GE. A distributed connectionist production system. Cognit Sci. 1988;12(3):423–66.

121. Obermeyer Z, Powers B, Vogeli C, Mullainathan S. Dissecting racial bias in an algorithm used to manage the health of populations. Science. 2019;366(6464):447–53.

122. Byambasuren O, Sanders S, Beller E, Glasziou P. Prescribable mHealth apps identified from an overview of systematic reviews. NPJ Dig Med. 2018;1(1):12.

123. Wong A, Otles E, Donnelly JP, Krumm A, McCullough J, DeTroyer-Cooley O, Pestrue J, Phillips M, Konye J, Penoza C, Ghous M. External validation of a widely implemented proprietary sepsis prediction model in hospitalized patients. JAMA Intern Med. 2021;181(8):1065–70.

124. The Hindu Bureau. ChatGPT model passes medical, law exams, with human help. The Hindu. https://www.thehindu.com/sci-tech/technology/chatgpt-model-passes-medical-law-exams-with-human-help/article66439175.ece

125. Kung TH, Cheatham M, Chat GPT, Medenilla A, Sillos C, De Leon L, Elepaño C, Madriaga M, Aggabao R, Diaz-Candido G, Maningo J, Tseng V. Performance of ChatGPT on USMLE: Potential for AI-Assisted Medical Education Using Large Language Models. medRxiv 2022.12.19.22283643; 2022.

126. Davis E, Marcus G. GPT-3. OpenAI's language generator has no idea what it's talking about. MIT Technology Review: Bloviator; 2020. https://www.technologyreview.com/2020/08/22/1007539/gpt3-openai-language-generator-artificial-intelligence-ai-opinion/

127. Ryan Daws. Medical chatbot using OpenAI's GPT-3 told a fake patient to kill themselves. AI News; 2020. https://www.artificialintelligence-news.com/2020/10/28/medical-chatbot-openai-gpt3-patient-kill-themselves/

128. Greene T. DeepMind tells Google it has no idea how to make AI less toxic. The Next Web; 2021.

129. Weidinger L, et al. Ethical and social risks of harm from Language Models. arXiv 2112.04359; 2021.

130. Bender EM, Gebru T, McMillan-Major A, Schmitchel S. On the dangers of stochastic parrots: Can language models be too big? Proceedings of the 2021 ACM conference on fairness, accountability, and transparency, pp. 610–623; 2021.

131. Truven Health Analytics. https://www.ibm.com/watson-health/about/truven-health-analytics

132. OptumLabs. https://www.optumlabs.com/

133. TrinetX. https://trinetx.com/

134. Claris Life Sciences. https://www.carislifesciences.com

135. Spector-Bagdady K, Krenz CD, Brummel C, Brenner JC, Bradford CR, Shuman AG. "My Research Is Their Business, but I'm Not Their Business": patient and clinician perspectives on commercialization of precision oncology data. Oncologist. 2020;25(7):620–6.

136. Chiruvella V, Guddati AK. Ethical issues in patient data ownership. Interact J Med Res. 2021;10(2):e22269.

137. Cole CL, Sengupta S, Rossetti S, Vawdrey DK, Halaas M, Maddox TM, Gordon G, Dave T, Payne PR, Williams AE, Estrin D. Ten principles for data sharing and commercialization. J Am Med Inform Assoc. 2021;28(3):646–9.
138. Lazer D, Kennedy R, King G, Vespignani A. The parable of Google Flu: traps in big data analysis. science, 2014;343(6176), pp.1203–1205.
139. Goel S, Hofman JM, Lahaie S, Pennock DM, Watts DJ. Predicting consumer behavior with Web search. Proc Natl Acad Sci. 2010;107(41):17,486–90.
140. Devin Coldewey, Frederic Lardinois AI is eating itself: Bing's AI quotes COVID disinfo sourced from ChatGPT. Techcrunch.com; 2023. https://techcrunch.com/2023/02/08/ai-is-eating-itself-bings-ai-quotes-covid-disinfo-sourced-from-chatgpt/
141. Lin Y. Some asymptotic properties of the support vector machine. Technical Report 1044r, Department of Statistics, University of Wisconsin, Madison; 1999.
142. Hornik K, Stinchcombe M, White H. Multilayer feedforward networks are universal approximators. Neural Netw. 1989;2(5):359–66.
143. Universal Approximation Theorem. Wikipedia. https://en.wikipedia.org/wiki/Universal_approximation_theorem
144. Moreira MWL, Rodrigues JJPC, Korotaev V, Al-Muhtadi J, Kumar N. A comprehensive review on smart decision support systems for health care. IEEE Syst J. 2019;13:3536–45.
145. Yang Q, Steinfeld A, Zimmerman J. Unremarkable AI: fitting intelligent decision support into critical, clinical decision-making processes. In: Proceedings of the 2019 CHI conference on human factors in computing systems. Association for Computing Machinery, New York, NY, USA, pp. 1–11; 2019.
146. Kouri A, Yamada J, Lam Shin Cheung J, Van de Velde S, Gupta S. Do providers use computerized clinical decision support systems? A systematic review and meta-regression of clinical decision support uptake. Implement Sci. 2022;17:21.
147. FHIR Clinical Guidelines (v1.0.0) (STU 1). In: CPG-on-FHIR. https://hl7.org/fhir/uv/cpg/. Accessed 22 Jan 2023.
148. Lomotan EA, Meadows G, Michaels M, Michel JJ, Miller K. To share is human! Advancing evidence into practice through a national repository of interoperable clinical decision support. Appl Clin Inform. 2020;11:112–21.
149. Yin J, Ngiam KY, Teo HH. Role of artificial intelligence applications in real-life clinical practice: systematic review. J Med Internet Res. 2021;23(4):e25759.
150. Varghese J. Artificial intelligence in medicine: chances and challenges for wide clinical adoption. Visceral Med. 2020;36(6):443–9.
151. Chew HSJ, Achananuparp P. Perceptions and needs of artificial intelligence in health care to increase adoption: scoping review. J Med Internet Res. 2022;24(1):e32939.
152. Holden RJ, Karsh BT. The technology acceptance model: its past and its future in health care. J Biomed Inform. 2010;43(1):159–72.
153. Plana D, Shung DL, Grimshaw AA, Saraf A, Sung JJ, Kann BH. Randomized clinical trials of machine learning interventions in health care: a systematic review. JAMA Netw Open. 2022;5(9):–e2233946.

Characterizing, Diagnosing and Managing the Risk of Error of ML & AI Models in Clinical and Organizational Application

Constantin Aliferis, Sisi Ma, Jinhua Wang,
and Gyorgy Simon

Abstract

This chapter covers essential practical methods for examining models, reviewing their face validity, and characterizing and managing risk of errors of such models at development and at deployment stages. This chapter also briefly discusses broader methods and best practices for detecting and correcting issues with ML modeling and the emerging concept of debugging ML models and analyses. A "toolkit" for application safety measures is presented.

Keywords

Calibration · Reliable model decision regions · Debugging ML · Toolkit for safe model application

Essential Model Diagnostics and Model Characterization

Recall from chapter "Principles of Rigorous Development and of Appraisal of ML and AI Methods and Systems " that well-engineered AI/ML methods, have well-characterized properties (theoretical and empirical) across many relevant dimensions that ensure that produced models have appropriate: Representation power; Transparency and Explainability; Soundness; Completeness; Tractable computational complexity of learning models; Tractable computational complexity of using models; Tractable space complexity of learning models; Tractable space complexity of storing and using models; Realistic sample complexity, learning

C. Aliferis (✉) · S. Ma · J. Wang · G. Simon
Institute for Health Informatics, University of Minnesota,
Minneapolis, MN, USA
e-mail: constantinaibestpractices@gmail.com

© The Author(s) 2024
G. J. Simon, C. Aliferis (eds.), *Artificial Intelligence and Machine Learning in Health Care and Medical Sciences*, Health Informatics,
https://doi.org/10.1007/978-3-031-39355-6_13

curves, and power-sample requirements; Probability and decision theoretic consistency; Strong comparative and absolute empirical performance in simulation studies; Transparency and explainability; and Strong comparative and absolute performance in real data with hard and soft gold standard known answers.

These properties (and especially the empirical ones) however, must be further studied on a more granular level once specific models are constructed following the best practices described in chapter "The Development Process and Lifecycle of Clinical Grade and Other Safety and Performance Sensitive AI/ML Models". For example, whereas we know that SVM methods are particularly well suited theoretically and empirically to constructing omics classifiers, or DL methods for image recognition, and so on (chapter "An Appraisal and Operating Characteristics of Major ML Methods Applicable in Healthcare & Health Science"), the specific level of performance and risk of error for a particular model created by a specific dataset for a specific problem solving context requires additional analysis tailored to the particulars of that application.

Therefore, as we transition from method development/characterization to model fit/characterization and we further consider the stages and components of a particular model's lifecycle we move from general properties and lifecycle stages to very concrete understanding of precisely how well this particular model will perform for the problem solving context in hand.

We clarify that in the present chapter we almost exclusively deal with risks due to prediction and other model output errors, giving more operational post-hoc analysis details for the process described in chapter "The Development Process and Lifecycle of Clinical Grade and Other Safety and Performance Sensitive AI/ML Models". We do not deal with regulatory, ethical, reproducibility etc, risks which are discussed in chapters "Regulatory Aspects and Ethical Legal Societal Implications (ELSI)", and "Reporting Standards, Certification/Accreditation, and Reproducibility".

An important first diagnostic for predictive models is testing whether the model is **statistically significantly different than the null model** (i.e., one that does not have any predictive signal). This is typically conducted with a label reshuffling test (LRT, see chapter "The Development Process and Lifecycle of Clinical Grade and Other Safety and Performance-Sensitive AI/ML Models"). The LRT will also inform whether the whole modeling protocol has any **propensity to produce unduly optimistic performance generalization estimates** under the null hypothesis (i.e., the data not having any predictive signal for the response).

If additional validation datasets are available (other than the ones used in the primary error estimation procedures) they can inform about whether the model and its associated generalization error/performance estimates indeed generalize well in new datasets sampled from the same population. For protocols that have passed the LRT for propensity to produce biased generalization error estimates, observing "shrinkage" of the performance from the original estimates to the new ones may be due to the following factors: (a) normal sampling variation; (b) differences of the new validation data from the discovery data because they originate from a slightly (or radically) different population. The latter possibility warrants further investigation, if observed.

One of the most important diagnostics for new models is their **calibration.** Chapter "Evaluation" provides a thorough technical description. To summarize the key concepts, calibration refers to how close the predictions of a model are to the true values. A perfectly-calibrated model is not necessarily a perfectly accurate model since the model may output predictions with a wide confidence interval. If for example, a model outputs that the probability of outcome T taking value 1 for input instance i, is .8 and it is perfectly calibrated, then in 80% of identical cases in the future $T = 1$ and the model will be correct, whereas in 20% of cases it will be wrong. In applications where it is not possible to achieve very accurate predictions it is still essential that a high degree of calibration is achieved. **Recalibration** refers to the procedure where miscalibrated models' outputs are adjusted so that they are better calibrated without the need to rebuild the models. The **binning** method is a very simple but very useful method to recalibrate models. The analyst first estimates the model's calibration in ranges ("bins") of probability outputs and then maps the original predictions to the true (calibrated) probabilities. This same technique can be used for **converting a nonprobabilistic output to a calibrated probability output** (Fig. 1).

Probability conversion of non-probabilistic outputs can be accomplished by other methods, for example using a mapping function such as a sigmoid filter (Fig. 2).

Analysts have a wealth of calibration metrics to use. These are designed to align with the data design and loss functions used in the project. For example, calibration metrics have been developed that are appropriate for case-control binary classification, n-ary classification, regression, survival and time to event models, time series models, etc., see chapter "Evaluation" for details.

Models' reliable and unreliable decision regions. It is also possible to invert the logic of the calibration analysis and seek the **regions in the model's output space where acceptable or unacceptable prediction errors are** observed. This approach establishes the model output regions where the model's predictions are trustworthy (i.e. low-error) and regions where they are not. It is advisable in such an analysis to calculate the FPR, FNR, TPR, TNR or other loss functions and evaluation metrics of interest so that the model can be safely deployed (see chapter "Evaluation").

The above model characterizations remove limitations that are analogous to human cognitive limitations e,g, the famous Dunning-Gruger effect [2] where human decision makers believe that their performance compared to others is higher than what it is and this bias is stronger in decision makers of low ability. Establishing calibration, confidence intervals and credible intervals, and reliable decision regions, ML models can avoid these biases altogether and be equipped with the *functional equivalent of self-awareness of their limitations that promotes safe model application.*

Another useful post-hoc analysis is that of **stability** which measures the degree by which the structure of a model or the values of its parameters change as a function of sampling variation. For practical reasons, stability analyses are typically conducted by generating a large number of datasets re-sampled from the original

1. Train SVM classifier in the *Training set*.

2. Apply it to the *Validation set* and compute distances from the hyperplane to each sample.

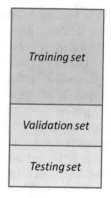

Training set

Validation set

Testing set

Sample #	1	2	3	4	5		98	99	100
Distance	2	-1	8	3	4	...	-2	0.3	0.8

3. Create a histogram with Q (e.g., say 10) bins using the above distances. Each bin has an upper and lower value in terms of distance.

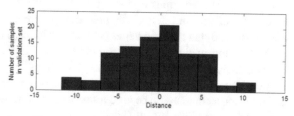

4. Given a new sample from the *Testing set*, place it in the corresponding bin.

   E.g., sample #382 has distance to hyperplane = 1, so it is placed in the bin [0, 2.5]

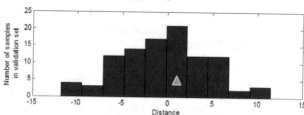

5. Compute probability P(positive class | sample #382) as a fraction of true positives in this bin.

   E.g., this bin has 22 samples (from the *Validation set*), out of which 17 are true positive ones , so we compute P(positive class | sample #382) = 17/22 = 0.77

Fig. 1 **Conversion of a non-probability model to a calibrated probability one, or a non-calibrated probability output to a calibrated one using the binning method.** *In the example, an SVM model is converted to calibrated probabilities however, the approach can be used on any classifier or regressor* [1]

dataset to simulate a sampling distribution. Then the modeling is conducted for each dataset and metrics on the model structures and parameter's stability are calculated. In common practice, highly unstable structures or parameter values are treated with

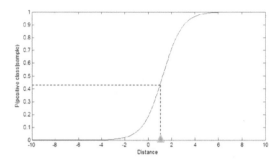

1. Train SVM classifier in the *Training set*.

2. Apply it to the *Validation set* and compute distances from the hyperplane to each sample.

Sample #	1	2	3	4	5	...	98	99	100
Distance	2	-1	8	3	4		-2	0.3	0.8

3. Determine parameters A and B of the sigmoid function by minimizing the negative log likelihood of the data from the *Validation set*.

4. Given a new sample from the *Testing set*, compute its posterior probability using sigmoid function.

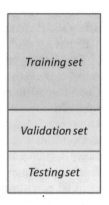

Fig. 2 **Conversion of a non-probability model to a calibrated probability one using the sigmoid filter (i.e., mapping function) method.** *In the example, an SVM model is converted to calibrated probabilities however, the approach can be used on any classifier or regressor* [1]

caution since they may be the result of variation due to small training sample size. We caution however that instability in modeling may be also caused by **structural properties of the distribution and/or the** learning algorithm operating characteristics and is not necessary proof that a model is unreliable or not generalizable [3]. The existence of equivalence classes in particular, may lead to *highly unstable features and models fitted from them by randomized algorithms, however if the unstable features are due to being members of an equivalence class they can still generalize well predictively.* See chapter "The Development Process and Lifecycle of Clinical Grade and Other Safety and Performance-Sensitive AI/ML Models" for a detailed discussion of equivalence classes and the importance to model them.

Equivalence classes are also very important for causal modeling since the causal discovery algorithms by necessity (imposed by learning theory) can learn the data generating function within the equivalence class. Whereas some algorithms (e.g., PC, or GES can score or learn representations of certain types of equivalence classes (e.g. due to latent variables or Markov equivalent structures), other algorithms (e.g., MMHC) learn a single member of the class and then the analyst has to generate the equivalence class of that member. See chapter "Foundations of Causal

ML" for more details about how these algorithms operate and what classes they output.

Similarly **equivalence classes for feature selection can also be critically important** since they can be used to investigate all possible sets of important optimal predictive model inputs for insights into the process that generates the data and for choosing the model with inputs that are most convenient, accessible and easier to deploy. Currently very few algorithms exist for inferring feature sets equivalence classes (see chapters "Foundations and Properties of AI/ML Systems", "An Appraisal and Operating Characteristics of Major ML Methods Applicable in Healthcare & Health Science", "The Development Process and Lifecycle of Clinical Grade and Other Safety and Performance-Sensitive AI/ML Models") and among them at this time only TIE* has a well-developed theory, wide applicability and reliable performance [4].

Establishing **credible intervals (CrIs)** of models' outputs is also an important model characteristic and diagnostic. The CrI is different than the common statistical **Confidence Interval (CI)** the latter measuring (e.g., the 95% or other) range of values for a model's parameters, accuracy or properties when models are built from a number of samples from the population. The 95% (or other width) CrI is the range that contains with probability 95% the true value of the model's parameter or predicted response. In a Bayesian framework it corresponds to a region of the posterior distribution for an estimated predicted response value or parameter value [5, 6].

In all cases especially after a model has been generated in, or converted to, a human readable form (using the many techniques and best practices discussed in chapter "The Development Process and Lifecycle of Clinical Grade and Other Safety and Performance-Sensitive AI/ML Models") **face validity tests** are very useful. Such tests are conducted by domain experts (and in some cases augmented by automated literature extraction and synthesis) who by using domain knowledge will seek to identify implausible patterns and relationships, or apparently dubious decision logic as possible errors in the model's construction.

If, as a trivial example, a model suggests that an inheritable genetic factor is caused by a lifestyle behavior that obviously denotes a reversal in causal order that is highly suspect. If, in a more sophisticated example, terminal outcomes (e.g., death) appear to have spouse variables (i.e., direct causes or direct effects of the outcome) this violates the data design and measurement constraints and has to be explained by the existence of unmeasured confounders (which is the most likely explanation in this example), by data errors, or by modeling errors.

Best Practice 13.1
Measure calibration and recalibrate as needed.

Best Practice 13.2
Convert scores to probabilities.

Best Practice 13.3
Test models for difference from null model.

Best Practice 13.4
Identify models' reliable and unreliable decision regions.

Best Practice 13.5
Measure stability and flag unstable models.

Best Practice 13.6
Extract and report model equivalence classes.

Debugging ML

In conventional programming, several techniques and tools exist for debugging programs to ensure that their behavior is the one intended by the programmer. "Bugs" are errors in coding that divert the original intension of the programmer to an unwanted or unanticipated program behavior. A variety of tools, techniques, and resources have been invented to help with conventional debugging. Such methods include interactive debugging, control flow analysis, unit testing, log file analysis, memory dumps, profiling and other techniques [7–9].

Debugging ML model building however involves many additional complexities and represents a higher order of difficulty for debugging, because of the following reasons:

1. **ML programs do not implement functions but functionals**. An ordinary programming function maps a set of inputs (the domain set) to a set of outputs (the codomain set). A ML functional is a function that takes a set of inputs (training and validation datasets) and maps them to a set of functions (i.e. decision models, which themselves are functions that take as inputs problem domain instances and output instance-specific decisions).

2. Whereas conventional programming admits a single or small number of correct solutions (e.g., a ranked list of numbers, all paths from point A to point B in a map, etc.) **ML programming admits an infinity of acceptable or even optimal outputs** (i.e., in predictive ML, any member of the whole equivalence class of models that exhibit optimal generalization performance) or the even larger set that exhibits near-optimal performance.

3. **ML algorithms are inherently stochastic** in terms of the inputs and may also involve stochastic operations on them. They have to accommodate infinite possible inputs and to be robust to noisy inputs.

4. **ML algorithms's properties interact with the data design** so that the quality of the output is not strictly a function of the data input but also a function of the alignment of the algorithm with the data generation and measurement design choices made by the analyst or user of the algortihm. The ML algorithms however seldom have built-in representations of the data design properties and how it affects their operation (which makes detecting related problems hard).

The process of debugging ML modeling is currently decidedly more of an art than a science. However this art is strongly informed by well-established scientific principles and properties from ML. The following are recommended approaches to tackle ML debugging to achieve model development error prevention and detection. They should be treated as starting point within a much larger and variable space of possibilities.

Best Practices 13.7. ML Debugging Strategies

1. **Start from conventional implementation debugging of ML algorithms**: e.g. trace step by step algorithms in simple but representative small scale problems; isolate and unit-test subroutines in data intake, model fitting and output. Same for conventional debugging of AI/ML model implementation.

2. **Debug real data**, e.g., :

    (a) Is the data conformant to expected format?
    (b) Is the data distributed according to distributional assumptions that underlie proper use of the algorithms/models used?
    (c) Is the data reflecting the sampling or data generation protocol? For example, for data supposed to be iid, is it? For data from randomized experiments can we predict the exposure? (if yes, then it was not properly randomized).
    (d) Are there outliers or other data abnormalities that violate ML algorithm data requirements?

3. **Debug simulations and resimulations**:

    (a) When artificial and semi-artificial data are used to test algorithm performance and the algorithm implementation does not behave according to theoretical expectations, test whether the simulated data conforms to the specification of the simulation.
    (b) If an algorithm or protocol is randomized, save any suspect random instantiations for debugging (because in subsequent runs the bug may not appear).

4. **Know well the behavior of algorithms** so that strange behaviors (for better or worse) are immediately apparent in complex analyses. For example:

   (a) If an algorithm is deterministic but outputs different results at each run on the same data this indicates a bug; conversely a randomized algorithm that outputs the same exact results indicates a bug.

   (b) If the algorithm is expected to have boundary behaviors (for example terminate upon meeting certain conditions) but does not, this indicates a bug;

   (c) If the algorithm is expected to converge monotonically toward a performance metric but it converges non-monotonically, this also indicates a bug, and so on.

   (d) If an algorithm is expected to converge and does not, investigate if it is normal non-convergence or systematic.

   (e) Investigate the root causes of happy accidents and surprises (see next section).

5. Build and use a set of benchmark datasets where the behavior of algorithms is known and new algorithms or new implementations can be readily compared.

6. Compare the implementation or instantiation and tuning of a ML algorithm or protocol to the same data *as published in reference-level prior literature*.

7. Examine the interactions of algorithms with embedding protocols and systems. If the same algorithm implementation behaves differently inside different implementations of the same protocol this indicates that the protocol implementation or interface with the ML algorithm is buggy.

Recognizing and Accommodating "Happy Accidents" & Surprises

In the practice of ML, we often encounter "happy accidents" and pleasant surprises. For example, when developing Markov Boundary algorithms (chapter "Principles of Rigorous Development and of Appraisal of ML and AI Methods and Systems") the developers were surprised that despite that the GLL algorithms were performing up to 100,000s of conditional independence tests per dataset without conventionally correcting for multiple comparisons, the resulting Markov Boundary sets did not contain significant numbers of false positives. Initially the developing team considered this as a likely bug that should be corrected with false positive rate control measures, however close inspection of the issue revealed that the variable elimination steps in the algorithms were eliminating the false positives. For example, when fed with 1000 random variables and no signal-carrying variables, and with conditional independence tests (CITs) set at minimal alpha of 5%, which would imply 50 false positives, the algorithm would output just 4 false positives [10, 11]. This gave valuable insights in the *self-regularizing behavior* of this class of algorithms and confirmed their robustness.

In another example, the same authors show that so-called epistatic functions, that is, extremely non-linear and discontinuous functions where only a specific subset of the inputs would reveal signal and all other lower order subsets were devoid of signal, can still be detected by linear learners and the classifier performance can grow arbitrarily close to perfect when the inputs are unbalanced (by data design)) or correlated (naturally). In addition, when the density of positive target is non uniform in the space of inputs, then arbitrarily strong signal can exist that is detectable by linear learners. For example, in the textbook XOR function which is a prime example of this class of functions, and T = XOR (A,B), neither A or B have univariate signal for T and must be considered together for the signal to become fully discoverable. This is a huge problem in high dimensional settings where the combinatorics become quickly intractable. This textbook version of the problem however is very unlikely to exist in practice because for signal to disappear in lower-order effects an unlikely arrangement of data has to exist [11].

In the benchmark of pathway reverse engineering study of [12] it was shown that basic correlation networks would perform well as long as the loss functions were tailored to their inductive bias. Specifically, despite that these techniques are not having causal discovery guarantees and can be shown to output massive numbers of false positives in many situations, in very low sample situations they may perform better in terms of sensitivity (trading off specificity) than causal algorithms simply because there is not enough sample to generate reliable results and proper causal algorithms are designed to avoid producing false positives.

In the domain of cancer genomics, random selection of biomarkers tends to give informative markers and strong signatures [13]. These are truly generalizable and robust and their existence is due to the wide propagation of cancer signal throughout the data generating transcriptomic network.

In a final example, while causal ML algorithms are designed to operate in faithful distributions (which do not have information equivalences), the designers of the Causal feature selection challenge [14] were surprised to discover that their resimulated data built using such algorithms exhibited information equivalencies (mostly as a result of statistical indistinguishability due to finite sample size). This increases the veracity of the resimulated data.

These examples show a common phenomenon in ML, i.e., that empirical results often perform better than expected due to **mitigation factors.** The modelers should investigate thoroughly any unexpected behaviors to find any errors, but should also keep an open mind about the possible validity of results due to error mitigating factors.

A Toolkit for Ensuring Safe Model Application

Best Practices 13.8. for Safe Model Deployment

1. **Outlier detection.** When encountering an application instance, determine whether it is an outlier with respect to the distribution where the model was validated and flag it as such [15, 16]. Refrain from making a prediction or decision for outliers.

2. **Region of reliable operation.** When encountering an application instance, determine whether it falls inside or outside the model's region of reliable operation (section "Essential Model Diagnostics and Model characterization"). Refrain from making a prediction or decision for cases outside the reliable region.

3. **Detect and address distribution shifts.** As application instances accumulate, determine if their distribution is different than the one used to validate the model (chapters "Data Design" and "Data Preparation, Transforms, Quality, and Management").

   (a) If yes, then alert the deployment and development teams for possible need to rebuilt the model because of distribution shifts.

   (b) When distribution shifts are observed, determine if they affect the model performance. If they do not, continue monitoring the shifts but do not withhold the model's decisions.

   (c) Characterize distribution shifts by seasonal trends, individual variables affected, emerging population mixture changes, etc., as appropriate for the application domain.

4. **When making a prediction or decision, also output the credible interval** for that input region (chapter "Overfitting, Underfitting and General Model Overconfidence and Under-Performance Pitfalls and Best Practices in Machine Learning and AI") as well as other loss function estimates applicable to the region.

5. **When explaining a model or a specific model's output also report the credible interval and stability of its structure and parameters.** Flag unstable and uncertain model characteristics.

6. **Apply continuous statistical process quality control metrics as predictions and decisions are prospectively validated** [16]. If predictions and actions are statistically significantly different than expected, then alert deployment and development teams for possible need to rectify or rebuilt the model.

7. **Make the above functions parametric** so that model operators can adapt the model deployment better to local application conditions (e.g., health care provider and patient preferences, organizational policies, evolving regulations etc.).

8. When more than one model are available, **apply the model that has best performance and safety profile for each application case** [17].

9. **When transferring a model developed from population P1 to population P2** analyze with existing historical data performance and safety before deployment. If operating characteristics are not satisfactory, then **consider rebuilding models from P2 data.**

10. **If some inputs are expected to be missing and decisions with partial input are desired,** consider using flexible input decision models, or dynamic imputation schemes at the design, fitting and validation stages (chapter "Foundations and Properties of AI/ML Systems"). **Do not apply models with partial or imputed inputs unless this is part of the models' design and validation.**

11. **If the quality of model data inputs changes** from the development and validation data to the application phase, apply appropriate detection mechanisms, flag such inputs and refrain from making predictions or other decisions (chapter "Data Preparation, Transforms, Quality, and Management").

12. **Develop and deploy ancillary alerting DSS** (geared to the model users and developers) that are designed to flag deviations from the conditions that guarantee safe and effective model performance *although it may not be directly detectable in data.* For example, for a COVID management model, deploy alerts related to new vaccines, population immunity, new variants, and other factors that may affect the model's validity but may not be detectable from the patient-level data before they create serious degradation in model performance.

Conclusions

Taken together the above practices are designed to establish several synergistic safety layers protecting models from falling off their "knowledge cliff". The listed safeguards comprise the functional equivalent of AI/ML "self-knowledge" of its limitations in order to avoid making hazardous decisions.

Key Concepts Discussed in This Chapter

Calibration

Recalibration and conversion of scores to probabilities

Reliable and unreliable model decision regions

Credible Intervals

Debugging ML: how is different than conventional code debugging; general strategies for ML debugging.

Model failure mitigation factors

Model deployment safeguards toolkit

Pitfalls Related to the Present Chapter

Pitfall 13.1. Models that are uncalibrated or with unknown calibration

Pitfall 13.2. Models with unknown correspondence of output to probabilities.

Pitfall 13.3. Not checking if model statistically significantly better than the null model.

Pitfall 13.4. Unknown model reliable and unreliable decision regions.

Pitfall 13.5.: Unknown stability and consequences for model safety and performance.

Pitfall 13.6. Being oblivious to model'sequivalence class

Pitfall 13.7. ML with bugs.

Pitfall 13.8. Falling over a model's "knowledge cliff" (i.e., succumbing to model deployment safety traps):
1. Outliers.
2. Falling outside model's region of reliable operation.
3. Distribution shifts.
4. Model decisions carry no information about its expected errors specific to that case.
5. Failing to flag, report and explain unstable and uncertain model characteristics.
6. Failing to detect and alert deployment and development teams for possible need to rectify or rebuilt the model.
7. Rigid specifications of safety functions, lack of adaptability to local application conditions.
8. Fail to exploit a plurality of tailored models to address the application cases.
9. Fail to safely transfer models developed from population P1 to population P2.
10. Fail to address missing inputs.
11. Failing to detect and manage drops in the quality of model data inputs.
12. Invisible deviations from the conditions that guarantee safe and effective model performance.

Summary of Best Practices Discussed in This Chapter

Best Practice 13.1. Measure calibration and recalibrate as needed

Best Practice 13.2. Convert scores to probabilities.

Best Practice 13.3. Test models for difference from null model.

Best Practice 13.4. Identify models' reliable and unreliable decision regions.

Best Practice 13.5. Measure stability and flag unstable models.

Best Practice 13.6. Extract and report model equivalence classes

Best Practice 13.7. Apply strategies for ML debugging:
1. Start from conventional debugging of ML algorithm implementation.
2. Debug with real data.
3. Debug simulations and resimulations.
4. Know well the behavior of algorithms so that strange behaviors (for better or worse) are immediately apparent in complex analyses. Investigate unusual behaviors (with respect to each algorithm's expected behavior).
5. Build and use a set of benchmark datasets.
6. Compare the implementation or instantiation and tuning of a ML algorithm to the literature.
7. Examine the interactions of algorithms with embedding protocols and systems.

Best Practice 13.8. Use safe model deployment toolkit:
1. Detect and manage outliers.
2. Detect and manage falling outside model's region of reliable operation.
3. Detect and manage distribution shifts.
4. Report Credible Interval and other loss function estimates applicable to the input region for every model decision.
5. Flag, report and explain unstable and uncertain model characteristics.
6. Apply continuous QC metrics as predictions and decisions are prospectively validated. Alert deployment and development teams for possible need to rectify or rebuilt the model.
7. Make the above safety functions parametric so that model operators can adapt the model deployment better to local application conditions.
8. When more than one model is available, choose the model that has best performance and safety profile for each application case.
9. Safely transfer models developed from population P1 to population P2, or rebuild models from P2 data.
10. Address missing inputs at the design, fitting and validation stages. Do not apply models with partial or imputed inputs unless this is part of the models' design and validation.

11. Manage drops in the quality of model data inputs from the development and validation data to the application phase.
12. Develop and deploy ancillary alerting DSS (geared to the model users and developers) that are designed to flag deviations from the conditions that guarantee safe and effective model performance.

Classroom Assignments & Discussion Topics in This Chapter

1. Which factors can you list that cause distribution shifts? Which ones may jeopardize decision models?

2. Give: (a) An example where highly unstable biomarker selection does not degrade model predictivity. (b) An example where highly stable biomarkers are not useful.

   HINT for (a): consider that markers BM1 and BM2 have exactly the same information for the response and the biomarker discovery procedure chooses them at random. Now increase the number of markers with such equivalent information.

3. Show how model instability may relate to sampling variation and to increased errors via the BVDE.

4. When conversion of scores to probabilities is desirable? When can it be superfluous? When detrimental?

5. (a) Describe how we can create models with high performance and accuracy by carving out input space regions of low performance/accuracy.
   (b) What are necessary preconditions for this to be successful?
   (c) What is the fundamental tradeoff involved?

6. If missing inputs are anticipated at model deployment, how would you choose among alternative options based on the tractability of running models? Compare for example BNs and KNN in this context.

7. [Advanced] Discuss the application of transductive learning methods to address successful model transference? What may be downsides of this approach?

8. Consider a situation where the data describing a patient population with disease D in region/health system H1 are radically different than those of region/health system H2.
   (a) What may cause these differences?
   (b) How would you go about building effective models for H1 and H2?

9. [Advanced] Is every degradation of model input data quality affecting the model's quality of outputs? How would you systematically incorporate this consideration in the design of robust models?

References

1. Statnikov A, Aliferis CF, Hardin DP, Guyon. A gentle introduction to support vector machines in biomedicine: theory and methods, vol. 1. World scientific; 2011.
2. Kruger J, Dunning D. Unskilled and unaware of it: how difficulties in recognizing one's own incompetence lead to inflated self-assessments. J Pers Soc Psychol. 1999;77(6):1121.
3. Ben-David, S., Von Luxburg, U. and Pál, D., 2006. A sober look at clustering stability. In Learning theory: 19th annual conference on learning theory, COLT 2006, Pittsburgh, PA, USA, June 22–25, 2006. Proceedings 19. Springer Berlin Heidelberg, pp. 5–19.
4. Statnikov A, Lemeir J, Aliferis CF. Algorithms for discovery of multiple Markov boundaries. J Mach Learning Res. 2013;14(1):499–566.
5. Harrell FE. Regression modeling strategies: with applications to linear models, logistic regression, and survival analysis, vol. 608. New York: Springer; 2001.
6. Steyerberg EW. Applications of prediction models. New York: Springer; 2009. p. 11–31.
7. Hailpern B, Santhanam P. Software debugging, testing, and verification. IBM Syst J. 2002;41(1):4–12.
8. Zhu H, Hall PA, May JH. Software unit test coverage and adequacy. ACM Comput Surv (CSUR). 1997;29(4):366–427.
9. https://en.wikipedia.org/wiki/Debugging#Techniques
10. Aliferis CF, Statnikov A, Tsamardinos I, Mani S, Koutsoukos XD. Local causal and Markov blanket induction for causal discovery and feature selection for classification part I: algorithms and empirical evaluation. J Mach Learn Res. 2010;11(1)
11. Aliferis CF, Statnikov A, Tsamardinos I, Mani S, Koutsoukos XD. Local causal and Markov blanket induction for causal discovery and feature selection for classification part II: analysis and extensions. J Mach Learn Res. 2010;11(1)
12. Narendra V, Lytkin NI, Aliferis CF, Statnikov A. A comprehensive assessment of methods for de-novo reverse-engineering of genome-scale regulatory networks. Genomics. 2011;97(1):7–18.
13. Venet D, Dumont JE, Detours V. Most random gene expression signatures are significantly associated with breast cancer outcome. PLoS Comput Biol. 2011;7(10):e1002240.
14. Guyon I, Aliferis C, Cooper G, Elisseeff A, Pellet JP, Spirtes P, Statnikov A. Design and analysis of the causation and prediction challenge. In Causation and prediction challenge. PMLR, pp. 1–33; 2008.
15. Hodge V, Austin J. A survey of outlier detection methodologies. Artif Intell Rev. 2004;22:85–126.
16. Oakland JS. Statistical process control. Routledge; 2007.
17. Statnikov A, Aliferis CF, Hardin DP, Guyon I. Gentle introduction to support vector machines in biomedicine, a-volume 2: case studies and benchmarks. World Scientific Publishing Company; 2013.

Considerations for Specialized Health AI & ML Modelling and Applications: NLP

Dalton Schutte and Rui Zhang

Abstract

Much information about patients is documented in the unstructured textual format in the electronic health record system. Research findings are also reported in the biomedical literature. In this chapter, we will discuss the background, resources and methods used in biomedical natural language processing (NLP), which will help unlock information from the textual data.

Keywords

NLP tasks · Deep learning in NLP · Graphical models in NLP · Large Language Models

Background

This section will cover some of the standard terminology, techniques, and resources that are essential to a variety of NLP tasks. A collection of terms that will appear frequently throughout will be defined and examples given where appropriate. Then, pre-processing techniques will be discussed followed by feature extraction. Finally, key biomedical NLP resources will be discussed.

D. Schutte · R. Zhang (✉)
Department of Surgery, University of Minnesota, Minneapolis, MN, USA
e-mail: zhan1386@umn.edu

© The Author(s) 2024
G. J. Simon, C. Aliferis (eds.), *Artificial Intelligence and Machine Learning in Health Care and Medical Sciences*, Health Informatics,
https://doi.org/10.1007/978-3-031-39355-6_14

Basic NLP Terminology

In general, NLP attempts to understand what the contents of a *corpus* is about. A **corpus** is a collection of text documents and often consists mostly of *unstructured data* (data without a formal structure). In the biomedical domain, a corpus may be a collection of physician's notes or reports (radiology reports or pathology reports) from an Electronic Health Record (EHR), journal abstracts or full-text articles in PubMed, etc. Large medical centers (academic or otherwise) naturally accumulate large volumes of unstructured text data where NLP techniques can be leveraged to extract relevant clinical information for a better understanding of the patient population or conducting observational studies.

Often a **document** refers to a single body of text, e.g. a single physician's note from a patient visit, an entire journal article, an individual tweet, etc. A document is comprised of words which may or may not be further decomposed into a string of characters called *tokens*. It is often the case that a word is the smallest semantic unit of a text while a token may be a part of a word or punctuation (i.e. "hasn't" is a word that could be decomposed to tokens "hasn" and "t").

Standard Pre-processing

There are some instances where it is useful to take raw text and use it in NLP tasks. However, it is often more useful to *preprocess* the text to some degree. Preprocessing text is applying techniques to prepare the text for ingestion in computational systems. There are a myriad of techniques to preprocess text that can be used together to prepare it for use. The ones that follow are some of the most common.

> Preprocessing is often required for many NLP tasks but the specific preprocessing techniques will vary by desired outcome. This includes any potential feature extraction that may be used.

Cleaning. Cleaning the text refers to removing unwanted characters or tokens from text and is often the first step in the preprocessing pipeline. Often, it is advantageous to remove characters that do not belong to a desired character set (i.e. UTF-8, ascii, etc.) or language (English, Mandarin, Spanish, etc.) as many tools and programs will have limitations on what type of text they can accept. Other times, it may be desirable to replace characters with phonetically similar characters (e.g. β → ss) or with unaccented characters (e.g. ü → u). Depending on the situation, it may also be useful to remove some non-alphanumeric characters (e.g. &, #, *) from text.

Once the documents are all using a shared character set, the next step is often to remove *stopwords*. A stopword is a frequently occurring word that carries little semantic value (e.g. "the", "a", "is", "of", etc.). It is well established that the word frequencies in languages have a Zipfian distribution: a small number of high-occurring words comprise the majority of most text. In English, these high-occurrence words are typically articles, some prepositions, pronouns, and variations of "to be" (i.e. "is", "was", etc.). Removing these from the text can significantly reduce the number of tokens that need to be used by models which can decrease training time and improve performance. Removing a large number of common words may seem counterintuitive, as in most machine learning problems it is desirable to keep common data points as they often indicate a trend or pattern of some sort, but, in the case of language, low semantic value translates to low information contribution to the model. These words are analogous to noise, in some sense.

Tokenization. The tokenization of text refers to decomposing a document into smaller computational pieces. This can be accomplished by one of many techniques. One of the most standard techniques for English is to perform simple *whitespace tokenization* where a string of text is divided based on whitespaces (e.g. spaces, tabs, new lines, etc.). This often produces tokens that are simply words, as the convention in English is typically to separate words with spaces. In the cases of words joined by a hyphen, how these are treated depends, in part, on how hyphens were handled in the preceding cleaning step.

Other methods for tokenization exist such as WordPiece, which is an example of a *subword tokenization* method. That is, it is splitting a word into smaller sub-word components to help avoid potential Out-of-Vocabulary (OoV) issues in downstream tasks, such as vector embedding.

Stemming & Lemmatization

It is very often the case that a single word will appear in a single document in various grammatical forms (i.e. "running", "ran", etc.). These words share a base meaning with some inflection induced for grammatical purposes. To reduce the number of distinct tokens or words in text, it may be useful to apply *stemming* or *lemmatization*. Both processes attempt to perform the same task, but in rather different ways.

Stemming works by simply dropping the ends of words in hopes that the base term is recovered. This works well for things that have simple endings such as "ends", "ending", "ended", etc. All of these are reduced to simply "end" by removing the various strings at the end of the base. This method fails when special spelling rules change the base term in some way. For example, "carry" and "carries", while having the same base, do not reduce to the same word by way of simply removing the ending characters due to English spelling conventions.

This is where lemmatization is useful. Lemmatization attempts to produce the base term but considers a vocabulary and morphological analysis of the words. In this way, lemmatization may return "carry" if given "carries" or "see" if given "saw".

Feature Extraction

Text contains a myriad of features that can be extracted for use in downstream tasks. These can be at a variety of levels from individual words, groups of words, entire sentences, parts of speech, term frequency, etc. Some key feature extraction methods will be discussed in the following sections. These can be used individually or in tandem and the discussion below is by no means exhaustive.

N-grams. An *n-gram* is simply a string comprised of n consecutive parts. These parts can be at the level of words, tokens, or even individual characters. These are extracted from text by, usually, padding the beginning and ending of the string with empty items to accommodate the first and last part, in the case where $n > 1$. For example, "She ran home" can be represented as:

unigram	{"she","ran","home"}
bigrams	{("","she"),("she","ran"),("ran","home"),("home","")}
trigrams (character level)	{" s", " sh", "she", "he ", "e r", " ra", "ran", "an ", "n h", " ho", "hom", "ome", "me ", "e "}

N-grams can be collected after cleaning or from raw (unprocessed) text depending on the use case. Stemming or lemmatization may also be performed before n-grams are extracted from text.

The collection of all unique n-grams are typically compiled into a table and assigned an index value for future use. Depending on the task and desired outcome, character level n-grams may provide more generalized morphological models than token level n-grams but at the cost of lost semantic meaning. Conversely, token level n-grams may provide more generalized semantic models but reduced morphological representation.

TF-IDF. While n-grams may show what tokens are present in a document, it does not, on its own, convey information regarding the relative importance of a token in a given document. This is where *term frequency-inverse document frequency (tf-idf)* can be useful. The TF-IDF is a statistic that reflects the relative importance of a token in a document or corpus.

Embeddings. Due to the large number of text features that may exist in a corpus, the features may often be sparse inputs that can make downstream machine learning difficult. As such, a common technique to reduce the dimensionality and sparsity of features is to embed the features in a Euclidean space. Three primary techniques exist to accomplish this embedding: an embedding layer, Word2Vec [1], and Global Vectors (GloVe) [2].

An embedding layer is a layer that is learned jointly with a neural network as the first layer in the network model. Because it is, often, trained from scratch, the embedded representation is going to be highly corpus and task specific. The drawback to this approach is that training is subject to the usual shortcomings of training neural networks and is also more data intensive than other techniques.

Word2Vec is a statistical model for learning embeddings in a more efficient manner. There are two primary training approaches to training a Word2Vec model: continuous bag-of-words (BoW) and continuous skip-gram. A continuous BoW model tries to predict a word given the context around the word and the continuous skip-gram model tries to predict the context of a word given the word. The core idea for this technique is that a word's meaning can be learned by the words that occur around it. This technique also tends to be faster and more efficient than training embedding layers.

The Global Vector (GloVe) technique is an extension of the Word2Vec model. A global word-word co-occurrence matrix is used in tandem with context methods (such as Word2Vec) to learn efficient models that scale well as the corpus size increases. Notably, it leverages statistical information contained in the co-occurrence matrix by using only the non-zero entries of the co-occurrence matrix. GloVe is able to obtain good results even on small corpora and often produces more informative embeddings.

> **Best Practice 14.1**
> Always test multiple preprocessing pipelines to find what works best for the desired goals.

Biomedical Resources for Clinical NLP

There are many resources specialized to the biomedical domain for NLP. Recent years have seen an explosion in databases, specially trained models, specialized tools and packages, various medical knowledge graphs, and much more. Below, we will focus on two resources that have several important tools that use them as a foundational component.

UMLS. The *Unified Medical Language System (UMLS)* [3] is a critical resource for many clinical NLP tasks. Ambiguity is present in all languages, and biomedical language is no exception. The medical realm is full of various terms that represent the same concept (e.g., "heart attack" and "myocardial infarction"). There is also a natural hierarchy that arises in biomedical terminology such as "transient ischemic attack" which is a type of "ischemic stroke" which is a type of "stroke". All of these relationships contain valuable information that can aid in a variety of NLP tasks and is where the UMLS comes in.

The UMLS is a collection of files containing a wealth of information but comprises three main components: the Metathesaurus, the Semantic Network, and the SPECIALIST Lexicon and Lexical tools. The Metathesaurus is the largest component and contains the concepts, semantic types and their identifies, such as the concept unique identifiers (CUIs). The Semantic Network contains information about the semantic relationships between concepts. The SPECIALIST Lexicon contains syntactic, morphological, and orthographic information about terms in the UMLS as well as more common English terms.

SemMedDB. The *Semantic MEDLINE Database (SemMedDB)* [4] is a repository of semantic predications extracted by applying a tool called SemRep to all PubMed citations (over 29 million citations). This results in over 96 million semantic predictions, which are triples of the form subject-predicate-object. SemRep will be further discussed in a later section. An example of a semantic predication is:

"Effects of Asian sand dust, Arizona sand dust, amorphous silica and aluminum oxide on allergic inflammation in the murine lung."

- Subject: C0002374 - Alumina
- Predicate: EFFECTS
- Object: C0021375—Inflammation, allergic
- Predication: Alumina EFFECTS Inflammation, Allergic

SemMedDB contains tables of predications, concept mentions, mappings of mentions and predications to source sentences, as well as the source sentences themselves. The database can be readily loaded into SQL for querying in various applications. The nature of predications also allows SemMedDB predications table to be loaded into a graph database to leverage relationships.

Clinical NLP Tasks

While many of the classic NLP tasks also exist in the clinical domain, there are often more specific applications of these tasks to clinical tasks. Often, high-level tasks include Named Entity Recognition (NER) for the purposes of identifying medications, procedures, etc. Relation extraction (RelEx) to identify why a treatment or course of action was decided on. Both of these are examples of *information extraction (IE)* tasks where the goal is to pull desired information from clinical free text. Some other tasks include text classification, text generation, and question answering. These can serve any number of purposes, but often are not instances of IE [5].

> Common NLP tasks that will be useful in a clinical setting include NER and RelEx as techniques of Information Extraction, Concept Normalization, Text Classification, Language Generation, and Question Answering. These can be used as means to ends (e.g. NER to extract entity mentions from patient notes, entity mention counts can be used to generate TF-IDF vectors which can be used in various machine learning models to predict outcomes) or as ends in themselves (e.g. RelEx to find if a patient had an adverse reaction to a particular substance).

Named Entity Recognition

Named Entity Recognition (NER) is the act of labeling specific terms or concepts in text, such as determining the part of speech for a token in text. In a clinical setting, this is often used to identify drugs or dietary supplements, procedures, symptoms, conditions, or other desirable information. A model that can identify these terms can be used for a variety of downstream tasks, such as recognizing a particular dietary supplement or an adverse event from clinical records [6].

A term or concept may have a single word or multiple. Using the example of drug recognition, the sentence "She has been taking aspirin for headaches" contains the drug "aspirin" that we would want identified. Alternatively given the sentence "The patient reports using black cohosh daily", we would want "black cohosh" to be extracted.

One of the most common forms of labeling for NER is BIO labeling. In this convention, "B-x" means beginning and is used to signify the first word of a named entity of type x in some text. In the examples above, "aspirin" would be labeled "B-drug", "headache" might be "B-symptom", and "black" from "black cohosh" would be labeled "B-supplement". "I-x" means the interior and is, similarly, used to signify a non-beginning term for a multi-word concept. Continuing from the example above, "cohosh" would be labeled "I-supplement" giving "black cohosh" the labels {"B-supplement", "I-supplement"}. O is used to represent any term outside of the defined labels. For example, "daily" from above is a frequency, but if we are only considering drugs, symptoms, and supplements, "daily" would be labeled O since we do not have a label defined for frequencies.

Concept Normalization

Concept normalization is the task of mapping multiple terms that have the same meaning to a common, standardized term. The UMLS attempts to do this by way of the Metathesaurus, for example, and often excels when doing so on text writing by medical professionals or appearing in scientific publications due to the nature of the vocabulary used by such individuals and in such contexts. However, this problem can be more complicated when the corpus includes text from individuals who are not medical professionals or writing without a more sophisticated medical vocabulary. This is prevalent when examining mainstream news articles or social media posts. An example of this would be mapping the phrase "head spinning" to "dizziness" or "feeling like I need to throw up" to "nausea". For tasks where the goal is to determine the prevalence of symptoms in tweets, for example, or what sort of side effects people experience when using dietary supplements, it is important that concepts are normalized unless specialized models are used [7].

Relation Extraction

Relation Extraction (RelEx) is the task of extracting terms and the interaction or relationship between them. In a clinical setting, this may be trying to determine what drug caused which side-effect in a patient. The relationships extracted can help identify incidence rates for side-effects, determine if a particular patient subpopulation is more likely to experience certain effects than another, etc. The results will often take the form of subject, relation, object between two entities and one of multiple pre-defined relationships. This type of result is essentially what is contained in SemMedDB. The tool used to generate SemMedDB, SemRep, is a rules-based tool that performs relationship extraction.

As an example, take the sentence "the patient reported nausea after his chemo-therapy treatment last week". One relationship that might be extracted is "chemotherapy-causes-nausea". Another might be "patient-experiences-nausea". It should be noted that prior to predicting the relationship between two concepts or terms, those terms first need to be properly identified. In other words, NER is neces-sary to perform RelEx.

Text Classification

Text classification is the act of classifying a collection of tokens with some label, such as determining if a movie review is positive or negative. In a clinical setting, this might be determining if a treatment was successful, if the patient has started using new medications, etc. Rather than operating on a token level, like most of the above tasks, this tends to consider a chunk of text in its totality. This might be n-grams, sentences, or entire documents depending on the particular task. A discrete collection of labels is often defined based on the goal for the task at hand.

For example, if we want to determine if a patient is stopping the use of a particu-lar medication [8], text classification may be an appropriate task. If we want to clas-sify a string of text as "started", "continuing", "discontinuing", or "unknown" with regards to a patient's use of a medication or supplement and are given the sentence, "the patient reports that he has not continued taking vitamin D supplements", the entire sentence would be labeled as "discontinued". This can help understand trends in patient treatment compliance or the effects starting/stopping a substance might have on health outcomes.

Natural Language Generation

Natural Language Generation (NLG) is the task of trying to produce text that has the appearance of something a human might produce. Famously, GPT-3 by OpenAI is known to be able to produce prose that has a high-degree of similarity to prose that has been written by poets, writers, reporters, and average internet users. In a medical setting, NLG may be used to help generate synthetic clinical notes without leaking any protected health information of patients, and thus can be used to develop clinical NLP systems [9]. NLG can also be used to generate answers to users' ques-tions [10].

Question Answering

Question Answering (QA) is selecting an answer from multiple choices given a query. Consumers increasingly are typing to find answers from the internet or smart device to their questions regarding medical conditions or medication usage. QA is a task to understand their questions and retrieve information and then generate answers automatically. The first component is the Natural Language Understanding, since the task at hand is to understand the question being asked as well as the available answer options in order to correctly determine which option answers the question. The second component is information retrieval, which is to find corresponding information from knowledge bases or the internet that may contain the contents to respond to their information. The final component is NLG, which is discussed above. CHiQA is an experimental AI-based QA system that is learning how to answer health-related questions using reliable sources for patients [11].

Symbolic Based Biomedical NLP

Symbolic NLP uses human-readable symbols and logic to create rules for a system. This is a subset of symbolic (also called Old-Fashioned AI). This process involves the explicit codification of human knowledge, behavior, and expertise into computer programs. While these systems may, at face, be easier to understand, they are often very difficult to construct and require considerable manual effort from domain experts to produce quality systems.

In the biomedical domain, there are a couple key tools that fall under the domain of symbolic NLP. Namely, MetaMap, SemRep, cTakes, and others are systems developed by groups of individuals with expertise in biomedical or clinical fields.

MetaMap [12] is a tool that performs NER and Concept Normalization of biomedical text. When given a body of text, MetaMap performs a number of preprocessing steps before attempting to identify medical terms and mapping them to standardized concepts in the UMLS. As such, MetaMap relies on the UMLS to function.

SemRep [13] is a tool that performs RelEx on biomedical text. SemRep is a rule-based system that uses MetaMap and the UMLS to handle NER before determining the relationship between the extracted concepts. Returning to the example:

"Effects of Asian sand dust, Arizona sand dust, amorphous silica and aluminum oxide on allergic inflammation in the murine lung."

- Subject: C0002374—Alumina
- Predicate: EFFECTS
- Object: C0021375—Inflammation, allergic
- Predication: Alumina EFFECTS Inflammation, Allergic

In this example, the subject and objects are identified by MetaMap in the UMLS Metathesaurus. SemRep then uses these identified concepts with a set of rules, with restrictions determined by the Semantic Network, to determine the relationship, or predicate, between the concepts. The result is the semantic predication Alumina EFFECTS inflammation, allergic.

cTAKES (clinical Text Analysis and Knowledge Extraction System) [14] is a system that extracts a variety of information from provided clinical documents. It performs NER, RelEx, negation detection, part-of-speech, tagging, normalization, sentence boundary detection, tokenization, and more. This tool also makes use of the UMLS for concept normalization.

There are many useful, freely available biomedical NLP resources. The UMLS, MetaMap, SemRep, and cTAKEs are good as tools in their own right or for use as baselines to compare newer methods against.

Pitfall 14.1
Implementing techniques from scratch when not necessary. It is unlikely that a hand-coded pipeline will be as fast as spaCy or cTAKEs when using multiple preprocessing steps.

Machine Learning for NLP

Due to the complexity of human language and the high-dimensional feature space, it is often advantageous to leverage machine learning models. These models often have a larger representational capacity than rule-based systems and often require less specialized expertise to develop. Most of the models that are used in non-NLP tasks can be readily used in NLP tasks. However, it will almost always be necessary to use some sort of a reduced input.

Consider a corpus that has 15,000 unique 1-grams (unigram) that were extracted during preprocessing. One could use a feature vector that simply has a 1 at the position of the desired unigram but this results in highly sparse input with a very high-dimension and it will be difficult, if not impossible, to train a decent model. As such, generating TF-IDF vectors or using vector embeddings will be essential to successfully training machine learning models.

Best Practice 14.2
Document rationale for design decisions. Provide performance metrics (speed and measures of accuracy) where possible.

Pitfall 14.2
Failing to document the results of all experiments can lead to frustration and repeating experiments. Include logging functions to document model parameters and performance metrics to avoid this.

Commonly Used ML Models in NLP

Supervised machine learning is the use of labeled training data to train models. Supervised models are often used in NLP for a variety of tasks. Things such as NER, RelEx, and text classification can be accomplished using models trained using labeled data. In the case of NER, for example, a sentence will have a corresponding BIO label for each token in the sentence and a model will learn to assign a label to each token.

The models typically used for supervised learning on non-NLP tasks can often be used for NLP tasks as well. Logistic regression, random forest, bagging, Naive-Bayes, etc. can all be used for classification and regression tasks in NLP.

Weakly supervised learning is a special case of supervised learning where the labels for the training set are generated using a simple heuristic or set of rules. The goal is to not generate perfect labels, or even good labels, but rather enough labels that sufficiently capture a general relationship between input text and some prediction.

For example, due to the absence of a comprehensive dietary supplement repository, or similarly specialized lexica, using a simple dictionary lookup to generate labels may be sufficient to generate a sizable labeled dataset for training. This also has the advantage of not requiring time consuming manual labeling by domain experts.

Unsupervised machine learning is the use of unlabeled training data to train models. Often, we think of clustering algorithms when unsupervised learning is discussed. While there can be a place for clustering, there are other specific instances of unsupervised learning that are more useful for language.

One such example is **token embedding**, where words are embedded into low-dimensional feature spaces. The key idea behind learning embedded representations of tokens is that semantically similar tokens are embedded more closely together in space than non-similar tokens. This also allows for an arithmetic of sorts to be learned on the embedded representation. The classical example of this is "king - man ~ queen - woman", and, in some instances, this approximation can be true for some embeddings.

Embedding can be done at the level of entire words or at the level of sub-word tokens. In other words, embedding n-character grams rather than complete words. This can help avoid one key issue that word-level embeddings can encounter, Out-of-Vocabulary (OoV) issues. This occurs when one tries to retrieve the embedding for a word that was not present in the training corpus. Since that word was not used, there is not a vector representation of that word in the embedding. This results in very rigid embeddings that require that OoV words be handled during preprocessing to avoid errors.

By embedding n-character grams, words that were not present may be decomposed into strings of characters that are present in the embedding. It is easy to reason that the space of all combinations of, say, 3-character grams is smaller than the space of words. This of course only holds up to a certain n before the space of character combinations exceeds the size of the space of unique words. As mentioned earlier, this is not without its tradeoffs but does come with the advantage of OoV not being as much of a potential issue provided the training set is sufficiently large.

> **Best Practice 14.3**
> Use a grid search over a reasonable set of hyper-parameters to produce the best model possible. This in combination with k-fold cross validation can increase the likelihood that the resulting model will be the strongest and most likely to generalize to unseen data.

Deep Learning in NLP

While traditional machine learning models may successfully perform some NLP tasks to a limited degree, there is an inherent limitation to how far these models can go. The complexity of language is better captured with highly non-linear models that have large representational capacity. This is where deep learning tends to excel. *Deep learning* is the use of neural network models as the model in machine learning tasks.

A *neural network*, in its simplest case, is a sequence of layers of matrix multiplication and non-linear activation functions with the output from one layer being input into the next. This iterative process allows neural networks to learn highly complex, high dimensional representations of the input data.

Models

A large number of the models that have enjoyed success in NLP tasks are models that learn via error back propagation to update model weights. The trends in research have pursued two main veins: increasing the model capacity or architectural innovations.

Increasing model capacity can be as simple as adding more layers or modules to increase the number of learnable parameters (weights) in a model. Innovations often occur in new training techniques, which are necessary in order to facilitate training such large models on massive volumes of data, and can take days or weeks to train on huge clusters of accelerated compute hardware. Architectural advances are actual changes in the ways the model can learn from the data. In the case of transformers, the use of multi-head attention mechanisms and encoder-decoder structures with positional encoding resulted in considerable gains over previous state-of-the-art NLP methods.

In some cases, the changes in training and architecture result in significant changes. As was the case with BERT, which used masked-language modeling pre-training and encoder units to produce a model that can be easily fine-tuned for a variety of tasks without needing to fully retrain a huge model from scratch every time a new task is introduced.

> **Best Practice 14.4**
> Apply appropriate rigor in analyzing the performance of machine learning models. Permutation tests, covariance analysis, etc. can be invaluable for diagnosing issues before deploying models.

RNN, LSTM, biLSTM

A *recurrent neural network* (RNN) [15] is a special type of neural network that passes its internal state (weights) forward as input for each computation in a sequence of data. This allows the network to learn using sequence data and makes them useful for NLP purposes. However, the vanilla RNN can be prone to suffering from vanishing and exploding gradients. This is when the gradients that are back propagated are either so small that the weights do not change enough to learn or are so large the weights change drastically and fail to converge.

While the vanishing and exploding gradient problem can be addressed using techniques such as gradient clipping, they can also be mitigated by using specialized RNN architectures. One such architecture is the **Long Short Term Memory** (LSTM) [16] network. The LSTM introduces "gates", namely, input, output, and forget gates. The forget gate is responsible for preventing gradients from vanishing or exploding.

The LSTM was a significant improvement over the vanilla RNN but can only process sequences in a single direction. To learn the context of a data point in a sequence, it is necessary to consider the points before and after in both directions, thus the **bi-directional LSTM** (biLSTM). The biLSTM is simply a LSTM layer that processes the sequence in the normal manner and a second LSTM layer that processes the reversed input sequence, the outputs are then combined into a single output. The two LSTMs have different sets of weights and internal states. It is often the case that a biLSTM will learn more quickly than an LSTM, depending on the task. In the case of language, where context is important, a biLSTM should often be preferred to an LSTM or RNN.

Transformers. In 2017, the *transformer* [17] architecture was introduced and has since become the basis for most state-of-the-art and fundamental models in NLP. The transformer is a neural transduction model that uses an encoder-decoder structure and self-attention. The use of the novel multi-head, scaled-dot product attention mechanism coupled with the unique architecture within the encoder and decoder layers helped set new state-of-the-art results.

Deep learning, transformer models in particular, can provide significant advantages over traditional machine learning methods, at some cost in terms of additional expertise and increased compute requirements.

BERT. In 2018, a new architecture and training methodology was proposed that used multiple layers of bi-directional transformer encoder layers as well as masked-language modeling and next sentence prediction training on massive amounts of data. The resulting model, Bi-directional Encoder Representations from Transformers (BERT) [18], achieved state-of-the-art results on several benchmarks.

A key advantage of BERT was the ability to extensively pre-train the model then fine-tune the pre-trained weights on individual NLP tasks in considerably less time. This meant that a single, large model could be trained over the course of days, but used indefinitely on any task by fine-tuning over hours or minutes.

For each task, a new prediction layer must be initialized to use the **contextual embedding**, the output from the main BERT model, as input. The weights inside BERT can be frozen or adjusted while training the new prediction layer. There has been work done to identify good fine-tuning procedures for BERT models such as a decaying learning rate with warm-up period, a range for learning rates, batch sizes, etc.

Some useful BERT models that have been trained on biomedical text to varying degrees include: Bio-BERT [19], BioClinical-BERT [20], PubMed-BERT [21], and Blue-BERT [22], to name a few. All of these models can be freely downloaded via huggingface for immediate use.

Best Practice 14.5

When using machine learning models, including deep learning models, always use a simple baseline for comparison. This can be as simple as some rules, a linear regression model, or as complex as a "vanilla" BERT model depending on the task at hand. It may be the case where a random forest will provide adequate performance and be faster at inference than a transformer!

Pitfall 14.3

Jumping straight to the most sophisticated, state of the art model can result in hours spent figuring out how to use a researcher's GitHub repository, or worse, implementing it from scratch based on a paper when a more simple model may have sufficed. Starting with a simple model can, critically, serve as a proof of concept for a product without the resource overhead that comes with many deep learning models.

Graphs

A *graph* is a collection of *vertices* and *edges*. Vertices, or nodes, represent some object or concept (drugs, proteins, diseases, etc.) and edges are relationships between them. A graph is unique in that it contains topological information that is absent in most other data structures. This topological information can be leveraged for NLP, particularly for medical NLP.

> Representing biomedical information with a graph structure can unlock insights via latent topological information that cannot be leveraged with other data structures. While this will not always be applicable, it can be powerful when it is.

Medicine is full of concepts and relationships between them. Drugs treat conditions, diseases affect particular organs, proteins are associated with biological processes. These relationships can be compiled into graph structures for use in tasks such as drug repurposing (a case of link prediction), predicting the type of relationship between nodes (edge classification), and interaction discovery (another case of link prediction).

Due to the special nature of graphs, specialized models have been developed called *graph neural networks* (GNN) [23]. These can come in a variety of flavors, but tend to leverage a mechanism called message passing between nodes to facilitate learning.

Tasks

Link prediction is attempting to determine the potential for two nodes to have some relationship where there currently is none, or rather, predicting the existence of an edge that does not exist. One example of this is to use a trained link prediction model to determine what the most likely connections are to a particular condition. The result of this could be filtered down to a ranked list of drugs that may not currently be used to treat that condition. This is an instance of drug repurposing and it can generate dozens of hypotheses to direct bench research.

Another example of link prediction is to try and predict links between drugs and dietary supplements. Given the lack of published research on drug-supplement interactions, such a task can help uncover potential interactions between a well-understood medication and a less-studied supplement [24].

Edge classification is attempting to determine what type of edge exists between two nodes. In the case of two drugs, for example, a trained edge classification model will attempt to predict the type of interaction between them (e.g. synergistic, opposite, etc.).

Graph Embeddings. A knowledge graph can be quite large and machine learning can be difficult if trying to work with the graph structure directly or one of its matrix representations. A *graph embedding* is a low-dimensional representation of the nodes of a graph. Each node gets associated with a learned vector representation in a low-dimensional vector space. Initial efforts in graph embedding worked in Euclidean or complex space and more recent efforts have explored hyperbolic space as well [25, 26].

Key Concepts in This Chapter

Preprocessing is often required for many NLP tasks but the specific preprocessing techniques will vary by desired outcome. This includes any potential feature extraction that may be used.

There are many useful, freely available biomedical NLP resources. The UMLS, MetaMap, SemRep, and cTAKEs are good as tools in their own right or for baselines to compare newer methods against.

Common NLP tasks that will be useful in a clinical setting include NER and RelEx as techniques of Information Extraction, Concept Normalization, Text Classification, Language Generation, and Question Answering. These can be used as means to ends (e.g. NER to extract entity mentions from patient notes, entity mention counts can be used to generate TF-IDF vectors which can be used in various machine learning models to predict outcomes) or as ends in themselves (e.g. RelEx to find if a patient had an adverse reaction to a particular substance).

Deep learning, transformer models in particular, can provide significant advantages over traditional machine learning methods, at some cost in terms of additional expertise and increased compute requirements.

Representing biomedical information with a graph structure can unlock insights via latent topological information that cannot be leveraged with other data structures. While this will not always be applicable, it can be powerful when it is.

Pitfalls in This Chapter

Pitfall 14.1 Implementing techniques from scratch when not necessary. It is unlikely that a hand-coded pipeline will be as fast as spaCy or cTAKES when using multiple preprocessing steps.

Pitfall 14.2 Failing to document the results of all experiments can lead to frustration and repeating experiments. Include logging functions to document model parameters and performance metrics to avoid this.

Pitfall 14.3 Jumping straight to the most sophisticated, state of the art model can result in hours spent figuring out how to use a researcher's GitHub repository, or worse, implementing it from scratch based on a paper when a simpler model may have sufficed. Starting with a simple model can, critically, serve as a proof of concept for a product without the resource overhead that comes with many deep learning models.

Best Practices in This Chapter

Best Practice 14.1 Always test multiple preprocessing pipelines to find what works best for the desired goals.

Best Practice 14.2 Document rationale for design decisions. Provide performance metrics (speed and measures of accuracy) where possible.

Best Practice 14.3 Use a grid search over a reasonable set of hyper-parameters to produce the best model possible. This in combination with k-fold cross validation can increase the likelihood that the resulting model will be the strongest and most likely to generalize to unseen data.

Best Practice 14.4 Apply appropriate rigor in analyzing the performance of machine learning models. Permutation tests, covariance analysis, etc. can be invaluable for diagnosing issues before deploying models.

Best Practice 14.5 When using machine learning models, including deep learning models, always use a simple baseline for comparison. This can be as simple as some rules, a linear regression model, or as complex as a "vanilla" BERT model depending on the task at hand. It may be the case where a random forest will provide adequate performance and be faster at inference than a transformer!

Questions and Discussion Topics in This Chapter

1. We want to try and determine what supplements patients undergoing surgical operations are using and correlate supplement use against outcomes.
   (a) The first step would be to identify supplements in patient notes. What type of task is this?
       (i) What existing tools might be used for this?
   (b) What types of preprocessing might be necessary?
   (c) How might weakly supervised learning be leveraged in the absence of a gold standard dataset?

2. We want to build a graph using biomedical research papers to investigate potential alternative uses for an existing drug.
   (a) What are some node types that would be of interest? (e.g. drug, gene, etc.)
       (i) What task would this be considered?
       (ii) What would be some advantages of applying concept normalization?
       (iii) What existing tools can help with this?
   (b) What are some edge types that would be of interest? (e.g. affects, treats, etc.)
       (i) What task would this be considered?
       (ii) What existing tools can help with this?
   (c) Assume we do not have annotated data to train a model with. How might a transformer model be leveraged in this case?

(d) Once the graph is constructed, what task are we now dealing with?
  (i) What would be a good baseline model for this task?
  (ii) How could the predictions of the trained model be evaluated?

3. Theoretically speaking, why might a feed-forward neural network outperform a SVM on a language related task? (Consider the capacity of each model)
  (a) What is the key difference between a feed-forward neural network receiving TF-IDF vectors and a LSTM receiving word embeddings? (Is there additional information contained in the sequential of specific tokens?)

4. Explain how the UMLS, MetaMap, SemRep, and SemMedDB are related.

References

1. Mikolov T, Chen K, Corrado G, Dean J. Efficient estimation of word representations in vector space. arXiv:1301.3781 [cs.CL]; 2013.
2. Pennington J, Socher R, Manning CD. GloVe: global vectors for word representation; 2014.
3. Bodenreider O. The Unified Medical Language System (UMLS): integrating biomedical terminology. Nucleic Acids Res. 2004;32(Database issue):D267–70. https://doi.org/10.1093/nar/gkh061.
4. Kilicoglu H, Shin D, Fiszman M, Rosemblat G, Rindflesch TC. SemMedDB: a PubMed-scale repository of biomedical semantic predications. Bioinformatics. 2012;28(23):3158–60. https://doi.org/10.1093/bioinformatics/bts591. Epub 2012 Oct 8.
5. Wang Y, Wang L, Rastegar-Mojarad M, Moon S, Shen F, Afzal N, Liu S, Zeng Y, Mehrabi S, Sohn S, Liu H. Clinical information extraction applications: a literature review. J Biomed Inform. 2018;77:34–49. https://doi.org/10.1016/j.jbi.2017.11.011. Epub 2017 Nov 21.
6. Fan Y, Zhou S, Li Y, Zhang R. Deep learning approaches for extracting adverse events and indications of dietary supplements from clinical text. J Am Med Inform Assoc. 2021;28(3):569–77. https://doi.org/10.1093/jamia/ocaa218.
7. Wang Y, Zhao Y, Schutte D, Bian J, Zhang R. Deep learning models in detection of dietary supplement adverse event signals from Twitter. JAMIA Open. 2021;4(4):ooab081. https://doi.org/10.1093/jamiaopen/ooab081.
8. Zhou S, Schutte D, Xing A, Chen J, Wolfson J, He Z, Fang Y, Zhang R. Identification of dietary supplement use from electronic health records using transformer-based language models. BMC Med Inform Decision Making. 2022;
9. Li J, Zhou Y, Jiang X, Natarajan K, Pakhomov SV, Liu H, Xu H. Are synthetic clinical notes useful for real natural language processing tasks: a case study on clinical entity recognition. J Am Med Inform Assoc. 2021;28(10):2193–201. https://doi.org/10.1093/jamia/ocab112.
10. Singh E, Bompelli A, Wan R, et al. A conversational agent system for dietary supplements use. BMC Med Inform Decis Mak. 2022;22:153. https://doi.org/10.1186/s12911-022-01888-5.
11. Demner-Fushman D, Mrabet Y, Ben AA. Consumer health information and question answering: helping consumers find answers to their health-related information needs. J Am Med Inform Assoc. 2020;27(2):194–201. https://doi.org/10.1093/jamia/ocz152.
12. Aronson AR, Lang FM. An overview of MetaMap: historical perspective and recent advances. J Am Med Inform Assoc. 2010;17(3):229–36. https://doi.org/10.1136/jamia.2009.002733.
13. Kilicoglu H, Rosemblat G, Fiszman M, Shin D. Broad-coverage biomedical relation extraction with SemRep. BMC Bioinform. 2020;21(1):188. https://doi.org/10.1186/s12859-020-3517-7.
14. Savova GK, Masanz JJ, Ogren PV, Zheng J, Sohn S, Kipper-Schuler KC, Chute CG. Mayo clinical Text Analysis and Knowledge Extraction System (cTAKES): architecture,

component evaluation and applications. J Am Med Inform Assoc. 2010;17(5):507–13. https://doi.org/10.1136/jamia.2009.001560.

15. Rumelhart DE, Hinton GE, Williams RJ. Learning internal representations by error propagation. Tech. rep. ICS 8504. San Diego, CA: Institute for Cognitive Science, University of California; 1985.

16. Hochreiter S, Schmidhuber J. Long short-term memory. Neural Comput. 1997;9(8):1735–80. https://doi.org/10.1162/neco.1997.9.8.1735.

17. Attention is all you need. NIPS'17: Proceedings of the 31st international conference on neural information processing systems; 2017, pp. 6000–6010

18. Devlin J, Chang M-W, Lee K, Toutanova K. BERT: Pre-training of deep bidirectional transformers for language understanding. NAACL-HLT. 2019;(1):4171–86.

19. Lee J, Yoon W, Kim S, et al. BioBERT: a pre-trained biomedical language representation model for biomedical text mining. Bioinformatics. 2020;36:1234–40.

20. Alsentzer E, Murphy J, Boag W, et al. Publicly available clinical BERT embeddings. In: Proceedings of the 2nd clinical natural language processing workshop; 2019, pp. 72–8.

21. Gu Y, Tinn R, Cheng H, et al. Domain-specific language model pretraining for biomedical natural language processing. ArXiv200715779 Cs Published Online First: 20 August 2020. http://arxiv.org/abs/2007.15779. Accessed 25 Sep 2020.

22. Peng Y, Yan S, Lu Z. Transfer learning in biomedical natural language processing: an evaluation of BERT and ELMo on ten benchmarking datasets. In: Proceedings of the 18th BioNLP workshop and shared task; 2019, pp. 58–65.

23. Scarselli F, Gori M, Tsoi AC, Hagenbuchner M, Monfardini G. The graph neural network model. IEEE Trans Neural Netw. 2009;20(1):61–80. https://doi.org/10.1109/TNN.2008.2005605. Epub 2008 Dec 9.

24. Schutte D, Vasilakes J, Bompelli A, Zhou Y, Fiszman M, Xu H, Kilicoglu H, Bishop JR, Adam T, Zhang R. Discovering novel drug-supplement interactions using SuppKG generated from the biomedical literature. J Biomed Inform. 2022;131:104120. https://doi.org/10.1016/j.jbi.2022.104120. Epub 20.

25. Choudhary S, Luthra T, Mittal A, Singh R. A survey of knowledge graph embedding and their applications. arXiv preprint arXiv:2107.07842; 2021.

26. Nickel M, Kiela D. Poincaré embeddings for learning hierarchical representations. Adv Neural Inform Process Syst. 2017;30

Considerations for Specialized Health AI & ML Modelling and Applications: Imaging—Through the Perspective of Dermatology

Dennis H. Murphree, Anirudh Choudhary,
Puneet K. Bhullar, and Nneka I. Comfere

Abstract

This chapter focuses on healthcare applications of deep learning in computer vision, specifically in the context of dermatology and dermatopathology.

Keywords

Convolutional neural networks · Computer vision tasks · Architectures for dermatology · Pathology

Introduction

Artificial intelligence and machine learning have made impressive progress in recent years, particularly in the realm of image analysis. In healthcare many specialties are image-centric in their data focus, with dermatology being a prime example. Other specialties that employ the astonishing power of deep neural networks when applied to images include radiology, cardiology and ophthalmology amongst others. Some non-image datasets have even been successfully recast as images in order to take advantage of the power of convolutional networks, for example treating the time series from 12-lead electrocardiograms as if they were images.

D. H. Murphree (✉) · N. I. Comfere
Department of Dermatology, Mayo Clinic, Rochester, MN, USA
e-mail: murphree.dennis@mayo.edu

A. Choudhary
Department of Computer Science, University of Illinois, Urbana-Champaign, IL, USA

P. K. Bhullar
Department of Dermatology, Mayo Clinic, Scottsdale, AZ, USA

In modern day (2022) dermatology, the intersection with artificial intelligence appears in several forms. In this chapter we will describe the dermatology AI landscape, providing an overview of the types of questions commonly asked and the data and processing needed to attempt to answer those questions.

We also suggest that while we warmly embrace the progress that AI in dermatology has made, in our opinion the most helpful frameworks going forward will likely fall under the category of "augmented intelligence", wherein humans and computers work synergistically to improve care delivery [1]. We also wish to direct the reader to Chapter '"From "Human versus Machine" to "Human with Machine"' for a discussion of AI-assisted decision making.

Please note that fully explaining many of the best practices and pitfalls identified in this chapter is beyond a reasonable scope. Rather they are intended to point the interested reader in the right direction.

Brief Review

Recent advances of AI in dermatology have primarily depended on leveraging so called **deep neural networks** (DNNs). This style of learning uses neural network-based computational models consisting of multiple processing layers. Traditional artificial neural networks (ANNs) are typically comprised of a limited number of layers built of a linear combination of "nodes". A node is similar to a linear regression model embedded inside a non-linear activation function. The weights both internal to the nodes as well as those in the combination of nodes are optimized from the data, and the network is trained to obtain supervised representations optimized for a specific task.

Deep neural networks have more complex architectures with a higher number of layers and connections, thus allowing them to learn data representations with multiple levels of abstraction. DNNs are usually trained in an end-to-end manner using backpropagation. In AI-based dermatology studies, the most common architecture employed is a special variety known as a **convolutional neural network (CNN)**.

> **Convolutional neural networks** are the primary AI tools in dermatology as of 2022.

CNNs are inspired by the visual cortex and leverage a convolution operator (a combination of matrix multiplication and summation) followed by feature pooling (averaging) to learn translation-invariant representations. They achieve superior performance due to their capacity to learn and extract deep and hierarchical features from skin image datasets. Current CNN architectures typically consist of multiple convolutional and pooling layers stacked together to model the input data space, where the output of one layer serves as the input to the following. Many state-of-the-art architectures used in dermatology have originally been developed by technology companies, and include examples such as ResNet, DenseNet121, EfficientNet and GoogleNet.

Best Practice 15.1
Always start with a known state-of-the-art network architecture rather than designing your own. EfficientNet is often a (relatively) fast way to see if your dataset has an extractable signal.

The most prevalent applications of AI in dermatology have been via traditional supervised learning, wherein a DNN is trained to learn the relationship between input data and known corresponding target labels. Examples of supervised learning include CNNs trained for skin cancer diagnosis, risk stratification of skin cancer (indolent vs aggressive), and general lesion identification.

DNNs require significant amounts of training data to perform well, and current dermatology datasets particularly pathology datasets are of limited size relative to massive troves of internet photographs, for example, ImageNet, used by major technology firms in training models. An important improvement therefore to the traditional training of DNNs for use in dermatology is transfer learning. In transfer learning, instead of starting from scratch, one begins with a network that is known to perform well on a similar problem. Transfer learning dramatically reduces the amount of training data required, and is particularly useful when examples with known outcomes can be challenging to acquire. Unsurprisingly, many of the published dermatology deep learning studies to date employ transfer learning to train their DNNs.

Best Practice 15.2
Use transfer learning any time you can find a dataset similar enough to yours.

Pitfall 15.1
When using transfer learning, if you cannot find a dataset naturally similar to yours and must start with weights from e.g. ImageNet, always try training from scratch as well. In pathology in particular sometimes it is better to just start over.

For a more complete description of these topics specific to dermatology, please see Murphree et al. [2] and Puri et al. [3]. For more general descriptions please consult [4] or [5].

Current Applications

Broadly speaking applications of computer vision in dermatology can be categorized either by input data or by problem type.

Categorizing application by input type. Input data is usually one of the following: clinical photographs, dermoscopic photographs, or digitized pathology slides (also known as whole slide images, or WSI). Dermoscopic photos are captured via special instruments known as dermatoscopes. These instruments are used by dermatologists to reduce reflections from the skin, and provide for a more uniform but very distinctive looking image. Dermoscopic images are immediately distinguishable from standard photographs by their unique circular appearance. Clinical photographs obtained by providers are often different enough in quality from those captured by patients that the two can be considered different data types.

Best Practice 15.3
Be alert to data differences in photographs acquired by patients vs those acquired by medical photographers or informed providers. If you mix them, be certain to check that there is balance among outcomes by origin. Are photographs acquired in a dermatologists office more likely to contain cases than controls?

Categorizing applications by problem type. Problem type is most typically supervised learning, where a label of interest is known for each observation, and can appear as classification or segmentation. For example, photographs of lesions may be labeled as malignant or benign. Similarly, regions of a pathology slide may be labeled (annotated) as epidermis, dermis, eccrine gland, etc. In the first case one might seek to classify the lesion in the photograph, while in the second one might seek to segment the slide into different regions of known tissue type. Often the two are combined, for example segmenting a slide to identify regions of tumor, then using those regions as training data input for e.g. a tumor risk classifier.

In addition to traditional supervised learning, in the pathology space in particular there is growing interest in weakly supervised learning, where expensive pixel-level annotations can be replaced in favor of slide-level labels. Slide level labels are often able to be extracted in an automated fashion from electronic health records, thus do not require manual effort by pathology specialists.

Best Practice 15.4
Weakly supervised learning may be a promising future direction to alleviate the burden of acquiring costly and time-consuming pixel level annotations.

Here we discuss different current or recent applications divided by problem type, with a special section on dermatopathology.

Classification

In a **classification problem**, the goal is to learn a label (or set of labels) for an image in its entirety. For example, given a photograph of a skin lesion the classifier might distinguish between melanoma and benign nevus, and if melanoma then might further characterize it as aggressive or indolent.

Given the understandably pressing nature of the disease, the vast majority of AI applications in dermatology have focused on cancer, primarily cutaneous lesions. Comparatively less attention has been paid other categories of skin disease such as inflammatory dermatoses (rashes). This may also be driven in part by the greater spatial uniformity of lesions in general. Here we will discuss only lesions.

Various AI-based approaches have been developed in the detection and diagnosis of skin cancer ranging from conventional low-level pixel processing methods using handcrafted features to more recent CNN-based deep learning approaches. CNNs have achieved state-of-the-art performance in skin lesion analysis along with superior performance to dermatologists in distinguishing between pigmented and non-pigmented skin lesions across multiple studies. For example, Esteva et al. [6] was the first to propose a CNN model to identify epidermal and melanocytic lesions, comparing its performance to 21 board-certified dermatologists on two specific tasks: distinguishing squamous cell carcinomas (SCC) from benign seborrheic keratoses (SK) and malignant melanomas from benign nevi. On a biopsy-proven test set of 135 epidermal, 130 melanocytic non-dermoscopy images and 111 melanocytic dermoscopy images, dermatologists were asked whether to biopsy, treat the lesion or reassure the patient without biopsy. In parallel, the CNN was tasked with classifying the same lesions. The network outperformed the average performance of the dermatologists in each case. The authors conclude by graphical inspection that the CNN's performance was comparable to that of the board-certified dermatologists. However, we note that no formal statistical test was applied. Concurrently, Han et al. (2019) [7] used a ResNet-based CNN to automatically classify 12 skin disorders, achieving a level of performance comparable to 16 dermatologists. The network determined coarse and irregular portions of the lesion as important features for malignant tumors, which was highlighted via gradient-based activation maps (Grad-CAM) generated from the CNN. The activation maps allowed interpretability of the CNN's classification output. Another study by Codella et al. [8] combined CNN with hand-coded features and sparse coding which could potentially achieve higher accuracy than dermatologists in melanoma detection. Brinker et al. (2019) [9] proposed an enhanced CNN architecture for skin lesion classification using 12,378 images. They did a thorough evaluation by comparing the classification performance of their CNN on 100 images and to that of 157 dermatologists across 12 university hospitals in Germany. This system was shown by some metrics to outperform the average dermatologist.

Haenssle et al. (2018) [10] similarly sought to compare the performance of a CNN trained to recognize melanoma in dermoscopic images to 58 international dermatologists with varying levels of experience in dermoscopy (29% beginner, 19% skilled, and 52% expert by self-report). The dermatologists were asked to classify lesions in two stages, including dermoscopy alone in the first stage and dermoscopy with clinical images and additional clinical information in the second stage. While the stage II performance of both beginner and skilled dermatologists improved significantly relative to stage I, the CNN, which was trained on images only still outperformed dermatologists of all experience levels in both the stages. This study highlights the importance of including a large group of dermatologists with varying levels of experience, as well as using open source datasets and lesions from different anatomic sites and of different histologic types during CNN training. They also demonstrate the importance of integrating clinical information and clinical experience when comparing human performance to algorithmic performance.

Recently, Soensken et al. (2021) [11] proposed a deep CNN which identifies early-stage melanoma by capturing wide-field photographs of patient bodies using mobile phones, subsequently ranking suspicious pigmented lesions (SPL) and flagging them for further examination. The AI tool achieved more than 90% sensitivity in distinguishing SPL from non-suspicious lesions and achieved comparable performance to board-certified dermatologists, thus highlighting its efficacy as a successful triage tool.

While the above studies are highlighted for their CNN performance in comparison to human dermatologists, there are numerous studies that address lesion identification. Most of these studies are focused on improved algorithmic performance with some of the recent studies focusing on improving model robustness. For example, Han et al (2018) [12] demonstrated that CNNs trained on images from Asian patients performed poorly on Caucasian patients and vice-versa, highlighting the importance of training CNNs with skin lesions from a wide range of age groups and ethnicities. Gessert et al. (2020) [13] used an ensemble of deep learning models including EfficientNets, SENet, and ResNeXt WSL using a search strategy for skin lesion classification. Maron et al. (2021) [14] proposed a benchmark out-of-distribution dataset for melanoma detection by adding artificial noise-based corruption and image perturbations to lesion images and observed that while DenseNet121 [15] showed the best corruption robustness, AlexNet achieved better perturbation robustness. Sayed, Soliman, and Hassanien (2021) [16] proposed an approach to tackle class-imbalance in existing melanoma classification datasets from ISIC challenges [17] and proposed a random over-sampling method followed by data augmentation achieving state-of-the-art accuracy using a simpler CNN architecture named SqueezeNet [18].

Although the mentioned studies demonstrate the richness and variety of applications of CNNs to classifying a variety of cutaneous lesions, including some that appear to perform well relative to non-specialists or trainees, at this time (2022) there appears to be only a single prospective clinical trial [19] utilizing AI for skin disease. We look forward to seeing more of these trials performed.

Segmentation

Segmentation is similar to classification, but rather than trying to predict a label for an image in its entirety it seeks to do so for each pixel in the image.

This problem is in many ways more challenging than classification. Nevertheless, deep learning has achieved promising success in skin lesion segmentation, in particular with melanoma. Lesion segmentation is still a challenging task for deep learning methods because of various complexities including regions of interest (ROIs) of varying shapes and sizes, fuzzy boundaries, capture-dependent color variation and the presence of hair. Due to these complexities, traditional "handcrafted" approaches such as those based on thresholding, region-based active contour models or clustering tend to underperform. In contrast, CNN-based methods can automatically create features that are maximally helpful, for example, to distinguish lesions from normal skin. Most segmentation frameworks leverage an encoder-decoder network wherein an "encoder" network consisting of convolution and pooling layers is used to extract features from the input image which are then passed to a "decoder" network which performs a series of unpooling and disconnection operations to construct the segmentation output. Goyal, Yap, and Hassanpour (2017) [20] used Fully Convolutional Networks (FCN) to learn hierarchical features and derive multi-class segmentation maps for three distinct forms of skin lesions: benign nevi, melanoma, and seborrheic keratoses. Yuan and Lo (2019) [21] achieved the highest segmentation accuracy (Jaccard (JAC) index of 76.5%) in the International Skin Imaging Collaboration's (ISIC) 2017 challenges [17] by using a 19-layer convolutional-deconvolutional neural network to segment skin lesions by training their model with different color spaces of dermoscopy images. Sarker et al. (2018) [22] proposed an architecture combining skip-connections, dilated residual and multi-scale pyramid pooling networks to extract additional contextual information. They also leveraged End Point Error as a content loss function to preserve melanoma boundaries.

The most popular architecture which has achieved state-of-the-art performance in skin lesion segmentation is U-Net [23].

U-Net was proposed for biomedical image segmentation and is based on Fully Convolutional Networks (FCN) for natural object detection. It has a U-shaped architecture which concatenates the feature maps from the encoder layer with corresponding upsampled decoder feature maps using "skip-connections", thus allowing it to retain fine-grained details required for segmentation. Lin et al. (2017) [24] did the initial study highlighting the efficacy of U-Net based histogram equalization (dice coefficient of 77%) over C-means clustering (dice coefficient of 61%) for skin lesion segmentation. Various architectures combining U-Net with alternate CNN architectures have been proposed subsequently. For instance, Zafar et al. (2020) [25] proposed a fully automatic skin lesion segmentation combining U-Net and ResNet achieving an average JAC Index of 77.2% on ISIC-2017 dataset. Recently, Ashraf et al. (2022) [26] highlighted that a JAC Index above 80% in lesion segmentation guarantees that the approach is reliable and appropriate for subjective clinical assessment. They proposed three deep learning models, including U-Net, deep residual U-Net (ResUNet), and improved ResUNet (ResUNet++) along with an improved pre-processing pipeline employing an inpainting algorithm to eliminate unnecessary hair structures. They also leveraged test time image augmentation and a conditional random field (CRF) in the postprocessing stage achieving state-of-the-art 80.73% Jaccard index on ISIC 2017 dataset.

Dermatopathology

Deep learning in dermatopathology is centered around traditional pathology slides that are digitized into images (WSIs) by scanners. Histology whole slides provide a much greater amount of cellular-level information highlighting morphological and spatial arrangement, thus making them attractive for deep learning-based biomarker extraction.

> Due to their immense size, special technical considerations are critically important when working with digitized pathology slide images. Currently the best practice is to divide the slide into smaller patches of tissue, often chosen to match a given neural network architecture.

> **Best Practice 15.5**
> A common paradigm for deep learning on pathology slides is to first divide the slide into small patches of tissue. Then one trains a tissue-level classifier, typically a deep neural network. This predicts the type of tissue in the patch using labels from pixel-level annotations. Afterwards, a slide-level classifier can be trained to predict using the tissue-level predictions as input and the slide labels as output. The slide-level classifier is typically a model such as logistic regression, often chosen to avoid overfitting.

Pitfall 15.2

While important in all applications of ML in healthcare, deep learning on whole slide images is especially prone to inadvertently learning biases in the dataset rather than actual physiology. A pernicious example is that of scanner effects. In a scanner effect, the model learns which scanner was used to aquire an image. This causes problems when one outcome of interest is more frequently acquired on one model of scanner, something common in multicenter studies. A red flag is if many examples of a single (potentially rare) disease need to be supplied by a single institution. Similar biases can occur if images are acquired using different staining protocols or scanning parameters.

The majority of applications of AI in dermatopathology to date have focused on the traditional formalin-fixed paraffin embedded tissue that is the mainstay of modern pathology. However, there is growing interest in also utilizing the fresh frozen tissue common in dermatologic surgery.

A prototypical AI project in dermatopathology focuses on extracting several features from WSI for diagnostic prediction tasks such as cancer grading or cancer subtyping. Moreno-Andrés et al. [27] developed a diagnostic support tool to identify mitotic cells within detected tumor regions for whole slide images (WSI). The authors report a diagnostic accuracy of 83% for their model trained on 59 WSIs. This tool could augment a dermatopathologist's practice by identifying areas of the slide with the highest density of mitotic figures, and could also potentially reduce the need for the immunohistochemical stains for mitosis.

Olsen et al [28] similarly trained a CNN using 450 WSI to classify basal cell carcinomas, dermal nevi, and seborrheic keratoses. Their Visual Geometry Group (VGG) network achieved an AUC of 0.99 for basal cell carcinomas, 0.97 for dermal nevi, and 0.99 for seborrheic keratoses. Hart et al [29] developed a CNN to differentiate between Spitz and conventional melanocytic lesions on histopathology. They trained their model on 100 curated whole slide images and first evaluated their model on curated image sections. Their model demonstrated 99% accuracy in this experiment. They then conducted a second experiment evaluating the model's performance on noncurated image patches of the entire slide. In contrast to the curated experiment, the model achieved a significantly lower accuracy of 52.3% on the noncurated patches. Hekler et al [30] built a similar CNN trained on 695 whole slide images to classify images as melanoma or benign nevi. They compared the performance of their CNN to dermatopathologists. Performance was evaluated on randomly cropped 10× magnification sections. The CNN achieved a melanoma sensitivity/specificity/accuracy of 76%/60%/68% respectively, while the 11 dermatopathologists achieved a mean sensitivity/specificity/accuracy of 51.8%/66.5%/59.2% respectively. However, these results should be interpreted with caution—in a normal clinical setting, pathologists have the ability to evaluate the whole slide and are not restricted to randomly cropped segments.

Sankarapandian et al. [31] presented a deep learning-based triaging system which performs hierarchical melanocytic specimen classification into low (MPATH I-II), Intermediate (MPATH III), or High (MPATH IV-V) diagnostic categories, enabling prioritization of melanoma cases. They leverage transfer learning using a pretrained ResNet50 network for extracting patch-level features from WSI and formulate the classification problem in a weakly-supervised multiple instance paradigm using tissue-level labels only. By combining patch features using max-pooling, their tool is able to classify suspected melanoma without requiring pixel-level annotations and could substantially reduce diagnostic turnaround time for melanoma by ensuring that suspected melanoma cases are routed directly to subspecialists.

Thomas et al. [32] proposed an interpretable deep learning method to classify several common skin cancers (basal cell carcinoma, squamous cell carcinoma and intraepidermal carcinoma) using WSI. Using manual labelling they characterised the tissue into 12 meaningful dermatological classes, including hair follicles, sweat glands as well as identifying the well-defined stratified layers of the skin. Subsequently, they trained a classifier to classify the sub-regions of WSI into the 12 classes thus representing the WSI with a segmentation map similar to a pathologist. By analysing the tissue context using the segmentation map obtained from the classifier, they achieved high accuracy of WSI classification as well as ensured interpretability.

One notable limitation in the dermatopathology literature is the limited work on leveraging AI to predict patient prognosis and response to therapy based on the morphological slide features. While existing approaches have tried to link pathological features, such as tumour grade and subtype, to effective patient prognosis, none of the methods have demonstrated a direct link between pathology images with multiscale features as well as patient's genetic profiles with survival outcomes and treatment response for adjuvant/neoadjuvant therapy.

Datasets and Challenges

All of the approaches described here depend critically on sufficient quantities of appropriate data, ideally free of biases and representative of a wide variety of patients. While this is unlikely to ever be achieved in practice, dermatology benefits from several large, publicly available datasets. Many of these datasets have been partially combined under the auspices of the International Skin Imaging Collaboration (ISIC) Archive [17]. Although the ISIC Archive has several known limitations [33], it is an invaluable resource for advancing AI research in dermatology. The collaboration also hosts challenges [17] each year, typically associated with prominent computer vision conferences, that provide an engaging opportunity for computer scientists to apply new techniques to relevant dermatologic problems.

Best Practice 15.6
Keep an up-to-date list of publicly available datasets so that you can use them when appropriate.

Conclusion

As an image-centric specialty dermatology has become an area of particular interest for applications of artificial intelligence and computer vision in healthcare. While many approaches have focused on pigmented and non-pigmented lesions, melanoma in particular, the field is vast, encompassing some 3000 known skin diseases and affecting approximate one third of the global population [34–36]. The opportunity this presents to ease the global disease burden, particularly by enhancing remote access to specialty care, is incredibly exciting and we look forward to its bright future.

Key Concepts in This Chapter

Deep Neurual Networks, especially convolutional neural networks, are the primary AI tools in dermatology as of 2022.

Broadly speaking applications of computer vision in dermatology can be categorized either by input data or by problem type.

Input data is usually one of the following: clinical photographs, dermoscopic photographs, or digitized pathology slides (also known as whole slide images, or WSI).

Problem type is most typically supervised learning, where a label of interest is known for each observation, and can appear as classification or segmentation.

In a classification problem, the goal is to learn a label (or set of labels) for an image in its entirety. For example, given a photograph of a skin lesion the classifier might distinguish between melanoma and benign nevus, and if melanoma then might further characterize it as aggressive or indolent.

Segmentation is similar to classification, but rather than trying to predict a label for an image in its entirety it seeks to do so for each pixel in the image.

The most popular architecture which has achieved state-of-the-art performance in skin lesion segmentation is U-Net.

Due to their immense size, special technical considerations are critically important when working with digitized pathology slide images. Currently the best practice is to divide the slide into smaller patches of tissue, often chosen to match a given neural network architecture.

Pitfalls in This Chapter

Pitfall 1. When using transfer learning, if you cannot find a dataset naturally similar to yours and must start with weights from e.g. ImageNet, always try training from scratch as well. In pathology in particular sometimes it is better to just start over.

Pitfall 2. While important in all applications of ML in healthcare, deep learning on whole slide images is especially prone to inadvertently learning biases in the dataset rather than actual physiology. A pernicious example is that of scanner effects. In a scanner effect, the model learns which scanner was used to aquire an image. This causes problems when one outcome of interest is more frequently acquired on one model of scanner, something common in multicenter studies. Similar biases can occur if images are acquired using different staining protocols or scanning parameters.

Best Practices in This Chapter

Best Practice 15.1. Always start with a known state-of-the-art network architecture rather than designing your own. EfficientNet is often a (relatively) fast way to see if your dataset has an extractable signal.

Best Practice 15.2. Use transfer learning any time you can find a dataset similar enough to yours. See pitfall below however.

Best Practice 15.3. Be alert to data differences in photographs acquired by patients vs those acquired by medical photographers or informed providers. If you mix them, be certain to check that there is balance among outcomes by origin.

Best Practice 15.4. Weakly supervised learning may be a promising future direction to alleviate the burden of acquiring costly and time-consuming pixel level annotations.

Best Practice 15.5. A common paradigm for deep learning on pathology slides is to first divide the slide into small patches of tissue. Then one trains a tissue-level classifier, typically a deep neural network. This predicts the type of tissue in the patch using labels from pixel-level annotations. Afterwards, a slide-level classifier can be trained to predict using the tissue-level predictions as input and the slide labels as output. The slide-level classifier is typically a model such as logistic regression, often chosen to avoid overfitting.

Best Practice 15.6. Keep an up-to-date list of publicly available datasets so that you can use them when appropriate.

Questions and Discussion Topics in This Chapter

1. Discuss: Are photographs acquired in a dermatologists office more likely to contain cases than controls?

2. Describe a red flag to look for when being alert to scanner effects.

3. What is the primary difference between supervised learning and weakly supervised learning?

4. Noise and artifacts may be present in images that are not visible to the human eye. Read this blog post by Andrew Janowczyk: http://www.andrewjanowczyk. com/the-noise-in-our-digital-pathology-slides/
   (a) How might this affect a study?
   (b) What approaches could you take to mitigate it?

5. What are some of the ways that published studies have compared machine performance to dermatologist performance? Do any study designs have particular advantages or disadvantages?

References

1. Kovarik C, Lee I, Ko J. Ad Hoc Task Force on Augmented Intelligence. Commentary: position statement on augmented intelligence (AuI). J Am Acad Dermatol. 2019;81(4):998–1000. https://doi.org/10.1016/j.jaad.2019.06.032. Epub 2019 Jun 25.
2. Murphree DH, Puri P, Shamim H, Bezalel SA, Drage LA, Wang M, Pittelkow MR, Carter RE, Davis MDP, Bridges AG, Mangold AR, Yiannias JA, Tollefson MM, Lehman JS, Meves A, Otley CC, Sokumbi O, Hall MR, Comfere N. Deep learning for dermatologists: Part I. Fundamental concepts. J Am Acad Dermatol. 2022;87:1343–51. https://doi.org/10.1016/j.jaad.2020.05.056.
3. Puri P, Comfere N, Drage LA, Shamim H, Bezalel SA, Pittelkow MR, Davis MDP, Wang M, Mangold AR, Tollefson MM, Lehman JS, Meves A, Yiannias JA, Otley CC, Carter RE, Sokumbi O, Hall MR, Bridges AG, Murphree DH. Deep learning for dermatologists: Part II. Current applications. J Am Acad Dermatol. 2022;87, 6:1352–60. https://doi.org/10.1016/j.jaad.2020.05.053.
4. LeCun Y, Bengio Y, Hinton G. Deep learning. Nature. 2015;521:436–44. https://doi.org/10.1038/nature14539.
5. Goodfellow I, Bengio Y, Courville A. Deep learning. Cambridge, Massachusetts: The MIT Press; 2016.
6. Esteva A, Kuprel B, Novoa RA, Ko J, Swetter SM, Blau HM, Thrun S. Dermatologist-level classification of skin cancer with deep neural networks. Nature. 2017;542(7639):115–8. https://doi.org/10.1038/nature21056.
7. Han SS, Park GH, Lim W, Kim MS, Na JI, Park I, Chang SE. Deep neural networks show an equivalent and often superior performance to dermatologists in onychomycosis diagnosis: automatic construction of onychomycosis datasets by region-based convolutional deep neural network. PLoS One. 2018;13(1):e0191493. https://doi.org/10.1371/journal.pone.0191493.
8. Codella N, Cai J, Abedini M, Garnavi R, Halpern A, Smith JR. Deep learning, sparse coding, and SVM for melanoma recognition in dermoscopy images. In: Machine Learning in Medical Imaging (Lecture Notes in Computer Science), pp. 118–126; 2015. doi: https://doi.org/10.1007/978-3-319-24888-2_15
9. Brinker TJ, Hekler A, Enk AH, von Kalle C. Enhanced classifier training to improve precision of a convolutional neural network to identify images of skin lesions. PLOS One. 2019;14(6):e0218713. https://doi.org/10.1371/journal.pone.0218713.
10. Haenssle HA, Fink C, Schneiderbauer R, Toberer F, Buhl T, Blum A, Kalloo A, Hassen ABH, Thomas L, Enk A, Uhlmann L, Reader study level-I and level-II Groups, Alt C, Arenbergerova M, Bakos R, Baltzer A, Bertlich I, Blum A, Bokor-Billmann T, Bowling J, Braghiroli N, Braun R, Buder-Bakhaya K, Buhl T, Cabo H, Cabrijan L, Cevic N, Classen A, Deltgen D, Fink C, Georgieva I, Hakim-Meibodi L-E, Hanner S, Hartmann F, Hartmann J, Haus G, Hoxha E, Karls R, Koga H, Kreusch J, Lallas A, Majenka P, Marghoob A, Massone C, Mekokishvili L, Mestel D, Meyer V, Neuberger A, Nielsen K, Oliviero M, Pampena R, Paoli J, Pawlik E, Rao B, Rendon A, Russo T, Sadek A, Samhaber K, Schneiderbauer R, Schweizer A, Toberer F, Trennheuser L, Vlahova L, Wald A, Winkler J, Wölbing P, Zalaudek I. Man against machine:

diagnostic performance of a deep learning convolutional neural network for dermoscopic melanoma recognition in comparison to 58 dermatologists. Ann Oncol. 2018;29(8):1836–42. https://doi.org/10.1093/annonc/mdy166.

11. Soenksen LR, Kassis T, Conover ST, Marti-Fuster B, Birkenfeld JS, Tucker-Schwartz J, Naseem A, Stavert RR, Kim CC, Senna MM, Avilés-Izquierdo J, Collins JJ, Barzilay R, Gray ML. Using deep learning for dermatologist-level detection of suspicious pigmented skin lesions from wide-field images. Sci Transl Med. 2021;13, 581:eabb3652. https://doi.org/10.1126/scitranslmed.abb3652.

12. Han SS, Kim MS, Lim W, Park GH, Park I, Chang SE. Classification of the clinical images for benign and malignant cutaneous tumors using a deep learning algorithm. J Invest Dermatol. 2018;138(7):1529–38. https://doi.org/10.1016/j.jid.2018.01.028.

13. Gessert N, Nielsen M, Shaikh M, Werner R, Schlaefer A. Skin lesion classification using ensembles of multi-resolution EfficientNets with meta data. MethodsX. 2020;7:100864. https://doi.org/10.1016/j.mex.2020.100864.

14. Maron RC, Schlager JG, Haggenmüller S, von Kalle C, Utikal JS, Meier F, Gellrich FF, Hobelsberger S, Hauschild A, French L, Heinzerling L, Schlaak M, Ghoreschi K, Hilke FJ, Poch G, Heppt MV, Berking C, Haferkamp S, Sondermann W, Schadendorf D, Schilling B, Goebeler M, Krieghoff-Henning E, Hekler A, Fröhling S, Lipka DB, Kather JN, Brinker TJ. A benchmark for neural network robustness in skin cancer classification. Eur J Cancer. 2021;155:191–9. https://doi.org/10.1016/j.ejca.2021.06.047.

15. Huang G, Liu Z, Van Der Maaten L, Weinberger KQ. Densely connected convolutional networks. In Proceedings of the IEEE conference on computer vision and pattern recognition; 2017, pp. 4700–4708.

16. Sayed GI, Soliman MM, Hassanien AE. A novel melanoma prediction model for imbalanced data using optimized SqueezeNet by bald eagle search optimization. Comput Biol Med. 2021;136:104712. https://doi.org/10.1016/j.compbiomed.2021.104712.

17. ISIC Challenge. https://challenge.isic-archive.com/. Accessed 24 Dec 2022

18. Iandola FN, Han S, Moskewicz MW, Ashraf K, Dally WJ, Keutzer K. SqueezeNet: AlexNet-level accuracy with 50x fewer parameters and< 0.5 MB model size. arXiv preprint arXiv:1602.07360; 2016.

19. Han SS, Kim YJ, Moon IJ, Jung JM, Lee MY, Lee WJ, Won CH, Lee MW, Kim SH, Navarrete-Dechent C, Chang SE. Evaluation of artificial intelligence–assisted diagnosis of skin neoplasms: a single-center, paralleled, unmasked, randomized controlled trial. J Invest Dermatol. 2022;142(9):2353–2362.e2. https://doi.org/10.1016/j.jid.2022.02.003.

20. Goyal M, Yap MH, Hassanpour S. Multi-class semantic segmentation of skin lesions via fully convolutional networks. *arXiv preprint arXiv:1711.10449*; 2017.

21. Yuan Y, Lo Y-C. Improving dermoscopic image segmentation with enhanced convolutional-deconvolutional networks. IEEE J Biomed Health Inform. 2019;23(2):519–26. https://doi.org/10.1109/JBHI.2017.2787487.

22. Sarker MMK, Rashwan HA, Akram F, Banu SF, Saleh A, Singh VK, Chowdhury FUH, Abdulwahab S, Romani S, Radeva P, Puig D. SLSDeep: skin lesion segmentation based on dilated residual and pyramid pooling networks. In *Medical image computing and computer assisted intervention—MICCAI 2018* (Lecture Notes in Computer Science), pp. 21–29; 2018. doi: https://doi.org/10.1007/978-3-030-00934-2_3

23. Ronneberger O, Fischer P, Brox T. U-Net: convolutional networks for biomedical image segmentation. In *Medical image computing and computer-assisted intervention—MICCAI 2015* (Lecture Notes in Computer Science), pp. 234–241; 2015. doi: https://doi.org/10.1007/978-3-319-24574-4_28

24. Lin BS, Michael K, Kalra S, Tizhoosh HR. Skin lesion segmentation: U-nets versus clustering. In *2017 IEEE symposium series on computational intelligence (SSCI)*, pp. 1–7; 2017.

25. Zafar K, Gilani SO, Waris A, Ahmed A, Jamil M, Khan MN, Kashif AS. Skin lesion segmentation from dermoscopic images using convolutional neural network. Sensors. 2020;20(6):1601. https://doi.org/10.3390/s20061601.

26. Ashraf H, Waris A, Ghafoor MF, Gilani SO, Niazi IK. Melanoma segmentation using deep learning with test-time augmentations and conditional random fields. Sci Reports. 2022;12(1):3948. https://doi.org/10.1038/s41598-022-07885-y.

27. Moreno-Andrés D, Bhattacharyya A, Scheufen A, Stegmaier J. LiveCellMiner: A new tool to analyze mitotic progression. PLoS One. 2022;17(7):e0270923. https://doi.org/10.1371/journal.pone.0270923.

28. Olsen TG, Hunter Jackson B, Feeser TA, Kent MN, Moad JC, Krishnamurthy S, Lunsford DD, Soans RE. Diagnostic performance of deep learning algorithms applied to three common diagnoses in dermatopathology. J Pathol Inform. 2018;9(1):32. https://doi.org/10.4103/jpi.jpi_31_18.

29. Hart SN, Flotte W, Norgan AF, Shah KK, Buchan ZR, Mounajjed T, Flotte TJ. Classification of melanocytic lesions in selected and whole-slide images via convolutional neural networks. J Pathol Informatics. 2019;10(1):5. https://doi.org/10.4103/jpi.jpi_32_18.

30. Hekler A, Utikal JS, Enk AH, Solass W, Schmitt M, Klode J, Schadendorf D, Sondermann W, Franklin C, Bestvater F, Flaig MJ, Krahl D, von Kalle C, Fröhling S, Brinker TJ. Deep learning outperformed 11 pathologists in the classification of histopathological melanoma images. Eur J Cancer. 2019;118:91–6. https://doi.org/10.1016/j.ejca.2019.06.012.

31. Sankarapandian S, Kohn S, Spurrier V, Grullon S, Soans RE, Ayyagari KD, Chamarthi RV, Motaparthi K, Lee JB, Shon W. A pathology deep learning system capable of triage of melanoma specimens utilizing dermatopathologist consensus as ground truth. In *Proceedings of the IEEE/CVF international conference on computer vision*, pp. 629–638; 2021.

32. Thomas SM, Lefevre JG, Baxter G, Hamilton NA. Interpretable deep learning systems for multi-class segmentation and classification of non-melanoma skin cancer. Med Image Anal. 2021;68:101915. https://doi.org/10.1016/j.media.2020.101915.

33. Cassidy B, Kendrick C, Brodzicki A, Jaworek-Korjakowska J, Yap MH. Analysis of the ISIC image datasets: usage, benchmarks and recommendations. Med Image Anal. 2022;75:102305. https://doi.org/10.1016/j.media.2021.102305.

34. Bickers DR, Lim HW, Margolis D, Weinstock MA, Goodman C, Faulkner E, Gould C, Gemmen E, Dall T. The burden of skin diseases: 2004: a joint project of the American Academy of Dermatology Association and the Society for Investigative Dermatology. J Am Acad Dermatol. 2006;55(3):490–500. https://doi.org/10.1016/j.jaad.2006.05.048.

35. Hay RJ, Augustin M, Griffiths CEM, Sterry W, The Board of the International League of Dermatological Societies and the Grand Challenges Consultation Groups. The global challenge for skin health. Br J Dermatol. 2015;172(6):1469–72. https://doi.org/10.1111/bjd.13854.

36. Hay RJ, Johns NE, Williams HC, Bolliger IW, Dellavalle RP, Margolis DJ, Marks R, Naldi L, Weinstock MA, Wulf SK, Michaud C, Murray CJL, Naghavi M. The global burden of skin disease in 2010: an analysis of the prevalence and impact of skin conditions. J Invest Dermatol. 2014;134(6):1527–34. https://doi.org/10.1038/jid.2013.446.

Regulatory Aspects and Ethical Legal Societal Implications (ELSI)

Steven G. Johnson, Gyorgy Simon, and Constantin Aliferis

Abstract

This chapter reviews the context of regulating AI/ML models, the risk management principles underlying international regulations of clinical AI/ML, the conditions under which health AI/ML models in the U.S. are regulated by the Food and Drug Administration (FDA), and the FDA's Good Machine Learning Practice (GMLP) principles. The GMLP principles do not offer specific guidance on execution, so we point the Reader to the parts of the book that discuss bringing these principles to practice via concrete best practice recommendations. Intrinsically linked with regulatory aspects are the Ethical, Legal, Social Implications (ELSI) dimensions. The chapter provides an introduction to the nascent field of biomedical AI ethics covering: general AI ELSI studies, AI/ML racial bias, and AI/ML and Health equity principles. Contrary to conventional risks/harms (data security and privacy, adherence to model use as stated in consent), ethical AI/ML involves model effectiveness and harms that *can exist within the intended scope of consent*. On the positive side, in the case of biomedical AI, these risks are in principle measurable and knowable compared to hard-to-quantify risks/harm due to data breaches. The chapter discusses (and gives illustrative examples) of the importance of causality and equivalence classes for practical detection of racial bias in models. The chapter concludes with a series of recommended best practices for promoting health equity and reducing health disparities via the design and use of health AI/ML.

S. G. Johnson (✉) · G. Simon · C. Aliferis
Institute for Health Informatics, University of Minnesota, Minneapolis, MN, USA
e-mail: joh06288@umn.edu

© The Author(s) 2024
G. J. Simon, C. Aliferis (eds.), *Artificial Intelligence and Machine Learning in Health Care and Medical Sciences*, Health Informatics,
https://doi.org/10.1007/978-3-031-39355-6_16

Keywords

AI/ML Risk management · ISO 14971 · FDA's AI Guidance · Health equity · disparities · Racial bias and the Causal-Path-to-Outcomes Principle · ELSI factors for health AI/ML

Model Implementation in the Context of Regulation

Model predictions, in order to have an impact on healthcare outcomes, must be deployed in patient care settings and used by clinicians so that they affect their decisions or actions. The results of models can be presented to clinicians in the form of a report, as part of a real-time dashboard or within worklists that get updated frequently. But the best method, *clinical decision support* (CDS), is to present the information from the model at the precise time during a clinical workflow when it is most useful to the clinician and patient.

> **Clinical Decision Support** provides clinicians, staff, patients, or other individuals with knowledge and person-specific information, intelligently filtered or presented at appropriate times, to enhance health and health care.[1]

The best CDS addresses the following 5 "rights": The right *information*, to the right *person*, in the right *format*, through the right *channel*, at the right time in the *workflow*.[2]

EHR vendors have historically provided their own proprietary methods for implementing CDS within clinical workflows, but there are standards that are slowly being adopted that could make model implementation easier and more portable across systems. CDS Hooks has emerged as a vendor-agnostic way to implement models.[3] The architecture supports the AI/ML models running on a server external to the EHR itself, which allows more flexibility in the maintenance and sharing of the model. The AI/ML model itself must be written in the programming language it was developed with and run in a suitable environment. EHR vendors are starting to create model execution environments (i.e. Epic Nebula, Cerner Project Apollo), but they are not currently very interoperable.

Once models are implemented within production clinical workflows, they must be monitored and their performance evaluated (chapter "Characterizing, Diagnosing and Managing the Risk of Error of ML & AI Models in Clinical and Organizational Application"). It is also important to select the appropriate performance metrics that depend on the problem the CDS models are solving (chapter "Evaluation"). Model performance in production may not match the performance estimated during model development. Model performance may also change over time due to **input data drifts, and model drifts**. Data drifts occur when the data distribution in the application population changes, or when additional terminology codes are adopted, or EHR documentation methods change thereby potentially changing input data expectations. Model drifts occur as a result of model outputs causing practice changes leading to changes in the validity of the models. In both of these cases, model retraining eventually becomes necessary.

ISO 14971 Standard on Risk Management of Medical Devices

After an AI or ML model has been fit, its performance is evaluated in controlled conditions, and the model is refined according to clinical-grade model *technical* criteria of performance and reliability, as described in chapter "The Development Process and Lifecycle of Clinical Grade and Other Safety and Performance-Sensitive AI/ML Models", after it is implemented in care. There are several regulations that govern clinical grade AI/ML models and systems. This chapter describes current regulatory requirements.

While the exact rules and regulations surrounding the use of clinical decision support tools may change, regulations in many countries, including the USA, European Union, Canada, and Australia, are informed by the ISO 15971 standard [4]. Conversely, several revisions to the standard were made to better align it with regional law. This standard, entitled "*Application of risk management to medical devices*", describes the process of risk management for medical devices throughout its entire life cycle. After reading this section, the Reader should be able to define key concepts related to risk management, be familiar with the related terminology, describe risk management in broad strokes, and understand the key decisions to make.

> The ISO 14971 standard describes the process of risk management for medical devices through their entire life cycle. https://www.iso.org/standard/72704.html

> The central thesis of risk management is that the expected benefits from using the device must outweigh the risk of potential harms.

To expand on this central thesis, we have to establish some definitions.

> A **medical device** is defined as "an instrument, apparatus, implement, machine, implant, software, or related article to be used alone or in combination for the diagnosis, prevention, treatment, monitoring or alleviation of disease, injury", or for supporting or sustaining life.

ISO 14971 provides a broad definition of a medical device with an extensive open-ended list of potential purposes. Given the context of this book, the medical device will most commonly be an AI/ML model assisting with or making clinical decisions, for example in the form of a risk or prognostic model, or as a decision support tool estimating risks under various treatment options.

An AI model is not a medical device if it is running as *part of* a device.

> **Benefit** is defined as the positive impact or desirable outcome stemming from the use of the medical device in question.
>
> **Harm** is injury or damage to the health of people, property or environment.
>
> **Risk** quantifies harm. It has two components: the probability of risk and the severity of said harm.
>
> **Risk management** is a process that consists of (i) establishing the intended use and foreseeable misuse of a medical device, (ii) identifying potential sources of harm and estimating the associated risks, (iii) determining whether the risks are acceptable, (iv) taking measures to reduce these risks, and (v) monitoring the device during the remainder of its life cycle and repeating the risk assessment as needed.

Let us look at these steps in more detail. Phrases in quotation marks are the terminology used by the standard.

(i) The process starts by **establishing the intended use and the foreseeable misuse of the device**. The "intended use" (also known as "intended purpose" in the EU) provides a description of how the device is intended to be used, including its purpose, the description of the target patient population, as well as a description of the users of the device, of the environment in which it will be used, and of the process of how the device is to be used. Moreover, the standard mandates that characteristics (quantitative as well as qualitative) that can affect the safety of the device be considered and limits need to be defined on these characteristics for safe use.

(ii) Next, **potential sources of harm ("hazards") are identified**. Sequences or combinations of events that could lead to harm should be considered and documented. For each source of harm, the associated risks, both their probabilities and their severities, are estimated. This step is referred to as "risk analysis" in the standard, which consists of "risk assessment", where the potential sources of harm are identified and "risk estimation" where the risk probabilities and severities are estimated.

> **Best Practice 16.1**
> Consider all relevant risks in different phases of the life cycle. Risks can change over time, e.g., the probability or severity of risk can change due to advancements in treatments or due to patient population drift.

As far as the scope of risk analysis is concerned, risks related to data and system security are explicitly included, as are risks stemming from the malfunction of the device.

Risks are not always estimable. For example if a set but very rare sequence of operations causes a fault deterministically, its risk may be hard to estimate with certainty. Similarly, some harms, such as the emergence of antibiotic-resistant pathogens caused by antibiotic overuse, may be impractical to estimate (quantify) in the context of infection risk models. In such cases, the potential harms themselves should be listed (without quantified risks).

(iii) The next step is called **"risk evaluation"**. In this step, it is determined whether the risks are acceptable.

Under some circumstances, the risk from using the device cannot be reduced to acceptable levels. In such cases a "risk-benefit analysis" can be carried out, proving that the expected benefit outweighs (the high) risk. For example, the use of a life-support device could fall into this category. In case of a "risk-benefit analysis", the benefits cannot include economic or business advantages (cost-benefit analysis can serve that purpose).

Risk evaluation for clinical decision support, that is when the device is applied to a particular patient, is excluded from the scope, because the tradeoff between the benefits and risks is very patient-dependent. Business decision making is also excluded from the scope.

(iv) **If the risks are not acceptable (too high), then "risk control" is performed.** As part of risk control, measures to reduce risk are developed, implemented, and verified. After the implementation and verification of these risk reduction measures, the remaining risk ("residual risk") is evaluated. If it is still deemed unacceptably high, further risk reduction measures are implemented and the residual risks are re-evaluated. These steps are repeated until the residual risk becomes acceptable.

If, in spite of all the risk control measures, the residual risk remains too high, the device may be abandoned, or the device itself or its intended use may be revised and the whole risk management process must be repeated from the beginning.

If the residual risk is acceptable and the expected benefits outweigh the potential harms, then a risk management report is produced detailing the above steps.

The "verification" of a measure is the provision of objective evidence proving that the measure successfully meets certain pre-defined objectives. This refers to distinct processes: proving that the measure is actually implemented and also proving that the measure reduced the risk. The level of effort should be commensurate with the level of risk.

Note that the risk control measures themselves can introduce new and different risks.

(v) The device enters the **post-production phase of its life cycle and post-production monitoring of the device commences.** Information about the use and misuse of the device is collected, and a decision is made whether the risk evaluation should be repeated. This may lead to the need for additional risk control measures and re-evaluation of the residual risks.

> **Pitfall 16.1**
> The ISO 14971 is not an implementation standard. It mandates that certain actions be taken but does not prescribe exactly how they will be carried out.

> **Best Practice 16.2**
> The rationale for the risk management plan is that having a plan produced ahead of time makes it less likely that a risk management step is overlooked or accidentally skipped.

FDA Regulation of AI/ML Use

In this section, we will focus on the regulatory framework developed by the United States Food and Drug Administration (FDA) for the regulation of Clinical Decision Support Software.[5] We will review a history of the evolution of the regulations and examine characteristics for what the FDA considers a medical device and therefore what needs to go through the FDA regulatory approval process. These regulations and processes will likely evolve over time and the information in this section may eventually be out of date. But the underlying reasons for the regulatory review should still be valid and it is important that these reasons are considered during the development of an AI/ML model.

The US Congress passed the 21st Century Cures Act in December of 2016 [6]. The Cures Act exempted certain software from regulation as long as (1) the healthcare provider could independently review the basis of the recommendation and (2) they didn't rely on it to make a diagnostic or treatment decision. But it wasn't very clear about which types of medical software could be exempted. In this timeframe, health systems developed algorithms and CDS, and they generally didn't seek FDA approval.

The FDA has monitored the evolution of how software was being used in medical decisions, and especially how software was developed, how AI/ML algorithms were trained on new data and how they evolved over time. In 2019, the FDA released a draft guidance on CDS software [7] in which it proposed a risk-based approach based on the International Medical Device Regulators Forum (IMDRF) Framework which could be used to categorize CDS as a medical device CDS or a non-device CDS. Based on feedback and comments, the FDA released its Final Guidance on September 22, 2022 [5]. This guidance abandoned the risk-based approach and provides a more detailed definition of which types of CDS are considered devices and should therefore be regulated. To clarify: the decision, whether a model needs to be regulated or not is no longer based on risks, however, risk management is still the central tenet of regulation (for the devices that need to be regulated).

> The FDA's Final Guidance defined four criteria and if the CDS meets all four criteria, then it is not considered a device CDS and is not regulated by the FDA [5]. If the model fails to meet any one (or more) of these criteria, then it is subject to FDA regulations. The four criteria are as follows:
>
> 1. the model is not intended to acquire, process, or analyze a medical image or a signal from an in vitro diagnostic device or a pattern or signal from a signal acquisition system;
> 2. the model is intended for the purpose of displaying, analyzing, or printing medical information about a patient or other medical information (such as peer-reviewed clinical studies and clinical practice guidelines);
> 3. the model is intended for the purpose of supporting or providing recommendations to a health care professional about prevention, diagnosis, or treatment of a disease or condition; and
> 4. the model is intended for the purpose of enabling such health care professional (HCP) to independently review the basis for such recommendations that such software presents so that it is not the intent that such health care professional rely primarily on any of such recommendations to make a clinical diagnosis or treatment decision regarding an individual patient.

The Final Guidance provides a detailed explanation for each of the criteria and uses examples to illustrate what is and is not considered a medical device.

Criterion 1: the FDA makes it clear that any software that analyzes medical images or device signals is a device. Then it goes further to define a pattern as multiple, sequential, or repeated measurements of a signal. They specifically give examples of patterns as electrocardiograms (ECG), continuous glucose monitors (CGM) and next generation sequencing (NGS). Examples of software that do not meet Criterion 1 and are therefore devices, include software that uses CT images to estimate fractional flow reserve, software that performs image analysis for diagnostically differentiating between ischemic and hemorrhagic stroke and software that analyzes multiple signals (e.g., perspiration rate, heart rate, eye movement, breathing rate) from wearable products to monitor whether a person is having a heart attack. But software that uses physiologic signals for biometric identification (i.e. retinal scan) is not a medical device since it is not being used for a medical purpose.

Criterion 2: the FDA describes *medical information about a patient* to be "the type of information that normally is, and generally can be, communicated between health care professionals in a clinical conversation…". The information's relevance to a clinical decision must be well understood and accepted. *Other medical information* includes "information such as peer-reviewed clinical studies, clinical practice guidelines, and information that is similarly independently verified and validated as accurate, reliable…". By this definition a single glucose measure (lab result) is *medical information about a patient*, but multiple glucose measurements over a period of time would be considered a pattern. Examples of non-devices are providing order sets, displaying evidence-based practice guidelines, drug-drug interactions and reminders for preventive care. Examples of a regulated device is software that analyzes patient-specific medical information (e.g., daily heart rate, SpO_2, blood pressure, etc.) to compute a score that predicts heart failure hospitalization because the score is not generally communicated between health care professionals and its relevance to a clinical decision is not well understood.

Criterion 3, addresses providing recommendations to HCPs. In particular, the FDA considers that if the software provides a specific diagnosis or treatment or provides a time-critical recommendation, then it may replace the HCPs clinical judgement (because the HCP is not given enough time to consider the recommendation and they are not given alternatives with supporting evidence). In that case, the CDS should be regulated. If a HCP is given a list of preventative, diagnostic or treatment options or a list of next steps (as long as it is not done in a time-critical manner), then that is allowable non-device CDS. On the other hand, examples of device CDS include software the predicts opioid addiction (it is a specific diagnosis) or software that alerts to potential for a patient to develop sepsis (requires a time-critical response). The FDA also considers automation bias, in which an HCP may rely too much on the output of the software for their decisions since it is coming from a (presumed infallible) computer.

Criterion 4, lastly, seeks to ensure that the HCP can review the basis for the recommendations so that they do not solely rely on the recommendation but use their clinical judgement. In support of this, the FDA recommends that the software (1) labels its intended use; (2) describes all inputs, their relevance and expected data quality; (3) lists applicable patient population; (4) provides a summary of the algorithm logic and methods; (5) presents results from clinical studies and validations to evaluate the model performance and (6) shows relevant patient-specific information and any missing, corrupted, or unexpected inputs that will enable the HCP to independently review the basis for the recommendations. The Final Guidance gives examples of software that provide recommendations (i.e. mammography treatment plan, depression treatment options) in a non time-critical manner but that do not provide all six aspects described above. Therefore, they are considered devices and should be regulated.

Over the past 25 years, only 521 AI software devices have been approved by the FDA, mostly in radiology[8]. The Final Guidance has only recently been published and it explicitly states that it is a non-binding recommendation. It remains to be seen how the FDA will enforce these recommendations and what actions the CDS and health AI/ML community will take to comply.

FDA's "Good ML Practice"

The U.S. Food and Drug Administration (FDA), Health Canada, and the United Kingdom's Medicines and Healthcare products Regulatory Agency (MHRA) have jointly identified 10 guiding principles that can inform the development of Good Machine Learning Practice (GMLP) [9]. These principles are primarily meant for clinical AI/ML models that will influence the health of patients. However, some of these guidelines are broader in scope, and are also applicable to knowledge discovery or healthcare operations and business models.

> **Caution:** The GMLP principles are just that—*principles*; they offer no concrete guidance on best practices that can help satisfy these principles.

In order to help with converting the principles to action, in this section, we will present the ten GMLP principles, quote from FDA's commentary about the principles and cross-reference with the chapters in the current book that discuss best practices that relate to each GMLP principle.

> **FDA GMLP 1. Multi-Disciplinary Expertise Is Leveraged Throughout the Total Product Life Cycle.**

This principle advocates for "in-depth understanding of a model's intended integration into clinical workflow, and the desired benefits and associated patient risks, can help ensure that ML-enabled medical devices are safe and effective and address clinically meaningful needs over the lifecycle of the device." (The quoted text is directly adopted from the FDA document.) This resonates with our BP practice recommendations in chapter "Principles of Rigorous Development and of Appraisal of ML and AI Methods and Systems", which advocate for having a concrete clinically-motivated problem formulation; our best practice recommendations in chapter "Evaluation" help with the evaluation of the model in terms of clinical effectiveness; and chapter "Characterizing, Diagnosing and Managing the Risk of Error of ML & AI Models in Clinical and Organizational Application" helps with risk characterization and management.

> **FDA GMLP 2. Good Software Engineering and Security Practices Are Implemented.**

"Model design is implemented with attention to the `fundamentals': good software engineering practices, data quality assurance, data management, and robust cybersecurity practices."

Data management and quality assurance are addressed in chapter "Data Preparation, Transforms, Quality, and Management" and good software engineering principles are described in chapters "Principles of Rigorous Development and of Appraisal of ML and AI Methods and Systems", "The Development Process and Lifecycle of Clinical Grade and Other Safety and Performance-Sensitive AI/ML Models" and "Characterizing, Diagnosing and Managing the Risk of Error of ML & AI Models in Clinical and Organizational Application" (i.e., relevant to method and model development, and mitigating the risks associated with clinical ML/AI). Although cyberattacks can cause damage and disruption through ML/AI models, we note that cybersecurity requires a holistic approach on the healthcare institution's part and the onus of defending a system from cyberattacks should not, under typical circumstances, be placed exclusively on ML/AI developers.

FDA GMLP 3. Clinical Study Participants and Data Sets Are Representative of the Intended Patient Population.

We extensively covered the concept of generalization/validity in the chapter on "Data Design" as inferring knowledge from the study sample through the available population about the target population.

FDA GMLP 4. Training Data Sets Are Independent of Test Sets.

The model performance estimators (leave out validation, cross-validation, bootstrap, external validation) in chapter "Evaluation" and the guidelines for avoiding over-fitting, under-fitting and model over/under confidence errors in chapter "Overfitting, Underfitting and General Model Overconfidence and Under-Performance Pitfalls and Best Practices in Machine Learning and AI" follow and elaborate on this principle.

FDA GMLP 5. Selected Reference Datasets Are Based Upon Best Available Methods.

Accepted, best available methods for developing a reference dataset (that is, a reference standard) ensure that clinically relevant and well characterized data are collected and the limitations of the reference are understood. If available, accepted reference datasets in model development and testing that promote and demonstrate model robustness and generalizability across the intended patient population are used. Chapters "Principles of Rigorous Development and of Appraisal of ML and AI Methods and Systems", "The Development Process and Lifecycle of Clinical Grade and Other Safety and Performance-Sensitive AI/ML Models", and especially "Data Design" address the issue of proper data for development and validation.

FDA GMLP 6. Model Design Is Tailored to the Available Data and Reflects the Intended Use of the Device.

Selecting the best modeling algorithms for the task and data is a fundamental tenet of this book. In earlier chapters, we drew attention to the perils of ignoring the vast selection of existing methods in favor of some particularly popular methods. Chapters "Foundations and Properties of AI/ML Systems", "An Appraisal and Operating Characteristics of Major ML Methods Applicable in Healthcare & Health Science", "Foundations of Causal ML" explained the characteristics of commonly used and state-of-the-art methods so that they can best be matched to the clinical problem at hand. Chapter "The Development Process and Lifecycle of Clinical Grade and Other Safety and Performance-Sensitive AI/ML Models" discusses the importance of deeply understanding and formally describing the clinical problem to be solved, as well as the capabilities of available algorithms, so that models can be developed that serve the intended use. Chapter "Data Design" describes how the training data can be designed and sampled so that it supports these needs. Finally, chapters "Evaluation", "Overfitting, Underfitting and General Model Overconfidence and Under-Performance Pitfalls and Best Practices in Machine Learning and AI" provide detailed guidance on how the model can be evaluated both in terms of performance, risk and other factors related to the intended use.

FDA GMLP 7. Focus Is Placed on the Performance of the Human-AI Team.

"Where the model has a 'human in the loop,' human factors considerations and the human interpretability of the model outputs are addressed with emphasis on the performance of the Human-AI team, rather than just the performance of the model in isolation." Chapter "Foundations and Properties of AI/ML Systems" places semantic clarity and model interpretability/explainability as a major desired property. Chapters "Foundations and Properties of AI/ML Systems", "An Appraisal and Operating Characteristics of Major ML Methods Applicable in Healthcare & Health Science", "Foundations of Causal ML" discuss interpretability of many AI/ML models and algorithms. Chapters "Principles of Rigorous Development and of Appraisal of ML and AI Methods and Systems", "The Development Process and Lifecycle of Clinical Grade and Other Safety and Performance-Sensitive AI/ML Models" and "Characterizing, Diagnosing and Managing the Risk of Error of ML & AI Models in Clinical and Organizational Application" discuss the role of explainable AI and interpretable ML methods. Finally, chapter "From 'Human versus Machine' to 'Human with Machine'" describes human cognitive biases as they related to decision making and computer interaction, and discusses ways to effectively combine the strengths of human and computer decisions while minimizing their weaknesses.

FDA GMLP 8. Testing Demonstrates Device Performance during Clinically Relevant Conditions.

"Statistically sound test plans are developed and executed to generate clinically relevant device performance information independently of the training data set. Considerations include the intended patient population, important subgroups, clinical environment and use by the Human-AI team, measurement inputs, and potential confounding factors."

This principle is addressed in the evaluation methods, and error management material in chapters "Evaluation", "Overfitting, Underfitting and General Model Overconfidence and Under-Performance Pitfalls and Best Practices in Machine Learning and AI" and "Characterizing, Diagnosing and Managing the Risk of Error of ML & AI Models in Clinical and Organizational Application".

FDA GMLP 9. Users Are Provided Clear, Essential Information.

FDA Principle 9 is that "users are provided ready access to clear, contextually relevant information that is appropriate for the intended audience (such as health care providers or patients) including: the product's intended use and indications for use, performance of the model for appropriate subgroups, characteristics of the data used to train and test the model, acceptable inputs, known limitations, user interface interpretation, and clinical workflow integration of the model. Users are also made aware of device modifications and updates from real-world performance monitoring, the basis for decision-making when available, and a means to communicate product concerns to the developer."

Chapter "Reporting Standards, Certification/Accreditation, and Reproducibility" describes the latest minimal information reporting standards for health AI/ML and related models, critically reviews gaps, and proposes that additional information across the range of best practices in the book is included in such reporting.

FDA GMLP 10. Deployed Models Are Monitored for Performance and Re-training Risks are Managed.

Specifically that: "deployed models have the capability to be monitored in "real world" use with a focus on maintained or improved safety and performance. Additionally, when models are periodically or continually trained after deployment, there are appropriate controls in place to manage risks of overfitting, unintended bias, or degradation of the model (for example, input data drift) that may impact the safety and performance of the model as it is used by the Human-AI team." Monitoring the real-world performance of models, re-training them, and the known risks of continuous model training are discussed in chapter "Characterizing, Diagnosing and Managing the Risk of Error of ML & AI Models in Clinical and Organizational Application".

Additional Regulatory Frameworks and Initiatives of Relevance

Recently, governments in the United States, European Union, and other countries have sought to create policy and legal frameworks governing the deployment and the use of AI/ML models and systems. The goal of these regulatory frameworks is to expand the digital economy while providing safety, quality, and ethical use standards for software that is employed for all high-risk purposes, including clinical decision support and other purposed affecting health [10, 11].

The **AI Act is a landmark EU legislation** to regulate Artificial Intelligence based on its capacity to harm people [12]. Among other provisions, it enforces an obligation for each EU country (or groups of countries) to set up at least one regulatory sandbox, a controlled environment, where AI technology could be tested safely. One of the ways for an AI to fall into the high-risk category is if it is used in one of the sectors listed under AIA Annex III, such as health, and would "pose a risk of harm to the health, safety or fundamental rights of natural persons in a way that produces legal effects concerning them or has an equivalently significant effect".

The final definition of AI in the AIA will have immense consequences as to which systems are regulated and which can bypass regulation [13].

Moreover under the EU's draft AI Act, open source developers would have to adhere to guidelines for risk management, data governance, technical documentation and transparency, as well as standards of accuracy and cybersecurity (reinforcing the commentary in the present volume related to the risks associated with open source code) [14].

The US National Institute of Standards and Technology (NIST) following a direction from the US Congress, issued recently [15, 16], the *Artificial Intelligence Risk Management Framework* (**AI RMF 1.0**), a guidance document for voluntary use by organizations designing, developing, deploying or using AI systems to help manage the many risks of AI technologies.

NIST points out that this is a "voluntary framework aiming to help develop and deploy AI technologies in ways that enable the United States, other nations and organizations to enhance AI trustworthiness while managing risks". Also that "AI systems are 'socio-technical' in nature, meaning they are influenced by societal dynamics and human behavior. AI risks can emerge from the complex interplay of these technical and societal factors, affecting people's lives in situations ranging from their experiences with online chatbots to the results of job and loan applications."

The AI RMF is divided into two parts. The first part discusses how organizations can frame the risks related to AI and outlines the characteristics of trustworthy AI systems. The second part, the core of the framework, describes four specific functions—govern, map, measure, and manage—to help organizations address the risks of AI systems in practice. These functions can be applied in context-specific use cases and at any stages of the AI life cycle.

In addition, NIST plans to launch a *Trustworthy and Responsible AI Resource Center* to help organizations put the AI RMF 1.0 into practice.

In general, the landscape of AI/ML policy and law, both broadly and in health sciences and healthcare, is fluid, rapidly evolving and organizations should closely monitor relevant developments and develop compliance readiness for adhering to laws and regulations, and for aligning with voluntary frameworks promoting safe and accountable AI/ML.

Concepts of Ethical and Social Implications of Health AI/ML

We open this section with the observation that traditional Ethical, Legal and Social Implications (ELSI) concerns, related to advanced Big Data technologies, emphasized the risks associated with the use of data for secondary research *outside the scope of informed consent.* Data privacy risks in particular (e.g. because of unauthorized uses, or data breaches [17]) describe an *out-of-consent scope* set of problems where potential harm to patients is often hard to quantify or predict and may even be unknowable in some cases.

As AI/ML is becoming more poised to affect human patients' well-being, a new set of ELSI challenges has emerged related to the performance, efficiency, risk, interpretability, governance, and acceptance of this technology. Models may underperform or have high margins of error, or preferentially benefit or harm a group of individuals, or create a set of risks that may exist *within the scope of consent and intended* use. As we will see in this section, some of these newer risks are, at *least in principle,* directly measurable and addressable. Significant challenges exist, however, in formulating the goals of ethical AI/ML as it relates to problems of bias and equity, and in operationalizing it.

Overall the emerging field of ethical health AI/ML represents a fruitful ground of scientific collaboration between ethicists, policy scholars, patient/group advocates, and biomedical data scientists, where best practices can eliminate ethical and social risks in systematic, measurable and controllable ways.

Important Definitions & Concepts Related to Ethical Social Justice Implications of Health AI/ML

Definition: Minority health (MH) "refers to the distinctive health characteristics and attributes of racial and/or ethnic minority groups, as defined by the U.S. Management and Budget Office (OMB), that can be socially disadvantaged due in part to being subject to potential discriminatory acts" [18, 19]

Definition: Minority Health Populations. NIH uses the racial and ethnic group classifications determined by the OMB. Currently the minority racial and ethnic groups are American Indian or Alaska Native, Asian, Black or African American, and Native Hawaiian or other Pacific Islander. The ethnicity used is Latino or Hispanic. Although these five categories are minimally required, the mixed or multiple race category should be considered in analyses and reporting, when available. Self-identification is the preferred means of obtaining race and ethnic identity [18, 19].

Definition. Health equity means social justice in health (i.e., no one is denied the possibility to be healthy for belonging to a group that has historically been economically/socially disadvantaged) [20]. Margaret Whitehead defined **health inequalities as health differences that are avoidable, unnecessary, and unjust** [21, 22].

Definition. Health Disparity. A health disparity (HD) is a health difference that adversely affects disadvantaged populations, based on one or more of the following health outcomes:
- Higher incidence and/or prevalence and earlier onset of disease.
- Higher prevalence of risk factors, unhealthy behaviors, or clinical measures in the causal pathway of a disease outcome.
- Higher rates of condition-specific symptoms, reduced global daily functioning, or self-reported health-related quality of life using standardized measures.
- Premature and/or excessive mortality from diseases where population rates differ.
- Greater global burden of disease using a standardized metric [18, 19].

Health disparities are the metric we use to measure progress toward achieving health equity. A reduction in health disparities (in absolute and relative terms) is evidence that we are moving toward greater health equity. Moving toward greater equity is achieved by selectively improving the health of those who are economically/socially disadvantaged, not by a worsening the health of those in advantaged groups [20, 21].

Definition. Populations with Health Disparities. For NIH, populations that experience health disparities include:
- Racial and ethnic minority groups.
- People with lower socioeconomic status (SES).
- Underserved rural communities.
- Sexual and gender minority (SGM) groups.

Definition. Health Determinants. Factors that impact an individual's health and the risk of experiencing health disparities. Each of these health determinants plays an important role in health disparities and interacts in complex ways to impact an individual's health. Health Determinants capture areas that go beyond the social determinants and include factors, such as individual behaviors, lifestyles, and social responses to stress; biological processes, genetics, and epigenetics; the physical environment; the sociocultural environment; social determinants; and clinical events and interactions with the health care and other systems [18, 19].

General Studies on ELSI for Health AI/ML

The ELSI literature on health AI is nascent but growing rapidly. Among other efforts, various factors have been studied and used in order to establish parameters for the ethical use of health AI/ML. We will highlight here a few studies as being indicative of this emerging scholarship.

Cartolovni et al. [23] conducted a scoping review that included 94 AI ELSI related publications. They identified four "main clusters of impact": AI algorithms, physicians, patients, and healthcare in general. The most prevalent issues were found to be patient safety, algorithmic transparency, lack of proper regulation, liability & accountability, impact on patient-physician relationship, and governance of AI empowered healthcare.

Guan et al. [24] identified ethical risk factors of AI decision making from the perspective of qualitative research, constructed a risk-factor model of AI decision making ethical risks using rooting theory, and explored risk management strategies. They point to technological uncertainty, incomplete data, and management errors as the main sources of ethical risks in AI decision making and find that the intervention of risk governance elements can effectively block the social risks. Guan, in a different study, [25] highlighted the importance of the roles of governments in ethical auditing and the responsibilities of stakeholders in an ethical governance system of health AI.

Price et al. [26] focused on privacy in the context of Big Data related medical innovation. They discuss how to define health privacy; the importance of equity, consent, and patient governance in data collection; discrimination in data uses; and how to handle data breaches.

Martinez-Martin et al. [27] investigates the ethical aspects of ambient intelligence, a fast growing area of AI involving the use of contactless sensors and contact-based wearable devices embedded in health-care (or home) settings to collect data (e.g., images of physical spaces, audio data, or body temperature). These sensors and devices are coupled with machine learning algorithms to efficiently and effectively interpret these data. These researchers point to ethical challenges around privacy, data management, bias, fairness, and informed consent as prerequisites for acceptance of the field and success of its goals.

In another study Martinez-Martin et al. [28] examine the ethical challenges presented by direct-to-consumer (DTC) digital psychotherapy services that do not involve oversight by a professional mental health provider. They found that there is inadequate regulation in this area that exacerbates concerns over safety, privacy, accountability, and other ethical obligations to protect an individual in therapy. The types of DTC services that present ethical challenges include apps that use a digital platform to connect users to minimally trained nonprofessional counselors, as well as services that provide counseling steered by artificial intelligence and conversational agents.

Parviainen et al. [29] address the timely issues surrounding the health-related use of chatbots. Such technology is not sufficiently mature to be able to replace the judgements of health professionals. The COVID-19 pandemic, however, has significantly increased the utilization of health-oriented chatbots, for instance, as a conversational interface to answer questions, recommend care options, check symptoms, and complete tasks such as booking appointments.

They suggest the need for new approaches in professional ethics as the large-scale deployment of artificial intelligence may revolutionize professional decision-making and client-expert interaction in healthcare organizations.

Racial Bias and AI/ML

In a case that attracted national attention (see also chapter "Lessons Learned from Historical Failures, Limitations and Successes of AI/ML In Healthcare and the Health Sciences. Enduring Problems, and the Role of Best Practices" as a case study of AI/ML failures) a model was used to decide which patients have high severity of illness so that more resources would be allocated to their treatment. The underlying operating principle of allocating more resources to more seriously ill patients and less resources to patients with non-serious disease is generally sound. Unfortunately, the developers of the model decided to use health expenditures ("cost") as a proxy for the severity. Because expenditures/cost are driven not only by severity (through intensity of treatment) but also by access to healthcare, which itself is driven by racial disparities in health, using cost as a proxy for severity led to prioritizing less seriously ill patients of one racial group with better access to care over another racial group with less access to care. The analysis of [30] demonstrates the importance of not carelessly substituting important variables with correlates, because this can lead to systematic harm to populations of a particular race (or other characteristic that *should not be linked to the quality of care received*).

In a study aiming at revealing racial biases [31] the investigators examined whether a ML model's decisions were sensitive to the inclusion of race as a predictive variable and found no biases in the examined model. Without challenging the results of [31] (which would require re-analysis of the data), we take the opportunity to point out a general pitfall: the strategy employed for racial bias detection is fraught with pitfalls and is not recommended for broad use. This is because of at least three reasons:

Pitfall 16.2

Using race variable's effect on model decision as a flawed criterion for detecting racial bias:

1. Race may have no effect in a model because other variables have the same information content as race. In other words, this bias detection strategy can systematically generate false negatives in certain distributions.
2. Race may be a justifiable predictor variable if biological reasons (or, more broadly, well-justified standard of care) suggest its appropriateness. For example, if members of a racial group carry a genetic mutation that increases risk for a disease, then a diagnostic or risk model for that disease should use race (in the absence of genotyping information) without this being a negative bias. In other words this bias detection strategy can also generate systematic false positives.
3. The Berkson bias (see chapter "Data Design") can induce spurious correlations if in the hospital (or other selected) populations, race correlates with diagnosis, treatment, and/or other decisions that influence outcomes. In such cases, diagnosis, treatment, etc. models may benefit (improve in accuracy) from the inclusion of race, but this is a reflection of selection bias of the hospitalized population, rather than racial bias. This is another systematic false positive scenario for the race variable inclusion-exclusion strategy.

It is useful to illustrate the importance of incorporating race in AI/ML models with the following example in Fig. 1. As demonstrated by this example, it is generally a good idea to incorporate race (or other group) variables in the models and optimize decisions for each group separately.

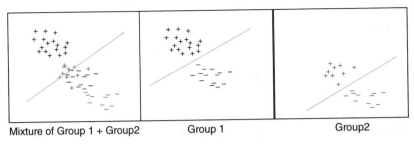

Fig. 1 Importance of incorporating racial group indicator variables. A classification problem with two classes (outcomes), '+' and '−', in a population consisting of two racial groups (depicted in red and blue), using two hypothetical variables (the horizontal and vertical axes) is presented. In the panel in the left, classification is performed in the mixture of the two racial groups. Having the mixture of the two groups represents the situation, where the race (group) variable is not included in the classification model. Perfect classification, separation of the '+'s from the '−'s, cannot be achieved. Moving the threshold of the classifier (depicted as a green line) to reduce errors for Group 1, increases errors for Group 2, and vice versa. In the middle panel the racial group variable RG is included in the model and we set RG = Group 1, perfect classification can be achieved for Group 1. In right panel RG = Group 2 and, again, perfect classification can be achieved for Group 2. Notice that health equity with respect to the benefit from the ML model (i.e. correct classification) in the left panel may be possible but at the expense of both groups under the optimal classifier (i.e., combination of middle and right panels). Also in the model of the left panel, equity in aggregate terms creates inequity on an individual level and vice versa due to differences in the sizes of the two groups. Surprisingly, certain authors examine balancing AI/ML errors across groups and not optimizing accuracy within groups assuming that in an AI/ML context, the harm of one equals to the benefit of the other. This may be true for resource allocation problems, but AI/ML decisions (and related benefits) are not generally a zero-sum game. See later in this chapter for cases where AI/ML deployment faces zero-sum dilemmas

Principles of Health Equity and AI/ML

The literature on AI/ML and health equity is growing. The current crop of studies is pointing to several important common themes, but, as we will see, it is occasionally not precise or technical enough to be readily operationalized.

For example, [32] found that various AI/ML reporting standards do not mention or do not have provisions for reporting how "fairness" is achieved in AI/ML models. These authors also proposed a set of recommendations:

- Engage members of the public and, in particular, members of marginalized communities in the process of determining acceptable fairness standards.
- Collect necessary data on vulnerable protected groups in order to perform audits of model function (e.g., on race, gender).
- Analyze and report model performance for different intersectional subpopulations at risk of unfair outcomes.
- Establish target thresholds and maximum disparities for model function between groups.

– Be transparent regarding the specific definitions of fairness that are used in the evaluation of a machine learning for healthcare (MLHC) model.
– Explicitly evaluate for disparate treatment and disparate impact in MLHC clinical trials.
– Commit to post-market surveillance to assess the ongoing real-world impact of MLHC models.

Chen et al. [33] provide a social-justice based framework and analysis of all stages of ML creation and deployment. They make the following recommendations:

1. Problems should be tackled by diverse teams and using frameworks that increase the probability that equity will be achieved. Further, historically understudied problems are important targets to practitioners looking to perform high-impact work.
2. Data collection should be framed as an important front-of-mind concern in the ML modeling pipeline, clear disclosures should be made about imbalanced datasets, and researchers should engage with domain experts to ensure that data reflecting the needs of underserved and understudied populations are gathered.
3. Outcome choice should reflect the task at hand and should preferably be unbiased. If the outcome label has ethical bias, the source of inequity should be accounted for in ML model design, leveraging literature that attempts to remove ethical biases during preprocessing, or with use of a reasonable proxy.
4. Reflection on the goals of the model is essential during development and should be articulated in a preanalysis plan. In addition to technical choices like loss function, researchers must interrogate how, and whether, a model should be developed to best answer a research question, as well as what caveats are included.
5. Audits should be designed to identify specific harms and should be paired with methods and procedures. Harms should be examined group by group, rather than at a population level. ML ethical design checklists are one possible tool to systematically enumerate and consider such ethical concerns prior to declaring success in a project.

Gianfrancesco et al. [34] identify several potential problems in implementing machine learning algorithms in health care systems with a strong focus on equity and propose suggested solutions as follows:

• Problem1: Overreliance on Automation
  Solution:

  – Ensure interdisciplinary approach and continuous human involvement.
  – Conduct follow-up studies to ensure results are meaningful.

• Problem 2: Algorithms Based on Biased Data
  Solution:

  – Identify the target population and select training and testing sets accordingly.
  – Build and test algorithms in socioeconomically diverse health care systems.
  – Ensure that key variables, such as race/ethnicity, language, and social determinants of health, are being captured and included in algorithms when appropriate.
  – Test algorithms for potential discriminatory behavior throughout data processing.
  – Develop feedback loops to monitor and verify output and validity.

- Problem 3: Non-clinically Meaningful Algorithms
  Solution:

  - Focus on clinically important improvements in relevant outcomes rather than strict performance metrics.
  - Impose human values in algorithms at the cost of efficiency.

McCradden et al. [35] provide recommendations for ethical approaches to issues of bias in health models of machine learning. These authors sharply criticize efforts to impose equal outputs of ML models ("neutral" models; e.g. [36]) given that underlying medical reasons may warrant such differences (see also Pitfall 16.1 (2) above). These authors also stress the importance of model transparency, model development transparency, good model goals and data design, model auditing post-deployment and "engaging diverse knowledge sources". The last recommendation means that *"Ethical analysis should consider real-world consequences for affected groups, weigh benefits and risks of various approaches, and engage stakeholders to come to the most supportable conclusion. Therefore, analysis needs to focus on the downstream effects on patients rather than adopting the presumption that fairness is accomplished solely in the metrics of the system"*.

Some Technical Observations on the Importance of Causal Modeling, Equivalence Classes, and System-Level Thinking

Causal modeling for detecting and correcting racial bias. Prosperi et al. [37] emphasize the importance of using causal modeling for health AI. We will use an example motivated by the general parameters of the racial bias case study incident analyzed in [30]. This example demonstrates the generally-applicable suitability of causal approaches for avoiding and detecting racial bias (also discussed in section "General Studies on ELSI for Health AI/ML" and chapter "Lessons Learned from Historical Failures, Limitations and Successes of AI/ML In Healthcare and the Health Sciences. Enduring Problems, and the Role of Best Practices"). Figure 2 shows the scenario where a racial group has limited access to healthcare compared to other groups. In that (socially unjust) environment, race determines health access. The differential access to care, for the same level of illness severity, leads to less treatment intensity received than other groups who have better access. Treatment intensity determines health expenditures (cost incurred by the health care provider). The left side of the graph depicts recent history and on the right side, present time where decisions have to be made about allocating scarce resources (i.e., the treatment intensity variable). Present-time treatment intensity is affected by severity of illness and determines health expenditure/cost. Severity of illness and treatment intensity determine medical outcomes.

Figure 3 now switches attention to the same scenario with some variables unobserved (as commonly happens in real-life modeling). It also shows how a spurious

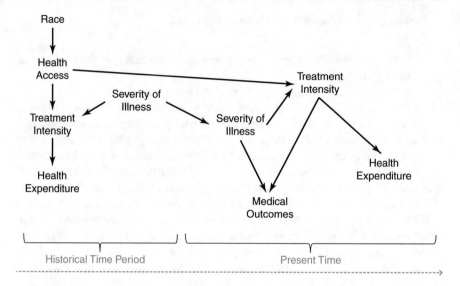

Fig. 2 Causal graph showing a racial health disparity scenario

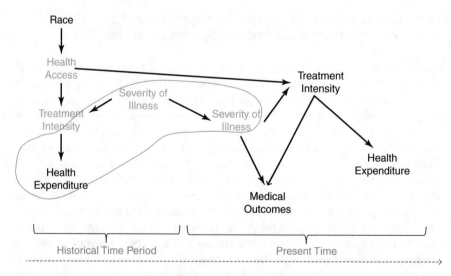

Fig. 3 Causal graph showing the same racial health disparity scenario with some variables unobserved. Correlation of health expenditures with Severity of illness

correlation develops between past health expenditure and present severity of illness (through past severity of illness).

Finally, Fig. 4 shows how the present day picture (with several variables unobserved) looks to the analyst. A **striking characteristic** of the model is that race causally influences treatment intensity. There is *no medical reason for this to*

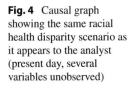

Fig. 4 Causal graph showing the same racial health disparity scenario as it appears to the analyst (present day, several variables unobserved)

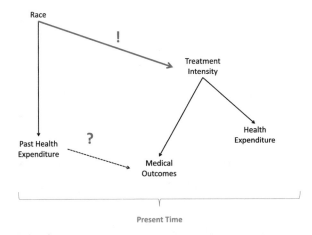

happen, and thus this should alert the analyst to investigate why such a racial bias exists in the process that generated the data. Moreover, past health expenditure will be flagged by latent variable detection algorithms as confounded or possibly confounded and is not detected as definitively causal for medical outcomes. *Using past health expenditures as proxy for the severity of illness (which is causal) will therefore not be warranted by the model.*

By comparison, if the same analyst builds a (optimally predicitve and compact) predictive model for medical outcomes, such a model would look like a function of {Past Health expenditures, and current intensity of treatment}. Race would most likely drop out of such a model because it is independent of medical outcomes given past expenditures and treatment intensity. The model would also tend to predict medical outcomes well. The analyst would be blinded by a purely predictive model to the role of race and may also be led to falsely believe that such a model can be used to guide health resource allocation (treatment intensity) to the patient who need it the most and expect that outcomes will improve.

This example is paradigmatic of a general rule useful for applied analysis which exploits algorithmic detection of causal paths to reveal racial biases and inequitable practices.

> **Causal-Path-to-Outcomes Principle of Bias Detection:** If there are one or more causal paths from race or other minority, marginalized or underserved population indicator variables to medical decisions that affect outcomes *and* they are not medically justified, this indicates an unethical bias that should be addressed (in the modeling, and/or in the practice that the model captures).

Ethical implications of equivalence class modeling for racial and other bias detection. If a large equivalence class exists for predictively optimal models, it is entirely possible for measured factors indicative of racial or other bias to escape detection by being replaced in the model by information equivalent variables. This can happen maliciously or accidentally, if the equivalence class is large and algorithms used cannot model the equivalence class but instead choose a random member.

To illustrate, consider a data distribution where race (or any other variable indicative of bias) is equivalent with many proxy variables *with respect to its influence to an important decision or outcome.* Then it is entirely possible for modelers and auditors to miss that a seemingly innocuous feature (or set of features) are information equivalent with race or encapsulate its information with respect to the outcome.

Pitfall 16.3

Standard statistical practices such as measuring collinearity are not sufficient solutions for detecting information equivalence, since collinearity measures whether variable set S is highly correlated with race (or other bias factor) *rather than whether race and S have the same information content with respect to sensitive decisions and outcomes.*

For more information on equivalence classes refer to chapter "Lessons Learned from Historical Failures, Limitations and Successes of AI/ML In Healthcare and the Health Sciences. Enduring Problems, and the Role of Best Practices" (and for algorithms capable of discovering them in chapters "An Appraisal and Operating Characteristics of Major ML Methods Applicable in Healthcare & Health Science" and "Principles of Rigorous Development and of Appraisal of ML and AI Methods and Systems").

Ethical implications of system-level thinking when designing AI/ML models. Oftentimes, AI/ML models are created within a narrow context and without having access to the "big picture" of a health system. For example, consider a hypothetical model designed to calculate risk of death for patients with acute pneumonia if admitted or not admitted in the Pulmonary ICU of a hospital. Assume that the model is highly accurate and can identify all patients that will receive significant benefit from the ICU and those who will not. Further assume that for the target population of this model the expected admissions (if the model's recommendation is followed) will not exceed ICU capacity. Unfortunately, the model cannot be deployed on those grounds alone, if we consider that other patients' needs may "compete" for the same pulmonary ICU beds, such as patients with acute asthma or other life-threatening pulmonary diseases. Assume further that a second model is built to decide who should be admitted from this second class of patients and is similarly accurate. However, it may well be the case that the combined recommended admissions by the two models now exceed the ICU's capacity. This scenario points to an obvious incongruity between the two models. Like any scarce resource allocation problem that may affect patient's welfare, this scenario is paradigmatic of serious ethical dilemmas that must be managed carefully and responsibly.

In a complex health system much more numerous, complex and subtle such interactions may combine and sabotage successful deployment and use of the health system's AI/ML ecosystem.

To use an electrical engineering analogy, the ML models function as components of a larger system that presently lacks protections against overloading the system. Well-designed electrical devices are engineered in such a way that their input and output obeys specifications ensuring that a system of interconnected such units will function properly.

What are the protections that can be enforced to make a complex system of AI/ML and human processes work harmoniously with one another? **Technical approaches** to solving this problem include:

(a) Develop models for locally optimized decisions and then use operations research, multi-objective optimization, and other integrative planning and management optimization frameworks to optimize their combined outputs [38–40]. AI/ML planning and ML systems can also help in optimizing such higher-level systems [41].

(b) Build in the AI/Ml models, from the ground up, the interactions among the various components of the health system so that the models are aware of, and are designed to satisfy, the higher level "objective functions".

(c) Pursue a hybrid approach where some problem solving areas are narrowly addressed and others jointly.

In general, the first approach is more modular and scalable, assuming that interactions can be managed by the subsequent combination/optimization. The second approach can capture important decision interactions that may be invisible at a higher level. These distinctions are analogous to stacking individual model outputs versus building combined models (chapter "An Appraisal and Operating Characteristics of Major ML Methods Applicable in Healthcare & Health Science"). The third approach is more flexible and should be advantageous, if implemented correctly.

Non-technical approaches, include:

(a) Appropriate governance and oversight of the AI/ML that has the large-scale view of the role and function of the AI/ML models in a system context.

(b) Initiating the creation of AI/ML by not only local problems (e.g., the needs of a small specialty unit), but these same local problems informed by larger perspectives and considerations, as well. Or conversely initiating large-scale goals for the AI/ML that is then addressed in a divide-and-conquer focused-model/system manner.

Guidelines for Ethical Health AI/ML (with a Focus on Health Equity)

We will conclude this chapter with recommended guidelines toward the overarching goals of using AI to create benefit to individuals and populations and not harm. A particular focus here will be on use of health AI/ML to reduce disparities and improve health equity.

Within these general directions we differentiate between AI/ML modeling that seeks to understand weaknesses and areas of improvement in the healthcare system and health science research (i.e., models geared toward uncovering and detecting factors compromising health or health equity), versus models for optimizing decisions, changing practices, individualizing decisions, and influencing policy.

We will call the first type of models **Models for Understanding** and the latter category, **Action Models**. As the guidelines show, these two models require different treatment. We will also interleave rationale for some of the recommendations (when such rationale is not obvious from prior discussion).

Best Practice 16.3
Health AI/ML should strive to always benefit and never cause harm to any individual or group of individuals. Do not design, develop or deploy models that make unnecessary and avoidable errors, or are grossly inefficient, or harmful in any way to any individual or group of individuals.

This book has described, across many chapters, many recommended practices toward implementing the above goal. *In the remainder we will present best practices that support the above goal but specifically strengthen it for health equity, fairness and social justice.*

Best Practice 16.4
AI should strive to decrease, and ensure that it does not increase health disparities. Do not design, develop or deploy models that may increase health disparities or systematically benefit or harm specific groups over others. Whenever possible seek to design, develop or deploy models that increase health equity.

Best Practice 16.5
Importance of an ethical, equity and social justice-sensitive culture of health AI/ML.
1. Cultivate a culture promoting health equity values and is broadly ethics-sensitive within the data science team.
2. Ensure proper training in health equity and overall biomedical ethics of all data scientists working on the project.
3. Participate in organizational efforts to build and sustain an organizational culture promoting strong biomedical ethics values.
4. Seek advice and active involvement from ethics experts, patients, patient advocates, and community representatives regarding possible harm of the contemplated AI/ML work to individuals, and threats to health equity. Seek to obtain insights, guidance and community support on how the AI/ML work can lead to reduction of disparities.
5. Hold yourself and others accountable to the above principles and aims.

Best Practice 16.6
Data Design must support health equity. Always collect data on health determinants especially those intertwined with health disparities and use them in modeling along with all other data relevant to the problem at hand. Ensure that representation of underserved and minority groups is adequate and well-aligned with ethical and health justice principles.

Best Practice 16.7
Model development and evaluation must support health equity.

1. Always, during problem formulation, data design, and model development, validation and deployment stages, consider and actively pursue modeling that does not compromise (and ideally benefits) equity.
2. Analyze the model decisions with respect to health determinant variables. Use interpretable/explainable models, causal modeling, and equivalence class modeling in order to develop a robust understanding of how the model's output may affect health equity and what related biases the model may exhibit. Fix problems related to bias.
3. If medical outcomes are not part of the model, and only intermediate proxies are modeled, examine their suitability. Also examine how model decisions affect outcomes post model deployment. Study how health determinants affect outcomes via the model's function.

Best Practice 16.8
Revealing racial bias and discriminatory practices. Use AI/ML to reveal harmful biases in health care, and health science practices (in aggregate and individually). Use the models to flag such biases and suggest ways to remove them. Models that reveal biases in order to correct them, by necessity capture the bias variables, their effects and interactions. "Sterilizing" these models from the bias they model, defeats the purpose of their existence and their value.

The **"Causal-Path-to-Outcomes Principle of Bias Detection"**. If there are one or more causal paths from race or other minority population indicator variables, to outcomes *and* they are not medically justified, this indicates an ethical bias that should be addressed (either in the modeling, or in the practice that the model captures).

Best Practice 16.9
Equitable access to beneficial AI. Ensure that all who would benefit from an AI/ML model have access to it.

Best Practice 16.10
System-level interactions and their ethical implications. AI/ML models, when deployed, will not operate in a vacuum. Different models designed for different populations when optimized separately for the individual populations, may be non-enforceable because they may "hit a wall" of limited resources. In such cases, system-level planning, goal-setting, and technical solutions must be brought to bear to optimize multi-objective functions and systems of local AI/ML respecting ethical principles and factors.

Key Concepts Discussed in This Chapter

Clinical Decision Support
ISO 14971 standard for risk management for medical devices
Medical Device
Benefit, Harm, Risk, Risk management
FDA's Final Guidance for AI-based clinical decision support
Minority health
NIH Minority health populations
Health equity, health inequity, health disparity
Populations with health disparities
Health determinants
Causal-Path-to-Outcomes Principle of bias detection

Pitfalls Discussed in This Chapter

Pitfall 16.1. The ISO 14971 is not a implementation standard. It mandates that certain actions to be taken but does not prescribe exactly how they will be carried out.

Pitfall 16.2. Using race variable's effect on model decision as a flawed criterion for detecting racial bias:

1. Race may have no effect in a model because other variables have the same information content as race. In other words, this bias detection strategy can systematically generate false negatives in certain distributions.

2. Race may be a justifiable predictor variable if biological reasons (or, more broadly, well-justified standard of care) suggest its appropriateness. For example, if members of a racial group carry a genetic mutation that increases risk for a disease, then a diagnostic or risk model for that disease should use race (in the absence of genotyping information) without this being a negative bias. In other words this bias detection strategy can also generate systematic false positives.

3. The Berkson bias (see chapter "Data Design") can induce spurious correlations if in the hospital (or other selected) populations, race correlates with diagnosis, treatment, and/or other decisions that influence outcomes. In such cases, diagnosis, treatment, etc. models may benefit (improve in accuracy) from the inclusion of race, but this is a reflection of selection bias of the hospitalized population, rather than racial bias. This is another systematic false positive scenario for the race variable inclusion-exclusion strategy.

Pitfall 16.3. Standard statistical practices such as measuring collinearity are not sufficient solutions for detecting information equivalence, since collinearity measures whether variable set S is highly correlated with race (or other bias factor) *rather than whether race and S have the same information content with respect to sensitive decisions and outcomes.*

Best Practices Discussed in This Chapter

Best Practice 16.1. Consider all relevant risks in different phases of the life cycle. Risks can change over time, e.g., the probability or severity of risk can change due to advancements in treatments or due to patient population drift.

Best Practice 16.2. The rationale for the risk management plan is that having a plan produced ahead of time makes it less likely that a risk management step is overlooked or accidentally skipped.

Best Practice 16.3. Health AI/ML should strive to always benefit and never cause harm to any individual or group of individuals. Do not design, develop or deploy models that make unnecessary and avoidable errors, or are grossly inefficient, or harmful in any way to any individual or group of individuals.

Best Practice 16.4 AI should strive to decrease, and ensure that it does not increase health disparities. Do not design, develop or deploy models that may increase health disparities or systematically benefit or harm specific groups over others. Whenever possible seek to design, develop or deploy models that increase health equity.

Best Practice 16.5. Importance of an ethical, equity and social justice--sensitive culture of health AI/ML.

1. Cultivate a culture promoting health equity values and is broadly ethics-sensitive within the data science team.
2. Ensure proper training in health equity and overall biomedical ethics of all data scientists working on the project.
3. Participate in organizational efforts to build and sustain an organizational culture promoting strong biomedical ethics values.
4. Seek advice and active involvement from ethics experts, patients, patient advocates, and community representatives regarding possible harm of the contemplated AI/ML work to individuals, and threats to health equity. Seek to obtain insights, guidance and community support on how the AI/ML work can lead to reduction of disparities.
5. Hold yourself and others accountable to the above principles and aims.

Best Practice 16.6 Data Design must support health equity. Always collect data on health determinants especially those intertwined with health disparities and use them in modeling along with all other data relevant to the problem at hand. Ensure that representation of underserved and minority groups is adequate and well-aligned with ethical and health justice principles.

Best Practice 16.7 Model development and evaluation must support health equity.

1. Always, during problem formulation, data design, and model development, validation and deployment stages, consider and actively pursue modeling that does not compromise (and ideally benefits) equity.
2. Analyze the model decisions with respect to health determinant variables. Use interpretable/explainable models, causal modeling, and equivalence class modeling in order to develop a robust understanding of how the model's output may affect health equity and what related biases the model may exhibit. Fix problems related to bias.
3. If medical outcomes are not part of the model, and only intermediate proxies are modeled, examine their suitability. Also examine how model decisions affect outcomes post model deployment. Study how health determinants affect outcomes via the model's function.

Best Practice 16.8. Revealing racial bias and discriminatory practices. Use AI/ML to reveal harmful biases in health care, and health science practices (in aggregate and individually). Use the models to flag such biases and suggest ways to remove them. Models that reveal biases in order to correct them, by necessity capture the bias variables, their effects and interactions. "Sterilizing" these models from the bias they model, defeats the purpose of their existence and their value.

The "Causal-Path-to-Outcomes Principle of Bias Detection". If there are one or more causal paths from race or other minority population indicator variables, to outcomes *and* they are not medically justified, this indicates an ethical bias that should be addressed (either in the modeling, or in the practice that the model captures).

Best Practice 16.9. Equitable access to beneficial AI. Ensure that all who would benefit from an AI/ML model have access to it.

Best Practice 16.10. System-level interactions and their ethical implications. AI/ML models, when deployed, will not operate in a vacuum. Different models designed for different populations when optimized separately for the individual populations, may be non-enforceable because they may "hit a wall" of limited resources. In such cases, system-level planning, goal-setting, and technical solutions must be brought to bear to optimize multi-objective functions and systems of local AI/ML respecting ethical principles and factors.

Questions and Discussion Topics in This Chapter

1. Explain the relationship between "intended use" and the concepts of target population, accessible population, study sample, inclusion and exclusion criteria from chapter "The Development Process and Lifecycle of Clinical Grade and Other Safety and Performance-Sensitive AI/ML Models".

2. What is the difference between risk assessment, risk estimation, risk evaluation, and risk control?

3. Consider the risk model (from chapter "Data Design in Biomedical AI/ML") used in diabetic patients that helps assess patients' risk of major cardiac events. The risk assessed by this model can be used for determining whether the patient should receive more aggressive treatment.
   (a) What are the potential benefits?
   (b) What are the potential harms?
   (c) Are the risks of these harms estimable? If so, how would you estimate them?

4. What potential problems can you think of when AI models are used for risk evaluation?

5. The ISO standard requires "risk evaluation", which is the step that determines whether a risk is acceptable, but does not provide guidance on how to perform this step. Explain how measures of clinical utility from chapter "Evaluation" relate to "risk evaluation". Explain how the decision curve (chapter "Evaluation") can be used for "risk evaluation".

6. Risk assessment includes the malfunction of models in its scope.

   (a) Can you think of malfunctions that an AI-based prognostic model could experience?
   (b) More generally, what kind of malfunctions can AI-based models experience?

7. Describe how you would go about using ML to model a care provider's decisions in such a way that the model may reveal biased treatment of certain groups of patients. Use ideas from explanation methods described in chapter "The Development Process and Lifecycle of Clinical Grade and Other Safety and Performance-Sensitive AI/ML Models" and the "Causal-Path-to-Outcomes Principle of Bias Detection". In particular, such a model can be thought as "global surrogate model" for a black box AI (which is the human care provider in this case).

   (a) What kind of data would you need?
   (b) What would be the technical challenges and pitfalls in creating such a model?
   (c) What would it mean for such a model to be high fidelity?
   (d) Assuming that an accurate model is created, how would you put it in practice to alert against biased care provider decisions or actions.
   (e) How would you use the model to help in the education of the care provider?

8. This is a self-introspective exercise – no need to report to class. What are your personal knowledge, attitudinal, or experiential gaps regarding a better understanding and practice of health equity and other ethical issues that once addressed will make a you a better health care or health sciences professional?

9. This is a self-reflective exercise – no need to report to class. Going back to prior work of yours, what limitations do you see in light of this chapter in terms of ELSI dimensions? How would you improve past work if you would do it anew today?

References

1. Osheroff JA, Teich JM, Middleton B, Steen EB, Wright A, Detmer DE. A roadmap for national action on clinical decision support. J Am Med Inform Assoc. 2007;14:141–5.
2. Campbell RJ. The five rights of clinical decision support: CDS tools helpful for meeting meaningful use. J AHIMA. 2013;84:42–7. (web version updated February 2016)
3. McCallie D, Mandel J, Shekleton K, Strasberg H, Narus S, Marshall P, DeVault P, Vetter I. Beyond SMART remote decision support with CDS hooks. AMIA annual symposium proceedings 2016; 2016.
4. ISO 14971:2019, Medical devices—application of risk management to medical devices. Paragraph 3.10
5. FDA. Clinical decision support software guidance for Industry and Food and Drug Administration Staff. In: U.S. Food and Drug Administration; 2022. https://www.fda.gov/media/109618/download. Accessed 12 Dec 2022.
6. 21st Century Cures Act. H.R. 34, 114th Congress; 2016. https://www.gpo.gov/fdsys/pkg/BILLS-114hr34enr/pdf/BILLS-114hr34enr.pdf. Accessed 12 Dec 2022

7. FDA. Clinical decision support software; draft guidance for Industry and Food and Drug Administration Staff; 2019. https://www.federalregister.gov/documents/2019/09/27/2019-21000/clinical-decision-support-software-draft-guidance-for-industry-and-food-and-drug-administration. Accessed 12 Dec 2022.

8. FDA. Artificial intelligence and machine learning (AI/ML)-enabled medical devices; 2022. https://www.fda.gov/medical-devices/software-medical-device-samd/artificial-intelligence-and-machine-learning-aiml-enabled-medical-devices. Accessed 12 Dec 2022.

9. FDA, Health Canada, UK MHRA. Good machine learning practice for medical device development: guiding principles; 2021. https://www.fda.gov/medical-devices/software-medical-device-samd/good-machine-learning-practice-medical-device-development-guiding-principles

10. AI Act: co-rapporteurs seek closing high-risk classification, sandboxes. Euractiv.com. https://www.euractiv.com/section/artificial-intelligence/news/ai-act-co-rapporteurs-seek-closing-high-risk-classification-sandboxes/

11. Online collection of all of the official EU AI Act documents. https://artificialintelligenceact.eu/documents/

12. European Commission: proposal for a regulation laying down harmonised rules on artificial intelligence; 21 April 2021. https://digital-strategy.ec.europa.eu/en/library/proposal-regulation-laying-down-harmonised-rules-artificial-intelligence

13. Bryson JJ. Europe is in danger of using the wrong definition of AI. Wired Magazine; 2022. https://www.wired.com/story/artificial-intelligence-regulation-european-union/

14. Engler A. The EU's attempt to regulate open-source AI is counter productive. Brookings.edu; 2022. https://www.brookings.edu/blog/techtank/2022/08/24/the-eus-attempt-to-regulate-open-source-ai-is-counterproductive/

15. NIST risk management framework aims to improve trustworthiness of artificial intelligence. NIST January 26, 2023. https://www.nist.gov/news-events/news/2023/01/nist-risk-management-framework-aims-improve-trustworthiness-artificial

16. AI Risk Management Framework. NIST. https://www.nist.gov/itl/ai-risk-management-framework

17. U.S. Department of Health and Human Services Office for Civil Rights. Breach portal. https://ocrportal.hhs.gov/ocr/breach/breach_report.jsf

18. National Institute on Minority Health and Health Disparities. Minority health and health disparities: definitions and parameters. https://www.nimhd.nih.gov/about/strategic-plan/nih-strategic-plan-definitions-and-parameters.html

19. Executive Office of the President, U.S. Management and Budget Office. Standards for maintaining, collecting, and presenting federal data on race and ethnicity; 2016. https://www.federalregister.gov/documents/2016/09/30/2016-23672/standards-for-maintaining-collecting-and-presenting-federal-data-on-race-and-ethnicity

20. Braveman P. What are health disparities and health equity? We need to be clear. Public Health Reports. 2014;129(1_suppl2):5–8.

21. Whitehead M, Dahlgren G. Concepts and principles for tackling social inequities in health: Levelling up Part 1. World Health Organization: Studies on social and economic determinants of population health, 2, pp. 460–474; 2006.

22. Whitehead M. The concepts and principles of equity and health. Health Promotion Int. 1991;6(3):217–28.

23. Čartolovni A, Tomičić A, Mosler EL. Ethical, legal, and social considerations of AI-based medical decision-support tools: a scoping review. Int J Med Inform. 2022;161:104738.

24. Guan H, Dong L, Zhao A. Ethical risk factors and mechanisms in artificial intelligence decision making. Behav Sci. 2022;12(9):343.

25. Guan J. Artificial intelligence in healthcare and medicine: promises, ethical challenges and governance. Chin Med Sci J. 2019;34(2):76–83.

26. Price WN, Cohen IG. Privacy in the age of medical big data. Nat Med. 2019;25(1):37–43.

27. Martinez-Martin N, Luo Z, Kaushal A, Adeli E, Haque A, Kelly SS, Wieten S, Cho MK, Magnus D, Fei-Fei L, Schulman K. Ethical issues in using ambient intelligence in health-care settings. Lancet Digital Health. 2021;3(2):e115–23.

28. Martinez-Martin N, Kreitmair K. Ethical issues for direct-to-consumer digital psychotherapy apps: addressing accountability, data protection, and consent. JMIR Mental Health. 2018;5(2):e9423.

29. Parviainen J, Rantala J. Chatbot breakthrough in the 2020s? An ethical reflection on the trend of automated consultations in health care. Med Health Care Philos. 2022;25(1):61–71.

30. Obermeyer Z, Powers B, Vogeli C, Mullainathan S. Dissecting racial bias in an algorithm used to manage the health of populations. Science. 2019;366(6464):447–53.

31. Kostick-Quenet KM, Cohen IG, Gerke S, Lo B, Antaki J, Movahedi F, Njah H, Schoen L, Estep JE, Blumenthal-Barby JS. Mitigating racial bias in machine learning. J Law Med Ethics. 2022;50(1):92–100.

32. Gichoya JW, McCoy LG, Celi LA, Ghassemi M. Equity in essence: a call for operationalising fairness in machine learning for healthcare. BMJ Health Care Inform. 2021;28(1)

33. Chen IY, Pierson E, Rose S, Joshi S, Ferryman K, Ghassemi M. Ethical machine learning in healthcare. Annu Rev Biomed Data Sci. 2021;4:123–44.

34. Gianfrancesco MA, Tamang S, Yazdany J, Schmajuk G. Potential biases in machine learning algorithms using electronic health record data. JAMA Intern Med. 2018;178(11):1544–7.

35. McCradden MD, Joshi S, Mazwi M, Anderson JA. Ethical limitations of algorithmic fairness solutions in health care machine learning. Lancet Digital Health. 2020;2(5):e221–3.

36. Fletcher RR, Nakeshimana A, Olubeko O. Addressing fairness, bias, and appropriate use of artificial intelligence and machine learning in global health. Front Artif Intell. 2021;3:561802.

37. Prosperi M, Guo Y, Sperrin M, Koopman JS, Min JS, He X, Rich S, Wang M, Buchan IE, Bian J. Causal inference and counterfactual prediction in machine learning for actionable healthcare. Nat Mach Intell. 2020;2(7):369–75.

38. Winston WL. Operations research: applications and algorithms. Cengage Learning; 2022.

39. Rais A, Viana A. Operations research in healthcare: a survey. Int Trans Operat Res. 2011;18(1):1–31.

40. Marler RT, Arora JS. Survey of multi-objective optimization methods for engineering. Struct Multidiscip Optimiz. 2004;26:369–95.

41. Pianykh OS, Guitron S, Parke D, Zhang C, Pandharipande P, Brink J, Rosenthal D. Improving healthcare operations management with machine learning. Nat Mach Intell. 2020;2(5):266–73.

Reporting Standards, Certification/ Accreditation, and Reproducibility

Gyorgy Simon and Constantin Aliferis

Abstract

This chapter covers the interrelated topics of (a) enhancing the quality, safety and reproducibility of clinical AI/ML via reporting standards frameworks; (b) recent efforts for accrediting health care provider organizations for AI readiness and maturity; (c) professional certification; and (d) education and related accreditation in the space of educational programs of data science and biomedical informatics specific to AI/ML.

Keywords

Reporting Standards · TRIPOD (and other common standards) · Certification · Accreditation

Reporting Standards

An essential element of successful application of a previously developed and validated model is to have documented exactly the intent of the model, its method of construction, the data used, the analytical modeling, the characteristics of the intended application population and the expected generalization performance and safety characteristics. These pieces of information can enable third parties, independent of the developers, to evaluate the rigor of the models, determine the appropriateness of their application to their settings, and perform further evaluations, refinements and enhancements as needed. For all the above to be feasible, sufficient documentation and reporting of the model development and validation process must

G. Simon (✉) · C. Aliferis
Institute for Health Informatics, University of Minnesota,
Minneapolis, MN, USA

exist. Certain narrower subsets of the above functions fall also under the rubric of *scientific reproducibility,* which is a major indicator of reliable science, of AI/ML models with a high likelihood of successful application in additional populations and settings. Reporting standards have been devised in the scientific publication sphere to facilitate these goals. However, these reporting standards can also be applied to *internal* organizational documentation practices.

The publication reporting standards prescribe a minimal set of information that different types of scientific publications in health sciences must include. They are not designed to improve research quality, study design or any aspect of research and development other than reproducibility. Even when publication is not a primary goal, these reporting standards can be useful as a guide for internal documentation of AI/ML model development.

In this chapter, we review and synthesize several existing reporting standards, and comment on their usefulness and applicability to AI/ML development.

> **Reporting standards** prescribe a minimal set of information that needs to be included in the model description.

Problems with reporting has been recognized as early as 1929 [1], and several guidelines have been proposed. The first evidence-based recommendations, CONSORT, have been published for clinical trials in 1996. These guidelines have established a protocol for developing reporting standards, for disseminating these guidelines, and recognized the need for collaboration among various stakeholders, including the researchers and the journals. The most established organization for reporting guidelines is the **E**nhancing the **QUA**lity and **T**ransparancy **O**f heath **R**esearch, EQUATOR [2]. In their own words, "The EQUATOR Network is an 'umbrella' organization that brings together researchers, medical journal editors, peer reviewers, developers of reporting guidelines, research funding bodies and other collaborators with mutual interest in improving the quality of research publications and of research itself."

The EQUATOR Network has over 250 reporting standards, covering a multitude of study types and settings. There are core reporting standards for several areas relevant to this book, including randomized trials (CONSORT), observational studies (STROBE), diagnostic accuracy (STARD), genetic risks prediction (GRIPS), and others. The most relevant standard is the Transparent Reporting of a Multivariable Prediction Model for Individual Prognosis or Diagnosis (TRIPOD).

Purpose and Value of Documenting AI/ML Models

Decision makers at health care provider organizations may appraise published models to determine appropriateness for particular clinical applications. Researchers may wish to replicate the same modeling process to compare the resulting model with alternatives. AI/ML data scientists may want to improve upon the model, etc. The publication of the model must contain sufficient information so that readers (i) can determine whether the research is sound, (ii) can determine whether the model has clinical utility in the intended or other contexts and (iii) test whether they can reproduce the results.

Moreover, changes in healthcare are constant; among many changes, demographics shift, practice patterns improve, diagnostic criteria are updated and new treatments are introduced. As a result, models need to be re-evaluated, updated, extended regularly. Complete documentation can help anticipate which elements need to be updated. The model or its predictors may have to be completely reconstructed for example due to changes in the underlying technologies or the model may have to be recomputed to prove the correctness of the development process to determine liability. Proper documentation of the model is necessary for these purposes and the reporting standards provide help in ensuring that at least a minimal set of required elements have been included in the documentation.

Pitfall 17.1
Poorly documented AI/ML models and their development and evaluation processes make independent review and replication efforts difficult.

Pitfall 17.2
Information required by reporting standards is a minimal set; additional information is often necessary.

Best Practice 17.1
Document the model, its development, validation and deployment process.

Best Practice 17.2
Document AI/ML models using reporting standards and extend with problem and technology-specific necessary information even if not part of the standard. Such extensions can be based on the various development stages and Best Practices in the present volume.

Relation to Reproducibility

Reproducibility is a cornerstone of science. Research is reproducible if independent scientists can recreate the findings (e.g., AI/ML models and their performance characteristics) based on the reported information. In the last decade, several large studies have been conducted to measure the reproducibility of published studies. In an attempt to reproduce results from 100 manuscripts in the psychology literature, a research team found that while 97% of the original studies reported a significant effect, only 36% of replication studies found that effect [3]. Replication efforts in biomedical and other fields found that approximately only 50% of the research studies was reproducible [4–6]. Failure of the studies to replicate was found to be predictable; e.g., predictions by peers about whether a study would replicate were highly correlated with the actual replication results [7]. The purpose of the reporting standards in this context is not to advocate for a particular modeling methodology, but to include information in the AI/ML model documentation that allows readers to decide whether the model development process used in the manuscript was sound and to test the reproducibility if needed.

> The key purpose of reporting standards/guidelines is to remind researchers what information to include in the manuscript and to remind peer-reviewers what information to look for. **Reporting guidelines do not prescribe how research should be done.**

Reporting Standards Adoption

In terms of current adoption of reporting standards, a 2022 study [8] examined 152 articles published in the year 2019 to determine which of the 22 key pieces of information recommended by the TRIPOD reporting standard were included. They found that some information, such as interpretation of the results and source of data were included in almost all publications, while others such as the flow of subjects and the predictive performance of the model were included in less than 10%. According to the TRIPOD authors, a model cannot be appraised properly without these pieces of information (we will appraise these claims and describe the TRIPOD standard later in the chapter).

Appraisal of the TRIPOD Standard

Among general purpose reporting standards, TRIPOD is the most applicable to AI/ML models. It comprises a checklist [9] of 22 items, a statement document [10], and an Explanation and Elaboration document [11]. Being a reporting standard for publications, the 22 items are organized by the section of the publication they must be included in: title, abstract, methods, results, etc.

At a high level, key information required includes the clinical context, the study objective, outcome (whether the outcome assessment was "blind"—carried out without knowing the predicted risk), data source, study setting (including the dates), participant information (eligibility, inclusion, exclusion criteria, treatments received), assessment of the predictors (including whether the assessment was "blind"—devoid of knowledge about the outcome), methods information (missing data, feature selection, model type), performance (calibration and discrimination), limitations, potential for clinical use, and funding information. As immediately obvious by examining the TRIPOD reportable elements, there is no guidance on how to pursue AI/ML modeling to ensure safety and effectiveness. Therefore full conformance with TRIPOD reporting does not lead to or guarantee these objectives.

Pitfall 17.3

TRIPOD does NOT guarantee that the resulting model is correct, free of bias and safe for clinical use.

TRIPOD is a reporting standard that seeks to bring to public view elements of proper construction of AI/ML models (e.g. population choice, outcomes and model accuracy, data used etc.). However, several fundamental limitations exist that include:

(a) TRIPOD assumes that the reader knows all appropriate best practices for the right design and execution of the above elements.
(b) TRIPOD is more of ex post factor forensic tool rather than proactive enabler of good AI/ML.
(c) The reporting entity may misrepresent the reported information and TRIPOD has no means of ensuring validity of reporting.
(d) TRIPOD reported elements are neither complete nor are they necessary to ensure high quality AI/ML models.
(e) TRIPOD does not aim to avoid biases and does not assess the risk of pertinent biases.

To address some of TRIPOD's limitations other reporting standards have been devised such as PROBAST [12] with a focus on bias reduction, and CHARMS [13] aiming to help reduce pitfalls in the study design, and provide checklists for this purpose.

We also note that TRIPOD is aimed at multivariate models, primarily regression models. Some of its items are not appropriate across machine learning methods. For example, not all machine learning methods have an intercept or a baseline hazard which are required by TRIPOD. At the time of this writing it has been announced that new AI-focused reporting standard versions of TRIPOD and PROBAST will be developed using a survey and Delphi methodology [14].

Synthesis of Reporting Recommendations from Multiple Existing Standards

Given that reporting standards are not tailored to AI/ML, it is useful to attempt a synthesis of recommendations adopting elements from multiple standards. Below we provide such an example, using items from four documentation standards for documenting ML models using EHR data. The standards are TRIPOD [T] (predictive models), PROBAST [P] (assessment tool for the potential of biases), CHARMS [C] (model appraisal and systematic reviews) and RECORD [R] (retrospective study using individual level data). We re-iterate that depending on the specifics of the models additional necessary documentation has to be provided in accordance with the Best Practices in the present volume.

In Table 1, we include the recommendation itself, organized by modeling steps, and denote which item it corresponds to in each standard.

The main purpose of this list is to demonstrate how multiple standards can be combined to arrive at a more complete documentation that helps the appraisal of the model, including the assessment of potential biases, and help determine the applicability of the model to another institution with different EHR data elements.

Throughout the book, we present a multitude of suggested best practices, designed to increase the likelihood of good modeling and reduce to a minimum the potential for error. These range from high level design down to fine-grain implementation details and can be used to provide complete reporting of critical factors affecting the quality of modeling. Such reportable dimensions and categories are, aspects of causal modeling, unstructured data modeling, diagnostics and assurances for overfitting and under performance avoidance, model selection strategies, modern feature selection, model explanation, regulatory conformance, equity and fairness considerations, and many other critical pieces of information not addressed in Table 1, and that should supplement and enhance the current reporting standards.

Table 1 Synthesis of four reporting standards. The columns correspond to the four reporting standards and the number to the corresponding item in each reporting standard

Item	T	P	C	R
Study Goals and Design				
1. Type of study	1		1	
(diagnostic, prognostic, treatment effect estimation, causal structure discovery, etc)				
2. Type of predictive modeling study			3	
(Model development with external validation, without external validation, external validation of an existing model)				
3. Objective	3b		2	3
4. Medical context; Rational for the study	3a		2	2
5. Intended moment of using the model			7	
Source of Data				
6. Source of data for training and validation	4a	1.1	8	1
(e.g. EHR, individual-level routinely collected, registry, randomized trial, etc)				
7. Key dates	4b		9d	
(start and end of accrual, start and end of follow-up, index date)				
Participants				
8. Study Setting	5a			5
(primary care, ICU, academic center, community hospital, etc) Number of locations and centers				
9. Eligibility criteria	5b	1.2	4, 9a	
10. Patient selection method				6.1,
(Codes, phenotype, algorithms, etc)				6.2
11. Linkage of databases				6.3

Table 1 (continued)

Item	T	P	C	R
12. Treatments received	5c		9c	
13. Study size	8		13	10
Flow diagram for sample selection	13a			13
14. Was there filtering of participants based on data quality?				13.1
15. Exclusion criteria		1.2		
16. Were all selected patients included in the analysis?		4.3		
17. Number of outcome events	14a	4.1	12a	15
18. Number of events in relation to the number of predictors			12b	
19. Participant characteristics (demographic, clinical features, missing predictors, missing outcome)	13b		9b, 13ab	14
20. Summary of follow-up				14c
Outcome				
21. Outcome definition	6a	3.1	5, 10a	7.1
22. Is the outcome pre-defined? Is it a standard outcome? (Composite outcomes can render predictors insignificant)		3.2	10c	
23. Were predictors excluded from the outcome definition? (Unless the predictor is the definition of the outcome)		3.3	10e	
24. How and when was the outcome assessed?	6a			
25. Was the outcome defined the same way for all participants?		3.4	10b	
26. Was the outcome assessment process blind to the model predictions?	6b	3.5	10d	
27. Time gap between predictor assessment and outcome determination		3.6	10f	
28. Time span of prediction (e.g. 7-year diabetes)	6a		6,10f	
Predictor Variables				
29. Definition of all predictors variables	7a		11ab	8
30. Time of the predictor variable assessment	7a		11c	
31. Was the predictor variable assessment process blind to the outcome?	7b	2.2	11d	
32. Were the predictor variables assessed the same way for all participants?		2.1		
33. Are all predictor variables available at the time the model is intended to be used?		2.3		
Modeling				
34. How was missing data handled? (Complete case analysis, imputation, etc)	9	4.4	13c	12c
35. How were the predictor variables handled?	10a		11e	11
36. Univariate association of the predictor variables with the outcome	14b			
37. Pre-selection based on univariate association (potential for bias by omission)		4.5		
38. Type of model, model construction process, feature selection	10b		14acd 14b	
39. Were the model assumptions satisfied?			14b	
40. Were complexities considered? (informative censoring, competing risk, sampling of controls, etc) (RECORD 12d breaks this down by study type)		4.6		12d
41. How were confounders controlled for?				12a
42. Sensitivity analysis				12e

(continued)

Table 1 (continued)

Item	T	P	C	R
43. Subgroup analysis				12b
Evaluation				
44. Measures of model evaluation	10d	4.7	15ab	
Both calibration and discrimination reported for classification				
45. Method of model evaluation	10b	4.7	16a	
(bootstrap, cross validation, etc)				
46. Are confidence intervals reported	16			
47. Performance in the development and validation data	19a			
Is over- and underfitting taken into consideration?				
48. If the performance was poor, was the model updated?	10e, 17			
49. Model comparison	10d			
50. Was external validation performed?			16a	
(temporal, geographical, different investigators, etc)				
51. For validation, describe model updates incl. recalibration	16		16b	
52. Were risk groups defined? How?	11			
53. For external validation, document differences between the	12		17c	
development and validation data sets.	13c			
54. Is there an alternative presentation of the final model		4.8	17b	
(e.g. conversion into a score)		4.9		
Are all components of the model taken into consideration (incl. the intercept)				
Interpretation				
55. Limitations	18			19.1
(non-representative sample, few events, excessive missing data, informative missing data, data not collected for this purpose, unmeasured confounders, eligibility changing over time, etc)				
56. Performance in the development and validation data	19a		18a	
57. Discuss the performance in the context of the objective	19b		18b	20
58. Discuss potential clinical use	20			
Miscellaneous				
59. Study protocol in the supplements	21			

HIMSS Analytic Maturity Model

Another important aid in ensuring the safe, fair, effective and efficient use of AI/ML in clinical practice is the certification of healthcare institutions by professional associations or societies with credible expertise and well-designed, validated certification processes for health AI/ML.

Certification ensures that certified healthcare institutions satisfy a minimum core set of requirements that are set forth by a reputable professional association or society with expertise in the area.

High quality certification ensures that meeting these requirements guarantees organizational competences.

Certification bodies can also offer advice on how to achieve the certification goals in areas of weakness.

Currently there is no professional association specializing in clinical or research AI/ML. HIMSS (Healthcare Information and Management Systems Society), which focuses on Healthcare Information Technology, has developed an 8-stage model of analytic maturity, called the Adaptation Model of Analytic Maturity (AMAM) [15], measuring an institution's analytic capabilities. AMAM is also intended as a roadmap, which, in consultation with HIMSS experts, lays a path forward for organizations that wish to improve their analytic maturity. The eight stages, numbered 0–7, are as follows [15].

We caution the reader that while the intent is to help organizations grow their analytical capabilities, there is a vast distance between conventional analytic capabilities and AI/ML capabilities. While the AMAM framework is not explicitly designed for AI/ML, there is language that strongly implies AI/ML competencies. Such organization competencies require a deep level of advanced scientific and technological understanding that goes beyond conventional analytics and IT.

The high-level certification requirements of Table 2 for example, lack the level of testable technical rigor and specificity that will ensure safe and effective AI/ML technology deployment in a high-risk domain such as clinical medicine. For example, there is little in the stated requirements that ensures that deployed technology is performant, reliable and cost-effective or that it can generate trust in patients, providers, regulators and other stakeholders. Moreover, much needed protection against grave decision making errors that can be produced by poorly understood and applied AI/ML

Table 2 HIMSS Adoption model of analytic maturity stages

Stage	Capabilities
0	The organization does not have any analytic capabilities, but has the desire to develop them.
1.	The organization has started to collect data and stores it at a central location (e.g. in a data warehouse). They have a strategy for developing data governance and for building out the analytic capabilities.
2.	The organization has built a data warehouse and is maturing their data governance. They have established an analytic competency center, responsible for managing the organization's analytic skills, standards and education.
3.	The data quality in the data warehouse is stable, broadly accessible within the organization. Data access is well managed and tools to access the data are standardized. The institution has mastered basic reporting capabilities.
4.	The institution has started directing analytic capabilities towards improving clinical, financial and operational processes. They have started making efforts towards providing analytic support for evidence-based clinical practice, tracking and reporting care and operational variability, and identifying and minimizing clinical and operational waste.
5.	The institution has expanded point-of-care analytics. Analytic capabilities now support population health and have developed a thorough understanding of the economics of care. Quality based performance reporting is implemented.
6.	The institution has reached maturity of predictive analytics and have started focusing on advanced data, such as genetic or biometric information, in preparation of more individualized medicine.
7.	They have developed the ability to deliver mass customization of care along with prescriptive analytics. The institution is leveraging advanced data (e.g. genetic or biometric) to tailor treatment decisions to the individual for personalized medicine.

technology do not seem to be sufficiently addressed. In general, (outside the narrow discussion of the AMAM model) we caution against the following general pitfall:

Pitfall 17.4

There is a world of difference between conventional hospital analytics and AI/ML technology.

Significant dangers exist for certification processes that do not discriminate among these domains to create false confidence in the existence of deep institutional competency and mastery of technologies, the complexity of which, in reality, radically exceeds the technical capabilities of most healthcare institutions.

Such technologies have the potential to radically advance population health when designed correctly, but also to hurt patients if not properly developed and deployed.

Academic Accreditation and Professional Certification Efforts

Beside reporting standards that aim to promote the quality of AI/ML scientific and technological development, and the certification of healthcare organizations along the lines of AI/ML competencies, another pillar of ensuring safety, equity, efficiency and effectiveness is training a specialized workforce with deep expertise in the science and technology of health AI/ML. In this section, we briefly look at two functions: (i) The availability of formal educational programs that educate health data science specialists in health AI/ML at the graduate, and post graduate levels; (ii) The training and certification of the broader health care and health sciences workforce to a minimally necessary level of understanding of these technologies; and (iii) The accreditation of educational programs that provide the above training and certifications.

Currently there are few programs across the nation providing specialized undergraduate, or graduate degrees in health data science and health AI/ML. There is also no accreditation specific to health AI and ML. Elements of healthcare and health science-related AI/ML are often taught in health informatics programs. Very few institutions are offering health AI/ML-focused degrees. The Commission on Accreditation for Health Informatics and Information Management Education (CAHIIM) [16] currently offers accreditation at the Master's Degree level. The CAHIIM standard is based on AMIA's (American Medical Informatics Association) informatics competencies that span health, social and behavioral science, information science and technology, leadership, professionalism, and areas at the intersections of these competencies [17]. These requirements were neither designed to nor do they achieve a comprehensive standard for specialty professional knowledge and competencies in AI/ML.

In terms of continued certification of the broader healthcare workforce, no organization offers AI/ML-specific certification. HIMSS (discussed above) offers certification for health information management systems (Certified Associate/ Professional in Healthcare Information and Management Systems; CAHIMS/ CPHIMS) and digital transformation strategy (Certified Professional in Digital Health Transformation Strategy; CPDHTS). Alternatively, for board certified physicians engaging in health information technology, the clinical informatics subspecialty [18, 19], developed jointly with AMIA, is offered by the American Board of Preventive Medicine or American Board of Pathology but is not designed to develop deep competency in AI/ML.

Pitfall 17.5

There is no professional association/society specifically for health AI/ML.

Pitfall 17.6

There is no accreditation or certification specifically for heath AI/ML.

Pitfall 17.7

There is a dearth of academic programs for educating health data scientists and health AI/ML experts.

Conclusions

The field of health care and health science research is in dire need for development of focused educational programs, meaningful individual and institutional certification, and comprehensive reporting standards. Initial efforts along these lines are promising and directionally sound; however significant and intensive efforts and investments are needed in these areas.

Key Concepts Discussed in This Chapter

Reporting standards prescribe a minimal set of information that needs to be included in the model description.

The key purpose of reporting guidelines is to remind researchers what information to include in the manuscript and to remind peer-reviewers what information to look for. It does not prescribe how research is done.

We discussed the TRIPOD standard for publishing predictive models.

We discussed additional standards. These include the PROBAST, which is a tool for assessing the potential for biases, and CHARMS for appraisal of models and systemic reviews.

Certification aims to ensure that healthcare institutions satisfy a minimum core set of requirements toward developing technical competency.

Educational programs for specialists and certification for the broader workforce will need to be expanded greatly in order to meet the demand for experts necessitated by the explosive growth of AI/ML.

Pitfalls in This Chapter

Pitfall 17.1. Poorly documented AI/ML models and their development and evaluation processes make independent review and replication efforts difficult.

Pitfall 17.2. Information required by reporting standards is a minimal set; additional information is often necessary.

Pitfall 17.3. TRIPOD does NOT guarantee that the resulting model is correct, free of bias and safe for clinical use.

TRIPOD is a reporting standard that seeks to bring to public view elements of proper construction of AI/ML models (e.g. population choice, outcomes and model accuracy, data used etc.). However several fundamental limitations exist that include:

(a) TRIPOD assumes that the reader knows all appropriate best practices for the right design and execution of the above elements.
(b) TRIPOD is more of ex post factor forensic tool rather than proactive enabler of good AI/ML.
(c) The reporting entity may misrepresent the reported information and TRIPOD has no means of ensuring validity of reporting.
(d) TRIPOD reported elements are neither complete nor are they necessary to ensure high quality AI/ML models.
(e) TRIPOD does not aim to avoid biases and does not assess the risk of pertinent biases.

Pitfall 17.4. Significant dangers exist for imperfect or immature certification processes to create institutional false confidence in the existence of deep competency and mastery of technologies the complexity of which radically exceeds the technical capabilities of most healthcare providers. Such technologies have the potential to either radically advance population health when designed correctly, but also to hurt patients if not properly developed and deployed.

Pitfall 17.5. There is no professional association/society specifically for health AI/ML.

Pitfall 17.6. There is no accreditation or certification specifically for heath AI/ML.

Pitfall 17.7. There is a dearth of academic programs for educating health data scientists and health AI/ML experts.

Best Practices in This Chapter

Best Practice 17.1. Document the model, its development, validation and deployment process.

Best Practice 17.2. Document AI/ML models using reporting standards and extent with problem and technology-specific necessary information even if not part of the standard. Such extensions can be based on the various development stages and Best Practices in the present volume.

Questions and Discussion Topics in This Chapter

1. List some benefits of internally documenting a predictive model in a way that the model can be recreated, including the predictor variables, the outcomes, the training and validation data sets, and the model.

2. Discuss benefits and possible downsides of publishing models in peer-reviewed scientific journals.

3. Can you think of ways to publish a model other than a research article?

4. Consider the 22 items of the TRIPOD checklist and answer the following questions.
   (a) Which items are necessary and which can be omitted for the internal documentation of a model?
   (b) If you develop a deep learning model, which items in the checklist may not make sense? Would you change your answer if the model was a GBM?
   (c) Can you think of other data elements that you may want to record for a deep learning model?
   (d) The TRIPOD checklist is designed for diagnostic and prognostic models. Would a model that quantifies the effect of an intervention fall into the purview of TRIPOD?
   (e) Which of the TRIPOD items should be included for a model that quantifies the effect of an intervention for internal documentation? You can modify the item as necessary.
   (f) For the same model (that quantifies the effect of intervention), are there additional pieces of information you would include for (a) internal documentation and (b) for publication of the model in a journal?
   (g) If you were to build a multivariate regression model as a prognostic model based on genetic biomarkers, what additional information would you include?
   (h) Consult the GRIPS checklist (https://www.ncbi.nlm.nih.gov/pmc/articles/PMC3175742/) and refine your answer to question (g).

5. The PROBAST tool (https://www.probast.org/wp-content/uploads/2020/02/PROBAST_20190515.pdf) is designed to assess the risk of bias in predictive models. It is not intended as a reporting standard. Read the PROBAST items and propose new reporting items to add to the TRIPOD checklist that allows for assessing the risk of bias.

6. Suppose you conduct a study for discovering the causal relationships among risk factors in Alzheimer's disease. This is neither a diagnostic nor a prognostic study, so it falls outside the scope of TRIPOD. Which TRIPOD items are relevant and what additional information should be reported?

7. Your goal is to document a prognostic predictive model, e.g. 7-year diabetes risk, for internal use in a manner that allows you to re-construct the predictors, outcome, training and validation data, and the model itself. Create a reporting checklist based on TRIPOD, PROBAST and CHARMS.

8. The HIMSS certification has eight stages, while the CAHIIM accreditation is a pass/defer decision. Can you think of advantages to having multiple stages versus making a binary pass/fail decision?

9. When you look at the stages 1-7 of the AMAM, each stage requires several competencies. Which AMIA competency areas correspond to AMAM competencies?

References

1. Altman DG, Simera I. A history of the evolution of guidelines for reporting medical research: the long road to the EQUATOR Network. J Roy Soc Med. 2016;109(2). https://journals.sagepub.com/doi/pdf/10.1177/0141076815625599
2. EQUATOR network. https://www.equator-network.org/
3. Open Science Collaboration. Estimating the reproducibility of psychological science. Science. 2015;(6251):349. https://doi.org/10.1126/science.aac4716. https://www.science.org/doi/10.1126/science.aac4716
4. Camerer CF, Dreber A, Foresll E, Ho TH, et al. Evaluating replicability of laboratory experiments in economics. Science. 2016;351(6280) https://doi.org/10.1126/science.aaf0918.
5. Piper K. Science has been in a "replication crisis" for a decade. Have we learned anything? Vox; 2020.
6. Baker M, Penny D. Is there a reproducibility crisis? Nature. 2016;533
7. Camerer CF, Dreber A, Holzmeister F, Ho TC, et al. Evaluating the replicability of social science experiments in Nature and Science between 2010 and 2015. Nat Human Behav. 2018;2:637–42.
8. Navarro CLA, Damen JAA, Takada T, Nijman SW, et al. Completeness of reporting of clinical prediction models developed using supervised machine learning: a systematic review. BMC Med Res Methodol. 2022;22:12.
9. TRIPOD checklist. https://www.tripod-statement.org/wp-content/uploads/2020/01/Tripod-Checklist-Prediction-Model-Development-and-Validation-PDF.pdf
10. Collins GS, Reitsma JB, Altman DG, Moons KGM. Transparent reporting of a multivariable prediction model for individual prognosis or diagnosis (TRIPOD): the TRIPOD statement. BMJ. 2014:350. https://doi.org/10.1136/bmj.g7594. [TRIPOD statement].

11. Moons KGM, Altman DG, Reitsma JB, Ioannidis JPA, et al. Transparent reporting of a multivariable prediction model for individual prognosis or diagnosis (TRIPOD): Explanation and Elaboration. Ann Intern Med. 2015;162:W1–W73. https://doi.org/10.7326/M14-0698. [TRIPOD E&E].
12. Moons KGM, Wolff RF, Riley RD, Whiting PF, Westwood M, Collins GS, Reitsma JB, et al. A tool to assess the risk of bias and applicability of prediction model studies: explanation and elaboration. Ann Intern Med. 2019; https://doi.org/10.7326/M18-1377. [PROBAST].
13. Moons KGM, de Groot JAH, Bouwmeester W, Vergouwe Y, Mallett S, Altman DG, et al. Critical appraisal and data extraction for systematic reviews of prediction modelling studies: the CHARMS checklist. PLoS Med. 2014;11(10):e1001744. [CHARMS].
14. Collins GS, Dirman P, Navarro CLA, Ma J, Hooft L, Reitsma JB, Logullo P, Beam AL, et al. Protocol for development of a reporting guideline (TRIPOD-AI) and risk of bias tool (PROBAST-AI) for diagnostic and prognostic prediction model studies based on artificial intelligence. BMJ Open. 2021;11:e048008. https://doi.org/10.1136/bmjopen-2020-04800.
15. [AMAM] HIMSS. Adoption Model for Analytics Maturiy (AMAM). URL: https://www.himss.org/what-we-do-solutions/digital-health-transformation/maturity-models/adoption-model-analytics-maturity-amam
16. [CAHIIM] CAHIIM. URL: cahiim.org
17. AMIA Board. AMIA 2017 core competencies for applied health informatics education at the master's degree level. JAMIA. 2018;25(12):1657–68. [AMIA competencies] https://www.cahiim.org/docs/default-source/about-cahiim/history/final-amia-health-informatics-core-competencies-for-cahiim.pdf?sfvrsn=fed062b8_4
18. Gardner RM, Overhage JM, Steen EB, Munger BS, Holmes JH, Williamson JJ, Detmer DE, for the AMIA Board of Directors. AMIA Board White Paper: core content for the subspecialty of clinical informatics. JAMIA. 2009;16:153–7. https://doi.org/10.1197/jamia.M3045.
19. Safran C, Shabot MM, Munger BS, Holmes JH, Steen EB, Lumpkin JR, Detmer DE, for the AMIA Board of Directors. AMIA Board White Paper: program requirements for fellowship education in the subspecialty of clinical informatics. JAMIA. 2009;16:158–66. https://doi.org/10.1197/jamia.M3046.

Synthesis of Recommendations, Open Problems and the Study of BPs

Constantin Aliferis and Gyorgy Simon

Abstract

This chapter assembles a list of all best practices (BPs), and pitfalls, discussed in the previous chapters. These are codified in a single hierarchical structure and assistive checklists intended to make them operationally useful. We differentiate between macro-, meso- and micro-levels of pitfalls and corresponding best practices-roughly corresponding to high-level principles, concrete differentiations of the above and granular/detailed tools and techniques for implementation. The recommended BPs are cross-referenced across the volume and key corresponding literature and other sources. Several open problems remain and the evolution of BPs for biomedical AI/ML is certain to become in the years to come a field of inquiry with explosive growth and value.

Keywords

Macro-, Meso-, Micro-level guidelines and best practices · Maturity level of guidelines and best practices · Impact level of guidelines and best practices · Continuous evolution of guidelines and best practices · Open problems in best practices of health AI/ML

Bringing Best Practices Together

With all components of understanding pitfalls and codifying corresponding best practices in place, we can now attempt a synthesis of all the material in this volume in a unified framework represented in Fig. 1. As can be seen, background

C. Aliferis (✉) · G. Simon
Institute for Health Informatics, University of Minnesota,
Minneapolis, MN, USA
e-mail: constantinaibestpractices@gmail.com

© The Author(s) 2024
G. J. Simon, C. Aliferis (eds.), *Artificial Intelligence and Machine Learning in Health Care and Medical Sciences*, Health Informatics,
https://doi.org/10.1007/978-3-031-39355-6_18

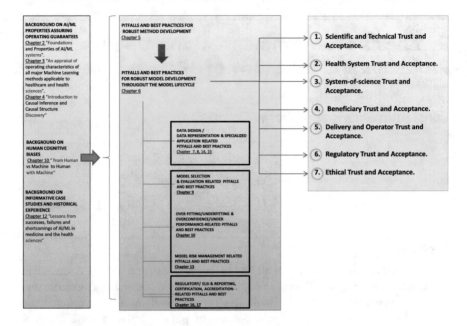

Fig. 1 Synthesis of the book sources and material

knowledge on methods' properties, human cognitive biases, and cases studies (left, grey background) informs the identification of pitfalls and the codification of corresponding best practices (blue background, middle). These address method development, model development, and components such as data design and encoding, model selection, error estimation, over fitting and under fitting avoidance, managing risk of model use are deployment and addressing regulatory and ELSI requirements. Taken together and when properly followed, these can enable the 7 dimensions of AI/ML trust, adoption and acceptance (on the right, green color).

The many pitfalls and best practices we presented throughout the present volume can be thought as belonging to 3 levels which are obvious to the reader by the context of their presentation and discussion:

> **Macro Level Guidance:** corresponds to correct specification of high-level design, in which a problem is mapped to AI and ML modeling, broad objectives, high level principles.
>
> **Micro Level Guidance:** corresponds to lower-level (but still significant) implementation details.
>
> **Meso Level Guidance:** corresponds to conceptual and implementation elements in-between the high (macro) and low (micro) levels. It encompasses neither too broad (and abstract), nor too narrow (and minute) details.

Moreover it is important to appreciate that some of the pitfalls and best practices are more immutable and unlikely to change than others as the field of AI/ML progresses. It is useful to appreciate the differences in maturity levels across pitfalls and guidelines presented in this book and the literature.

Maturity level:
- A **mature** designation denotes immutable, perennial or otherwise robust recommendation.
- An **evolving** designation denotes a recommendation that is work-in-progress, evolving or otherwise subject to likely modifications in the future.

Finally, not all guidance has the same gravity. Some best practices are critical and should be always adhered to according to their **impact level**:

- **High Impact:** corresponds to an action that must be addressed, otherwise serious pitfalls may follow with significant probability. If not addressed, because of special circumstances of a particular problem context, then an explicit rationale must be developed to support the exception.

- **Medium Impact:** corresponds to recommendations that ideally should be addressed. If, however, resource constraints or other factors preclude addressing, then milder pitfalls may ensue, or serious pitfalls with very small probability. In this category we will also include recommendations that can be addressed at a later stage of developing the AI/ML solution.

In APPENDIX 3 of the present book, we collected all best practices of the present volume and characterized them according to maturity and importance. Indicative examples are given in the table below.

Best Practice	Maturity	Impact
10.1: [Context: model development and validation]. Deploy procedures that prevent, diagnose and remedy errors of overconfidence in, or over fitting of, models	MATURE	HIGH
10.2.6: [Context: benchmarking of methods] follow theoretically and empirically proven specifications of reference (i.e., prototypical or official use of employed method)	MATURE	MEDIUM
10.5.7: Models for individual patients: use dense time series data, leverage population models, search for and model abrupt distribution shifts of the individual (including learning and modeling shifts at the population level).	EVOLVING	MEDIUM

Notice that this synthesis is enabled by examining these recommendations across multiple stages and aspects of the AI/ML R&D process and thus the reader can appreciate this final consolidated view with the benefit of having accumulated diverse knowledge about the various scientific and technical aspects of health AI/ML addressed in the book's chapters.

Open Problems, Unknowns & Future Directions

We discuss next, some of the open problems and future directions in the study of best practices for biomedical AI/ML.

Adapting best practices to novel or unanticipated contexts of use. *"Rules are for the obedience of fools and the guidance of wise men"*[1]. This famous quote captures the notion that as user expertise grows the need for strict adherence to rules reduces.

For example, as we saw throughout the present volume, the context of use may influence the validity or application scope of a guideline. Every best practice recommendation is stated with a set of use cases and contexts in mind. It is important to consider if a particular R&D or AI/ML technology deployment project has special characteristics that may subtly or overtly affect the appropriateness of a particular guideline. See for example the discussion of genomics and overfitting in chapter "Lessons Learned from Historical Failures, Limitations and Successes of AI/ML In Healthcare and the Health Sciences. Enduring Problems, and the Role of Best Practices". It is up to the project team to establish that deviations from best practices, especially ones designated as critical in the above checklists is appropriate. Conversely, if a recommended best practice is assessed to be too lax for a problem at hand, it may be necessary to incorporate additional restrictions, safeguards, performance requirements etc. that go beyond the ones presented here.

Related to the above, **newer technology may (and should) render manual safeguards of today, automatic,** and indeed this is a trend in ML, for example many newer algorithms that incorporate multiple protections against overfitting, or sampling variation (see chapter "An Appraisal and Operating Characteristics of Major ML Methods Applicable in Healthcare & Health Science"). This is also the case for statistical techniques that incorporate regularization/shrinkage and do not require pre-processing data with PCA or other dimensionality reduction. Systems that are designed around protocols and stacks that implement best practices will also advance the ease of use and reduce the need for manual enforcement of best practices.

Sufficiency vs necessity and assumption-mitigating factors. Often techniques that are designed to work well under specific sufficient assumptions *surprise the research community by working well in settings that violate these assumptions.* Perhaps the most classic example in the history of data science is the success of linear models even when deployed in domains with non-linear data generating

---

[1] Attributed to Harry Day, the Royal Flying Corps First World War fighter ace.

functions (for example, due to bias-variance reasons, see chapter "Foundations and Properties of AI/ML Systems"). Another example is the mitigation of the hardness of large scale causal models despite the fact that worst case computational complexity for even small networks is intractable (see chapter "Foundations and Properties of AI/ML Systems"). Benchmarks have shown that methods whose sufficient assumptions are violated, manage in some situations to outperform better–designed methods (for example, in very small samples simple univariate association strategies may outperform more complex modeling strategies; or in another example XOR parents of a response have non-zero first order effects if they are correlated, i.e., they do not exhibit the worst-case behavior of the textbook XOR function). These considerations suggest that data scientists should operate with an open mind and employ a plurality of techniques as these may yield good but unexpected results. They must walk the fine line between allowing for empirical happy surprises on one hand, and avoiding wishful thinking or not prioritizing methods according to their fit to the problem, on the other.

Ramifications of tampering with validated codes. It takes lengthy, costly and demanding efforts to build methods that meet specific performance criteria with guaranteed properties (as detailed in chapter "Principles of Rigorous Development and of Appraisal of ML and AI Methods and Systems"). At the same time, changes to original specifications that on the surface may appear insignificant can have major effects on these properties and performance (see chapter "Lessons Learned from Historical Failures, Limitations and Successes of AI/ML In Healthcare and the Health Sciences. Enduring Problems, and the Role of Best Practices" - text categorization benchmark study). This issue becomes of great relevance in light of open science frameworks in which anyone can access and modify codes and algorithms with potentially uncontrollable consequences to quality due to the modifications. Establishing unique identifiers for algorithm and code versions with associated properties, benchmarks and other performance properties, may serve as a possible solution to this problem.

Transparency of algorithms and codes is desirable in many ways especially for validating methods and tools, however it opens up the possibility for abuse, unintended damage or even "gaming" of models and systems. **Black box** methods and systems are utterly undesirable when not operating as intended or to the standard of safety and performance that generates trust and adoption. On the opposite side of things, black box systems that are "locked" to avoid tampering and degrading alterations may be desirable under many circumstances. Also as it has been advocated in the AI literature, if the well-validated statistical advantage of a black box model is so superior to the performance of the best transparent model, it may be impractical or even unethical to not use the best performing model. Navigating these tradeoffs is certainly a challenge.

Developing a culture that values and strives for performant and responsible AI/ML is of paramount importance for wide spread adoption of BPs. Such culture can be developed in key places: education (health science and professional health schools), ethics training, engagement with community, government, health systems, tech industry. This culture should be built around guiding principles with sound scientific basis and broad acceptance.

Over-engineering and over-regulating. As with every aspect of science and technology, if best practices are enforced in very prescriptive, bureaucratic or superficial ways lacking thoughtfulness, there is the danger to stifle innovation and render progress slow. The need to ensure safety and performance by adhering to best practices designed to support these goals has to be carefully balanced against the very real **opportunity costs** inherent in unnecessarily delaying deployment of useful AI/ML both in healthcare and the health sciences.

Need for evolving best practices systematically. Undoubtedly, the recommendations and codified best practices in this volume and elsewhere will evolve as the science and technology of AI/ML advance and as new use cases in health care and health science research emerge. It is important that this evolution is informed by prior generations of best practices and that the various stakeholders who will be called to adopt and advance the state of the art in BPs will do so without re-inventing the wheel. There is a body of knowledge in particular that we cannot imagine to require radical re-design or abandonment in any point in the foreseeable future. For example, we will always need to have health care models and decision support systems with precise goals guiding their design and deployment. We will always need reliable estimators of model performance. We will always need to design data capture, sampling and measurements in ways that support the modeling objectives. We will always need to manage the trade-offs of model bias and sampling variance. We will always need to pay particular attention to the distinction between causal and associational models and their strengths and limitations. We will always need to equip AI/ML models and systems with protective measures against operating outside their knowledge and safe performance boundaries. We will always need to ensure against unethical and biased operation of such technology. These are just a few examples of essentially immutable objectives stemming from fundamental laws of statistics and learning theory, computer science, statistical risk management, computability, and ethics.

Bypassing regulations by claiming exploratory intent. It is all too easy to disguise a decision model that guides user actions as one that merely advises or informs the user. This has been a problem throughout the history of health AI/ML. Regulation must address such abuses, otherwise they can render regulation perfunctory and ineffective but also because they can grossly distort the performance and safety requirements at the design stages of AI/ML systems.

Misaligned sentiment and technical reality. As we saw in chapter "Lessons Learned from Historical Failures, Limitations and Successes of AI/ML In Healthcare and the Health Sciences. Enduring Problems, and the Role of Best Practices" a large distance between the reality of AI/ML capabilities and the over-promising of results led to multiple and deep crises in the history of the field. This danger is always present and should be taken very seriously. It is the position of the present book that rational and careful R&D and deployment facilitated by appropriate best practices can accelerate passage thru the precarious terrain of the hype cycle.

Need to conduct R&D with limited resources. For reasons of simplicity we presented feasibility and mission-critical development as discrete and mutually exclusive approaches. However even when mission-critical models and systems are sought, "ideal" development, validation and deployment of AI/ML not only is not always possible, but it could also be economically unwise. A phased approach where R&D can be abandoned once sufficient evidence against feasibility is gathered, is a more economically realistic approach. This **phased model of feasibility → iterative development until mission-critical goals are met**, is a worthy direction that is also congruent with established models of industrial R&D. However at this time the precise mechanisms to optimally manage such phased development in the health AI context, is an open problem.

We finally ask:

Do best practices need to be universally accepted? Should there be a single set of acceptable and/or effective best practices for health AI/ML? We can conceptualize health AI/ML BPs as comprising a *necessary shared core criteria,* and a component corresponding to additional *sufficient criteria with multiple alternatives of equal outcomes.* In other words to the extent that BPs abide by the laws of statistics, data science, and so forth, they may vary in various details (of sufficient criteria). What has to be present in all useful guidelines is an underlying shared core of necessary criteria. Finally, there is value in establishing BPs that further *specialize the general rules to narrow fields of application* with more or less restrictive requirements. We expect that such variations will become a topic of fruitful research.

Conclusion

It is our hope that the specific guidances presented here, especially when focused on persistent and immutable desiderata and laws of biomedical data science, will be a useful basis for both the growing success of biomedical AI/ML, and for assisting in the study of best practices as its own worthwhile subfield of AI/ML.

Key Concepts Discussed in This Chapter

Macro, Meso, and Micro Level Guidelines and Best Practices
BP Maturity levels: Mature vs Evolving
BP Impact levels: High vs Medium Impact

Key Messages Discussed in This Chapter

- Bringing Best Practices together. From background knowledge on methods' properties, to the identification of pitfalls and the codification of corresponding best practices to enable the 7 dimensions of AI/ML trust, adoption and acceptance.
- A checklist that integrates and characterizes all discussed BPs (Appendix 3).
- Best practices may need to be adapted to novel or unanticipated contexts of use.
- In the future, newer technology may (and should) render manual safeguards automatic.
- Mitigating factors can exist that can overcome lack of sufficient assumptions for correctness or other properties.
- Tampering with validated codes may have unwanted ramifications.
- There are pros and cons of transparent algorithms and codes vs Black Box technology.
- Developing a culture that values and strives for performant, ethical and accountable AI/ML is of paramount importance for wide spread adoption of BPs
- Over-engineering and over-regulating AI/ML are dangers that need be recognized and addressed.
- Improving BPs is unavoidable but needs to be done systematically.
- Bypassing regulations by claiming exploratory intent may hinder successful regulation and AI/ML based solution design.
- Misaligned expectations and technical reality is a problem that may be mitigated by BPs.
- Phased feasibility to iterative development may allow more economically efficient R&D.
- Multiple sets of BPs that achieve equal outcomes are conceivable.

Classroom Assignments & Discussion Topics Chapter "Synthesis of Recommendations, Open Problems and the Study of Best Practices"

1. Choose 3 of the listed BPs in the book that you think are most likely to change in the future and explain why you chose those.

2. Choose 3 of the listed BPs in the book that you think are least likely to change in the future and explain why you chose those.

3. Give 2 examples where an unusual context of use may override a listed guideline of your choice.

4. Should systems that incorporate BPs give users the option to turn the BPs off? Discuss.

5. How can generative algorithm specifications enable safe alterations of core algorithms?

6. Provide 3 examples of algorithms that embed the following BPs: managing model complexity, managing sampling variance, differentiating between causal and predictive modeling.

7. Have you encountered positive and negative examples of attitudes toward AI/ML safety? Discuss.

8. Give an example of over-engineering AI/ML.

9. Give an example of over-regulating AI/ML.

10. Can you think of ways to ensure that a stated exploratory intent is genuine?

11. What generates in your view misaligned of societal sentiment about biomedical AI/ML with technical reality? Can you think of solutions?

12. Assume that two sets of BPs exist and give different guidance for a particular context or use case. How would you resolve this situation?

Appendix A: Models for Time-to-Event Outcomes

Time-to-Event Outcomes

Survival data, (aka **time-to-event data**), describes the distribution of time until an event occurs. This **event** can be the failure of a device, incidence of a disease, a recurrence of a disease, an adverse event, or death. **Time** is the number of days, weeks, months, years, etc. from the beginning of follow-up until the event. Alternatively, it can also be calendar time such as the subject's age at the time of the event. We tend to think of events as negative, such as death (after all, the field of survival analysis is named after studying survival time, the time to death), but it can also be a positive event, such as discharge from hospital. In the following, we use the terms "survival" and "time-to-event" interchangeably as long as context clarifies the use, and we also use the terms "event", "failure" and "death" interchangeably, unless this causes confusion.

Analytic tasks involving a time-to-event outcome are analogous to most other outcome distributions. The main tasks are (1) estimating the time-to-event (or the survival probability distribution $S(t)$); (2) testing whether two time-to-event distributions are statistically different; and (3) assessing whether one or more covariates (e.g. exposures) significantly affect the survival distribution.

The need for survival analysis. At first glance, time-to-event could be viewed as a continuous quantity and be modeled as one of the many known non-negative distributions, however, this approach breaks down for the following reasons. First, some subjects never experience the event of interest within the practical time frame of the study. Discarding these patients (with unknown time-to-event) leads to loss of information, because we know that these patients did not experience an event until the end of the study. In other words, time-to-event is not missing completely, it has been bounded. Second, some subjects are lost to follow-up before the study ends. Again, discarding such patients because their time-to-event is missing, discards useful information (i.e., that they had not experienced an event until the time they were lost to follow-up). Both of these situations are referred to as *right censoring* (see terminology section below). Third, in a study where the outcome is not death, many enrollees may have already experienced the event before enrollment. If this is allowed, cases with time-to-event = 0 can have high probability. Moreover,

© The Editor(s) (if applicable) and The Author(s) 2024
G. J. Simon, C. Aliferis (eds.), *Artificial Intelligence and Machine Learning in Health Care and Medical Sciences*, Health Informatics,
https://doi.org/10.1007/978-3-031-39355-6

parametric distributions handle the general properties of time-to-event modeling poorly. As an example, fourth, outliers (extreme survivors) are common, and they have potential to become an *influential point* for some distributions. Also, fifth, many parametric distributions have parameters that mathematically relate to their moments (mean, variance). Censored data can make the estimation of moments on which model parameters depend, difficult, thus compromising the model.

Pitfall A.1.1 In most practical settings, it is a significant pitfall to model time-to-event/survival using ordinary predictive modeling classification or regression.

Best Practice A.1.1 When modeling time-to-event outcomes, specialized methods, such as the ones described in this section, should be used, at minimum as comparators with conventional techniques.

Terminology

Let T be a random variable with T_i denoting the time at which an event happened to subject i. Let $f(t)$ denote the density of T and let $F(t)$ denote the cumulative density of T. The cumulative density is referred to as the **failure** function and is defined as

$$F(t) = \Pr(T \le t) = \int_0^t f(\tau)d\tau.$$

The **survival** (or survivor) function is the complement of the failure function and is defined as the probability that a subject survives beyond a particular time t

$$S(t) = \Pr(T > t) = \int_t^\infty f(\tau)d\tau = 1 - F(t).$$

Properties of the survival function. The survival function is monotonic, non-increasing, equals 1 at time 0 and decreases to 0 as time approaches infinity [44].

Often, instead of the survival function, we model the instantaneous "probability" of an event. The **hazard** function is the instantaneous "probability" per unit time that an event occurs exactly at time t given that the patient has survived at least until time t,

$$h(t) = \lim_{\Delta T \to 0} \Pr(T \le t \le T + \Delta T | T > t).$$

Properties of the hazard function. The hazard function can be thought of as the "velocity" of the failure function or the rate of change in the failure function. Since the survival function is non-increasing, the failure function is non-decreasing and $h(t)$ is non-negative. The hazard is not a true probability, it is a rate [44].

The **cumulative hazard** is

$$H(t) = \int_0^t h(\tau)d\tau.$$

The hazard and survival functions are linked to each other through the following relationship [45]. By taking the derivative of ln $S(t)$, we get

$$\frac{d \ln S(t)}{dt} = \frac{dS(t)/dt}{S(t)} = -\frac{f(t)}{S(t)} = -h(t),$$

which leads to

$$S(t) = \exp(-H(t)).$$

Figure A.1 shows the survival (left) and the hazard (right) functions for the diabetes dataset in [46]. The horizontal axis corresponds to the follow-up time (in years). For visualization purposes we show points (in grey color) on the actual hazard "curve". There is one point every follow-up day. The hazard estimates can change frequently in any direction as long as they remain non-negative. To further improve interpretability, a smoothed version of the hazard curve is also presented in black. The survival curve is a non-increasing step function starting at 1 at time 0 and ends at 0 at time infinity. It appears smooth in this figure because of the high resolution (daily) and large sample size, but it is nonetheless a step function. Note that the survival function relates to the *lack of* event (probability of *not having* an event), while the hazard function relates to experiencing an event (the rate of *having* an event).

Censoring

When a patient is lost to follow-up and is no longer observable, the time-to-event beyond the time of the patient dropping out cannot be observed. This is not a typical missing data problem as it first appears, because we have partial observations: the event did not occur while the subject was under observation. This partial observability is called **censoring**.

Left censoring happens, when the event takes place before the subject enters observation. We know that the event has already occurred at time 0, but we do not know when. **Right censoring** happens when the event takes place after the subject

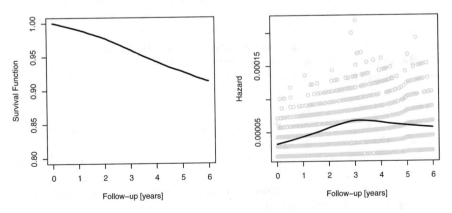

Fig. A.1 Illustration of the survival and hazard functions. The left panel shows the survival function, while the right panel shows the smoothed hazard function for the diabetes data set in [46]

is no longer observed. We know that the event did not take place during the observation period but we do not know when/whether it occurred afterwards. Common reasons for right censoring are that the study ended, the subject is lost to follow-up or the subject withdrew from the study. Finally, **interval censoring** brackets the time of the event between two time points. We know that the event did not take place before the first time point and that it already occurred by the second time point.

Let C denote the time to censoring with density $g()$ and cumulative density $G()$. With $\tilde{T}$ denoting the true time-to-event, the subject's **follow-up time** T is $T = \min\left(C, \tilde{T}\right)$. Let δ denote the event type: $\delta = 1$ if an event took place ($\tilde{T} \, '' \, C$); and $\delta = 0$ if the subject got censored ($\tilde{T} > C$).

Censoring is **random**, if $\tilde{T}_i$ is independent of C_i given X_i, where X_i is the covariate vector of observation i. Random censoring assumes that subjects who are censored at time t are similar in terms of their survival experience to the subjects remaining in the study. **Independent censoring** is a related concept. When a study has subgroups of interest, **independent censoring** is satisfied if censoring is random in all subgroups. **Uninformative censoring** happens when the distribution of C_i and $\tilde{T}_i$ do not share parameters [45, 47].

Competing risks arises when we have multiple outcomes of interest and the occurrence of one outcome prevents us from observing another outcome. As an example, consider heart disease and mortality as two outcomes of interest. If a patient dies (from a cause other than heart disease) we can no longer observe the patient's time to heart disease. In this case, we may have complete observation of the time-to-death, but we only have partial information about the time to heart disease: we only know that it is greater than the time-to-death.

Inference About Survival

In this section, we discuss methods to summarize the time-to-event distribution of a population. First, the time-to-event distribution can be summarized into a statistic (a single number) much in the same way as the mean or median summarizes aspects of a typical distribution. The fundamental difference is censoring: some subjects may not experience an event and thus their exact time-to-event is unknown. Next, we describe the time-to-event distribution as a function of time. We show methods to estimate the survival function and equivalently the cumulative hazard function. Finally, we present methods of constructing confidence intervals around the survival and cumulative hazard functions.

Summary Statistics of Survival

A concise way of describing the survival distribution is by presenting summary statistics. Often used summary statistics of common statistical distributions include the mean, the standard deviation, and the median. However in survival analysis, in the presence of censoring, it is desirable to account for the follow-up times when we compute summary statistics. Below, In Table A.1, we describe some of the commonly used survival statistics [44].

Table A.1 Common statistics to summarize survival time distributions

Statistic	Definition	Remark
Average survival time	$\bar{T} = 1/N \sum_i T_i$	Ignores censoring
Average hazard rate	$\bar{h} = \dfrac{\sum_i \delta_i}{\sum_i T_i}$	Uses hazard instead of survival to account for censoring
Median survival time	Survival time t, where $S(t) = 0.5$	Lessens the impact of outliers
k-year survival rate	Percentage of patients surviving k-years after their diagnosis [48]	Common choices for k include 5, 7, 10

Estimating the Survival Function

We present two estimators of the survival function: the Kaplan–Meier and the Nelson–Aalen estimator. They yield very similar results, with, the Kaplan–Meier estimator is more commonly used for estimating survival itself, while the Nelson–Aalen estimator estimates the cumulative hazard function, which is converted into the survival function.

Kaplan–Meier (Product Limit) Estimator

Let the index j iterate over the distinct time points t_j when an event took place. Let us assume that there are J such time points. The product limit formula is

$$\hat{S}(t_j) = P(T > t_j) = P(T > t_j | t > t_{j-1}) P(T > t_{j-1})$$
$$= \left[1 - P(T = t_j | T > t_{j-1}) \right] P(T > t_{j-1})$$
$$= (1 - h_j) S(t_{j-1}),$$

where h_j is the hazard at time t_j. Expanding this formula yields the Kaplan–Meier estimate

$$\hat{S}(t_j) = \prod_j (1 - \hat{h}_j) = \prod_j \left(1 - \frac{d_j}{n_j} \right),$$

where d_j is the number of events and n_j is the number of patients at risk at time t_j.

Nelson–Aalen Estimator

The Nelson–Aalen estimator estimates the cumulative hazard as

$$\hat{H}(t) = \sum_{j:t_j \leq t} \frac{d_j}{n_j}.$$

The relationship between the cumulative hazard and the survival function can be used to estimate survival, yielding the Breslow formula

$$\hat{S}(t_j) = \exp(-\hat{H}(t)) = \prod_{j:t_j \leq t} \exp\left(-\frac{d_j}{n_j} \right).$$

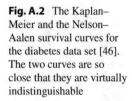

Fig. A.2 The Kaplan–
Meier and the Nelson–
Aalen survival curves for
the diabetes data set [46].
The two curves are so
close that they are virtually
indistinguishable

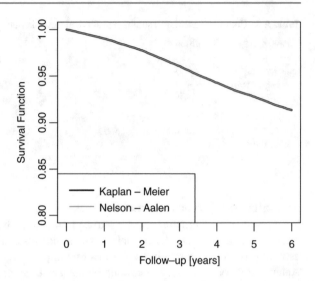

Comparison of the Kaplan–Meier and the Breslow (Nelson–Aalen) estimators (Fig. A.2). Since $exp\,(-h_j) \sim 1 - h_j$ for small h_j, the Kaplan–Meier and the Breslow estimates are very similar and asymptotically equal. The Breslow estimate has uniformly lower variance but is upwards biased [45]. When ties are present in the data, the Kaplan–Meier estimate is more accurate. **Fleming and Harrington** proposed a modification to the Breslow estimate by introducing a small jitter to break the ties in the follow-up times.

Confidence Intervals for the Survival Curves

Whenever conducting a survival analysis it is imperative to present confidence intervals. Statistical packages routinely offer such estimates. However when survival analysis is conducted with modified conventional predictive methods often there are no facilities for CI estimation. We thus present here the fundamentals of estimating CIs for survival curves and hazard curves.

There are two fundamentally different approaches to constructing the confidence intervals. First, the confidence interval can be constructed in survival space, which requires the variance of the survival estimate. A second approach is to build the confidence interval in a transformed space and map the upper and lower limits back into survival space. Common transformations include log, where the confidence interval is constructed in essentially the cumulative hazard space, log–log, log–logit, etc.

Greenwood's Formula First we consider constructing the confidence interval in survival space. The variance of the log survival function can be estimated using Greenwood's formula

$$\text{Var}\left(\log \hat{S}(t)\right) = \sum_{j:t_j \le t} \frac{d_j}{n_j\left(n_j - d_j\right)},$$

where d_j and n_j are defined previously as the number of events at t_j and the number of patients at risk at time t_j, respectively. The *delta method* can be used to derive the variance of the (non-log) survival function, which yields the **plain-scale** confidence interval

$$\hat{S}(t) \pm z \sqrt{\hat{S}(t)^2 \sum_{j:t_j \le t} \frac{d_j}{n_j\left(n_j - d_j\right)}},$$

where z is the normal quantile corresponding to the confidence level.

Alternatively, the confidence interval can be constructed in log-survival space and exponentiated back into (non-log) survival space, yielding

$$\hat{S}(t)\exp\left(\pm z\sqrt{\text{Var}\left(\log \hat{S}(t)\right)}\right).$$

Recommendation When estimating the confidence interval for a survival function, use the Kaplan–Meier estimator for the survival function, construct the confidence interval in log-survival space using the Greenwood formula and exponentiate the limits back into survival space [45].

One caveat is that the limits of the confidence interval can fall outside the [0, 1] range for both the plain-scale and the log-scale. Formulating the confidence interval on the complementary log–log scale, i.e. log[−log S(t)], ensures that the limits are within the 0–1 range, but offers little additional benefit.

Confidence Interval Through the Nelson–Aalen Estimator

Confidence intervals can also be constructed using the Nelson–Aalen estimator of cumulative hazard. Since the Nelson–Aalen estimator has a binomial likelihood, it yields the same confidence interval as above.

Alternatively, the connection to the Poisson likelihood can be exploited, yielding a different (lower) variance for the Nelson–Aalen estimator

$$\text{Var}\left(\hat{H}(t)\right) = \sum_{j:t_j \le t} \frac{d_j}{n_j^2}.$$

This variance can be directly used to construct a confidence interval for the cumulative hazard, but using the log-cumulative hazard scale is recommended. By the delta method,

$$\text{Var}\left(\log \hat{H}(t)\right) = \frac{\text{Var}\left(\hat{H}(t)\right)}{\hat{H}(t)^2},$$

yielding a confidence interval of

$$\hat{H}(t)\exp\left(\pm z\sqrt{\mathrm{Var}\left(\hat{H}(t)\right)/\hat{H}(t)^{2}}\right).$$

Although the cumulative hazard and the survival function are tightly linked, when the goal is to build a confidence interval for the survival function, the recommended method is to use the Kaplan–Meier estimate with Greenwood's formula in log-survival scale; but when the goal is to build a confidence interval for the cumulative hazard, the recommended method is the Nelson–Aalen estimator of the cumulative hazard, its Poisson-based variance estimator and using log-cumulative-hazard scale [45].

Method label: Kaplan–Meier (KM) estimator of survival curves	
Main use	– Estimate survival curves – Visualization of survival curves
Context of use	– Non-parametric modeling – Predict survival probability at time t – The data does not meet the assumptions of more sophisticated (e.g., Cox regression) survival modeling
Secondary use	– Checking the proportional hazards assumptions
Pitfalls	**Pitfall A.1.1.1.** Estimating the effect of covariates is difficult. A separate curve is computed for each covariate combination. Does not scale to more than a very small number of covariates
Principle of operation	– Non-parametric estimator
Theoretical properties and empirical evidence	– In biomedicine is practically expected and used in every publication involving survival
Best practices	**Best Practice A.1.1.1.** Plotting the KM curve can reveal data problems. Consider the complementary log–log plot of the KM curve
References	Recommended textbooks include [44, 45, 47]

Comparing Survival Curves

Comparing the Estimated Survival Curves from Two or More Populations Two survival curves are considered statistically equivalent when the data supports the hypothesis that the true survival curves of the underlying populations are the same and any apparent difference between them is merely due to random variations in the samples that were used to estimate the curves. Testing for differences of survival curves is essential in order to establish that any nominal or apparent differences are not due to random sample variation.

Consider a group variable, which divides the population into G groups. At each unique event time, $j = 1,...,J$, the association between grouping and survival can be assessed. The null hypothesis is that the hazard at time t_j is the same across all groups for all j. The alternative hypothesis is that the hazard differs between the groups at least one j.

Let n_{gj} denote the number of subjects at risk in group g at time t_j and let d_{gj} denote the number of failures in group g at time t_j. For simplicity, we concentrate on the two-sample test, where $G = 2$. The expected number of failures in group 1 at time t_j is

$$e_{1j} = \frac{n_{1j}}{n_{1j} + n_{2j}}\left(d_{1j} + d_{2j}\right).$$

The observed number of failures across time in group g is $O_g = \sum_j d_{gj}$ and the expected number of failures is $E_g = \sum_j e_{gj}$. The **log-rank statistic** becomes

$$Z = \frac{\left(O_g - E_g\right)^2}{\mathrm{Var}\left(O_g - E_g\right)},$$

and the variance can be estimated from the hypergeometric distribution. Z follows a X^2 distribution with 1 degree of freedom and can be used as test of curve equivalence.

Extensions of the Log-Rank Test

The log-rank test in its original form considers the difference between the number of observed and expected events at the jth failure time with equal weight for all j. By using different weights over time, one can emphasize different parts of the survival curve. The test statistic with weights $w(t_j)$ is

$$Z = \frac{\left(\sum_j w\left(t_j\right)\left(d_{gj} - e_{gj}\right)^2\right)}{\mathrm{Var}\left(\sum_j w\left(t_j\right)\left(d_{gj} - e_{gj}\right)\right)}.$$

Several weighing schemes have been devised and each provides a different emphasis. Below we summarize some of the most common tests. In case of the Wilcox test, the weight at each unique failure time is the number of subjects at risk, $w(t_j) = n_j$. Since usually there are more patients at risk at the beginning, this weighing scheme emphasizes the beginning of the survival curve, namely the early failures. The Tarone–Ware test is similar, except it uses $w(t_j) = \sqrt{n_j}$. The Peto test uses $w(t_j) = \underline{S}(t)$, where weights are proportional to the survival probability and the Flemington–Harrington weight is a more general version, assigning weights that depend on a weighted product of the survival and failure probabilities [47].

Effect of Covariates on Survival

We use regression models to assess the effect of covariates on the hazard. Models we consider fall into two categories: semi-parametric and parametric models. The semi-parametric models are extensions of the Cox proportional hazards regression. The Cox model is semi-parametric; it models the hazard as a product of a non-parametric baseline hazard and a multiplicative effect of the covariates. The covariates thus have a proportional (multiplicative) effect on the baseline hazard, resulting in the proportional hazards assumption. The second class of models are fully parametric. They make a distributional assumption about the cumulative hazard (as a function of time) and model the location parameter of this distribution as a linear additive function of the covariates. The location parameter shifts time, accelerates or decelerates the passing of time, thus these models are referred to as accelerated failure time models.

Cox Proportional Hazards Regression

The key idea behind the proportional hazards model is to model the hazard through a regression model composed of a time-dependent baseline hazard and a proportional (multiplicative) covariate effect.

Figure A.3 illustrates the proportional hazards assumption using the diabetes example from [46]. The left panel shows the cumulative hazard of diabetes as a function of years of follow-up time. The orange curve in the plot corresponds to patients with impaired fasting glucose (IFG) and the blue line corresponds to patients with healthy glucose. At all time points, the ratio of cumulative hazard along the orange line versus the blue line is constant, 6.37. In other words, having IFG (versus not having IFG) confers a proportional, 6.37-time increase in diabetes risk upon the patients, and it remains constant across time.

Let X be the covariate matrix, and let X_i denote the covariate vector for subject i. The hazard at time t is

$$h_i(t) = h_0(t)\exp(X_i\beta), \qquad (A.1)$$

where $h_i(t)$ is the hazard of the ith subject at time t, $h_0(t)$ is the baseline hazard (common across all subjects) at time t, and β are regression coefficients. The cumulative hazards can be expressed as

$$H_i(t) = H_0(t)\exp(X_i\beta) = \exp(X_i\beta)\int_0^t h_0(\tau)d\tau,$$

showing that the covariates increase (or decrease) the cumulative hazard proportionally relative to the baseline cumulative hazard.

In the diabetes example in Fig. A.3, the cumulative baseline hazard $H_0(t)$ is the blue curve in the left panel, X_i denotes whether the patient presents with impaired

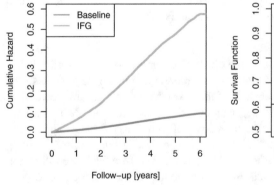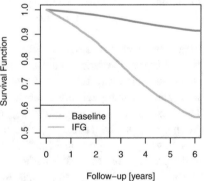

Fig. A.3 Proportional hazards assumption. The left panel shows the cumulative hazard of patients with normal glucose (in blue) and impaired fasting glucose (IFG) (in orange) as a function of follow-up time (in years). The ratio of the underlying hazards of the orange line to the blue line is constant: the hazard along the orange line versus the blue line has the same proportion. The right panel transforms the cumulative hazard into survival probability

fasting glucose (IFG) and the cumulative hazard $H_i(t)$ for patients with IFG is the orange curve.

Comparing the hazards of two subjects, i and j, we obtain

$$\frac{H_i(t)}{H_j(t)} = \frac{H_0(t)\exp(X_i\beta)}{H_0(t)\exp(X_j\beta)} = \frac{\exp(X_i\beta)}{\exp(X_j\beta)}.$$

The resulting quantity is the **hazard ratio** and is constant with respect to time. The name *proportional hazard* reflects the fact that the hazards of two patients are proportional to each other. Continuing with the diabetes example, if patient i has IFG ($X_i = 1$) and patient j does not ($X_j = 0$), with $\beta = 1.85$, the hazard ratio is $\exp(1.85) = 6.37$. Therefore, the ratio of the hazard between the orange and the blue curves in Fig. A.3 is 6.37.

When fitting a proportional hazards regression model, the partial likelihood is maximized in terms of the coefficients

$$\prod_i \prod_t \left(\frac{R_i(t)\exp(X_i\beta)}{\sum_j R_j(t)\exp(X_j\beta)} \right)^{\delta_i(t)},$$

where i iterates over the subjects, t over the time points, $R_i(t)$ indicates whether subject i is in the risk set at time t, and $\delta_i(t)$ indicates whether subject i had an event at time t. This formula assumes no ties in event times. The likelihood is "partial" in the sense that the baseline hazard remains unspecified.

From the fundamental equation of the proportional hazards model (formula (A.1)) it follows that if the base hazard is known or can be estimated, then the absolute hazard can be estimated by multiplying the base hazard with the proportional estimate effect of the modeled covariates.

Assumptions
(i) The proportional hazards assumption: the covariates have a proportional (multiplicative) effect on the hazard relative to the baseline hazard.
(ii) Independence. Observations with an event are independent of each other. Only observations with an event are multiplied in the partial likelihood.
(iii) The effect of the covariates is linear and additive on the log–log survival.

Testing the significance of the covariates
Generally, in regression, we have two ways to test the significance of a coefficient. The first method is the **likelihood ratio test** and the second one is the **Wald test**. Although the proportional hazards regression maximizes a partial likelihood (as opposed to a full likelihood) as it leaves the baseline hazard unspecified, this does not affect the likelihood ratio test and both methods remain applicable.

Estimating the Baseline Hazard
Fitting a Cox proportional hazards model does not require the estimation of the baseline hazard. After the model has been fitted, the baseline hazard function is

estimated using a variant of the Nelson–Aalen estimator that incorporates effects of covariates

$$\hat{H}_0(t) = \sum_{j:t_j \le t} \frac{\delta_j}{\sum_k R_k(t_j) \exp(X_k\beta)},$$

where $R_k(t)$ indicates whether subject k is in the risk set at time t_j. Notice, that when $\beta = 0$, this reduces to the Nelson–Aalen estimator from the earlier "Estimating the Survival Function" section.

The variance of the baseline hazard is also based on the Nelson–Aalen estimator

$$Var\left(\hat{H}_0(t)\right) = \sum_{j:t_j \le t} \frac{d_j}{\left(\sum_k R_k(t_j) \exp(X_k\beta)\right)^2}.$$

Making Predictions
For an individual i, hazard can be estimated as

$$\hat{H}_i(t) = \hat{H}_0(t) \exp(X_i\beta)$$

and the corresponding survival can be computed using the Breslow estimator

$$\hat{S}_i(t) = \exp\left(-\hat{H}_i(t)\right).$$

Testing the Proportional Hazards Assumption
There are three methods for testing the proportional hazards assumption.

(i) Visual Inspection

The first method is visual inspection of the log–log survival plot. Since under the proportional hazards assumption,

$$\hat{S}_i(t) = \exp\left(-\hat{H}_0(t) \exp(X_i\beta)\right),$$

its log–log transform is

$$\log\left(-\log \hat{S}_i(t)\right) = \left(\log \widehat{H}_0(t)\right) + X_i\beta.$$

The log–log transform of two survival curves, corresponding to two different values of X_i, (say) X_1 and X_2, only differ in the $X_i\beta$ term, which is not a function of time t, thus the two curves should be parallel with a distance of $(X_2 - X_1)\beta$ between them.

To check the validity of the proportional hazards assumption, we plot the log–log transform of the Kaplan–Meier survival curves for two different values of X_i and expect these curves to be parallel.

A benefit of visual inspection is that we can see where (at what t) the violation of the proportional hazards assumptions happens and we may also see patterns that suggest the functional forms to correct the violation. *However, the decision whether*

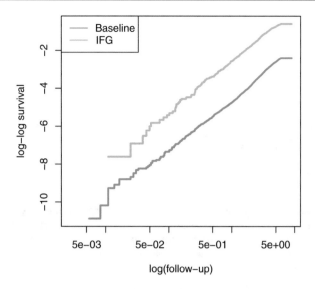

Fig. A.4 Log–log survival plot of the diabetes dataset. The blue line corresponds to patients with healthy glucose levels, and the orange line to patients with impaired glucose levels. The log–log plots for the two levels of glucose status (normal versus impaired glucose) are parallel, suggesting that the proportional hazards assumption is acceptable

the proportional hazards assumption is violated is subjective, no test statistic or p-value is provided to guide the visual comparison.

Figure A.4 shows the complementary log–log plot of the diabetes data set. The blue line corresponds to patients without impaired fasting glucose (IFG) while the orange line corresponds to patients with IFG. Since the two lines, corresponding to the two levels of glucose status, are parallel, the proportional hazards assumption appears to hold for glucose status. Although a formal test reports significant departure from the proportional hazards assumption, the lines look reasonably parallel and it is safe to assume the reported violation is merely a result of the large sample size (54,700 patients).

Figure A.5 shows two synthetic examples where the proportional hazards assumption is violated. In both examples, the blue line represents the baseline hazard and the orange line corresponds to some exposure. In the left panel, the effect of the exposure changes from beneficial to harmful at about 2 years. In the right panel, the effect of the exposure (orange line) is quadratically related to (log) time.

(ii) Time-Dependent Covariates

The second method is based on time-dependent covariates. Under the proportional hazards assumption, adding regression terms involving interactions between the covariates and functions of time should not improve the fit. To check the validity of the proportional hazards assumption, we fit models of the form

$$h(t) = h_0(t)\exp\left(X\beta + \left(X \times g(t)\right)\gamma\right),$$

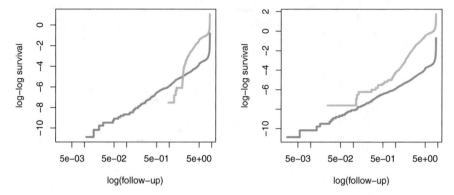

Fig. A.5 Violations of the proportional hazard assumption. The blue line is the baseline hazard, while the orange line corresponds to some treatment. The left panel shows a violation where the treatment effect "switches over": while it is beneficial initially, it becomes harmful after some time. The right panel shows a violation, where the treatment line is a function of time. The curve suggests a function form (quadratic)

where $g(t)$ are vectors of function of time, $X \times g(t)$ are covariate-time interactions and γ is the coefficient vector of the covariate-time interaction terms. Under the proportional hazards assumption, we expect $\gamma = 0$.

A benefit of this method is that a statistical test is performed, a p-value is obtained, and thus the decision is objective. A weakness is the need for choosing an appropriate function $g(t)$. Different choices of $g()$ can lead to different conclusions. Common choices include the identity:$g(t) = t$; the log transform of time: $g(t) = log\ t$; and the heaviside function, where $g(t) = 1$ if t exceeds a threshold τ and $g(t) = 0$ otherwise.

(iii) Schoenfeld Residuals

The third method is based on the Schoenfeld residuals. The Shoenfeld residual at the jth event (which occurred at time t_j) is defined as

$$s_j = \sum_i \left[X_i - X_i \frac{R_i(t_j)\exp(X_i\beta)}{\sum_k R_k(t_j)\exp(X_k\beta)} \right] \delta_i(t_j).$$

The notation is the same as before: $R_i(t_j)$ denotes whether patient i is in the risk set at time t_j, and $\delta_i(t_j)$ denotes whether patient i had an event at time t_j.

Typically, in regression, we estimate some outcome y using predictors X. We can use the resulting regression model to predict $\hat{y}$ based on the predictors X. The residual is the difference between the predicted and actual outcomes, $\hat{y} - y$.

The Schoenfeld residual turns this process on its head. At a particular value of y, we predict X, and the residual is the difference between the predicted and actual X.

In the context of Cox models, the residual at time t_j, measures the difference between X_i and its expectation given the model and the outcome (at time t_j). To see this, consider that $\dfrac{R_i\left(t_j\right)\exp\ \exp\left(X_i\beta\right)}{\sum_k R_k\left(t_j\right)\exp\ \exp\left(X_k\beta\right)}$ is the probability of an event given the risk set at t_j and the sum $\sum_i X_i \dfrac{R_i\left(t_j\right)\exp\ \exp\left(X_i\beta\right)}{\sum_k R_k\left(t_j\right)\exp\ \exp\left(X_k\beta\right)}$ is the expectation of X_i. The Schoenfeld residual can thus be thought of as an observed-expected residual.

There is a Schoenfeld residual for each covariate at each event time. The Schoenfeld residuals can be combined into a $D \times p$ matrix, where D is the total number of events and p is the number of predictors.

Consider a model for hazard with time-varying coefficients

$$h(t) = h_0(t)\exp\left(X_i\beta(t)\right).$$

This model allows for the coefficient β to change over time. This formulation can account for example for a treatment to have a burn-in period before it reaches its full efficacy or for the treatment to lose efficacy over time. The proportional hazards assumption states that $\beta(t) = \beta$ for all t.

Therneau and Grambsch showed that

$$E\left(s_{jk}^*\right) + \hat{\beta}_k = \beta_{k(t_j)},$$

where $\hat{\beta}$ is obtained from a Cox model, $\hat{\beta}_k$ is its kth component, and s_{jk}^* is the scaled Schoenfeld residual (for the jth event and the kth covariate). The scaling factor is the variance of X_k. Recall that X_k is being "predicted" based on the outcome and thus it has variance [45].

The model fit can be visualized by plotting the Schoenfeld residual as a function of t (or some function $g(t)$ of t). Under the proportional hazards assumption, $\beta_k(t_j) = \beta_k$ and thus $E\left(s_{jk}^*\right) + \hat{\beta}_k$ should be independent of time or a function thereof, so the line should be horizontal. Deviations both in terms of the location (which t) and the extent can be seen from the graph.

A formal test for the violation of the proportional hazards assumption can be obtained by fitting a regression line to the plot of form

$$\beta_k(t) = \beta_k + \gamma\left(g(t) - \underline{g}\right),$$

where $\underline{g}$ is the mean value of the transformed time. Under the proportional hazards assumption, γ should be 0.

Addressing the Violations of the Proportional Hazards Assumption

The consequences of violating the proportional hazards assumption are usually not dire. Violations do not usually affect the predictions, they mostly affect the error estimates. Workarounds for the violations exist, however, they end up answering a question that is different from the original research question. When the data set is large, violations are almost unavoidable. Thus depending on the extent of the violation and purpose of the study, we may opt to ignore the violation.

Accordingly, when a test reports a proportional hazards violation, we start by verifying that the non-proportionality is substantial. Not all non-proportionalities are substantial. Statistically significant non-proportionality can arise from large sample sizes, where even small deviations from proportionality can become significant; or violation can arise also from influential points. The former can be ignored, the latter can be removed. To assess whether a non-proportionality is substantial, the key method is visualization. Not only can visualization show whether the non-proportionality is substantial, but it can also suggest a functional form to correct it. Once we verified that the violation is substantial and decided to address it, we have several options.

The first option is stratified Cox models. If the covariate with the non-proportionality is a factor with relatively few levels, it can be used as a stratification factor in a stratified Cox model. The non-proportional effect now becomes part of the baseline hazard. If the covariate is a quantitative variable, stratified Cox models can still be constructed, but the variable needs to be categorized (into a few categories) before it can be used as a stratification factor.

If the non-proportionality is present in a relatively short timeframe and not in the entire timeline, the timeline can be partitioned into segments in which the proportional hazards assumption holds and separate Cox models can be constructed in each time segment.

Finally, if the non-proportionality was detected through methods (2) or (3), using time or a transformation of time, $g(t)$, adding an interaction term with the appropriate time-transformation can resolve the non-proportionality.

Method label: Cox proportional hazards regression	
Main use	– Regression models for time-to-event outcomes
Context of use	– Right-censored data
	– Interest is the effect of covariates and making predictions
	– Same interpretability as classical regression models for other outcome types
Secondary use	N/A
Pitfalls	**Pitfall A.1.3.1.** The key assumption is the proportional hazards assumption. Often, violation of the proportional hazards assumption is a non-issue, occasionally it can lead to problems
	Pitfall A.1.3.2. The models assume linearity and additivity. Not appropriate if these assumptions are violated
	Pitfall A.1.3.3. High dimensionality is a problem for the unregularized model
Principle of operation	– It is a semi-parametric regression model
	– The effect of covariates is a proportional (multiplicative) increase/decrease relative to a time-dependent baseline hazard
	– Coefficient estimates are obtained from maximizing a partial likelihood
Theoretical properties and empirical evidence	– Although a partial likelihood is maximized, the favorable properties of maximum likelihood estimation are preserved: estimates are consistent, efficient and asymptotically normally distributed
	– Partial likelihood is convex and thus easy to solve

Method label: Cox proportional hazards regression	
Best practices	**Best Practice A.1.3.1.** First-choice model for time-to-event data
	Best Practice A.1.3.2. Consider, additionally, whether the problem can be solved as a classification problem, or using survival modeling versions of ML predictive models
	Best Practice A.1.3.3. In the presence of substantial violations, different models, including extensions of the Cox PH, may be more appropriate
	Best Practice A.1.3.4. Consider the Markov Boundary feature selector for survival analysis that results from using Cox proportional hazards models as conditional independence testing within the Markov Boundary algorithm
	Best Practice A.1.3.5. For high-dimensional data, consider regularized Cox proportional hazards models. Also consider the Cox Markov Boundary method described above
References	Kleinbaum DG, Klein M. Survival Analysis. A Self-Learning Text. 2020, Springer
	Therneau T, Grambsch P. Modeling Survival Data. Extending the Cox Model. 2000, Springer

Extensions of the Cox Proportional Hazards Regression

Several extensions to the Cox PH model have been proposed [45]. In this section, we review some of them.

1. Stratified Cox Model

   Stratified Cox models allow the population to be divided into different non-overlapping groups, called "strata". Each stratum has its own baseline hazard and each group may also have its own coefficient vector. The standard form of a stratified Cox models is

$$h_i(t) = h_{0k}(t)\exp(X_i\beta),$$

which assumes a common covariate effect across all strata that is proportional to the stratum-specific baseline hazard, $h_{0k}(t)$ for the kth stratum. The coefficients represent an "average" hazard ratio across the population (regardless of strata). This is the most flexible way of incorporating effects that violate the proportional hazards assumption, but stratified cox models offer no direct way of assessing the significance of the stratifying factor. An alternative form of the stratified Cox models considers the possibility of some covariates in a stratum (or some of the strata) having an effect that differs from its effect in other strata. Such effects are incorporated as interaction effects between the covariate and the stratum. If all covariates have interactions with the strata, then the resulting Cox model is the same as fitting separate Cox models for each stratum. Naturally, having to estimate separate baseline hazards and interaction terms requires sufficient sample size.

2. Recurring Events and Counting Process Cox Model

So far, time-event data was described by the triplet $\{T_i, \delta_i, X_i\}$, where T_i denotes the time to event, δ_i the event type (event or censoring), and X_i is the covariate vector. Alternatively, each subject's timeline can be divided into multiple segments and each segment can be described by a quartet $\{start_i, end_i, \delta_i, X_i\}$, where $start_i$ and end_i are the two end points of the time segment, δ_i denotes whether an event occured in the time segment, and X_i is the covariate vector. This format is called the **counting process format**. Many applications of the counting process format exist, here we highlight a few.

The first application is the change of the time scale. The term time scale refers to the way time is measured. The triplet format measures time on the *study scale*, and, specifically, time 0 is when subjects entered the study. The counting process format allows for different time scales. For example, time can be measured as patients' age, where $start_i$ is the age when they entered the study and end_i is the age when they experienced an event. We discuss different time scales in more detail later.

Another commonly used application of the counting process format is **time-dependent covariate Cox models**. Time-dependent covariate Cox models allow for modeling under the assumption that the covariates can change over time. The time scale is divided into multiple segments and each segment can have its own covariate vector. As long as the subjects experience at most one event, the time-dependent covariate Cox model does not cause any complications, even though each subject can contribute multiple observations (rows). This stands in contrast to longitudinal data analysis (Section "Longitudinal Data Analysis" in Chapter "An Appraisal and Operating Characteristics of Major ML Methods Applicable in Healthcare & Health Science"), where observations from the same subject are correlated and this causes estimation issues. The key assumption to avoid such estimation problems is that the subjects have at most one event.

A third application of the counting process format is when subjects can experience multiple events. The timeline can be divided into multiple segments when subjects experience an event. Now, each subject can enter the partial likelihood function multiple times, every time they have an event. Several remedies exist. First, we can consider only the first even of all patients. Second, we can use longitudinal data analysis techniques. Analogues of both GEEs and mixed effect models exist for time to event outcomes. A third, commonly used option is to initially fit a model ignoring the correlation due to the possibly multiple observations per subject (with event) and then re-computing the error estimates, taking the correlation into account. Chapter 8.2.2 of [45] describes three popular variations of this option in detail.

3. Age-Scale Models

The term **time scale** refers to the way time is measured for a time-to-event outcome. Typically, time is measured from a particular event, e.g. enrollment into the study, to the end of study. This is the **study time scale**. An alternative is **calendar scale**, where time is measured based on a calendar, e.g. the age of the participant.

Changing the time scale has two important effects. First, the risk sets are different. At first sight it may appear that age scale can be easily converted into a study-scale by $T_i = end_i - start_i$, however, the risk sets are different. Consider two patients. The first one enters the study at the age of 40 and suffers a heart attack (event of interest) at the age of 51. The second one enters the study at 55 and suffers a heart attack 5 years later at the age of 50. On the study-time scale, we have two events, one at 5 and one at 11 years. At the time of the first event, at year 5, we have a risk set of two patients. In contrast, on the age scale, we have two events, one at 51 and one at 60. At both events, the risk set contains only one patient. Since the risk sets are different, the survival estimates (or equivalently the hazard estimates) are different, as well. These two time-scales yield different results and admit different interpretations.

The second effect of age-scale relates to how age is entered into the model. One option is to use study-scale and add a covariate that represents age; and the other option is to use age-scale. In case of using age scale, age is modeled completely non-parametrically; the baseline hazard is a function of age. As such, the statistical significance of the age effect is difficult to assess. Conversely, when age is added as a covariate, the usual assumptions (linear, additive effect) apply and the baseline hazard is based on time in the study. Whether we use age-scale or study-time scale can also be determined based on whether the model assumptions about age as a covariate are reasonable.

Parametric Survival Models

In this section, we model the time-to-event variable T using parametric distributions. Consider X, a covariate matrix and β the regression coefficients. Rather than modeling T directly, we model its natural logarithm as

$$\log T = \mu + X\beta + \sigma W.$$

Terminology

In this model, μ is called a **location parameter**, σ is called the **scale parameter** and W is the error term. Similarly to linear regression, we assume a distribution for the error term W which implies a distribution for $\log T$. The distribution of W is assumed to be a location-scale distribution. **Location-scale distribution**s have two parameters, a location and a scale. For example, the normal (Gaussian) distribution is a location-scale distribution, with the mean μ being the location and σ the scale. When W follows a location-scale distribution, $\log T$, as defined above, follows the same distribution as W, but with different location and scale parameters. The distribution of T is typically different, but related.

This shift in location μ accelerates or decelerates the passing of time and thus this class of models is referred to as **accelerated failure time (AFT)** models. Let $S_0(t)$ denote the survival time distribution when all covariates are 0. The survival time distribution for a subject with covariates X is

Fig. A.6 Illustration of an accelerated failure time model on the diabetes data set

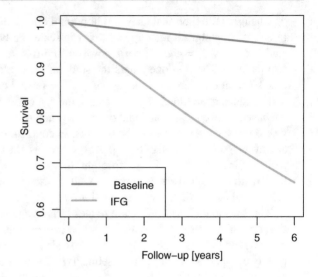

$$S(t) = \Pr(T > t) = \Pr(\log T > \log t)$$
$$= \Pr(\mu + X\beta + \sigma W > \log t)$$
$$= \Pr(\mu + \sigma W > \log t - X\beta)$$
$$= \Pr(\exp(\mu + \sigma W) > t \exp(-X\beta))$$
$$= S_0(t)(t \exp(X\beta))$$

The covariates, depending on the sign of $X\beta$, accelerate or decelerate the passing of time by a factor of $exp(-X\beta)$.

Figure A.6 shows an AFT model fitted to the diabetes dataset. The outcome is diabetes-free survival, the horizontal axis is follow-up years. The orange line represents patients with impaired fasting glucose (IFG) and the blue represents patients with normal fasting glucose. Patients with normal fasting glucose have higher diabetes-free survival probability. If we draw a horizontal line at a particular (diabetes-free) survival probability, and compute the ratio of the time it takes to get to that probability along the blue line versus the orange line, we would find that this ratio is constant, exp(−2.08) = .12 in this example. In other words, the time it takes for the diabetes-free survival to drop to a probability P is much shorter (takes 0.12 times as long) for patients with IFG than without.

Different AFT models differ in the distribution of W and T. In what follows, we will describe some of the most commonly used AFT models and their specific assumptions and conclude the section by describing how to select the most appropriate model based on the assumptions.

Log-Normal Survival Model

Suppose that we assume a standard normal distribution for the noise, $W \sim N(0, 1)$. The log of survival time (log T) is then distributed as $N(\mu + X\beta, \sigma^2)$ and T itself follows a log normal distribution. The survival function is

Fig. A.7 Example exponential survival curves corresponding to different rate parameters

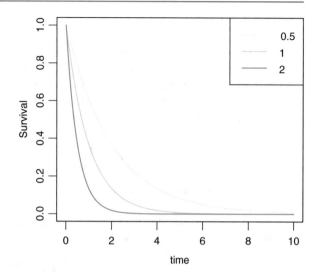

$$S(t) = 1 - F(t) = 1 - \Phi\left(\frac{\log T - \mu - X\beta}{\sigma}\right),$$

where Φ is the cumulative density of the standard normal distribution.

Exponential Survival Model

One commonly used survival time distribution is the exponential distribution. The exponential distribution yields a survival function

$$S(t) = \exp(-\lambda t), \quad \lambda > 0,$$

where λ is a location parameter, often called the *rate parameter*. The exponential distribution does not have a scale parameter. Figure A.7 shows exponential survival curves corresponding to different rate parameters.

If T follows an exponential distribution, $\log T$ and thus W follows an extreme value distribution. The extreme value distribution can be re-parameterized to become a location-scale distribution, yielding a density of

$$f_{EV}(x; \mu; \sigma) = \frac{1}{\sigma}\exp\left(\frac{x-\mu}{\sigma} - e^{\frac{x-\mu}{\sigma}}\right),$$

where μ is the location and σ is the scale parameter. If T follows an exponential distribution, the scale is set to 1.

In the exponential survival model, we assume that the error term W follows extreme value distribution with location 0 and scale 1, $W \sim EV(0, 1)$. Then $\log T = \mu + X\beta + \sigma W$ follows $EV(\mu + X\beta, \sigma)$. If $\sigma = 1$, T follows exponential distribution with $\lambda = \exp(\mu + X\beta)$, yielding an exponential survival function of

$$S(t) = \exp(-\lambda t) = \exp(-\exp(X\beta)t).$$

This leads to the following assumptions:

(i)   The exponential survival model is an accelerated failure time model.
      This follows from the model construction $log\ T = \mu + X\beta + \sigma W$ and it also
      implies that for fixed quantile of the survival ($S(t) = q$), changing a covariate X
      scales the survival time by a fixed ratio, $exp(X\beta)$.
(ii) The exponential survival model is a **constant hazard model**:

$$h(t) = \frac{f(t)}{S(t)} = \lambda.$$

The hazard does not depend on time.

(ii) The exponential survival model is a proportional hazard model, because the
      hazard ratio of two observations, X_1 and X_2, is

$$\frac{h_1(t)}{h_2(t)} = \frac{\lambda_1}{\lambda_2} = \frac{exp(\mu)exp(X_1\beta)}{exp(\mu)exp(X_2\beta)} = \frac{exp(X_1\beta)}{exp(X_2\beta)}$$

and is a constant with respect to time.

(iv) Assumptions of the linear regression model continue to apply: observations
      are assumed independent, and the effects of the covariates on the hazard are
      linear and additive. This also means that log–log of the survival function
      should be linear, allowing for graphical checking of the model suitability.

Weibull Survival Model

The Weibull distribution is a generalization of the exponential distribution. Its survival function is

$$S(t; \lambda, \alpha) = exp(-\lambda t^{\alpha}), \quad \alpha > 0, \lambda > 0,$$

where α is called the *shape parameter*. If time T follows a Weibull distribution, log
T follows an extreme value distribution. Figure A.8 shows Weibull distributions
with various parametrizations.

Similar to the exponential distribution, we assume that the error term W follows
standard extreme value distribution $W \sim EV(0, 1)$. The log survival time then follows
$EV(\mu + X\beta, \sigma)$ and the survival time itself follows Weibull with

$$\lambda = exp\left(-\frac{\mu + X\beta}{\sigma}\right), \quad \alpha = \frac{1}{\sigma}.$$

This yields a survival function

$$S(t) = exp(-\lambda t^{\alpha}) = exp\left(-exp\left(-\frac{\mu + X\beta}{\sigma}\right)t^{\frac{1}{\sigma}}\right).$$

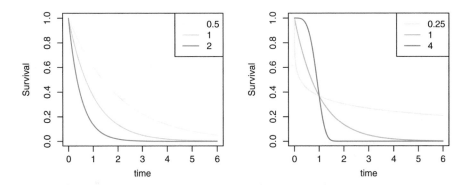

Fig. A.8 Weibull distributed survival probabilities using different parameterizations. The left panel shows curves with varying λ and the right panel with varying α parameter

From this, the following assumptions follow.

(i) By construction, the Weibull model is an AFT model.
(ii) The Weibull model is a proportional hazards model. The hazard function is

$$h(t) = \lambda \alpha t^{\alpha-1} = \alpha t^{\alpha-1} \exp\left(-\frac{\mu}{\sigma}\right) \exp\left(-\frac{X\beta}{\sigma}\right) = h_0(t) \exp\left(-\frac{X\beta}{\sigma}\right),$$

where $h_0(t)$ is the hazard when all covariates are 0. The hazard ratio of two observations i and j is

$$\frac{h_i(t)}{h_j(t)} = \frac{\exp\left(-\dfrac{X_i\beta}{\sigma}\right)}{\exp\left(-\dfrac{X_j\beta}{\sigma}\right)},$$

which does not depend on time.
(iii) The covariates are linear and additive in terms of log–log survival.

Log-Logistic Survival Model
Another commonly used distribution for survival time is the log-logistic distribution. Its survival function takes the form

$$S(t) = \frac{1}{1 + \lambda t^{\alpha}}, \quad \lambda > 0, \; \alpha > 0.$$

Figure A.9 shows examples of log-logistic survival curves. The log-logistic distribution has two parameters. Changing λ (left panel) accelerates/decelerates the passing of time and changing α, the "shape" parameter, (right panel) changes the shape of the survival curves. For reference, a survival curve following the exponential distribution is included as a dashed gray line.

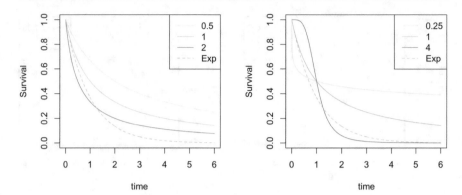

Fig. A.9 Example log-logistic distributions. The left panel shows log-logistic survival functions with varying λ parameter. The right panel shows the effect of varying the α parameter. For comparison, the exponential distribution is included in dashed lines

In the log-logistic survival models, the error term W follows the standard logistic distribution. The logistic distribution can be re-parameterized into a location-scale distribution with density

$$f(x; \mu; \sigma) = \frac{\exp\left(\dfrac{x - \mu}{\sigma}\right)}{1 + \exp\left(\dfrac{x - \mu}{\sigma}\right)}.$$

When we model survival time as a log-logistic distribution, the error term is assumed to follow standard logistic ($\mu = 0$, $\sigma = 1$). Log survival time (log T) then follows logistic with location $\mu + X\beta$ and scale σ.

Time itself follows log-logistic distribution with parameters

$$\lambda = \exp\left(-\frac{\mu + X\beta}{\sigma}\right), \quad \alpha = \frac{1}{\sigma}.$$

The survival function then becomes

$$S(t) = \frac{1}{1 + \exp\left(\lambda t^{\alpha}\right)} = \frac{1}{1 + \exp\left(t^{1/\sigma} \exp\left(-\dfrac{\mu + X\beta}{\sigma}\right)\right)}.$$

This leads to the following assumptions.

(i) The log-logistic survival model is an accelerated failure time model, which follows from its method of construction.
(ii) It is a proportional odds model. The odds of survival is

$$O(t) = \frac{S(t)}{1 - S(t)} = \frac{1}{\lambda t^{\alpha} \exp\left(\dfrac{X\beta}{\sigma}\right)} = \frac{1}{\lambda t^{\alpha}} \exp\left(-\frac{X\beta}{\sigma}\right).$$

Consider two observations, i and j. Their odds ratio is

$$\frac{O_i(t)}{O_j(t)} = \frac{\exp\left(-\dfrac{X_i\beta}{\sigma}\right)}{\exp\left(-\dfrac{X_j\beta}{\sigma}\right)},$$

which is constant over time.

It is worth noting that the log-logistic model is *not* a proportional hazard model.

The usual assumptions about the linear and additive effect of the covariates on the hazard remain.

Method label: accelerated failure time (AFT) models	
Main use	– Regression models for time-to-event outcomes
Context of use	– Right-censored data
	– Interest is the effect of covariates and making predictions
	– Same interpretability as regression models for other outcome types
Secondary use	
Non-recommended uses and pitfalls	**Pitfall A.1.4.1.** The key assumption is the accelerated failure time (AFT) assumption. Not appropriate if this assumption is violated
	Pitfall A.1.4.2. The models assume linearity and additivity. Not appropriate if these assumptions are violated
	Pitfall A.1.4.3. High dimensionality is a problem
Principle of operation	– Fully parametric model that specifies the full likelihood
	– The error term is assumed to have a location-scale distribution. This ensures that the log survival time has the same distribution. Covariates change the location parameter, accelerating/decelerating the passing of time
Theoretical properties and empirical evidence	– Parameter estimates are obtained using maximum likelihood estimation. They are consistent, unbiased, efficient and asymptotically normally distributed
	– AFT is a family of distribution with different properties
	Exponential survival model—constant hazard assumption
	Weibull survival model—AFT and PH
	Log-logistic survival model—AFT and proportional odds assumption
Best practices	**Best Practice A.1.4.1.** Use AFT if the assumptions are met
	Best Practice A.1.4.2. Use Cox PH if only the PH assumption is met
References	Klein JP, Moeschberger ML. SURVIVAL ANALYSIS Techniques for Censored and Truncated Data. 2003, Springer
	Kleinbaum DG, Klein M. Survival Analysis. A Self-Learning Text. 2020, Springer

Parametric Survival Models Versus Cox PH Models

If the model assumptions of the parametric models are met, the parametric models are more efficient. If the assumptions are not met or if we are in doubt, the semi-parametric model is more robust to model misspecification and only requires the proportional hazards assumption. Below we look at methods to determine whether a particular parametric model is appropriate.

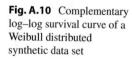

Fig. A.10 Complementary log–log survival curve of a Weibull distributed synthetic data set

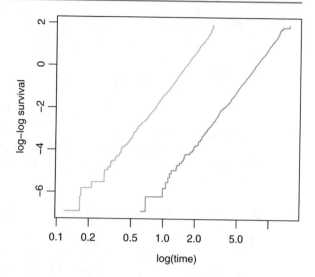

Weibull model. If the survival times follow a Weibull distribution, they form a straight line on the complementary log–log plot. The complementary log–log plot plots the log–log survival function $\log(-\log(S(t))$ against the log of time. The slope of this line is the shape (α) parameter of the Weibull distribution. If the slope is one, then the survival times follow an Exponential distribution.

If for a covariate, two lines, corresponding to two different values of the covariate, are straight and parallel, then we meet both the AFT and the proportional hazards (PH) assumptions. For the Weibull distribution, if either the AFT or PH assumptions is met, the other is assumption is automatically met.

Figure A.10 shows the complementary log–log plot of a synthetic Weibull distributed survival data set. The orange and blue lines correspond to two different values of a covariate. Both lines are straight and parallel, indicating that the Weibull distribution is appropriate for modeling the data and that both the AFT and PH assumptions are met.

The left panel in Fig. A.11 shows the complementary log–log plot of the diabetes data set. We continue to use impaired fasting glucose (IFG) as the sole covariate and the two survival curves were computed using the Kaplan–Meier estimator. The two lines corresponding to the two values of this covariate, IFG in orange and non-IFG in blue, are reasonably straight and parallel for the first 6 years. Beyond 6 years, the curves turn and become horizontal. They remain parallel but they no longer continue to have the same slope. The turn signals a violation of the AFT assumption, however, they remain parallel, indicating that the PH assumption is still met. This appears to be a small violation, however, a large portion of the population have a follow-up time in excess of 6 years.

The right panel in Fig. A.11 shows the Weibull fit (in dashed lines) and the Kaplan–Meier survival curve (in solid line) for the IFG patients (orange) and non-IFG patients (blue). We can see that the lack of events beyond 6 years caused a substantial bias in the Weibull estimates. We expected this bias based on the

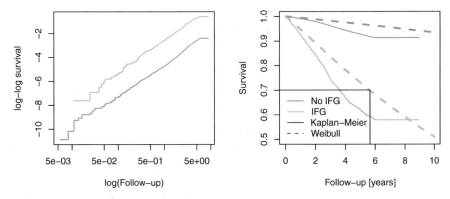

Fig. A.11 Weibull survival model on the diabetes data set. The right panel shows the complementary log–log survival curve. The orange line corresponds to patients with IFG and the blue line without. The right panel shows the survival curves. The solid lines are estimated using the Kaplan–Meier estimator, while the dashed lines are computed from a Weibull model. Orange corresponds to patients with IFG, while blue corresponds to patient with healthy fasting glucose

violation of the AFT assumption. Since the PH assumption is still met, a Cox model would be a better fit for this data.

Log-logistic model. The assumption underlying the log logistic model is the proportional odds assumption. If the event time distribution follows a log logistic distribution, the log(time) versus log odds of failure curve should be straight. For two values of a covariate, if the model follows the proportional odds assumption, the lines should be parallel.

Figure A.12 shows a synthetic data set that has log-logistically distributed event times. The two colors represent log-odds-failure curves corresponding to two values of the sole covariate. Except for the very early follow-up times (time < 1e−1), where data is sparse, the lines are reasonably straight and parallel.

Figure A.13 shows the log-odds-of-failure plot of the diabetes data set. Up to 6 years, the lines representing IFG and non-IFG patients are straight and parallel, however after 6 years, the lines turn horizontal. This indicates that the log logistic model is not appropriate for this data set.

Non-linear Survival Models

The regression models in the previous sections all assume that the covariates have an additive linear relationship with the log hazard or log survival time. To overcome this limitation, the original features X can be transformed through a non-linear non-additive transformation to serve as the input to the partial or full likelihood function of the above models. Deep-learning based survival models and the Gradient Boosting Machine (GBM) for time-to-event outcome have taken this approach. The $X\beta$ term in the Cox partial likelihood is replaced by a non-linear non-additive function $f(X)$. This function is an ANN for deep learning and a GBM for Cox GBM.

A Random Survival Forest (RSF) consists of a collection of B trees. This collection does not directly maximize a likelihood function like the previously discussed

Fig. A.12 Log odds-
failure time curves for
synthetic log-logistic data

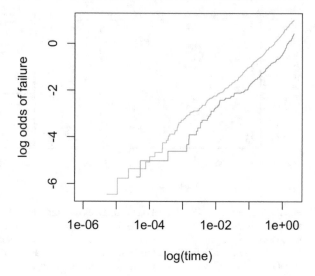

Fig. A.13 Log-odds-
failure time plot of the
diabetes data set

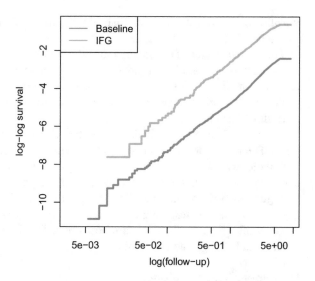

methods, so RSF works slightly differently. In RSF, each of the B trees models the
cumulative hazard of a patient using the Nelson–Aalen estimator. The cumulative
hazard estimates from the B trees are then averaged to obtain an overall prediction
for the cumulative hazard [49].

One key in time-to-event modeling is censoring. The partial likelihood automatically takes censoring into account, but the full likelihood may not. Deep learning
models based on the full likelihood, assuming a Weibull distributed survival time,
have been proposed. An alternative to the partial likelihood in the presence of censoring is the censoring unbiased loss (CUL), which is a general method for

bias-correcting the unobservable loss. Censoring unbiased deep learning (CUDL) follows this strategy [50, 51].

High-dimensional data. Similar to non-survival regression models, high dimensionality, when the number of predictor variables is large relative to the number of observations, poses a challenge. In non-survival regression, regularizing the likelihood function was one of the solutions. Analogous solutions by regularizing the partial likelihood function of the survival models has been proposed in the form of an elastic-net style Cox model.

Survival models for longitudinal data. When we have longitudinal data, the covariates and the outcome can change over time. We have already discussed extensions to the Cox model that allow for changing predictors (time-dependent covariates) and recurring events. In the general regression setting, longitudinal data is handled through marginal models or through mixed effect models, because the observations become correlated. We have also discussed that in the Cox model, as long as we only have one event per patient, marginal or mixed effect models are not required [45].

Apart from providing the correct error estimates in the longitudinal setting, mixed effect models are also used for separating subject-specific and population effects. Frailty models are the time-to-event outcome analogues of the mixed effect regression models and allow for modeling subject-specific effects.

References
The references are the same as in Chapter 3.

Appendix B: Models for Longitudinal Data

Longitudinal Data Analysis

Longitudinal data is generated when measurements are taken for the same subjects on multiple occasions. For example, EHR data of patients is longitudinal as the same measurements, e.g. vitals, are taken at multiple encounters. Longitudinal data stands in contrast with single cross-sectional data, where measurements are taken (or aggregated) at a single particular time point. It also contrasts with **time series** data, where measurements are taken for a single subject (or for few subjects) for a long period of time and inference is conducted within the subject.

Using longitudinal data offers several advantages. (1) It can provide more information about each subject than data from a single cross-section since we observe the subject over a time span. (2) It also allows for a crossover study design, where a patient can be a control patient for himself: When a subject experiences an exposure during the study period, he/she is a "control" subject before the exposure and is an "exposed" patient after the exposure. (3) it also allows for separating aging effects from intervention effects. Finally, (4) it allows for separating subject-specific effects from population effects [5, 53].

Figure B.1 shows an illustrative synthetic data set. Five subjects are followed over 10 time periods and a measurement is taken in each time period. The left panel shows a plot of the data set. The horizontal axis represents time, and the vertical axis is the measurement. We can see an overall upward trend: as time increases the measured values increase. We fitted a linear regression model to the entire data, which is shown as the bold black line. This model is a **population-level** model and it confirms this increasing trend. We also fitted a regression line, shown as dashed gray lines, to each individual subject. These are called **individual-level** lines. We can see that most (all five in this sample) subjects also exhibit an increasing trend, but their initial points (y-intercepts) vary, and their slopes also vary. Some methods allow for modeling individual effects such as the per-subject intercept and per-subject slope.

These advantages of longitudinal data analysis, however, come at a price. The multiple observations of the same patients are correlated with each other, which violates the i.i.d. (independent, identically distributed) assumption that most analytic methods make.

© The Editor(s) (if applicable) and The Author(s) 2024   749
G. J. Simon, C. Aliferis (eds.), *Artificial Intelligence and Machine Learning in Health Care and Medical Sciences*, Health Informatics,
https://doi.org/10.1007/978-3-031-39355-6

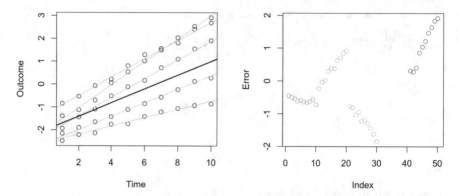

Fig. B.1 Longitudinal data illustration. Five subjects are followed over 10 time periods and a measurement is taken in each time period. The left panel shows a plot of the data set. The horizontal axis represents time and the vertical axis is the measurement. The bold black line depicts an overall trend (population trend) and the 5 dashed lines represent the (individual) trends of the five subjects. The right panel shows the error relative to the population trend. The horizontal axis is an index, grouped by subject. Different colors represent different subjects

The right panel in Fig. B.1 shows the error relative to the population-level regression model (the bold black line in the left panel). The horizontal axis is simply an observation index and the vertical axis is the (signed) error (residual). Observations from the five subjects are grouped together along the horizontal axis in increasing order of time: index 1–10 corresponds to the ten time points of the first subjects, etc. Different subjects are depicted in different colors. We can see that the errors of each subject (errors depicted in the same color) tend to form clusters. Within a subject, once we know the error of one observation, errors of the other observations will typically not differ as much as errors from a different subject. This means that errors of the same subject are correlated with each other. There is also a trend within each subject: as time increases, the errors tend to increase or decrease. This is due to the differences in the growth rates of the different subjects (the differences across the slopes of the gray lines in the left panel).

When we assume that the errors in the right panel are generated from 50 independent observations, we would estimate the variance of the outcome to be about 1 (ranging between −2 and 2). Once we account for the fact that the observations came from 5 different subjects, the spread of the error becomes the range covered by the same color, and the variance becomes approximately 0.57; and after accounting for the differences in individual growth rates, the error variance drops to (approx.) 0.1. Such reduction in the noise variance leads to much improved error estimates and is very beneficial for detecting significant effects from exposures.

The data is **balanced** when measurements for all subjects are taken at the same time points. When the data is balanced, coefficient estimates, whether they are computed using methods for longitudinal data or for cross-sectional data, will be similar albeit with substantially different errors. If the purpose of the analysis is prediction for previously unseen subjects, no individual effect estimates will be available, thus the results obtained from the regular regression models will be very similar to those obtained from the longitudinal models.

Conversely, methods designed for longitudinal data should be used when the design is not balanced, the significance of the coefficients needs to be estimated, estimating errors is important, individual (within-subject) effects are of interest, or if predictions are to be made for previously seen patients (whose individual effect sizes are already estimated).

All methods in this section can address the correlation in the errors among observations of the same subject by assuming a variance–covariance structure within a subject. As a result, they provide more statistical power and reduced errors as compared to methods that assume that the observations are independent. Additionally, the error can be decomposed into subject-level errors, including a subject-level intercept and a subject-level growth rate (slope). Linear mixed models (LMMs) in "Regression Models for Longitudinal Data" and generalized LMMs in "Generalized Linear Mixed Effect Models (GLMM)" have this ability.

Terminology and Notation

The sampling unit of the analysis is a subject or a patient and we index the sampling units $i = 1, \ldots, N$. The analytic units are observations. Each patient can have multiple observations, indexed by $j = 1, \ldots, n_i$, taken at n_j different occasions (time points). The time of these occasions are denoted by t_{ij}, the time of the jth occasion for the ith patient. The design is **balanced**, if all subjects share the same time points.

Let y_{ij} denote the response variable (of patient i at occasion j) and let X be covariates. The covariates for subject i can be time-invariant (constant across time) or it can vary across time. The vector of time-invariant covariates for subject i are denoted by X_i and the vector of time-varying covariates form subject i at occasion j is denoted by X_{ij}.

The questions we ask about longitudinal data are similar to and are a superset of the questions we ask about cross-sectional data. These questions include:

(i) Are two sets of observations ($y_{i1}, y_{i2}, \ldots, y_{in}$ and $y_{k1}, y_{k2}, \ldots, y_{kn}$), one for patient i and the other one for patient k, different?

(ii) Are observations at different time points j and k different ($y_{\cdot j} =^? y_{\cdot k}$)? Or more broadly, describe the changes in observations over time.

(iii) Making predictions. We may wish to predict the value of the observation at a particular time point for a subject we have observed before; or we may want to predict the value of an observation for a subject that we have not seen before.

(iv) Estimate the effect of exposures.

(v) Estimate subject-specific effects.

ANOVA and MANOVA for Repeated Measures

Consider a cohort of patients. For each patient, we measure some aspect of their health, e.g. their blood glucose level, at multiple occasions. These patients are subject to an intervention, e.g. blood glucose control, at three different levels: standard of care, aggressive and very aggressive. Methods in this section aim to answer the following kind of questions:

(i)   Does the blood glucose level in patients change over time? Namely, does the set of blood glucose measurements taken from the cohort at one time point differ from the set of blood glucose measurements taken from the same cohort at a different time point?

(ii) Does different levels of glucose control result in different glucose levels? Does the average glucose measurement in the "standard of care" group differ from the glucose measurement in the (say) "aggressive" group?

We can approach this analysis in two ways, which we can illustrate through describing how we would organize the data for the analysis. The first organization is the **person-period (PP)** organization, where each row in our data table corresponds to the outcome (blood glucose) measured at a particular time point. The second organization is a **person-level (PL)** organization, where there is one row for each person and this one row contains the entire measurement vector for that person. **ANOVA** assumes the PP format and **MANOVA** assumes the PL format [52].

   If the sole interest is the change of the outcome over time, we only have a time effect. This corresponds to a **single-sample** analysis. If we are also interested in the treatment effect, we have a **multiple-sample** analysis: each treatment level corresponds to a "sample". Both ANOVA and MANOVA can be single or multiple-sample.

ANOVA

ANOVA models the person-period observations y_{ij}. We start our discussion with the one-sample ANOVA, where the sole interest is the effect of time. The model is

$$y_{ij} = \mu + \pi_i + \tau_j + \varepsilon_{ij},$$

where μ is the grand mean, π_i is the subject-effect and τ_j is the time effect. The time effect τ_j, the effect of interest, is a *fixed effect* and the subject-effect π_i is a *random effect*, and is modelled as $\pi_i \sim N\left(0,\sigma_\pi^2\right)$, where σ_π^2 is the between-subject variance.

   Random effects are effect estimates that are computed for observation units that are thought of as a random sample from a population. In contrast, **fixed effects** are effect estimates computed for specific observation units. The subject effects π_i are random effects, because the corresponding units, namely the patients, are thought of as a (hopefully) representative random sample (the study cohort) from a population of patients. We could have conducted our study with a different random sample from the same population and we would expect similar results. Conversely, the time effects τ_j are fixed effects, because we wish to know the effect of time period j on the outcome. The time points are not a representative random sample from a population of time points, they represent periods of exposure to the intervention. If we conducted our study using different time periods, say 2 months exposures as opposed to 2 days, we would certainly expect to get different results.

Model assumptions
(i) The subject effect is assumed homogeneous over time and the time effect is assumed homogeneous over the subjects.
(ii) The within-subject error ε_{ij} is normally distributed with mean 0 and variance σ_e^2. Neither the mean nor the variance depends on the subject i or occasion j.
(iii) The time effects sum to 0 over time.
(iv) $E(y_{ij}) = \mu + \tau_j$
(v) $Var\left(y_{ij}\right) = \sigma_\pi^2 + \sigma_e^2$
(vi) Subjects are independent, $Cov(y_{ij}, y_{kj}) = 0$ for all patients $i \neq k$ on all occasions j.
(vii) Covariance among the observations of the same subject is constant, σ_π^2, over time.

This set of assumptions lead to a variance–covariance matrix of

$$\Sigma_i = \begin{bmatrix} \sigma_\pi^2 + \sigma_e^2 & \sigma_\pi^2 & \sigma_\pi^2 & \cdots & \sigma_\pi^2 \\ \sigma_\pi^2 & \sigma_\pi^2 + \sigma_e^2 & \sigma_\pi^2 & \cdots & \sigma_\pi^2 \\ \sigma_\pi^2 & \sigma_\pi^2 & \sigma_\pi^2 + \sigma_e^2 & \cdots & \sigma_\pi^2 \\ \vdots & \vdots & \vdots & \ddots & \vdots \\ \sigma_\pi^2 & \sigma_\pi^2 & \sigma_\pi^2 & \cdots & \sigma_\pi^2 + \sigma_e^2 \end{bmatrix},$$

which is referred to as **compound symmetry**.

The importance of the compound symmetry structure is the assumption that the covariance (and correlation) among the observations from the same patient is constant. Typically, this assumption is unrealistic, observations closer together in time tend to be more correlated than observations further apart in time.

Under this model, we can test the hypothesis that

$$H0 : \tau_1 = \tau_2 = \cdots = \tau_n = 0.$$

By using contrasts, more detailed tests of the time effect can be derived. The interested reader is referred to Chapter 2 in [52] for details.

Multiple-Sample ANOVA

Assume that a treatment is applied to groups of patients, one group per treatment level. The model now needs to be extended to accommodate group effects

$$y_{ij} = \mu + \pi_{i(k)} + \tau_j + \gamma_k + \left(\gamma\tau\right)_{kj} + \varepsilon_{ijk}.$$

The group effects are γ_k and group-specific time effects $(\gamma\tau)_{kj}$ are also included. The $i(k)$ notation signals that subject i is nested in group k and ε_{ijk} is now a within-group, within-subject variance. Additional assumptions are that (1) the group effects must sum to 0, $\sum_k \gamma_k = 0$,, and that (2) group-specific time effects must also sum to 0,

$\sum_k \sum_j (\gamma\tau)_{jk} = 0$. The group effect and its interaction with time are fixed effects, so the variance–covariance matrix remains unchanged.

With this model, we can test whether time effects exist, whether group (treatment) effects exist and whether their interaction effects exist. The interested reader is referred to [52] for the details of these tests.

Method label: repeated measures ANOVA	
Main use	– ANOVA for repeated measures data
Context of use	– Single-sample or multiple-sample ANOVA
	– Assumes the data to be in the PP (person-period) format
	– Assessing the significance of time effects and treatment effects
Secondary use	
Pitfalls	**Pitfall A.2.2.1.** Repeated Measures ANOVA is not a predictive model
	Pitfall A.2.2.2. Repeated Measures ANOVA assumes compound symmetry; not appropriate when this assumption is violated
Principle of operation	– Operates on the same principle as most ANOVA methods
	– See the text for detailed models
Theoretical properties and empirical evidence	– Requires balanced design
	– Assumes the compound symmetry
	– Performs statistical tests of time effect and treatment effects
	– Contrasts can be used to perform specific tests (e.g. difference between two treatment levels)
Best practices	**Best Practice A.2.2.1.** Also consider the random intercept LMM. The LMM is more flexible and contains the ANOVA specification as a special case
References	Hedeker D, Gibbons RD. Longitudinal Data Analsyis. Wiley, 2006. Chapter 2

MANOVA

Multivariate ANOVA (MANOVA) treats the observations of a subject over time as a single outcome vector. The model then becomes

$$y_i = \mu + \varepsilon_i,$$

where y_i, μ, and ε_i are vectors of length n (the number of time points). $Var(y_i) = \Sigma$ is an arbitrary variance–covariance matrix—no assumption about its structure is made. The lack of assumptions about the structure of the variance–covariance matrix is the main benefit of MANOVA, however, its disadvantage is that the study design has to be balanced and no missing values are allowed.

Similarly to the multivariate ANOVA, MANOVA can be used when multiple treatment groups are compared. For each group k, an observation vector y_{ik} is produced and the single-sample model is extended to

$$y_{ik} = \mu + \gamma_k + \varepsilon_{ik}.$$

The γ_k vector (of length n) is the treatment effect of treatment level k across the n time points. The variance–covariance matrix Σ is shared by all groups.

MANOVA allows for testing the same hypothesis as ANOVA.

Method label: repeated measures MANOVA	
Main use	– MANOVA for repeated measures data
Context of use	– Single-sample or multiple-sample MANOVA
	– Assumes the data to be in the PL (person-level) format
	– Assessing the significance of time effects and treatment effects
Secondary use	
Pitfalls	**Pitfall A.2.2.3.** Repeated Measures MANOVA is not a predictive model
	Pitfall A.2.2.3. Repeated Measures MANOVA in its original form, does not allow for missing observations
Principle of operation	– Operates on the same principle as most ANOVA/MANOVA methods
	– See the text for detailed models
Theoretical properties and empirical evidence	– Requires balanced design
	– In contrast to ANOVA, it does not make the compound symmetry assumption, but it does not allow missing values
	– Performs statistical tests of time effect and treatment effects
	– Contrasts can be used to perform specific tests (e.g. difference between two treatment levels)
Best practices	**Best Practice A.2.2.2.** Also consider LMMs
References	– Hedeker D, Gibbons RD. Longitudinal Data Analysis. Wiley, 2006. Chapter 3

Regression Models for Longitudinal Data

The key difference between methods developed for longitudinal data and for cross-sectional data lies in the ability to take within-subject correlations into account. The methods described in this section take two approaches to account for the within-subject correlation. First, Linear Mixed Effect Models (LMM) aim to partition the variance–covariance matrix into within-subject and between-subject variances. If the source of variance is of interest, then the Mixed Effect Models should be used. The second approach, Generalized Estimating Equations (GEE) [69], assumes a parametric form for the variance–covariance matrix. It treats this as a nuisance parameter and marginalizes it out. As such, this method is more computationally efficient than the LMM, but does not distinguish between the within-subject and between-subject effects.

Mixed Effects Regression Models for Longitudinal Data

Regular regression models model the outcome as a combination of deterministic "fixed" effects and a random noise

$$y_i = \beta_0 + X_i\beta + \varepsilon_i,$$

where β_0 is an intercept, β is a vector of coefficients for the fixed effects imparted by the covariates X_i and ε is a normally distributed noise term with mean 0 and variance σ^2.

Mixed effects regression models, similarly to regular regression models, allow for fixed effects, but they further partition the "noise" into different anticipated random effects. Different types of LMM models differ in the random effects they anticipate, which in turn, confers different structures on the variance–covariance matrix.

Let the subscript i correspond to the subject and j to the (index of) the occasion when the subject was observed. Let X_{ij} denote the covariate vector and y_{ij} the response of subject i at occasion j. The time point of this occasion is t_{ij}.

Mixed effect models are often expressed in the hierarchical format. The first-level model is on the level of the population

$$y_{ij} = \beta_{0i} + X_{ij}\beta + t_{ij}\beta_{ti} + \varepsilon_{ij},$$

and the second-level (subject-level) models define the models for the intercept β_{0i}, the (time) trend β_{ti} for subject i. Mixed effect models are a family of models that chiefly differ in the way β_{0i} and β_{ti} are defined. Different definitions lead to different variance–covariance matrices based on different assumptions, however, all mixed effect models share some common assumptions.

First, as in all linear models, the fixed effects, X_{ij}, are assumed to have a linear additive relationship with y_{ij}. This assumption can be relaxed by including a priori known interactions and nonlinearities.

Second, time enters the mixed effect models explicitly (t_{ij}). This allows for observation times to vary across subjects. In many models, time has a linear additive effect on the response, however, models with curvilinear relationships will be discussed later.

Third, the structure of the variance–covariance matrix is specified through a random intercept and/or trend. This allows for the dimension of the variance–covariance matrix to vary across patients, which in turn, allows for a differing number of observations across subjects. The second and third properties combined make mixed effect models appropriate for the analysis of longitudinal data that is not of repeated measures design (observation times vary) or for repeated measures design with missing observations.

Fourth, models in this chapter assume an outcome with Gaussian distribution, but mixed effect models have been extended to the exponential family outcomes through a linkage function that linearizes these outcomes. These models, Generalized Mixed Effect Models, are the mixed-effect analogues of GLMs.

In the following sections, we describe specific mixed effect models, their assumptions, relationships between covariates, time and outcome they can represent, and the variance-covariance matrix forms these assumptions yield.

Random Intercept Models
Random intercept models are mixed effect models with a subject-specific random intercept effect but only with a population average trend effect. The second level models are thus

$$\beta_{0i} = \beta_0 + \upsilon_i$$
$$\beta_{ti} = \beta_t.$$

The subject-specific intercept β_{0i} is decomposed into a population average effect β_0 and a subject-specific random effect v_i. The time effect β_{ti} is simply the population average trend (slope) β_t (without a subject-specific random effect). Thus the random intercept model decomposes the "noise" into a subject-specific random effect v_i and the actual noise at the jth occasion ε_{ij}.

It is further assumed that

$$v_i \sim N\left(0, \sigma_v^2\right)$$

$$\varepsilon_i \sim N\left(0, \sigma_e^2\right).$$

This yields a block-diagonal variance–covariance matrix. Each block corresponds to a subject and is of the form

$$\Sigma_i = \begin{bmatrix} \sigma_v^2 + \sigma_e^2 & \sigma_v^2 & \sigma_v^2 & \cdots & \sigma_v^2 \\ \sigma_v^2 & \sigma_v^2 + \sigma_e^2 & \sigma_v^2 & \cdots & \sigma_v^2 \\ \sigma_v^2 & \sigma_v^2 & \sigma_v^2 + \sigma_e^2 & \cdots & \sigma_v^2 \\ \vdots & \vdots & \vdots & \ddots & \vdots \\ \sigma_v^2 & \sigma_v^2 & \sigma_v^2 & \cdots & \sigma_v^2 + \sigma_e^2 \end{bmatrix}.$$

This form of variance–covariance matrix is referred to as compound symmetry. It assumes that the covariance between observations of the same subject are constant over time. This is often unrealistic: observations closer to each other in time are typically more correlated than observations further away in time.

Random Growth Models

Random growth models, in addition to the subject-specific random intercept, also have a random slope for time. This allows (1) for changes (slopes) to vary across subjects and (2) for time to enter the variance–covariance matrix. The second-level model is

$$\beta_{0i} = \beta_0 + v_{0i}$$

$$\beta_{ti} = \beta_t + v_{ti}.$$

Similarly to the way the intercept was decomposed into a subject-specific effect v_{0i} and a population-level effect β_0 in the random intercept model, in the random growth model the time effect is also decomposed into a subject-specific effect v_{ti} and a population-level time effect β_t. It is assumed that

$$v_{0i} \sim N\left(0, \sigma_{v_0}^2\right), v_{ti} \sim N\left(0, \sigma_{v_t}^2\right)$$

$$\varepsilon_i \sim N\left(0, \sigma_e^2\right).$$

With subjects i and k being independent, the variance–covariance matrix is block-diagonal, with each block representing a patient and taking a form of

$$\Sigma_i = \sigma_e^2 I + T_i \Sigma_v T_i^T,$$

where

$$T_i^T = \begin{bmatrix} 1 & 1 & \cdots & 1 \\ t_1 & t_2 & \cdots & t_{n_i} \end{bmatrix},$$

and

$$\varsigma_i = \begin{bmatrix} \sigma_{v_0}^2 & \sigma_{v_0 v_t} \\ \sigma_{v_0 v_t} & \sigma_{v_t}^2 \end{bmatrix}.$$

With time entering the covariance matrix, the covariance among the observations of the same patient can change over time.

Polynomial Growth Model

To model non-linear time effects, the level-1 model can be extended with polynomials of time.

Specifically, in vector notation, it becomes

$$y_i = \beta_{0i} + X_i \beta + T_i v_i + \varepsilon_i,$$

where T_i contains polynomial of t_i. To be able to model a quadratic time effect, T_i would be (Fig. B.2)

$$T_i = \begin{bmatrix} 1 & t_1 & t_1^2 \\ 1 & t_2 & t_2^2 \\ 1 & \vdots & \vdots \\ 1 & t_{n_i} & t_{n_i}^2 \end{bmatrix}.$$

Comparison of the Various Model Assumptions

Figure B.3 illustrates the difference among the three model types. Four synthetic data sets were generated using four different assumptions. In all four data sets, five subjects were observed at 10 time points. The four data sets are plotted in the four panels. For all four panels, the horizontal axis is the index j of the observations, grouped by subject. The vertical axis is the error relative to a population-level model.

The first assumption is the random intercept. This causes errors to cluster by subject. The mean of the error in each subject is the subject's random intercept β_{0i}. No other structure can be observed: the scale of the errors remains the same over time.

The second assumption corresponds to the growth model. In addition to clustering due to the random intercept, the plot also shows that the errors consistently increase over time, at a rate that differs across patients. This growth rate is the random slope v_{it}. Observations of the same subject closer together in time have more similar errors (and thus observations) than observations of the same subject further apart in time. This is a violation of the compound symmetry structure, but the random growth model can handle this situation correctly.

The third assumption is quadratic time, random intercept. The data has both linear and quadratic population-level time effect but only a random intercept. We only removed the linear time effect, thus the errors (residuals) form a per-subject parabola, indicative of a quadratic effect. The parabolas have similar shape across patients (although different parts of the same parabola are visible), which suggests that this is a (quadratic) population-level effect, but the parabolas have different foci along the y axis, suggesting a subject-level random intercept.

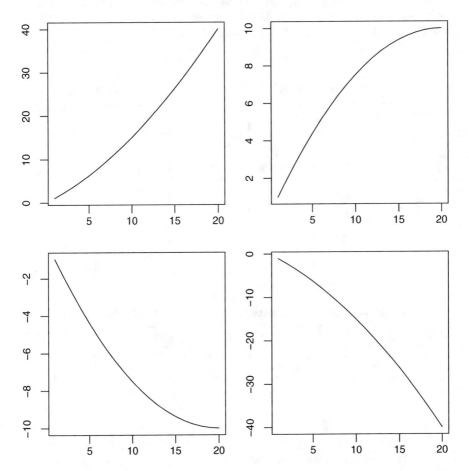

Fig. B.2 Polynomial time effects. For illustration purposes, quadratic polynomials are used, but higher order polynomials are also allowed. The horizontal axis is time and the vertical axis is its effect. In the top row, the effect of time is positive ($v_{it} > 0$) and in the bottom row it is negative. In the left column, the quadratic effect is positive ($v_{it}^2 > 0$) and in the right *column, it is negative*

Finally, the quadratic growth model has both population-level as well as a subject-level quadratic time effect. The quadratic structure is apparent in the parabolic shapes of the within-subject errors, however, the shape of the parabolas change across the patients, suggesting a subject-level effect. Because of the strong population-level quadratic time-effect, it is difficult to see whether the subject-level time effect is only linear or quadratic. The parabolas are located at different positions along the vertical axis, which indicates a subject-level random intercept.

Generalized Linear Mixed Effect Models (GLMM)

Generalized Linear Mixed Effect Models related to LMMs the same way as Generalized Linear Models (GLMs) relate to linear regression models. GLMMs allow for a link function to link the expectation of the outcome with the linear predictor. Similarly to GLMs, GLMMs can thus be used to solve regression problems with non-Gaussian dependent variables, such as classification problems (logistic outcome), counting problems (Poisson outcome), etc.

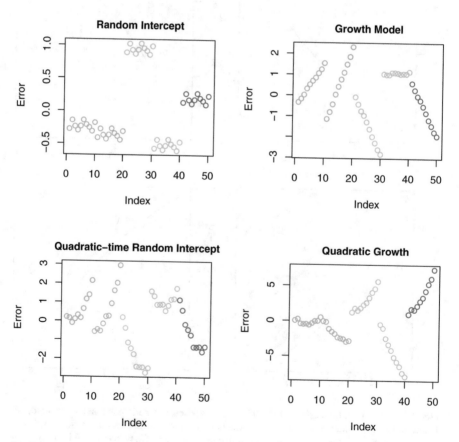

Fig. B.3 Comparison of the various model assumptions

Method label: linear mixed effect models (LMM)	
Main use	– Regression models for longitudinal data
Context of use	– Longitudinal data with balanced or unbalanced design
	– Separates subject-level effects from population-level effects
	– Predictive modeling with within-subject predictions
	– Accurate error estimates are required or the interest is the statistical significance of covariates
Secondary use	– Generalized LMM has been developed for non-Gaussian response variables
Pitfalls	**Pitfall A.2.3.2.** GEEs can be computationally more efficient and may produce better predictive models. Use LMM when the goal is to identify subject-level effects
Principle of operation	– Partitions the error into subject-level and population-level components
	– Random intercept model: assumes a subject-specific intercept
	– Random growth model: assumes a subject-specific intercept and time-trend
	– Polynomial growth model: assumes a subject-specific curvilinear time effect
Theoretical properties and empirical evidence	– See the text for the detailed assumptions
	– ML estimator. Coefficient estimates are consistent, asymptotically normal
Best practices	**Best Practice A.2.3.1.** Use LMM when the goal is to identify subject-level effects
	Best Practice A.2.3.2. If the main purpose is estimating the effect size of covariates or making predictions for previously unseen subjects, GEE can be more computationally effective
References	– Hedeker D, Gibbons RD. Longitudinal Data Analysis. Wiley, 2006. Chapter 4

Generalized Estimating Equations

As discussed earlier, the key statistical challenge with longitudinal data is the correlation among the observations of the same subject. This challenge is addressed by assuming a variance–covariance matrix for the error when the regression parameters are estimated. In "Mixed Effects Regression Models for Longitudinal Data" section, we described a method for constructing such a matrix by separating the error variation into a set of subject-specific and a set of population-level effects. These effects define the form of the variance–covariance matrix. An alternative strategy is to assume a functional form for the variance–covariance matrix. This second strategy is the subject of the current section.

In this approach, the parameters that define the variance–covariance matrix are treated as nuisance parameters and the main interest is the coefficients of the covariates, including time. The variance–covariance parameters are marginalized (integrated out) and hence this type of models are referred to as **marginal models**.

The development of the generalized estimating equations models proceeds similarly to the generalized linear models. Given a covariate matrix X, the following components are defined.

(i) Linear predictor: $\eta_{ij} = X_{ij}\beta$;
(ii) Linkage function that links the mean of the linear predictor to the expectation of the outcome $g(E(Y_{ij})) = \mu_{ij}$;
(iii) A variance function relating the mean of the outcome to its variance:

$$Var\left(y_{ij}\right) = \phi V\left(\mu_{ij}\right);$$

(iv) A working variance–covariance matrix parameterized by a: R(a)

The first three components are shared with the generalized linear models; GEEs add the fourth component.

Several variance–covariance matrix forms are implemented by statistical software packages and the most common matrices are described below.

(i) Identity: $R(a) = I$. This assumes that the observations of a subject are independent of each other and thus it reduces a GEE to a regular GLM.
(ii) Exchangeable: $R(a) = \rho$. Observations of the same subject have constant covariance ρ, which does not depend on time. This matrix form is the same as the compound symmetry in the random intercept models.
(iii) Autoregressive: $R(a) = \rho^{|j-j'|}$. With j and j' denoting two time steps, the covariance among observations of the same subject depends on time. If $\rho < 1$, then the further away the observations are in time, the smaller the covariance.
(iv) Unstructured. Each element of the matrix is estimated from data.

Among the four matrices, we have already seen the identity and the exchangeable structures and the unstructured matrix is straightforward to imagine. The autoregressive matrix will take the following form

$$R(\rho) = \begin{bmatrix} 1 & \rho & \rho^2 & \rho^3 & \cdots \\ \rho & 1 & \rho & \rho^2 & \cdots \\ \rho^2 & \rho & 1 & \rho & \cdots \\ \vdots & \vdots & \vdots & 1 & \ddots \end{bmatrix}.$$

When $|\rho| < 1$, increasing powers of ρ become smaller, thus the more distant two observations are in time, the smaller their covariance.

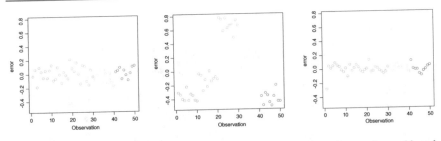

Fig. B.4 Illustration of the error distributions corresponding to the independent, exchangeable and autocorrelated variance/covariance structures

Figure B.4 shows three types of error distributions. For 5 subjects, 10 observations were generated using independent error (left panel), exchangeable error (middle panel) and autocorrelated error (right panel). The 5 subjects are shown in different colors and their 10 observations are ordered by time along the horizontal axis. The noise has standard normal distribution with $\sigma = .1$ in all three cases. The error in the left panel is noise and all errors, regardless of which subject they came from, are independent: knowing the error of an observation for a patient does not provide any information about the error of another observation of the same patient or about any observation of any other subject. In the middle panel, the error has a noise component and a random intercept component. Errors are correlated within each subject and subjects are independent of each other. We have seen this correlation structure earlier. Finally, in the right panel, we have autocorrelated errors. Two errors of the same subject are more similar to each other the closer they are to each other in time.

Method label: generalized estimating equations (GEE)	
Main use	– Regression models for longitudinal data – A linkage function can be specified
Context of use	– Longitudinal data with unbalanced design – Most used when the focus is on coefficient estimates and making predictions for previously unseen patients
Secondary use	
Pitfalls	**Pitfall A.2.4.1.** No individualized effects are estimated. Consider the LMM if separation of the individual effects from the population effect is desired

Method label: generalized estimating equations (GEE)	
Principle of operation	– Uses estimating equations
	– It is a marginal model. Assumes a parametric form for the working variance/covariance matrix and marginalizes it out
Theoretical properties and empirical evidence	– Uses M estimation. Specification of the likelihood is not required
	– Solving estimating equations very computationally efficient
	– Even if the structure of the variance/covariance matrix is misspecified, it yields good results
Best practices	**Best Practice A.2.4.1.** Use GEE when predictions for previously unseen subjects is needed
	Best Practice A.2.4.2. Use LMM when subject-specific effects are of interest
References	– Hardin, J.W. and Hilbe, J.M., 2002. *Generalized estimating equations*. Chapman and Hall/CRC
	– Hedeker D, Gibbons RD. Longitudinal Data Analysis. Wiley, 2006. Chapter 3

References

The references are the same as in Chapter 3.

Appendix C: Best Practices and Pitfalls

Chapter 2. Foundations of AI

2.1. Pursue development of AI/ML algorithms, programs or systems that have tractable complexity.	Mature	High impact
2.2. Do not rely on parallelization to make intractable problems tractable. Pursue tractable algorithms and factor in the tractability analysis any parallelization.	Mature	High impact
2.3. Do not rely on Moore's law improvements to make an intractable problem algorithm or hard program practical. Pursue tractable algorithms and factor in the tractability analysis any gains from Moore's law.	Mature	High impact
2.4. When faced with intractable problems, consider using strategies for mitigating the computational intractability by trading off with less important characteristics of the desired solution	Mature	High impact
2.5. As much as possible use models and systems with established properties (theoretical + empirical). Work within the maturation process starting from systems with unknown behaviors and no guarantees, to systems with guaranteed properties.	Mature	High impact
2.6. When using Decision Analysis (DA) and Maximum Expected Utility (MEU)-based reasoning: 1. Ensure that the structure of the problem setting is completely/accurately described by the DA tree. Omit known or obvious irrelevant factors. 2. Elicit utility estimates in a way that captures patients' true preferences using standard utility-elicitation methods. 3. Accurately calculate probabilities of action-dependent events and action-independent events. 4. In most conditions, and whenever applicable, data-driven approaches should be preferred to subjective probability estimates. Use probability-consistent statistical or ML algorithms to estimate the probabilities. 5. Ensure that the decision analysis is applied to the correct population. 6. Conduct sensitivity analyses that reveal how much the estimated optimal decision is influenced by uncertainty in the specification of the model. 7. Whenever possible, produce credible intervals/posterior probability distributions for the utility expectations of decisions.	Mature	High impact
2.7. Pursue ML solutions with the right inductive bias for the problem at hand.	Mature	High impact

G. J. Simon, C. Aliferis (eds.), *Artificial Intelligence and Machine Learning in Health Care and Medical Sciences*, Health Informatics,
https://doi.org/10.1007/978-3-031-39355-6

2.8. Create a data generating or data design procedure that matches well the requirements of the problem at hand and works with the inductive bias to achieve strong results.	Mature	High impact
2.9. Do not misinterpret the No Free Lunch Theorem! Cross validation and independent data validation, as well as their cousin reproducibility, are robust pillars of good science and good ML practice and are not challenged by the NFLT.	Mature	High impact
2.10. Clustering should not be used for predictive modeling.	Mature	High impact
2.11. A very useful form of clustering is post-hoc extraction of subtypes from accurate predictor models.	Mature	High impact
2.12. The choice of generative vs discriminative modeling affects quality of modeling results and has to be carefully tied to the problem domain characteristics. All else being equal discriminative models confer efficiency (computational and sample) advantages.	Mature	High impact

Chapter 3. Appraisal of ML Techniques

Chapter 3.2. Foundational Techniques

3.2.1.1. Unless a generalized linear model is more appropriate, OLS is a good baseline technique.	Mature	Medium impact
3.2.1.2. Building an OLS, even if it is known not to produce optimal predictive performance, can reveal data problems, biases, etc.	Mature	Medium impact
3.2.2.1. Use GLM as first pass, or main comparator classifier.	Mature	Medium impact
3.2.2.2. Building a GLM, even if it is known not to produce optimal predictive performance, can reveal data problems, biases, etc.	Mature	Medium impact
3.2.4.1. Deep learning is most recommended for predictive modeling in large imaging datasets. Other domains may also be good candidates. In all cases additional (alternative and comparator) methods should be explored at this time within the same error estimation protocols (see "The Development Process and Lifecycle of Clinical Grade and Other Safety and Performance-Sensitive AI/ML Mode").	Evolving	High impact
3.2.4.2. At this time, ANNs are not suitable for causal discovery and modeling. Formal causal methods should be preferred (see chapter "Foundations of Causal ML").	Evolving	High impact
3.2.4.3. ANNs are not suitable for problems where explainability and transparency are required, or when large reduction of the feature space is important to model application.	Evolving	High impact
3.2.5.1. SVMs are primary choice for omics, text classification, and combined clinical/molecular/text tasks.	Evolving	High impact
3.2.5.2. SVMs are secondary choice for feature selection (with Markov Boundary methods being first choice). In very small sample situations where Markov Boundary methods may suffer, SVM feature selection can be first choice.	Mature	Medium impact

3.2.5.3. SVM weights, features or models should not be interpreted causally.	Mature	High impact
3.2.5.4. Explain SVMs by converting them to interpretable models via meta-learning or other approaches; and convert scores to probabilities when needed.	Mature	High impact
3.2.6.1. Naïve Bayes has limited utility in modern health applications and is not a recommended method in usual circumstances.	Mature	High impact
3.2.6.2. Use Bayes Networks when flexible classification is needed.	Mature	High impact
3.2.6.3. Use causal network models when causal structure discovery and causal effect estimation are needed.	Mature	High impact
3.2.6.4. Causal probabilistic graphs, and local causal and Markov Boundary methods have important equivalence class modeling capabilities not found in other methods.	Evolving	High impact
3.2.6.5. Markov Boundary induction (identified via specialized algorithms) is typically the feature selection method of choice.	Mature	High impact
3.2.6.6. Use Causal Bayes Networks for modeling full joint distributions (e.g., for simulation or re-simulation purposes) while also preserving causal structure.	Mature	High impact
3.2.6.7. Use Causal BNs for guiding experiments in the presence of information equivalences.	Evolving	High impact
3.2.7.1. Use k-Nearest Neighbors (KNN) as comparator not as primary predictive modeling methods.	Mature	High impact
3.2.7.2. In KNN predictive modeling, optimize k with model selection.	Mature	High impact
3.2.7.3. Use adaptive KNN for high dimensional data, and combine with strong feature selection.	Mature	High impact
3.2.7.4. For KNN, explore the right distance metric for the data at hand via model selection.	Evolving	Medium impact
3.2.8.1. Use Decision Trees for interpretable modeling, alone or in conjunction with other methods.	Mature	High impact
3.2.8.2. Use Decision Trees for target variable-specific subpopulation discovery (alone or in conjunction with other methods).	Mature	High impact
3.2.8.3. Use Decision Trees as baseline comparator method for predictive modeling.	Mature	Medium impact
3.2.8.4. Use Decision Trees in ensembles (Boosting) or bagging (Random Forest) algorithms to improve predictivity.	Mature	High impact
3.2.9.1. Do no use clustering to discover causal structure.	Mature	High impact
3.2.9.2. Do not use clustering for predictive modeling.	Mature	High impact
3.2.9.3. Tailor the use of clustering algorithm and metric to the problem at hand.	Mature	High impact
3.2.9.4. Derive predictive subgroups from properly-built and validated classifiers (Decision Trees are particularly good candidates.)	Mature	High impact
3.2.9.5. Perform sensitivity analysis to study the impact of the choice of parameters, metrics and algorithms on clustering (and every other ML method).	Mature	High impact
3.2.9.6. Repeat and summarize multiple runs of randomized clustering algorithms.	Mature	High impact
3.2.9.7. Start from causal and predictive algorithms and use subgrouping and clustering to summarize, visualize, etc. their results.	Mature	High impact

Chapter 3.3. Ensemble Modeling

3.3.1.1. Consider stacking as a high priority choice of algorithm when high performance is needed, when base algorithms do not have optimal inductive bias, and interpretability is not a strong requirement.	Mature	Medium impact
3.3.3.1. Use random forests (RFs) as primary or high priority choice when high predictivity is required and interpretability is not of high importance.	Mature	High impact
3.3.3.2. When using RF, do not rely on the internal error estimation but use an independent unbiased error estimator. Similarly, nest the RF inside a model selection protocol, in order to optimize its hyper parameters.	Mature	High impact
3.3.3.3. When feature selection is important, combine RF with an external feature selection algorithm.	Mature	High impact
3.3.3.4. Control Decision Tree size in random forests by using the recommendations of the inventor in the original publication as the starting point.	Mature	High impact
3.3.4.1. Use boosting (GBM) as a primary or high priority choice when high predictivity is required and interpretability is not of high importance.	Mature	High impact
3.3.4.2. When feature selection is important, combine GBMs with an external feature selection algorithm.	Mature	High impact
3.3.4.3. Control overfitting by restricting the number of iterations in the GBM.	Mature	High impact
3.3.4.4. If data is noisy, prefer noise-robust GMBs.	Mature	High impact
3.3.4.5. Select an appropriate link function for exponential family outcomes in GBMs.	Mature	High impact

Chapter 3.4. Regularization

3.4.1.1. Consider using penalized regression in high-dimensional datasets that classic regression cannot handle at all. Otherwise, feature selection or dimensionality reduction have to be applied.	Mature	High impact
3.4.1.2. Use penalized regression as comparator method along with others as appropriate for the application domain.	Mature	High impact
3.4.1.3. Penalized regression may be useful for some types of feature selection, but not as first-choice feature selection method.	Mature	High impact
3.4.1.4. When non-linear regularized models are needed, select an appropriate link function. Also consider alternatives such as kernel SVMs or Kernel Regression.	Mature	High impact

Chapter 3.5. Feature Selection

3.5.1.1. Markov Boundary procedures are first choice for feature selection (FS) when modest sample size (or more) is available, regardless of how high is the dimensionality. They are particularly appropriate when (1) causal interpretation of findings is desired (2) we wish to have consistent and coherent predictive and valid causal models (3) we wish to find equivalence classes of optimal feature sets or optimal classifiers	Mature	High impact
3.5.1.2. SVM-RFE is a first choice in very small sample size and high dimensional settings when causal conclusions are not sought.	Mature	High impact
3.5.1.3a. Do not over interpret features selected by UAF. Contrary to common over-interpretation in common genomics practice, the top-ranked variables are not strongly suggestive of biological, mechanistic, or causal importance, nor are they the strongest predictive factors.	Mature	High impact
3.5.1.3b. Use UAF when sample sizes are extremely small.	Mature	High impact
3.5.1.4. Generic wrapping and stepwise feature selection procedures should be (and are increasingly) retired from practice.	Evolving	High impact
3.5.2.1. When eliminating expensive, dangerous and/or unnecessary inputs by predictor models is beneficial, then use features selection instead of dimensionality reduction.	Mature	High impact
3.5.2.2. For prediction of specific outcomes, feature selection targeting these outcomes (as opposed to unsupervised dimensionality reduction) should be the method of choice.	Mature	High impact
3.5.2.3. Using a data transform based on the top-2 principal components is a staple of visualization of data for exploratory purposes.	Mature	Medium impact
3.5.2.4. Neither principal component analysis (PCA) nor exploratory factor analysis (EFA) should be over-interpreted causally, predictively, or otherwise.	Mature	High impact
3.5.2.5. PCA for classification can be overfitted, so it needs to be treated like any other data operation by the model selection and error estimation protocol.	Mature	High impact

Chapter 3.6. Time-to-Event Outcomes

3.6.1. When modeling time-to-event outcomes, specialized techniques (such as survival analysis) should be used. Generic predictive modeling methods should be used as comparators or supplemental models.	Mature	High impact
3.6.1.1. Plot the Kaplan-Meier (KM) curve because it can reveal data problems. Consider the complementary log–log plot of the KM curve, as well (for checking modeling assumptions).	Mature	High impact
3.6.3.1. Cox PH is first-choice model for time-to-event data.	Mature	High impact
3.6.3.2. Consider, additionally, survival modeling versions of ML predictive models when they exist.	Mature	Medium impact
3.6.3.3. In the presence of substantial violations, different models, including extensions of the Cox PH, may be more appropriate than the standard Cox model.	Mature	High impact

3.6.3.4. Consider the Markov Boundary feature selector for survival analysis that results from using Cox proportional hazards models as conditional independence testing within the Markov Boundary algorithm.	Evolving	Medium impact
3.6.3.5. For high-dimensional data, consider regularized Cox proportional hazards models. Also consider the Cox Markov Boundary method (described above in 3.6.3.4) for feature selection.	Mature	High impact
3.6.3.6. If age is included in the model and has nonlinear relationship to a time-to-event response, consider an age-scale Cox PH model.	Mature	Medium impact
3.6.4.1. Use an accelerated failure time AFT model over a Cox model if its assumptions are met.	Mature	High impact
3.6.4.2. Use Cox PH instead of AFT if the AFT assumptions are not met but the proportional hazards assumption is.	Mature	High impact

Chapter 3.7. Longitudinal Data

3.7.2.1. When using ANOVA, also consider the random intercept LMM (linear mixed effect models). The LMM is more flexible and contains the ANOVA specification as a special case.	Mature	High impact
3.7.2.2. In general prefer LMMs instead of MANOVA.	Mature	High impact
3.7.3.1. Use LMM when the goal is to identify subject-level effects.	Mature	High impact
3.7.3.2. If the main purpose is estimating the effect size of covariates or making predictions for previously unseen subjects, GEE (generalized estimating equations) can be more efficient than LMM.	Mature	High impact
3.7.4.1. Use GEE when predictions for previously unseen subjects is needed.	Mature	High impact

Chapter 4. Causal AI/ML

4.1. For predictive tasks (i.e., without interventions contemplated) use of Predictive ML is sufficient and first priority. For causal tasks (i.e., with interventions contemplated) use of Causal ML is necessary.	Mature	High impact
4.2. In order to estimate unbiased causal effects, control variables that are sufficient to block all confounding paths. These variables can be identified by causal structure ML algorithms.	Mature	High impact
4.3. Often there is a choice of multiple alternative variable sets that block confounding paths. An applicable choice is to control/condition on the set Parents (exposure) in order to block all confounding paths connecting A and T. However this sufficient confounding blocking variable set is not necessarily the minimal one and it is recommended to use the minimal blocking variable set in order to maximize statistical power and minimize uncertainty in the estimation of the causal effect.	Mature	Medium impact

4.4. A protocol for health science causal ML	Evolving	High impact

1. Define the goal of the analysis
2. Preprocess the data
3. Conduct causal structure discovery
4. Conduct causal effect estimation
5. Assess the quality and reliability of the results
6. Implementation and enhancement of results

Chapter 5. Method Development and Evaluation

5.1. Methods developers should strive to characterize the new methods according to the dimensions of theoretical and empirical properties.	Mature	High impact
5.2. Methods developers should carefully disclose the known and unknown properties of new methods at each stage of their development and provide full evidence for how these properties were established.	Mature	High impact
5.3. Methods adopters and evaluators (users, funding agencies, editorial boards etc.) should seek to obtain valid information according to the dimensions of theoretical and empirical properties for every method, tool, and system under consideration.	Mature	High impact
5.4. Methods adopters and evaluators should map the dimensions of theoretical and empirical properties for every method, tool, and system under consideration to the problem at hand and select methods based on best matching of method properties to problem needs.	Mature	High impact
5.5. The properties of a ML algorithm can be negatively or positively affected by the ML protocol to extreme degrees (see "Lessons Learned from Historical Failures, Limitations and Successes of AI/ML In Healthcare and the Health Sciences. Enduring Problems, and the Role of BPs" for several important case studies that show the practical consequences). Similarly the data design can negatively or positively affect the ML protocol and its embedded algorithms to extreme degrees. Therefore, it is imperative to design AI/ML methods taking into account any positive or negative interactions of data design with the protocols and embedded algorithms employed.	Mature	High impact
5.6. The preferred design for validating AI/ML methods with real life data with known answers is the centralized benchmark design. Distributed benchmark designs, whenever feasible, add value by exploring natural variation in how methods are applied by experts. Competitions have several intrinsic limitations and can add value but have to be interpreted carefully.	Evolving	High impact

5.7. Develop and validate ML/AI methods using the following stages/ steps: Step 1. Rigorous problem definition (in precise mathematical terms and establishing how the mathematical goals map to the healthcare or health science discovery goal) Step 2. Theoretical analysis of problem (complexity, problem space characteristics, etc.) Step 3. First-pass algorithms solving problem Step 4. Theoretical properties of first pass algorithms: focus on representation power, soundness and completeness, transparency, interpretability Step 5. Algorithm refinements and optimizations Step 6. Empirically test algorithms in controlled conditions Step 7. Empirically test algorithms in real life data with known answers/ solutions Step 8. Empirically test algorithms in real life data without known answers/solutions but where future validation can take place	Mature	High impact
5.8. Avoid evaluating methods by employing persuasive expert narratives lacking validity.	Mature	High impact
5.9. Do not reinvent the wheel. Verify that the problem solved by a new method has not been previously solved by a better performing method.	Mature	High impact
5.10. Create open box methods to the full extent possible. Do not pursue weak justifications that fail to translate the models to accurate human readable representations.	Mature	Medium impact
5.11. Do not confuse "open source" for "transparent" and "closed source" for "black box".	Mature	Medium impact
5.12. Interpret results of application of a method at the level justified by its known properties.	Mature	High impact

Chapter 6. Model Development Lifecycle

6.1.1. Define the goals and process of AI/ML model building as either feasibility/exploratory or as clinical-grade/mission-critical and apply appropriate quality and rigor criteria and best practices.	Mature	High impact
6.2.1.1. When pursuing risk and performance-sensitive model development, specify concrete model performance targets for well-defined care or discovery settings.	Mature	High impact
6.2.1.2. When pursuing risk and performance-sensitive model development, engage all appropriate stakeholders.	Mature	High impact
6.2.1.3. When pursuing risk and performance-sensitive model development translate model accuracy to value, establish value targets and translate predictivity and other technical model characteristics into real-world value assessments.	Mature	High impact
6.2.1.4. When pursuing risk and performance-sensitive model development carefully consider and plan for system-level goals and interactions. Avoid too narrow ("tunnel vision") model development.	Mature	High impact
6.2.1.5. When pursuing clinical-grade and risk-sensitive model development, carefully consider ELSI and JEDI desiderata and consequences.	Mature	High impact

6.2.1.6. When pursuing feasibility, exploratory, or pre-clinical models relax stringency of requirements applicable to clinical-grade models.	Mature	Medium impact
6.2.1.7. When pursuing clinical-grade and risk-sensitive model development, interpret models and models' decisions exactly as their known properties justify.	Mature	High impact
6.2.2.1. When pursuing risk and performance-sensitive model development, create a rigorous and powerful data design which facilitates modeling that will meet performance and safety requirements.	Mature	High impact
6.2.2.2. When pursuing risk and performance-sensitive model development, judiciously interpret the limitations of convenience data/data designs on the performance and meaning of feasibility and exploratory models.	Mature	High impact
6.2.3.1. When moving from first pass modeling to optimized clinical grade models take into account: the problem space characteristics; data available for development and testing; prior literature on approaches and results previously explored both in terms of data design, algorithms and models; verification and reproducing prior literature findings/claims; and obtaining robust preliminary estimates of predictivity of the first pass models and whether they meet requirements.	Mature	High impact
6.2.3.2. Avoid overfitting caused by repeatedly analyzing same data from first pass to optimized modeling stages.	Mature	High impact
6.2.4.1. Everything else being equal, prefer interpretable model families when interpretability is desired.	Mature	Medium impact
6.2.4.2. Use standardized coefficients (if applicable) when comparing feature contributions in linear models.	Mature	High impact
6.2.4.3. Very large models, even when produced with intrinsically interpretable methods, may still be hard to interpret because of sheer scale. Isolating critical information from large models or simplification are recommended.	Mature	High impact
6.2.4.4. Apply feature selectors that maximally reduce dimensionality without loss of predictivity. Compact models are always easier to explain. Combine with interpretable model families or surrogate models as appropriate.	Mature	Medium impact
6.2.4.5. If accuracy is of paramount importance and if the black box models have significant accuracy advantage over the best interpretable models you can build, then use the black box model but apply explanation methods: • Global surrogate models aiming to have high fidelity everywhere in the input space over all patterns that will be classified by the model. Verify generalizable fidelity of surrogate model before using. • Local surrogate models aiming to have high fidelity in the local input space for every pattern that will be classified by the model. Verify generalizable fidelity of surrogate model before using. • Human expert surrogate models which must be high fidelity everywhere in the input space and be over-fitting resistant. Verify generalizability and fidelity of human expert explanations of models.	Evolving	High impact
6.2.4.6. Shapley values, Shapley value approximations and feature importance methods that try to summarize complex model behaviors in one or few values are not advised as general or routinely used methods for explaining ML models.	Evolving	High impact

6.2.4.7. (a) Use equivalence class modeling algorithms for discovering the equivalence class of optimally accurate and non-reducible predictive models. E.g. TIE* instantiated with GLL-MB or other sound Markov boundary subroutines (see "Foundations and Properties of AI/ML Systems" and "An Appraisal and Operating Characteristics of Major ML Methods Applicable in Healthcare and Health Science"). (b) Use equivalence class modeling algorithms for discovering the equivalence class of direct causes. E.g. TIE* instantiated with GLL-PC or other sound local causal neighborhood subroutines ("Foundations and Properties of AI/ML Systems" and "An Appraisal and Operating Characteristics of Major ML Methods Applicable in Healthcare and Health Science"). (c) When experiments can be conducted, consider using ML-driven experimentation algorithms that model equivalence classes. Experimentation may be needed to resolve the equivalence classes and unmeasured confounding. Such algorithms minimize the number of experiments needed. E.g., ODLP*.	Evolving	High impact
6.2.4.8. When pursuing risk and performance-sensitive model development, optimize model performance verifying that targets are met; otherwise, modify or enhance data design, algorithms, and protocols, or relax requirements; once modeling is complete, characterize error and other properties that are essential for safe and effective deployment and explain models and check their face validity.	Mature	High impact
6.2.5.1. Do not establish and exercise IP rights in ways that undermine fundamental principles of scientific reproducibility, openness to model and method scrutiny, and validation.	Evolving	Medium impact
6.2.5.2. Establish IP rights that are conducive to successful dissemination, and patients and society benefit from AI/ML innovation.	Evolving	Medium impact
6.2.5.3. Protect IP rights from "bypassing" that exploit model equivalence classes.	Evolving	High impact
6.2.6.1. When developing clinical-grade and mission-critical models address regulatory, legal, bias, ethical, social justice, and health equity issues.	Mature	High impact
6.2.7.1. When developing clinical-grade and mission-critical models address critical issues of implementation including: (1) conversion to practical, inexpensive, objective production models; (2) ensuring sustainability via reimbursement, cost reductions etc.; (3) demonstrating to stakeholders of meeting clinical or research needs and adding value; (4) providing user education and support; (5) ensuring community and patient buy-in; (6) sandboxing CDS while it is evaluated in care environment; (7) ensuring scaling of CDS; (8) integration into clinical, research and R&D workflows as appropriate.	Mature	High impact

6.2.8.1. When developing clinical-grade and mission-critical models ensure that the AI/ML models will stay within their knowledge boundaries by addressing: outliers, safe and unsafe decision regions, calibration and recalibration, incorporating patient preferences, managing data shifts and model performance shifts, address population mixture changes, seasonality and trends, epidemic dynamics, various interventional externalities (e.g., changes in standards of care, new vaccines, new populations, new treatments). Carefully consider how models can successfully generalize from the original data/populations used for model development and validation to other populations and settings and address pristine vs noisy inputs, model input mapping and harmonization, missing input values and rebuilding models.	Mature	High impact
6.2.9.1. When developing clinical-grade and mission-critical models ensure that ancillary and secondary objectives, benefits and work products are managed and preserved	Evolving	Medium impact
6.2.9.2. Documentation. Throughout the model development process complete and thorough documentation must be maintained. Key elements of this documentation include: (1) Model goals (2) Risk assessments (3) Key interactions and input from stakeholders (4) AI/ML governance and oversight committee deliberations (5) Software documentation (6) Data design documentation (7) Data documentation (8) IP documentation (9) Legal and compliance documentation (10) User guides and training documentation (11) Ancillary work products documentation (12) Checklists and worksheets (e.g., ones provided in this book to keep track of following relevant best practices)	Mature	High impact

Chapter 7. Data Design

7.1.1. The ML data design needs to take the operative setting of the ML models into account.	Mature	High impact
7.2.1. Seek to ensure validity and generalizability with good data design first. Resort to analytic corrections of biases only to the extent that optimal design is not attainable.	Mature	High impact
7.2.2. Ensure that the accessible population is representative of the target population.	Mature	High impact
7.2.3. Ensure that the discovery sample is representative of the accessible (and target) populations.	Mature	High impact
7.3.1. A cross-sectional study suffices if one can answer the analytic question with the *prevalence* of the outcome in the exposed and unexposed groups.	Mature	High impact

7.3.2. Use the easiest/most economical data design that can solve the problem. The mapping of the problem to a problem type can help find the best design.	Mature	High impact
7.3.3. Use cohort studies if the time gap between the index date and the outcome is important and the outcome is not very rare.	Mature	High impact
7.3.4. Use cohort studies if you need to estimate the prevalence and/or incidence of outcomes, separately for exposed and unexposed patients (if an intervention is considered).	Mature	High impact
7.3.5. Whenever possible, the use of clinical trial data is recommended as a replacement for case/control studies.	Mature	Medium impact
7.3.6. Case/control design is best suited when the outcome is rare, but the exposures are relatively frequent.	Mature	High impact
7.4.1. If you see an unexpected effect direction, always consider the possibility of Simpson's paradox and Berkson bias.	Mature	High impact

Chapter 8. Data Management, Transformation, Quality

8.2.1. Create and use a data dictionary in which each data element in the dataset that we are working with, is defined.	Mature	High impact
8.4.1. Whether the data need to be pivoted or not depends on the software that will be used for modeling. Almost always, the software will expect pivoted (wide) data.	Evolving	Medium impact
8.4.2. The choice between person-level and person-event format is driven by the analytic need and the analytic software (model) that is chosen accordingly.	Mature	Medium impact
8.4.3. If categorical variables with sematic relationships among their levels need to be converted into a set of indicator variables, design an encoding scheme (if possible) that makes this semantic relationship explicit to the learning algorithm.	Mature	Medium impact
8.5.1. EHR data can be used for discovery, but be aware of the quality issues and select modeling methods that can correct for the relevant and potentially consequential issues.	Mature	High impact
8.5.2. Provide a minimal set of data quality metrics for Completeness, Plausibility and Conformance.	Mature	High impact
8.7.1. It is a best practice to document all data transformations so that the entire process can be reproduced from scratch if necessary.	Mature	High impact
8.7.2. A minimum sufficient set of tools for learners: a common data model, at least one of the data science programming languages, and data access using SQL.	Evolving	Medium impact
8.7.3. Every project should create and maintain a data pipeline, which is a repeatable process that performs all of the steps required to transform data from the source data to the final analytic fact table that is used as input for the analytic and modeling part of the project.	Mature	High impact
8.7.4. Ensure that meta-data associated with phenotypes and variables contains enough information to allow for the re-creation of the phenotypes/variables from source data.	Mature	High impact

Chapter 9. Model Evaluation Methods and Metrics

9.1.1. Use evaluation metrics appropriate for the outcome type.	Mature	High impact
9.1.2. Multiple metrics are needed to cover different aspects of model performance. Use sets of measures that provide complementary information.	Mature	High impact
9.1.3. Common complementary pairs of classifier performance evaluation metrics include: (1) precision/recall; (2) specificity/sensitivity; (3) bias/discrimination.	Mature	High impact
9.1.4. The ROC is much more commonly used than the Lorenz curve and is more familiar to many readers.	Mature	High impact
9.1.5. Consider showing the Lorenz curve (possibly in combination with the ROC) when low-risk patients are of particular interest.	Mature	Medium impact
9.1.6. All of the measures in Table 9.1.6 (MSE, MAE, MAD, Pearson residual, R^2, adjusted R^2) are appropriate for Gaussian data.	Mature	Medium impact
9.1.7. MSE is more sensitive to outliers than MAD.	Mature	High impact
9.1.8. When evaluating predictive models with continuous outcomes that are heteroscedastic, consider using a residual that normalizes the expected variance (such as the Pearson residual for counts) or at least for the predicted value.	Mature	High impact
9.1.9. When the relationship between the predicted and actual values is not linear, consider using a rank-based measure such as Spearman or Kendall correlation.	Mature	High impact
9.1.10. The most common evaluation metric of a time-to-event model is Harrell's C statistic (survival concordance).	Mature	Medium impact
9.1.11. Time-dependent predictions can be summarized into a single value as (1) survival probability at the end of the study, (2) survival probability at the median survival time, (3) or survival probability at some clinically relevant time.	Mature	Medium impact
9.1.12. If an ROC is desired, time-to-event prediction can be converted into classification outcomes at a specific (clinically relevant) time point using the C/D strategy to plot the ROC.	Mature	Medium impact
9.2.1. For case/control designs, use OR.	Mature	High impact
9.2.2. Absolute and relative risk measures provide complementary information, so whenever possible, both should be reported.	Mature	High impact
9.2.3. Absolute risk reduction (ARR) and number needed to treat (NNT) convey the same information and differ in interpretation. ARR is dimensionless, while NNT is measured in number of patients and is preferred in clinical practice. Choose between the two based on the target audience.	Mature	Medium impact
9.3.1. Include *all* alternative interventions in a health economic evaluation.	Mature	High impact
9.3.2. Include the opportunity cost as cost of intervention/program in a health economic evaluation.	Mature	High impact
9.3.3 Do not use intermediate end-points unless they are very strongly linked to the outcome of interest.	Mature	High impact
9.4.1. In model evaluation and/or validation, consider the sampling unit carefully.	Mature	High impact
9.4.2. A typical leave-out validation size is 30% of the sample.	Mature	Medium impact

9.4.3. For cross validation, a typically number of folds is 10 in moderate sample size and 5 in large sample sizes.	Mature	Medium impact
9.4.4. When using the bootstrap estimator select a number of repetitions that is sufficient for the problem based on related literature. Reported minimum repetitions generally range from 100 to >500.	Mature	Medium impact
9.4.5. When using the bootstrap, estimate the bias and correct for it unless it is negligible. If the bias is unknown or cannot be corrected, then a different estimator must be used.	Mature	High impact
9.4.6. Use the least computationally expensive estimator that yields small enough bias and variance in the problem at hand. For very small sample size, consider as first choice Leave One Out Cross Validation (LOOCV). For small sample size, using a less-flexible classifier, the .632 bootstrap can offer the best performance but it can be biased. For medium sample sizes, repeated balanced ten-fold cross validation is recommended. For large samples sizes, holdout or five-fold Cross Validation or corrected bootstrap is recommended.	Mature	High impact

9.4.7. Applying data imputation procedures on training data and using the imputation model on the test data (in cross validation estimators):
  (a) Ensures that bias is avoided
  (b) Mimics practical implementation of the final model (which has to be eventually deployed without the benefit of seeing a large number of the application population).
	Mature	High impact

9.4.8. Tune the parameters of an algorithm separately on each fold/resample.	Mature	High impact
9.4.9. After error estimation has been accomplished and an optimal hyperparameter value assignment has been identified, the final model has to be built on the entire data set, with the hyperparameter values, that were found to be best on average, and without conducting further internal error estimation.	Mature	High impact
9.4.10. If the sample size allows, pseudo-prospective (temporal) validation is recommended in addition to the internal validation and other planned external validations.	Evolving	Medium impact
9.4.11. If your model was developed using public data, registry data, or other external data, always make sure that it is valid on the target institution's internal data.	Mature	High impact

Chapter 10. Overfitting, Overconfidence, Under Performance

10.1. Deploy procedures that prevent, diagnose and remedy errors of overconfidence in, or overfitting of models.	Mature	High impact

10.1.1. Manage model complexity with respect to data generating function complexity and to available sample size using:
  (1) Regularization
  (2) Dimensionality reduction
  (3) Feature selection
  (4) Bayesian Priors and Bayesian ensembles
  (5) Algorithm-embedded capacity control
  (6) Statistical model/data complexity measures
  (7) Model selection
  (8) Combination approaches
	Mature	High impact

10.1.2. Characterize and manage statistical uncertainty.	Mature	High impact
10.1.3. Use unbiased estimators of model performance or correct bias of biased estimates.	Mature	High impact
10.1.4. Lock models at predefined stages in the modeling process and not allow further tampering with locked models.	Mature	Medium impact
10.1.5. Correct multiple statistical hypotheses tests (explicitly or implicitly).	Mature	High impact
10.1.6. Thoroughly specify and report the entirety of procedures used to obtain models so that independent verification of generalizability is possible.	Mature	High impact
10.1.7. Conduct iterative or sequential modeling via unbiased protocols.	Mature	High impact
10.1.8. Use representative datasets, appropriate populations and make generalizability claims from appropriate datasets.	Mature	High impact
10.1.9. Coordinate analysis over many teams and same data via appropriate unbiased protocols.	Mature	High impact
10.1.10. Use reproducible, standardized data input steps.	Mature	High impact
10.1.11. Employ normalization/data transforms that do not require entirety of sample (or confine such transforms within discovery and validation datasets independently).	Mature	High impact
10.1.12. Prevent learners from learning the wrong patterns via spurious co-occurrence; control structural relations and biased sampling; and incorporate domain knowledge-based review that reveals spurious learning.	Mature	High impact
10.1.13. Control via nested model selection all (and not just a few) factors that can lead to overconfidence.	Mature	High impact
10.1.14. If possible combine modelling of individual patients with population modeling.	Evolve	High impact
10.1.15. Do not over-interpret the generalizability of bespoke hand-created AI models unless sufficient number of validation datasets can be obtained to support such claims. Consider creating computable versions of model hand-crafting modeling when possible.	Mature	High impact
10.1.16. Use label reshuffling testing for evaluating the overfitting/overconfidence bias of the whole analysis protocol.	Evolving	High impact
10.1.17. Apply with appropriate caution independent dataset validation and be mindful of dangers of over interpretation of positive and negative results.	Mature	High impact
10.1.18. Instead of pursuing strict and exact reproducibility across datasets, study the variant and invariant findings from these datasets.	Evolving	High impact
10.1.19. Whenever possible, use reanalysis (with both original and unbiased or otherwise improved protocols, including single coordinated protocols as needed) when verifying the validity of models produced by third parties.	Mature	High impact
10.1.20. Use domain knowledge and related face-validity tests by experts to flag potential model errors. The experts themselves may be prone to biases or domain theory may not cover models' new findings so do not over-interpret experts' objections.	Mature	High impact
10.1.21. Apply "safety net" measures for ensuring that a model is not applied to the wrong person or population.	Mature	High impact

10.1.22. Examine stability of models, parameters and other findings and examine more deeply unstable findings. Be aware that it is possible for unstable models to be perfectly valid.	Evolving	High impact
10.2. Deploy procedures that prevent, diagnose and remedy errors of model under-performance or underfitting.	Mature	High impact
10.2.1. To maximize predictivity deploy and explore all relevant learning method families during model selection.	Mature	High impact
10.2.2. To maximize predictivity and generalizability deploy and explore all relevant data preparation steps to the domain and task at hand.	Mature	Medium impact
10.2.3. To maximize predictivity systematically and sufficiently explore the hyper parameter space.	Mature	High impact
10.2.4. Anticipate several preliminary and refinement modeling stages and incorporate them into sequential nested designs to avoid overfitting and overconfidence.	Mature	High impact
10.2.5. Inform analyses by methods literature so that best known methods for task and data at hand are always explored along with novel methods.	Mature	High impact
10.2.6. Follow theoretically and empirically proven specifications of reference prototypical or official use of employed methods.	Mature	High impact
10.5.7. In models for individual patients: use dense time series data, leverage population models, search for and model abrupt distribution shifts of the individual (including learning and modeling shifts at the population level).	Evolving	Medium impact
10.5.8. Conduct power sample analysis and more generally characterize the effects of sample size on modeling. In the absence of knowledge of learning curves, use: (1) dynamic sampling schemes whenever appropriate (2) sensitivity analysis for results using convenience samples by iteratively reducing available sample size (sub-sampling on a convenience sample) (3) simulations (4) domain knowledge (5) network-scientific knowledge (6) reference to robust results in very similar domains (7) dynamic sampling schemes	Evolving	High impact

Chapter 11. From 'Human vs Machine' to 'Human with Machine'

11.1. Consider the possibility that a hybrid, "human in the loop" system may outperform human or computer decisions.	Mature	Medium impact
11.2. Examine the topology of errors in human and computer models.	Evolving	High impact
11.3. Explore ensemble learning as a strategy for building hybrid decision models.	Evolving	High impact
11.4. Work with implementation experts for bringing complex human/ AI decision making into the clinical or scientific settings.	Mature	High impact

Chapter 12. Case Studies (Pitfalls, Successes)

12.7.1. Follow the Institute of Medicine's (IOM's) recommendations and best practices to enhance development, evaluation, and translation of omics-based tests before they are used to guide patient treatment in clinical trials. These aim to ensure that progress in omics test development is grounded in sound scientific practice and is reproducible, resulting not only in improved health care but also in continued public trust.	Mature	High impact
12.9.1. Literature limitations imply (among other things) that readers should seek, read and interpret health AI/ML papers taking the following factors into consideration: disjointed expertise, publication bias, limited self-correction, level of risk of bias, literature disconnected across fields, Matthew effect, compounding of publication bias with Matthew effect, amplification of errors.	Evolving	High impact
12.11.1. Taken at face value, comparative studies of deep learning and ML vs simple statistical baselines, collectively support the following: (1) ML is not guaranteed to outperform classical simpler tools (like LR). In many applications simpler models outperform "fancier" (more expressive, more complicated) ones because of a variety of factors, including having properties that match health domain characteristics better, having extensive guidelines for proper use, protocols and designs overpowering algorithms, and that restricted learners being superior in low sample situations. (2) It is an excellent idea to always include baseline comparators such as LR and other methods in model building. (3) A significant portion of nominally very high DL performance is linked to highly-biased research designs (incomplete cross validation, possible overfitting and error estimation bias, and other methodological issues that lead to over confidence in models). In clinical studies with strong methodology and lower risk for bias, the DL does not seem to perform as well.	Evolving	High impact
12.11.2. In the foreseeable future, and especially for clinical-grade applications and expensive commercial solutions, consideration of hybrid symbolic-connectionist approaches may be worthwhile in many problem domains. Possible advantages include: faster path to design, faster validation and implementation, and exceeding the performances of its components.	Evolving	Medium impact
12.11.3. Large-scope systems are particularly suitable for human–computer hybrids and the corresponding practices described in 'From "Human Versus Machine" to "Human with Machine"', should be taken into account.	Evolving	Medium impact

12.12.1. Ten important principles to guide the responsible, ethically appropriate, and practical use and sharing of clinical data for the purposes of care and discovery 1. Mission-driven. Data sharing with external parties must be consistent with the organization's core missions of patient care, education, and research for the purpose of generalizable knowledge and the advancement of health 2. Payment for academic work. Financial compensation should be based on the value of the contribution (e.g., academic research, expertise, or invention) provided by the mission-driven organization; data alone and financial gain should not be primary drivers 3. Minimum necessary. Data sharing will be limited to the minimum data elements needed for the project 4. Limited agreements. Data sharing agreements should be nonexclusive, have defined time limits, and permission for data use should be revocable at any time 5. No transfer of ownership. Data sharing agreements confer stewardship; data ownership cannot be transferred and, as such, recipients cannot redistribute or sell the data 6. No reidentification. Data recipients should not attempt to reidentify deidentified data 7. Limited data association. Data cannot be associated with other data sets without explicit permission 8. Transparency. The key purpose of data sharing activities and engagements should be transparent to all stakeholders, including patients and study participants 9. Conflicts. Conflicts of interest must be transparent with appropriate governance of both employee and organization-level conflicts 10. Oversight. All decisions about data sharing should be overseen by appropriate representative stakeholders—much like an institutional review board overseeing human subjects research	Evolving	High impact
12.13.1. Equivalence classes should be modeled and considered in the interpretation of models 1. Use equivalence class modeling algorithms for discovering the equivalence class of optimally accurate and non reducible predictive models 2. Use equivalence class modeling algorithms for discovering the equivalence class of direct causes 3. When experiments can be conducted, consider using ML-driven experimentation algorithms that model equivalence classes. Experimentation may be needed to resolve the equivalence classes and unmeasured confounding	Evolving	High impact

Chapter 13. Managing AI Prediction Error Risk

13.1. Measure calibration and recalibrate as needed.	Mature	High impact
13.2. Convert scores to probabilities when needed.	Mature	Medium impact

13.3. Test models for difference from null model.	Mature	High impact
13.4. Identify models' reliable and unreliable decision regions.	Mature	High impact
13.5. Measure stability and flag unstable models.	Evolving	Medium impact
13.6. Extract and report model equivalence classes.	Mature	High impact
13.7. Apply strategies for ML debugging: 1. Start from conventional debugging of ML algorithm implementation 2. Debug with real data 3. Debug simulations and resimulations 4. Know well the behavior of algorithms so that strange behaviors (for better or worse) are immediately apparent in complex analyses. Investigate unusual behaviors (with respect to each algorithm's expected behavior) 5. Build or acquire and use a set of benchmark datasets 6. Compare the implementation or instantiation and tuning of a ML algorithm to the literature 7. Examine the interactions of algorithms with embedding protocols and systems 8. Understand and accommodate mitigation factors	Evolving	High impact
13.8. Use safe model deployment toolkit: 1. Detect and manage outliers 2. Detect and manage falling outside model's region of reliable operation 3. Detect and manage distribution shifts 4. Report Credible Intervals for relevant loss function estimates applicable to the input region for every model decision 5. Flag, report and explain unstable and uncertain model characteristics 6. Apply continuous QC metrics as predictions and decisions are prospectively validated. Alert deployment team for possible need to rectify or rebuilt the model 7. Make the above safety functions parametric so that model operators can adapt the model deployment better to local application conditions 8. When more than one model is available, choose the model that has best performance and safety profile for each application case 9. Safely transfer models developed from population P1 to population P2, or rebuild models from P2 data 10. Address missing inputs at the design, fitting and validation stages. Do not apply models with partial or imputed inputs unless this is part of the models' design and validation 11. Manage drops in the quality of model data inputs from the development and validation data to the application phase 12. Develop and deploy ancillary alerting DSS (geared to the model users and developers) that are designed to flag deviations from the conditions that guarantee safe and effective model performance	Evolving	High impact

Chapter 14. NLP

14.1. Always test multiple preprocessing pipelines to find what works best for the desired goals.	Mature	High impact
14.2. Document rationale for design decisions. Provide performance metrics (speed and measures of accuracy) where possible.	Mature	High impact
14.3. Use a grid search over a reasonable set of hyper-parameters to produce the best model possible. This in combination with k-fold cross validation can increase the likelihood that the resulting model will be the strongest and most likely to generalize to unseen data.	Mature	High impact
14.4. Apply appropriate rigor in analyzing the performance of machine learning models. Permutation tests, covariance analysis, etc. can be invaluable for diagnosing issues before deploying models.	Mature	High impact
14.5. When using machine learning models, including deep learning models, always use a simple baseline for comparison. This can be as simple as some rules, a linear regression model, or as complex as a "vanilla" BERT model depending on the task at hand. It may be the case where a random forest will provide adequate performance and be faster at inference than a transformer.	Mature	High impact

Chapter 15. Computer Vision

15.1. Always start with a known state-of-the-art network architecture rather than designing your own. EfficientNet is often a (relatively) fast way to see if your dataset has an extractable signal.	Evolving	High impact
15.2. Use transfer learning any time you can find a dataset similar enough to yours.	Evolving	High impact
15.3. Be alert to data differences in photographs acquired by patients vs those acquired by medical photographers or informed providers. If you mix them, be certain to check that there is balance among outcomes by origin.	Mature	High impact
15.4. Weakly supervised learning may be a promising future direction to alleviate the burden of acquiring costly and time-consuming pixel level annotations.	Evolving	Medium impact
15.5. A common paradigm for deep learning on pathology slides is to first divide the slide into small patches of tissue. Then one trains a tissue-level classifier, typically a deep neural network. This predicts the type of tissue in the patch using labels from pixel-level annotations. Afterwards, a slide-level classifier can be trained to predict using the tissue-level predictions as input and the slide labels as output. The slide-level classifier is typically a model such as logistic regression, often chosen to avoid overfitting.	Evolving	High impact
15.6. Keep an up-to-date list of publicly available datasets so that you can use them when appropriate.	Mature	High impact

Chapter 16. Regulatory and Ethical, Legal, Social Implications

16.1. Consider all relevant risks in different phases of the AI/ML life cycle. Risks can change over time, e.g., the probability or severity of risk can change due to advancements in treatments or due to patient population drift.	Mature	High impact
16.2. The rationale for the risk management plan is that having a plan produced ahead of time makes it less likely that a risk management step is overlooked or accidentally skipped. Have a risk management plan.	Mature	High impact
16.3. Health AI/ML should strive to always benefit and never cause harm to any individual or group of individuals. Do not design, develop or deploy models that make unnecessary and avoidable errors, or are grossly inefficient, or harmful in any way to any individual or group of individuals.	Mature	High impact
16.4. AI should strive to decrease, and ensure that it does not increase health disparities. Do not design, develop or deploy models that may increase health disparities or systematically benefit or harm specific groups over others. Whenever possible seek to design, develop or deploy models that increase health equity.	Mature	High impact
16.5. Importance of an ethical, equity and social justice—sensitive culture of health AI/ML: 1. Cultivate a culture that promotes health equity values and is broadly ethics-sensitive within the data science team. 2. Ensure proper training in health equity and overall biomedical ethics of all data scientists working on a project. 3. Participate in organizational efforts to build and sustain a broader organizational culture promoting strong biomedical ethics values. 4. Seek advice and active involvement from ethics experts, patients, patient advocates, and community representatives regarding possible harm of the contemplated AI/ML work to individuals, and threats to health equity. Seek to obtain insights, guidance and community support on how the AI/ML work can lead to reduction of disparities. 5. Hold yourself and others accountable to the above principles and aims.	Mature	High impact
16.6. Data Design must support health equity. Always collect data on health determinants especially those intertwined with health disparities and use them in modeling along with all other data relevant to the problem at hand. Ensure that representation of underserved, marginalized, and minority groups is adequate and well-aligned with ethical and health justice principles.	Mature	High impact

16.7. Model development and evaluation must support health equity. 1. Always, during problem formulation, data design, and model development, validation and deployment stages, consider and actively pursue modeling that does not compromise (and ideally benefits) equity. 2. Analyze the model decisions with respect to health determinant variables. Use interpretable/explainable models, causal modeling, and equivalence class modeling in order to develop a robust understanding of how the model's output may affect health equity and what related biases the model may exhibit. Fix problems related to bias. 3. If medical outcomes are not part of the model, and only intermediate proxies are modeled, examine their suitability. Also examine how model decisions affect outcomes post model deployment. Study how health determinants affect outcomes via the model's function.	Mature	High impact
16.8. Revealing racial bias and discriminatory practices. Use AI/ML to reveal harmful biases in health care, and health science practices (in aggregate and individually). Use the models to flag such biases and suggest ways to remove them. Models that reveal biases (in order to correct them), by necessity capture the bias variables, their effects and interactions. "Sterilizing" these models from the bias they model, defeats the purpose of their existence and their value.	Evolving	High impact
16.8b. The "Causal-Path-to-Outcomes Principle of Bias Detection". If there are one or more causal paths from race or other minority population indicator variables, to outcomes and they are not medically justified, this indicates an ethical bias that should be addressed (either in the modeling, or in the practice that the model captures).	Evolving	High impact
Best Practice 16.9. Equitable access to beneficial AI. Ensure that all who would benefit from an AI/ML model have access to it.	Mature	High impact
Best Practice 16.10. System-level interactions and their ethical implications. AI/ML models, when deployed, will not operate in a vacuum. Different models designed for different populations when optimized separately for the individual populations, may be non-enforceable because they may "hit a wall" of limited resources. In such cases, system-level planning, goal-setting, and technical solutions must be brought to bear to optimize multi-objective functions and systems of local AI/ML respecting ethical principles and factors.	Evolving	High impact

Chapter 17. Reporting Standards

17.1. Document the model, its development, validation and deployment process.	Mature	High impact
17.2. Document AI/ML models using reporting standards and extent with problem and technology-specific necessary information even if not part of the standard. Such extensions can be based on the various development stages and Best Practices in the present volume.	Mature	High impact

Index

Printed in the United States
by Baker & Taylor Publisher Services